HEALTH
INFORMATION
MANAGEMENT

HEALTH INFORMATION MANAGEMENT

Formerly *Medical Record Management*
by EDNA K. HUFFMAN, RRA

Tenth Edition, Revised by the

American Health Information Management Association

Jennifer Cofer, RRA - Editor

1994

PHYSICIANS' RECORD COMPANY

BERWYN, ILLINOIS

PREFACE AND ACKNOWLEDGEMENTS

As with previous editions, the tenth revision of *Medical Record Management,* now known as *Health Information Management,* is intended to be a basic textbook and reference for the field of medical records and health information management. Edna K. Huffman, the original author of this text, was one of the first educators in the field of medical record management and the seventh president of the American Health Information Management Association (then known as the American Association of Medical Record Librarians). Her dedication to the advancement of the profession through education has been the impetus for the Association to continue revising her book over the years. This revision provides general information on a broad range of topics. As a result, the editor must either have a vast knowledge of almost all aspects of health information management, or as in my case, rely on respected colleagues for their expertise in various areas.

The persons listed below graciously shared their time and knowledge. Several, including Kelli Marsh, Rebecca Sykes, Rose Lefkowitz, and Sherry Finkel Murphy, also provided forms, resources, graphics, and ideas. Joette Hanna completely rewrote Chapter 16 on the management of quality. L. Edward Bryant spent valuable vacation time helping me with Chapter 15. All are experts in their field; all gave their help generously, in the spirit of contributing to this respected book.

Chapter 1	Mildred St. Leger, RRA
Chapter 2	Joan Hayward, MS, RRA Susan Williams, RRA
Chapter 3	Eleanor Taylor, MS, RRA
Chapter 4	Richard Brown, RRA Teresa Ganser, MS, RRA Kelli Marsh, RRA Susan Miller, MBA , RRA
Chapter 5	Carol Roberts, RRA
Chapter 6	Joan Hayward, MS, RRA Susan Williams, RRA

Chapter 7	Evelyn M. Whitlock, RRA
Chapter 8	Monica Pappas, RRA
Chapter 9	Therese Jorwic, RRA, CCS Margaret Steward, RRA Andrea Albaum-Feinstein, MBA, RRA Pat Brooks, RRA
Chapter 10	Barbara Lee Peace, RRA
Chapter 11	Joan Hayward, MS, RRA Susan Williams, RRA
Chapter 12	Virginia Kelikian Coburn, MBA
Chapter 13	Rebecca Sykes, MBA, ART Jay Koefle Debbie Heile Rose Frances Lefkowitz, RRA, MPA Sherry Finkel Murphy
Chapter 14	Rebecca Sykes, MBA, ART Jay Koefle Bob Gibson
Chapter 15	L. Edward Bryant, Jr. Mary D. Brandt, MBA, RRA
Chapter 16	Joette Hanna, RRA
Chapter 17	Monica Pappas, RRA
Chapter 18	Amy B. Tate, MBA

Editing Health Information Management has been an interesting and challenging project. It is my continuing hope that the time and commitment given to this edition will be obvious to each person who uses it.

JENNIFER COFER, RRA, *EDITOR*

TABLE OF CONTENTS

chapter **1**

INTRODUCTION TO HEALTH INFORMATION MANAGEMENT

HEALTH INFORMATION MANAGEMENT

Information is the lifeblood of the health care delivery system. The medical record, in manual or automated form, houses the medical information that describes all aspects of patient care.

Physicians, nurses, and other health care providers require medical information for treating a patient. The medical record serves as a communication link among care-givers. Documentation in the medical record also serves to protect the legal interests of the patient, health care provider, and health care facility. Medical records are important to the financial well-being of the facility as they substantiate reimbursement claims. Other uses of medical records include provision of data for medical research, education of health care providers, public health studies, and quality review.

There are two health information management professionals: medical record administrators and medical record technicians. Both use a broad scope of knowledge in meeting their challenge. They must understand the health care delivery system and the flow of medical information within it. Fundamentals of medical science are used to process the content of the medical record. Human resource management is necessary for accomplishing the work of the health information department and working with others in the health care delivery system. Medical record technicians must also understand health care statistics, legal aspects, and computer data entry and retrieval. Medical record administrators utilize records management and information systems theory to design manual and computerized storage and retrieval systems. They also must possess basic knowledge of statistics and research methods, law, computer science, and finance to ensure complete and accurate medical records to fulfill the variety of purposes for which they are used.

This chapter describes the evolution of health care and medical records, describes the uses of the medical record, orients the reader to the health care delivery system, and describes the health information management profession in depth.

EVOLUTION OF HEALTH CARE IN THE UNITED STATES

EARLY AMERICA

When America was discovered nearly 500 years ago, medical care was almost nonexistent, and physicians of that day were few in number. There were no organizations or hospitals to assist them, and there were no medical records. Medical records have become increasingly important because medicine and health care have achieved very high standards. To appreciate how far these standards have come, one may consider America's beginnings.

History books tell us of how medicine has evolved through the centuries. Plagues were common, often following the routes of travelers. Lepers were isolated, and monks practiced medicine attending nearly all the hospitals that existed. In the New World, the arriving colonist was subjected to epidemic diseases, hostile attack, and severe winters. Smallpox, measles, yellow fever, influenza, scarlet fever, and diphtheria were just a few of the contagious diseases that threatened their existence.

RENAISSANCE PERIOD

The Renaissance in Europe in the 16th and 17th centuries brought about not only a revival of interest in the arts, literature, and philosophy, but the beginning of a new concept of society which was based on economic growth and care for its citizens. In England there was a growing awareness that a healthy population was a positive factor in economic growth. In America, settlements began to appoint commissions to control the spread of disease, although their chief functions at first were to care for the sick, provide for orphans, and bury the dead. Little was done to prevent disease except through isolation and quarantine.

18th AND 19th CENTURIES

Health care improved slowly during the early decades of the 18th century, but it wasn't until after the American Revolution that there was evidence of real progress. Benjamin Franklin was one of the leaders in a movement to establish the first incorporated hospital. This institution, now known as Pennsylvania Hospital, was established in Philadelphia in 1752. Franklin served as secretary of the hospital, and many of its earliest records, listing the patient's name, address, disorder, and dates of admission and discharge are in his handwriting. In 1803 it was ordered that a detailed record be kept of the interesting cases, and many of these are found to be illustrated with pen-and-ink sketches. In 1873 the hospital began to keep histories and has an unbroken file to the present day.

The New York Hospital opened in 1771 and started its first register of patients in 1791. This register gives interesting notes concerning the patients. Many of the histories follow a definite routine similar to that used today: stating diagnosis, age, date of admission, occupation, illness, treatment, and progress notes.

Massachusetts General Hospital in Boston opened in 1821 and has the distinction of having a complete file of clinical records for every patient admitted. From these records all diseases and operative procedures were cataloged, and the findings were used for patient care, research, and statistical purposes.

As the population of the United States increased and moved westward, the demand for medical practitioners far exceeded the supply. With the opening of hospitals and the increasing population, many private proprietary medical schools sprang up almost overnight. Called "diploma mills," they graduated students in as little as six months. By 1869 there were 72 such medical schools in the United States.

TWENTIETH CENTURY

In 1909-1911 Abraham Flexner, financed by the Carnegie Foundation, made a comprehensive study of the status of medical education in the United States. Flexner described the sad picture of inferior schools incapable of providing an acceptable medical education. After the appearance of this report, many of the inferior schools closed.

Improvement of Records Through Hospital Standardization

In 1913 the American College of Surgeons was founded under the leadership of Dr. Franklin H. Martin. One of the objectives of this new group was to raise the standards of surgery. To accomplish this objective, they felt a sound standard of surgical training would have to be adopted, and data on the training of the surgeon in the hospital as well as in the medical school would be crucial. The College felt it could elevate the standards of surgery by a continent-wide standardization of hospitals.

In order to properly evaluate the surgical work of their candidates for fellowship, the College required the submission of case records of patients upon whom the candidate had performed major surgery. It soon became apparent that these records were not adequate. The College thus realized that their Hospital Standardization Program would have to require better medical records for use not only by candidates for fellowship, but also for efficient care of the patient in present and future illnesses; for the medicolegal needs of the hospital, physician, and the patient; and for use in medical research. They, therefore, adopted as one of the minimum requirements for hospital standardization "that accurate and complete case records be written for all patients and filed in an accessible manner in the hospital." It is shocking to note that in 1918 only 1.6 percent, or 89 out of 5,323, registered hospitals met the standards of the first survey. Numerous other hospitals were not even registered. During one of the early years, the results of the survey were so poor that in the best interests of the public the records were burned.

Steady improvement in the quantity and quality of medical records began with the advent of hospital standardization. Each year on the initiative of Dr. Franklin H. Martin and Dr.

Malcolm T. MacEachern, Director of Hospital Activities of the American College of Surgeons, subjects pertaining to medical records were included in hospital standardization conferences.

Improvement of Records Through Organization

As these conferences had been successful in creating interest in the improvement of medical records, Dr. Malcolm T. MacEachern issued a special invitation to the medical record workers of the United States and Canada to attend a meeting in Boston during the Clinical Congress of the American College of Surgeons. The meeting was to be devoted exclusively to medical records and medical record keeping. He appointed Mrs. Grace Whiting Myers, librarian emeritus of Massachusetts General Hospital, as general chairman to organize committees, direct the preparation of a program, and plan exhibits. This was the first meeting lasting more than a day where problems concerned with medical record content, availability, and preservation were exclusively discussed and where exhibits of exclusive interest to medical record workers were shown.

As this meeting was drawing to a close on October 11, 1928, Mathew W. Foley, editor of *Hospital Management* and father of National Hospital Day, pointed out that organization had brought about improvements in many fields and would undoubtedly accomplish the same in medical records. A motion to organize resulted, and Mrs. Myers was elected first president. The new group called itself the Association of Record Librarians of North America and took as its main objective: "To elevate the standards of clinical records in hospitals, dispensaries, and other distinctly medical institutions." Fifty-eight medical record workers became charter members of the group.

Accreditation Replaces Standardization

The era in which the American College of Surgeons carried the primary responsibility for the establishment of standards for the hospitals of the United States and Canada came to an end on December 6, 1952. On that date the organization now known as the Joint Commission on Accreditation of Healthcare Organizations assumed the responsibility.

Since the inception of the Joint Commission, other accrediting agencies have also been created. Some of the common goals of accrediting agencies are to: develop and maintain standards by which health care facilities may measure and strengthen their programs; improve the quality of services offered by these facilities; and offer to the facility, community, and the consumer a mechanism of accountability and assurance of high quality care. The standards used in the survey process are developed by the respective accrediting agencies with the aid of experts in that particular field. These standards are revised as changes in the state of the art, government regulations, demand, or need of the public occur.

Joint Commission on Accreditation of Healthcare Organizations

The Joint Commission on Accreditation of Healthcare Organizations has as its mission improving the quality of care and services provided and the environment of care through the voluntary accreditation process. This commitment extends to care offered - all major types of organized health care settings.

The American Hospital Association, American Medical Association, American College of Surgeons, American College of Physicians, and American Dental Association sponsor the Joint Commission and each provides representatives who comprise the Joint Commission Board of Commissioners. These commissioners write and publish the standards and determine the accreditation status of various types of health care facilities.

The JCAHO has standards for and surveys a number of healthcare facilities, including the following:

- Acute care hospitals, including general, mental health, specialized, and rehabilitation hospitals.
- Home care agencies and organizations.
- Long-term care facilities.
- Facilities that offer services in mental health, chemical dependency, and mental retardation.
- Ambulatory health facilities, including outpatient surgery centers, physician group practices, and managed care providers.

Presently the Joint Commission grants accreditation for a maximum of three years if a facility is in substantial compliance with the standards. Approximately 18 months from the date of its survey, each accredited facility receives a letter from the Joint Commission stressing the importance of ongoing self-assessment and reminding the facility that correction of any recommendations it received in its last survey should be completed or well under way to avoid jeopardizing the accreditation award for the next full survey.

Facilities found to be in compliance with the JCAHO standards receive "accreditation," or for those few in almost total compliance, "accreditation with commendation." In both cases, however, the accreditation is not automatically renewable, so the facility must undergo the full accreditation process each time its accreditation status approaches expiration.

If the facility is not adequately in compliance with the Joint Commission's standards, it may receive "conditional accreditation." In that case, the Joint Commission expects that the facility can remedy its problems within six months. Each facility that receives provisional accreditation must develop a plan of correction and have a follow-up survey, which determines its ultimate accreditation status

If the facility continues to be out of compliance, or when there is an immediate threat to patient health or safety, the JCAHO gives the status of "non-accredited".

The Joint Commission accreditation survey may serve purposes other than the accreditation process. Many states have legislation or administrative arrangements enabling their hospital licensure agencies (see also next section on licensure) to recognize Joint Commission hospital accreditation in whole or in part for licensure purposes. The licensure agencies may require the hospital to submit evidence of accreditation in connection with their application for relicensure, and may even require a copy of the most recent recommendations.

In a few states, representatives of the state hospital licensure agency participate in the Joint Commission survey process to review licensure requirements not covered under Joint Commission requirements. In all cases the licensure and accreditation decisions are made independently by the respective organizations. Many agencies perform periodic validation inspections of a sample of hospitals with accredited status as a method to replace state licensure inspection.

These state-specific arrangements have resulted from initiatives by state hospital associations in order to reduce the number of surveys/inspections which member hospitals must undergo. The reason for providing these arrangements is that survey/inspection preparations and conduct of the survey divert hospital resources from patient care activities.

Hospitals accredited by Joint Commission (or the American Osteopathic Association) are also recognized as meeting the *Conditions of Participation* for receiving reimbursement for Medicare and Title XIX patients. The state certifying agency conducts random validation surveys of a sample of hospitals certified by virtue of accreditation and complaint investigations in such hospitals. The results of these surveys and investigations are reported annually by the Health Care Financing Administration to Congress.

To assist health care facilities to comply with accreditation standards, the Joint Commission publishes various guides, newsletters, periodicals and reference books.

American Osteopathic Association

Osteopathic hospitals voluntarily obtain accreditation from the American Osteopathic Association (AOA).

The AOA was founded in 1897 and is headquartered in Chicago. Members include osteopathic physicians (DOs), surgeons, and graduates of osteopathic medicine.

To qualify for accreditation by the AOA, hospitals with only doctors of osteopathy (DOs) on their medical staffs must use the term "osteopathic" in their titles and on hospital stationery. Hospitals in which the medical staff is composed of both osteopaths and medical doctors (MDs) are eligible for AOA accreditation but need not use the "osteopathic" designation in the hospital title.

The accreditation manual, *Accreditation Requirements of the American Osteopathic Association*, includes specific requirements for compliance along with interpretive remarks. The accreditation process itself is similar to that of the Joint Commission. The AOA may grant a hospital accreditation for either one, two, or three years. If a hospital receives accreditation for only one year, the AOA may mandate a consultation for deficient areas. The AOA may also withdraw or deny accreditation. A hospital must apply for accreditation annually. Hospitals applying for their first accreditation must have consultation.

Commission on Accreditation of Rehabilitation Facilities

The Commission on Accreditation of Rehabilitation Facilities (CARF), founded in 1966, was established to adopt and apply standards in these facilities throughout the United States.

To be eligible for a survey by CARF, the facility's major purpose must be rehabilitation of individuals requiring restorative and adjustive or employment services in an integrated and coordinated individualized program. In carrying out its program, the facility may place emphasis on one or more of the following: physical restoration, personal and social development, vocational development, sheltered employment, speech pathology, audiology, or work activity.

Accreditation Association for Ambulatory Health Care

The Accreditation Association for Ambulatory Health Care (AAAHC) was incorporated in 1979.

The purpose of the AAAHC is to assist ambulatory health care professionals in improving the quality of care provided in their organizations, to compare their performance with recognized standards, and to provide for sharing of expertise through consultation among members.

A health care facility must be formally organized and must provide primarily ambulatory care services to be eligible for an AAAHC accreditation survey. AAAHC has accredited single and multispecialty group practices, ambulatory surgery centers, health maintenance organizations, college and university health services, and community and neighborhood health centers. The AAAHC standards are very similar to those of the Joint Commission.

The Accreditation Survey Process

The method by which accrediting agencies determine compliance with their regulations or standards is generally the same. To be considered, the interested facility must submit an application and complete a comprehensive questionnaire including the numbers and types of clinical services performed.

These are reviewed to determine if the facility meets the basic accreditation requirements.

If it appears the facility is in compliance, an on-site survey is scheduled. The survey team consists of professionals in various health care disciplines. Hospital accreditation-survey teams usually include at least a practicing physician and hospital administrator. The surveyors review the survey documents and then conduct on-site observation. The on-site observation includes a review of the physical plant, discussions with key personnel and others with an interest in the facility, and review of medical records. A major component of the survey is review of records. Surveyors look at a sample of each facility's medical records to make sure they describe care fully and to make sure the facility follows its care policies.

At the end of their visit, these professionals provide a summation conference with representatives of the facility's governing body, administration, medical staff, and other staff members as appropriate. In this conference the surveyors report their findings, discuss major deviations from the regulations or standards, and make recommendations for correcting them. The representatives of the facility are given an opportunity to comment on any adverse findings.

The surveyors file their findings in a report to the accrediting agency for whom they conducted the survey. The report may also include information submitted by the public, state or federal agencies, or associations. The facility receives a copy of the report and is allowed to respond in writing regarding the findings. The appropriate authority in the accrediting organization, on written recommendations of the surveyors, makes the decision on accreditation. If a decision is contrary to what the facility believes to be appropriate, the facility may appeal the decision by submitting additional information supporting its view. The surveying organization will review this information along with all other pertinent information and make a final decision. Surveys for determining continued compliance with the standards for accreditation are conducted at specified intervals, according to the regulations of the various agencies.

Role of Medicare Certification

The Department of Health and Human Services (DHHS) is the Cabinet level department of the federal executive branch most involved with the nation's human concerns, including health. It has among its major subdivisions the: Social Security Administration (SSA); Health Care Financing Administration (HCFA); and the U.S. Public Health Service (USPHS). The Secretary of DHHS advises the President on health policies and programs and directs department staff to carry out programs approved by Congress.

In 1965 Congress enacted a health care program to provide hospitalization and medical insurance for the aged. Title XVIII of the Social Security Act contains the provisions for the Medicare program, officially titled "Health Insurance for the Aged and Disabled." At the same time, Title XIX, "Grants to States for Medical Assistance Programs," was enacted to form the basis for Medicaid.

Medicare had a profound effect on all health care institutions. At the outset, this law gave financial assistance under certain conditions to most of the nation's population 65 years of age and over. Since then other federal laws have been enacted to admit groups such as the handicapped and those with end-stage renal disease (ESRD). Over 25 million people in our 200 million plus population are federally insured.

Requirements for health care facilities' reimbursement under the Medicare program are contained in the reference *Regulation Number 5, Federal Health Insurance for the Aged*. Within this publication are subparts entitled "Conditions of Participation" for each of the various types of health care facilities. Regulations relative to the compilation and maintenance of patients' medical records are found throughout the regulations, emphasizing the concept that good medical records reflect that a health care institution is rendering good quality patient care.

As a major payer of health care, the federal government must ensure that it is paying for quality medical services necessary for treatment. To evaluate the necessity and quality of health care services, the government contracts with Peer Review Organizations (PROs). The PROs review many aspects of the care of Medicare patients, and they often base their judgments on what is in patient records.

Role of the States

As long as states do not conflict with federal requirements, they are free to enact their own laws, considering those areas which are important to that state.

Medicaid is the medical assistance program created by Title XIX of Public Law 89-97. It is designed to meet the needs of low income people. While it is subject to certain broad federal guidelines and is funded in part by the federal government, the program is operated and administered by each state. The individual states determine benefits covered beyond basic services required by federal law, the eligibility of individuals to receive benefits, and, in general, the allowed rate of payment to providers.

Licensure of health care facilities is also a state (or in some cases a local) governmental activity which gives legal approval for a facility to offer the services for which it is licensed. In order to obtain a license, the facility must meet certain specified requirements for physical aspects of the facility, services provided including medical records, and personnel employed to provide such services. Each licensing body develops the regulations used to evaluate facilities in their geographic area. Licensure is usually performed annually. Licensure standards are generally considered to be the minimum acceptable requirements a facility must meet to operate.

HEALTH CARE TODAY

Until the 20th century, emphasis was on the medical care of the sick and mainly involved physicians, nurses, and hospitals. In the last century significant progress has been made in learning about disease processes and all the factors that predispose one to disease and illness. Many new techniques and instruments have been developed to diagnose and treat diseases.

Where once health was defined simply as the absence of disease, health now is defined as the state of complete physical, mental, and social well-being. In this more comprehensive definition, consideration is given to health care which includes the prevention of disease and health maintenance, in addition to medical care which is curative or palliative. With these changing attitudes toward health, the public now considers

Essential Characteristics of Hospitals

1. The primary function of the institution is to provide diagnosis and treatment, both surgical and nonsurgical, for patients who have any of a variety of medical conditions.

2. Inpatient beds are maintained in the institution.

3. There is governing authority legally responsible for the conduct of the institution.

4. There is an administrator to whom the governing authority delegates the full-time responsibility for the operation of the institution in accordance with established policy.

5. There is an organized medical staff to which the governing authority delegates responsibility for maintaining proper standards of medical care.

6. Each patient is admitted on the medical authority of, and his care is under the direction of, a member of the medical staff.

7. The nursing services are under the direction of a full-time registered professional nurse.

8. Registered professional nurse supervision and other nursing services are continuous.

9. A medical record is maintained for each patient.

10. Pharmacy services are maintained in or by the institution and supervised by a licensed pharmacist.

11. Diagnostic x-ray services, with facilities and staff able to conduct a variety of procedures, are maintained in the institution.

12. Clinical laboratory services, with facilities and staff able to conduct a variety of tests and procedures, are maintained in or by the institution, and anatomical pathology services are regularly and conveniently available.

13. Operating room services, with facilities and staff, are maintained in the institution.

14. Food served to patients meets their nutritional requirements, and modified diets are regularly available.

FIGURE 1. ESSENTIAL CHARACTERISTICS OF HOSPITALS

health care to be a right to which everyone is entitled regardless of financial status.

Today the health care delivery system includes many different kinds of practitioners, facilities, and organizations working together to provide broad health care services to consumers.

There are many types of health care facilities. In general, the length of time in which patients stay at the facility for care serves to characterize the major types of facilities. This section will briefly describe them.

HOSPITAL (ACUTE) CARE

The acute care hospital has traditionally been the primary health care facility, and provides the most comprehensive and intensive medical care services. The hospital is an establishment that provides inpatient beds, medical services, and continuous nursing services for diagnosis and treatment by an organized medical staff. Hospitals are classified as acute, or short-term, because the average length of time patients stay is less than 30 days.

The general acute care hospital is one that provides general medical and surgical care. Figure 1 summarizes the characteristics of the general hospital. Other short-term hospitals may specialize in treating certain types of patients or illnesses. For example, short term psychiatric hospitals provide inpatient care for those suffering from mental health disorders. There are also children's hospitals, those specializing in heart disease, diseases of the eyes and ears, and so forth.

Ownership

While hospitals are generally short term, they may serve different types of patients and may have different types of ownership or sponsorship.

Single hospital ownership by a community, church, or government is the traditional kind of hospital ownership. In the past it has been financed primarily through funding by the sponsoring organization, and often assisted by endowments, gifts, and other funds obtained through public benefits and charities. Because the costs of medical care have risen so fast in the past few decades, many individually owned hospitals have joined forces with other hospitals and health care facilities to remain in business.

A multi-hospital system has been defined as "two or more hospitals that are leased, sponsored, or contract-managed by a central organization." This organizational pattern provides a means of consolidating many resources, such as capital, services, and personnel which has been shown to lower the costs of medical services. Figure 2 illustrates different ownership patterns.

U.S. HOSPITALS BY TYPE OF CONTROL

I. Government Owned
    A. Federal   Army/Air Force/Navy/
                          Veterans Administration

    B. State   Psychiatric/Chronic Disease/State
                          University/Medical School

    C. Local   Hospital District/County/City

II. Non-Government Owned
    A. Voluntary   Church Owned or Affiliated,
                          Community/Regional

    B. Proprietary   Individual Ownership
                          Corporation Owned/Single/
                          Chain (multi)

FIGURE 2. U.S. HOSPITALS BY TYPE OF CONTROL

Organizational Structure

In any form of hospital ownership, the organizational structure includes a sharing of power among the governing board, chief executive officer, and medical staff. Figure 3 displays a typical organizational chart.

Governing Board

The governing board, which is the ultimate authority in the institution, is made up of persons who are knowledgeable in their field and have a responsible standing in the community. In some instances governing boards include representatives of the medical staff, but this may not be legally possible in some states.

The major responsibility of the governing body is to provide

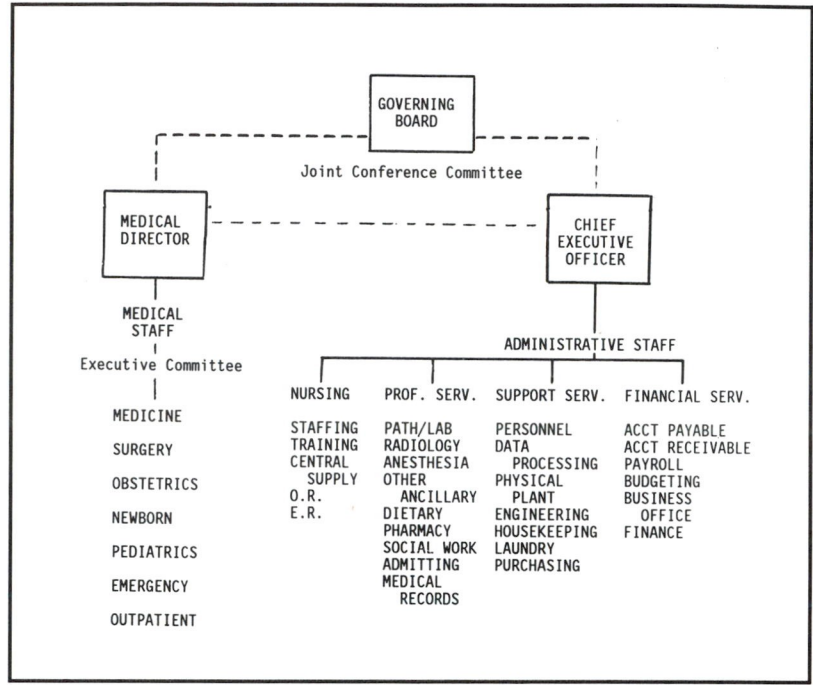

FIGURE 3. TYPICAL ORGANIZATION CHART

proper care to patients. This is done by selecting an efficient medical staff and chief executive officer (CEO). The medical staff provides the medical services, and the CEO employs and directs the staff needed to maintain the hospital and its services.

Medical Staff

The Joint Commission on Accreditation of Healthcare Organizations standards and state licensure laws require that every hospital have a single organized medical staff. The medical staff of the hospital has overall responsibility for the quality of professional services, and is accountable to the governing body. The Joint Commission further specifies that the medical staff includes fully licensed physicians and other individuals permitted by law and by the hospital to provide patient care services independently in the hospital. All medical staff members must have delineated clinical privileges that allow them to provide patient care services independently within the scope of their clinical privileges. All members of the medical staff are also subject to medical staff and departmental bylaws, rules, regulations, and review as part of the hospital quality program.

Medical staff bylaws are the principles and policies with which each medical staff member agrees to comply. Medical staff bylaws have legal standing and are accepted by the courts as a basis for legal decisions. Rules and regulations outline the mechanisms and the details implementing the principles contained in the bylaws. The bylaws, rules, and regulations adopted by the medical staff require approval from the governing body.

The Joint Commission requires the medical staff bylaws, rules, and regulations to specify medical staff membership categories and to delineate qualifications for granting clinical privileges. Physicians must apply for medical staff membership and/or clinical privileges from the governing body; and their applications are evaluated on the basis of education, experience, ethics, competence, physical health status, and current licensure.

Many hospitals maintain several categories of medical staff membership for which applicants may apply:

- Active staff deliver most of the medical services in the hospital and perform all significant organizational and administrative duties pertaining to the medical staff.
- Associate staff are members who are being considered for advancement to the active medical staff.
- Consulting staff are highly qualified practitioners who are available as consultants when needed to improve patient care.
- Courtesy staff are given the privilege to admit an occasional patient to the hospital.
- Honorary staff are former members honored with emeritus positions or other outstanding practitioners whom the medical staff desires to honor.

Appointment to the medical staff and duration of clinical privileges made for a period of not more than two years. A mechanism for reappointment to the medical staff and/or renewal of clinical privileges must be described in the medical staff bylaws and rules and regulations. Reappraisal of the individual physician includes information concerning current licensure, health status, professional performance, judgment, clinical skills as indicated by results of quality assurance activities, and challenges to licensure or registration, termination or limitation of membership or loss of privileges at another hospital, and other reasonable indicators of continuing qualifications.

Medical staff bylaws also provide a mechanism to elect officers to conduct the necessary hospital medical staff activities. In some institutions the title chief of staff is used instead of president, while in other institutions there may be a salaried chief of administrative duties, and a president of the medical staff who is responsible primarily for presiding at staff meetings, appointing medical staff committees, and communicating the views of the staff to the administration and governing board.

The medical staff framework established in the bylaws, rules, and regulations usually identifies several committees through which the responsibilities of the medical staff will be accomplished.

At a minimum, there must be an Executive Committee which acts for the medical staff between staff meetings. In small facilities the medical staff as a whole may serve as the Executive Committee. This committee is responsible for coordinating the activities and general policies of the various clinical departments, making recommendations to the governing body on appointments to medical staff membership and delineating clinical privileges for each eligible individual, and organizing and reviewing mechanisms for quality assurance activities. The Executive Committee receives and acts on reports and recommendations from medical staff committees and clinical departments. The chief executive officer attends each Executive Committee meeting as an ex-officio member.

Many hospitals have multiple committees with assigned charges. Common among them is the Credentials Committee, which is responsible for evaluating applicants for medical staff membership, making recommendations for initial appointments to the Executive Committee, conducting a regular review of each staff member's performance, and making rec-ommendations regarding reappointments and hospital privi-leges.

Another common committee is the Joint Conference Com-mittee, which serves as a liaison between the governing body, the chief executive officer, and the medical staff. By providing an opportunity for interchange of information and discussion, the committee promotes mutual understanding of each other's problems and activities. Thus the broad experience, knowl-edge, and responsibility of both groups can be utilized before major decisions are made.

In smaller hospitals, the medical staff is composed of rela-tively few physicians and specialty representatives, thus, there is no need to divide the staff into departments. Large medical staffs with many specialists may maintain several departments. These departments or services usually repre-sent clinical specialties such as Medicine, Surgery, Obstetrics, Gynecology and Pediatrics in a medium-sized facility; while a large teaching hospital may also have departments for many subspecialties such as urology, cardiology, and ophthalmology.

A departmentalized medical staff has a chairperson heading each service who is responsible for assuring the implementa-tion of a planned and systematic process for monitoring and evaluating the quality and appropriateness of patient care and the performance of all individuals with clinical privileges in the department.

Chief Executive Officer

The chief executive officer (CEO) is the manager of the hospital. This person must be able to take the elements of manpower, materials, technology, and capital, and integrate them into a desired whole that is best for the hospital. The role of CEO is often that of a change agent, and the adminis-trative responsibilities are extremely demanding.

The staff that is employed by the CEO consists of many types and kinds of allied health professionals, nursing person-nel, and support personnel. Their qualifications vary accord-ing to the facility's needs and patient care expectations.

AMBULATORY CARE

Ambulatory or outpatient care is one of the fastest growing areas in health care. When ambulatory care was first provided by hospitals, its purpose was to give medical care to the poor who could not afford a private physician. This concept is no longer true today, because ambulatory care has been found to be medically superior for many types of treatments, is generally more cost-effective for specific treatments, and improves accessibility to health care for all.

There are many types of ambulatory care facilities. Within a hospital, ambulatory care may be provided in an outpatient clinic, emergency department, day surgery area, or through diagnostic referral services. Free-standing ambulatory care may or may not be hospital affiliated: health maintenance organizations, surgicenters, emergicenters, neighborhood health centers, dialysis centers, and community mental health centers are examples. Ambulatory care is also provided in physician offices and private physician group practices.

LONG TERM CARE

Long term care facilities are generally defined as those in which patients receive care for a period of time longer than 30 days. There are several types of long term care facilities.

A nursing home is a facility that provides nursing care on a 24-hour basis as well as other support services. Individuals receiving such care are often referred to as residents instead of patients, as they remain in the nursing home for a relatively long period of time.

Physical medicine and rehabilitation facilities may also be characterized as long term, although such care may be given not only in an inpatient setting but to outpatients. Individuals receiving care in such facilities primarily require special support services in addition to varying levels of nursing care.

Long term care may also be provided in the home through a home health agency such as the Visiting Nurse Association, subdivision of a local or state health or welfare department, or a department of a hospital or other health care facility.

Finally, the hospice is another form of care sometimes classified as long term. It provides palliative and supportive care for terminally ill patients and their families. Emphasis is placed on the control of symptoms and preparation for and support before and after death. The hospice can be free-standing, hospital based, or home based. A hospice is really not a type of facility but a new concept of providing health care services where necessary.

HEALTH CARE PRACTITIONERS

Just as there are many types of health care facilities there are also many types of health care practitioners. Providing health care is no longer the sole responsibility of the physician. The physician relies on a great number of health care professionals whose contributions to patient care fulfill the physician's orders and complement the physician's service. The individuals who contribute to both direct and indirect patient care comprise the health care team.

PHYSICIANS

A physician is a person skilled in the art of healing. There are two types of physicians: The Doctor of Medicine (MD) and the Doctor of Osteopathy (DO).

An MD is an individual who has earned a doctor of medicine degree from an accredited medical school. Upon obtaining the degree and while applying for state licensure, a physician generally completes a year of internship at a hospital, practicing general medicine under the supervision of the medical staff. Most physicians wish to practice a specialty, such as internal medicine, surgery, cardiology, and so forth. Continued study in the chosen specialty is accomplished by completing a residency program (three to several years) in the specialty area. Collectively, physicians who are completing internships and residency programs are referred to as house staff in a health care facility. They are salaried by the facility and are closely supervised by members of the medical staff who are responsible for their performance.

Osteopathic physicians are physicians who obtain a doctor of osteopathy degree from an approved school of osteopathy. The literal meaning of osteopathy is "disease of the bone." The osteopath believes that disease is related to the structure of the body. The osteopath prefers treatments restoring the integrity of the musculoskeletal system to interventions such as drug therapy and surgery.

Other doctoral practitioners include podiatrists (DPM), dentists (DDS), chiropractors (DC), and optometrists (OD). Licensure limits practice, treatments, and drug prescriptions to their particular field of preparation. Hospitals may grant admitting privileges to dentists and podiatrists with the provision that a physician prepares the patient's history and physical examination and the physician is also responsible for the overall medical supervision of the patient.

NURSES

Nursing is one of the oldest, most well-established health care professions. The history of nursing shows a continually expanding role for its practitioners.

The registered nurse (RN) is a health care practitioner whose major task is coordinating the factors that influence the patient's health, such as observing symptoms and reactions, accurate recording of facts, carrying out treatments, and administering medications. In the inpatient setting the nurse carries out physicians' orders, helps the patient adjust to hospitalization, assists with discharge planning, and provides health care information and counseling to the patient. In the ambulatory setting the nurse interfaces with physicians, hospitals and clinics, as well as school authorities, social agencies, housing authorities, and the state health department.

RNs are graduates of approved schools of nursing and have passed a state licensure examination. Nursing programs may be in two-year junior colleges, three-year diploma schools, or in four year baccalaureate institutions. A few states have set minimum requirements for licensure at the baccalaureate level. Nurse anesthetists, nurse midwives, and nurse practitioners have special training in addition to a nursing degree. The nurse anesthetist has special training in anesthesia to assist the anesthesiologist (a physician who specializes in anesthesiology) and to administer anesthesia without direct supervision in certain pre-defined situations. The nurse midwife specializes in obstetrical care and has sufficient training to manage routine pregnancies and deliveries. The nurse practitioner performs diagnostic and therapeutic tasks under the direction of a physician.

A licensed practical nurse (LPN) is an individual who has received a formal course of instruction (usually nine months to a year) in practical nursing and who has taken a state examination to become a licensed practical nurse. Practical nursing is the performance of nursing duties which do not require the professional knowledge and skills of a registered nurse, including the care of convalescent, chronically ill, aged or infirm patients, and the carrying out of medical and nursing orders under the supervision of registered nurses or as directed by a licensed physician.

PHARMACISTS

A pharmacist is an individual who prepares, preserves, compounds, and dispenses drugs. Pharmacists are in many different settings, both within health care facilities and in health-related organizations. Pharmacists may own and manage pharmacies, they may hold positions in governmental regulatory agencies - for instance the Food and Drug Administration - and they may be involved in research, development, manufacturing, and distribution of drugs in a pharmaceutical company. Pharmacists play an important role in patient health care settings, educating physicians and nurses to recent developments in drug therapy, developing drug policies and control systems, upgrading distribution procedures, and counseling patients.

ALLIED HEALTH PRACTITIONERS

Allied health is a much newer concept than medicine and nursing. Although some of the occupations within allied health existed before the term allied health became popular such as medical social work, many are the result of technological advances. For example, the electron microscopist came into existence only after the electron microscope became commonly used in health care. "Allied health" applies to occupations whose primary function is to provide health services or promote health. Preparation for such occupations range from on-the-job training to postgraduate education. The occupations include those which have direct patient care responsibilities, such as physical therapists and occupational therapists, and those with little or no direct patient contact, such as medical laboratory technologists, community health educators, and health information practitioners. Figure 4 is a

EDUCATIONAL REQUIREMENT	PATIENT ORIENTED	LABORATORY ORIENTED	ADMINISTRATION ORIENTED	COMMUNITY ORIENTED	OTHER
Postbaccalaureate/Masters	Audiologist Clinical Psychologist Medical Social Worker Rehabilitation Counselor Speech Pathologist Psychiatric Social Worker Corrective Therapist Music Therapist Art Therapist Physical Therapist		Hospital Administrator Biostatistician	Public Healt Administrator Health Educator Nutritionist Engineering Specialties	Biomedical Engineer Health Physicist Medical Illustrator Medical Librarian
Baccalaureate (Some with Postbaccalaureate Clinical Training)	Dietitian Occupational Therapist Dental Hygienist Orthopedic Technologist Prosthetist	Medical Technologist	Medical Record Administrator	Sanitarian	Medical Writer Nuclear Medical Technologist
Associate Degree and Other Prebaccalaureate	Dental Assistant Dispensing Optician Food Service Supervisor Occupational Therapy Assistant Orthoptic Technician Emergency Medical Technician Dietary Technician Recreation Technician Therapeutic Recreation Technician Speech and Communication Aide Physical Therapist Assistant	Cytotechnologist Dental Laboratory Technician Medical Laboratory Technician Radiologic Technician	Medical Record Technician Medical Secretary Ward Manager		Environmental Technologist Biomedical Instrument Technician
1-Year	Respiratory Technician Dietary Aide	Certified Laboratory Assistant	Medical Assistant Medical Office Assistant Nursing Unit Clerk		

FIGURE 4. ALLIED HEALTH PRACTITIONERS

table of allied health occupations arranged by educational preparation.

HEALTH CARE ADMINISTRATORS

A chief executive officer (CEO) of a health care facility is responsible for providing the environment in which direct health care services are provided. The terms administrator or president are also used to describe these individuals. CEOs coordinate intrahospital resources, make decisions about expanding available facilities, incorporate new health care services, and maintain established programs for health care. The CEO works with external agencies and regulatory bodies for purposes of quality assurance, cost containment, accreditation, and licensure.

The CEO of a facility operates in a business environment, and often it is a competitive environment as well. CEOs usually have master's-level preparation in hospital or business administration. Licensure requirements vary according to the type of facility and state in which the administrator works. Several organizations, including the American College of Healthcare Executives and the American Health Care Association (for long-term care administrators) provide a form of certification and encourage standards of excellence among their members. Continuing education activities play a prominent role in the ongoing career development of administrators.

A chief financial officer (CFO), of a health care facility is responsible for overseeing all accounting and financial affairs of the health care facility. The background of this individual is often that of a certified public accountant but may also be that of master's preparation in business or finance. The Healthcare Financial Management Association offers a certifying examination which addresses the special issues of financial management in health care facilities.

Chief information officer (CIO) is a relatively new, senior level executive position in health care facilities. Often going by such titles as data services manager, health information manager, or vice president for information services, the CIO is an intermediary between the top business objectives of an organization and the information functions throughout. The CIO generally holds a master's degree prepared with experience and interest in broad applications and uses of various kinds of information. The CIO engages in strategic planning and marketing, and heads up information system development and automation planning.

Public health administrators are commonly found in health-related organizations which do not provide direct patient care, especially government. Public health administrators set policy and develop procedures for health care programs apart from individual health care facilities, such as those administered by state health departments, etc. Most of these individuals have a master's degree in public health.

HEALTH-RELATED ASSOCIATIONS, ORGANIZATIONS, AND AGENCIES

To further the goals of health care facilities and practitioners, many health-related organizations have been created. Their purposes are many and varied - from representing individual or institutional members to raising funds for medical research. In addition to accrediting, certifying, and licensing agencies, progress in achieving high standards of health care in the US must also be credited to the efforts of these groups. Some of the major groups are described here.

American Medical Association

This is the oldest of the medical associations. It was founded in 1847 and has its headquarters in Chicago, Illinois. Its components are state, county, and territorial groups of physicians.

The organizational structure is made up of several officers, a Board of Trustees, a House of Delegates, and several councils. Each council has its own purposes, projects, and responsibilities. The Council on Medical Education, for example, approves internship and residency programs for physicians and sets standards for medical schools throughout the country.

American College of Surgeons

The American College of Surgeons (ACS) was founded in 1913. This is a professional association for surgeons and was formed to establish standards of surgical education and practice.

As mentioned earlier in this chapter, the American College of Surgeons was the first association to become aware of the great need to improve the quality of medical care. Its Hospital Standardization Program, begun in 1918, was a major influence in improving medical care until the accreditation program of the Joint Commission on Accreditation of Healthcare Organizations took over.

Today the primary purpose of the ACS, which is headquartered in Chicago, is to improve the quality of care for surgical patients by elevating the standards of surgical education and practice. One way it achieves this purpose is by surveying and approving cancer programs and registries.

American College of Physicians

Founded in 1936, the American College of Physicians (ACP) has its headquarters in Philadelphia, Pennsylvania. The ACP certifies specialists in internal medicine through its certification board. The board determines the qualifications of candidates and administers examinations to physicians who meet its standards. These physicians must be doctors of medicine (MDs).

American Hospital Association

The American Hospital Association was founded in 1898 and is headquartered in Chicago. Its major purpose is to promote public welfare through its leadership and to provide better health services.

The AHA conducts research and educational projects in a wide variety of areas such as health care administration, hospital economics, hospital facilities and design, and community relations. It represents hospitals by speaking on their behalf on national legislative issues. It conducts many educational programs and seminars, maintains an excellent library, and publishes an annual survey of hospitals.

World Health Organization

The World Health Organization (WHO) was founded in 1948 and maintains its headquarters in Geneva, Switzerland. It functions through six regional offices located around the world.

Membership is open to any country. The WHO collaborates with the United Nations and assists governments in strengthening their health services wherever possible.

THE HEALTH CARE CONSUMER

As the concept of health has changed from the treatment and care of acute conditions to that of maintaining a state of well-being, the concept of the patient has changed as well. Once patients were merely recipients of direct services for the treatment of diseases. Consistent with this changing view, the public is increasingly concerned with prevention of disease, improved health conditions, safety of the work place, and safety of foods and products. In this role all Americans become consumers of health care whether direct or indirect.

Not only have the expectations of health care consumers changed but also the level of participation in their care. Consumers want to have a voice in selecting their health care services. They want explanations of their problems and knowledge of what is going to take place in their care plans. Health care providers are finding it necessary to reorient themselves to this more open and informed attitude. Medical record documentation takes on even greater importance in such an environment.

THE MEDICAL RECORD

The medical record today is a compilation of pertinent facts of a patient's life and health history, including past and present illness(es) and treatment(s), written by the health professionals contributing to that patient's care. The medical record must be compiled in a timely manner and contain sufficient data to identify the patient, support the diagnosis or reason for health care encounter, justify the treatment, and accurately document the results.

As a broader concept of health care has developed, the term "health record" has emerged and is often used interchangeably with "medical record." There are differences in the terms, however, just as there are differences between "medical care" and "health care."

The ideal concept of a health record is a single repository of all data on an individual health care consumer's health status. This would include birth records, immunization records, reports of all physical examinations, as well as records of all illnesses and treatments performed in any health care setting. Efforts are being made to define standards for such a longitudinal record, but records that exist in most health care facilities today are not nearly as comprehensive as the ideal health record described. In most health care facilities, records include only data compiled at that particular facility about specific episodes of medical care. Thus the term medical record is still used to accurately describe the content of present records. The term health record has come to be used more in facilities that provide health care services other than or in addition to acute, short term medical care, such as ambulatory care.

The health information practitioner must ensure that the medical record contains all of the pertinent information needed for patient care and other uses. The process of ensuring that the medical record is complete and useful requires a thorough knowledge not only of the medical record content, but also information concerning purpose, ownership, value, uses of, and responsibility for the medical record.

The role of today's patient records, however, goes far beyond individual patient care. In the competitive health care environment, medical information is key. Data, for example, on the number and types of operations a hospital performs, may help the hospital decide whether to expand services. Likewise, information on the quality of care helps the medical staff monitor and evaluate itself.

The need for comprehensive information on each patient, coupled with facilities' needs for aggregate data, is a compelling reason that facilities are computerizing their records. Computerization of patient information is the first step toward a record that reflects a patient's total care, not just one episode. Computerization also gives caregivers fast access to medical information, thus improving their ability to treat patients.

PURPOSE

The main purpose of the medical record is to accurately and adequately document a patient's life and health history, including past and present illness(es) and treatment(s), with emphasis on the events affecting the patient during the current episode of care.

OWNERSHIP

The medical record developed in a health care facility or under its auspices is considered to be the physical property of that facility. The information contained therein, however, is the property of the patient and thus must be available to the patient and/or the patient's legally designated representative upon appropriate request. Regulations regarding access to the medical record vary depending on state law. The fact that the facility owns the paper upon which the record is written does not prevent others from submitting legitimate claims to see and copy the information therein. Discussion of the release of medical record information is presented in Chapter 15, Legal Aspects of Medical Records.

USES OF THE MEDICAL RECORD

The document compiled as the medical record contains a wealth of information and has many uses, both personal and impersonal. Personal use refers to usage in which the identity of the patient is retained and is necessary. A request for copies of portions of a patient's hospital medical record by the insurance company which provides hospitalization coverage for the patient is an example of personal use. The copies are needed for the company to process the patient's claim and thus provide a service to the particular patient.

Impersonal use refers to the usage in which the identity of the patient is not retained and is not necessary. Use of data from 1,000 medical records for a research study is an example of impersonal use. The major reason the medical record department concerns itself with these differences is that a proper authorization by the patient or legal representative for release of information is required before information can be released for personal use.

The medical record is used in a number of ways:

Patient Care Management -

- to document the course of the patient's illness and treatment during each episode of care;
- to communicate between the physician and other health professionals providing care to the patient; and
- to inform health professionals providing subsequent care.

Quality Review - to evaluate the adequacy and appropriateness of care.

Financial Reimbursement - to substantiate insurance claims of the health care facility and patient.

Legal Affairs - to provide data to assist in protecting the legal interests of the patient, the physician, and the health care facility.

Education - to provide actual case studies for the education of health professionals.

Research - to provide data to expand the body of medical knowledge.

Public Health - to identify disease incidence so plans can be formulated to improve the overall health of the nation and world.

Planning and Marketing - to identify data necessary for selecting and promoting facility services.

VALUE OF THE MEDICAL RECORD

The data within the medical record are valuable to many users:

- To the Patient - A medical record contains data regarding a patient's past and present health and presents documentation by health professionals of the patient's current condition in the form of physical findings, results of diagnostic and therapeutic procedures, and the patient's responses.

Because health professionals provide care to a number of people during a given time period, they are not expected to remember the details of each patient's illness and response to treatment. The patient also may not remember the significant details of illnesses and treatment. Thus the record serves as a reference for both the patient and health professional. It provides substantiation of care given, which is needed for the processing of the patient's health insurance claims. The record also serves the patient by providing data to health professionals who treat the patient on subsequent episodes of care, so continuity of care is provided to the patient. The record provides data which may protect the legal interests of the patient in workers' compensation, personal injury, or malpractice cases.

- To the Health Care Facility - The medical record provides data to evaluate the performance of health professionals working in the health care facility and to evaluate use of the facility's resources, such as special diagnostic equipment and services offered by the facility. The record is used in surveys by licensing, certifying, and accrediting agencies in evaluating care which the facility provides and in determining compliance with the standards of the respective agency.

The record is relied upon more and more to substantiate claims submitted to third-party payers. Health care facilities extract data from the medical record to report the diagnoses or reasons for the health care encounter and procedures performed for a given patient in order to correctly file a payment claim. Because the record documents the care given, it can be used, if necessary, to protect the facility in lawsuits.

- To Health Care Providers - The medical record provides information to assist all professionals in caring for a patient during the current episode of care and during subsequent visits to a facility. The record documents the care given by each professional, thus protecting their legal interests. The record assists physicians, in particular, in providing continuity of care across different health care delivery levels. For their own education, all professionals may review records of patients for whom they have provided care.
- To Educators, Researchers, and Public Health Officials - Medical records contain data which assist health professionals and students in the health professions to learn about patient care and disease processes. Medical records are indispensable in furthering medical research by supplying a database for evaluating the effectiveness of treatments for specific diseases.

The medical record also provides data for reporting vital events such as births and deaths to the public health agency in each state. Requirements for reporting certain diseases, such as communicable diseases and gunshot wounds, also exist in each state to protect the health of the individual and the public. Statistics developed from data gathered in this manner may document the need for state, national, and world health programs.

- To Organizations Responsible for Health Care Claim Payments - Insurance companies and federal/state program reviewers scrutinize medical records to determine if documentation exists to substantiate the facility's claim for insurance benefits. For continued participation in federal/state health insurance programs, the medical records maintained by a facility are reviewed to determine compliance with standards regarding medical record content.

RESPONSIBILITY FOR THE MEDICAL RECORD

It is the responsibility of the facility to provide a record for each patient and safeguard the record and its content against loss, damage, tampering, and unauthorized use. Responsibility for providing, directly or indirectly, an adequate medical record is shared by many members of administration and the medical staff.

In almost all states, the governing body is held responsible for the proper care of the patient as well as for the proper selection of a qualified medical staff and chief executive officer. As the final authority, it is legally and morally responsible for determining that each patient receives high quality medical care, documented by a complete and accurate medical record. The governing body fulfills this responsibility by delegation of facility operations to the chief executive officer as its representative.

The authority to manage a health care facility is delegated to the chief executive officer by the governing body. Medical records generated by a facility are the property of that facility and thus are rightfully the concern of the chief executive officer. The CEO is responsible for ensuring that the medical staff adopts rules and regulations providing for the maintenance of complete medical records in a timely manner, and must see that such policies are consistently enforced. The CEO delegates to the staff of the health information department responsibility for processing, storing, and retrieving the medical record. However, administration is responsible for providing adequate direction, space, equipment, and personnel to perform these tasks effectively.

The director of the health information department works with physicians and the directors of other departments to educate the administrative and medical staff in proper documentation practices and to assist them in designing medical record systems which facilitate documentation.

The major responsibility for an adequate medical record rests with the patient's physician. Other physicians and health care professionals are responsible for correctly documenting the care they provide.

As a group, the medical staff is responsible for determining bylaws and rules and regulations by which it is governed. Licensure, certification, and accreditation agencies all have standards requiring that the medical staff rules and regulations address certain issues regarding the medical record.

Generally, these issues include:

- provisions for the keeping of accurate and complete clinical records
- delineation of individuals authorized to make entries in the medical record
- time limit following admission of the patient in which a history and physical examination must be entered in the patient's record
- time limit following discharge for completion of the record
- provisions for review of the quality of medical records

THE AMERICAN HEALTH INFORMATION MANAGEMENT ASSOCIATION

As previously discussed, the American Association of Record Librarians of North America was founded in 1928. Since then, it has grown in membership and services. Today it's known as the American Health Information Management Association (AHIMA), to better reflect the broad roles of members. The association's purpose is to improve the quality of health care through improving the quality of information.

Various membership categories are open to persons interested in promoting the purposes of the association. Active members receive all the association's services and may participate fully in association activities. Persons working in related fields may choose to join as associate members, while student membership is available for those enrolled in health information programs. For health information professionals in specialized areas, AHIMA offers membership in sections and societies.

State health information associations are integral parts of AHIMA, as they conduct educational workshops, influence state legislation, and assist members in practice issues.

Four groups are essential to the association's planning and operations:

- The House of Delegates is the association's legislative body, with members from each state association. At each annual convention, the House of Delegates helps the association make business decisions and plan for the future.
- The Board of Directors is responsible for the management of the business and professional affairs of the association. Members of the Board are volunteers elected from the AHIMA membership.
- Many volunteer teams participate in the association's activities and carry out important roles such as overseeing the accreditation of educational programs, guiding the certification process, and developing position statements for the association.
- The AHIMA headquarters is located in Chicago. An executive director conducts the day to day business of the association and sees that its many services are carried out. Services include accreditation of academic programs, offering educational activities and publications, influencing national legislation, offering certification examination and credentials maintenance, and answering members' professional questions.

The Foundation of Record Education (FORE) of AHIMA, is a non-profit corporation founded in 1962. Its purposes are to promote education by providing loans, engage in research, and engage in other educational activities. FORE provides low-interest loans to students and has an extensive specialized library of medical record and health information publications. The FORE library makes its resources available to members and to the public

AHIMA Code of Ethics

The health information profession has its own code of ethics, and like other medical ethics, it is based on the Oath of Hippocrates. That oath says, in part:

"Whatever, in connection with my professional practice or not in connection with it, I see or hear, in the life of men, which might not be spoken of abroad, I will not divulge, as reckoning should be kept secret."

Because of the trust placed in every person who works in health information management, each staff member should observe this code:

AHIMA

AMERICAN HEALTH INFORMATION
MANAGEMENT ASSOCIATION

919 NORTH MICHIGAN AVENUE, SUITE 1400, CHICAGO, ILLINOIS 60611-1683

CODE OF ETHICS

Preamble

The health information management professional abides by a set of ethical principles developed to safeguard the public and to contribute within the scope of the profession to quality and efficiency in health care. This code of ethics, adopted by the members of the American Health Information Management Association, defines the standards of behavior which promote ethical conduct.

Principles

1. The Health Information Management Professional demonstrates behavior that reflects integrity, supports objectivity, and fosters trust in professional activities.
2. The Health Information Management Professional respects the dignity of each human being.

3. The Health Information Management Professional strives to improve personal competence and quality of services.

4. The Health Information Management Professional represents truthfully and accurately professional credentials, education, and experience.

5. The Health Information Management Professional refuses to participate in illegal or unethical acts and also refuses to conceal the illegal, incompetent, or unethical acts of others.

6. The Health Information Management Professional protects the confidentiality of primary and secondary health records as mandated by law, professional standards, and the employer's policies.

7. The Health Information Management Professional promotes to others the tenets of confidentiality.

8. The Health Information Management Professional adheres to pertinent laws and regulations while advocating changes which serve the best interest of the public.

9. The Health Information Management Professional encourages appropriate use of health record information and advocates policies and systems that advance the management of health records and health information.

10. The Health Information Management Professional recognizes and supports the Association's mission.

Maint./Cert.7/93 *Amended October 1991*

THE HEALTH INFORMATION
MANAGEMENT PROFESSIONAL

HISTORY OF EDUCATIONAL GROWTH

For the first few years after organization of the Association, the founding members were busy bringing about needed changes in their own departments. As time went on, they realized that those trained by the apprenticeship method could not be expected to go out and organize departments that would meet the newer, more stringent requirements for health information services.

Under the leadership of Je Harned Bufkin, a curriculum was drawn up for the use of hospitals desiring to establish schools. The prerequisites for application, the content and length of the courses, and the procedures to be followed for approval of the schools were also established. By 1935 the educational program was ready to function, and schools were approved in Massachusetts General Hospital, Boston; Rochester General Hospital, Rochester, New York; St. Mary's Hospital, Duluth, Minnesota; and St. Joseph Hospital, Chicago.

St. Mary's Hospital in Duluth was affiliated with the College of St. Scholastica from the very beginning, and its program was the first to grant a baccalaureate degree in medical records. Other programs gradually made the transition from the hospital setting to the college or university.

Presently there are approximately fifty accredited educational programs in health information administration, all of which either grant degrees or require them for entrance. Accredited educational programs in medical record technology number nearly one hundred eighty.

Until 1942 the Association inspected and approved its own schools, but then it was felt that the educational experience of the Council on Medical Education of the American Medical Association (AMA) would be of great benefit. Upon approval of its House of Delegates, the AMA assumed responsibility for the approval of schools for health information administration and its Council on Medical Education was authorized to establish standards, inspect training programs, and publish lists of approved schools.

Until mid-1944, the Committee on Allied Health Education and Accreditation (CAHEA) of the AMA and AHIMA's Council on Accreditation (previously known as the Council on Education) jointly shared responsibility as accrediting agencies for these educational programs. In mid-1994, the CAHEA went out of existence and AHIMA's Council on Accreditation transitioned into joint specialized accreditation activity with a successor organization, the Commission on the Accreditation of Allied Health Educational Programs (CAAHEP). Educational standards embodied in the document currently entitled, "Essentials for an Accredited Program for the Medical Record Administrator and Medical Record Technician", are approved by the AHIMA House of Delegates and by the collaborating organization. These standards, and the accompanying document which specifies the entry level competencies (Domains,

Tasks, and Subtasks) for both types of practitioners (see Figure 5), serve as the minimum criteria for educational programs in this professional field seeking to prepare competent health information management practitioners.

Domain I: Assess institutional and patient-related information needs and department informational, service, and operational needs.

Domain II: Design and select departmental service and operational systems, and information systems for patient-related data.

Domain III: Implement departmental service and operational systems, and information systems for patient-related data.

Domain IV: Evaluate departmental, operational and service systems, and information systems for patient-related data.

FIGURE 5. MAJOR ENTRY-LEVEL COMPETENCY (DOMAIN) AREAS

THE HEALTH INFORMATION MANAGEMENT PROFESSIONAL

The term health information management professional is a general one, describing all types of professionals in a wide variety of settings. Currently, however, the AHIMA offers certification examinations in three specialized health information areas, described in this section. In 1994, the titles of the credentials continue to refer to medical records, even though course work and knowledge of these professionals is increasingly in the area of health information management.

MEDICAL RECORD ADMINISTRATOR

An approved educational program in medical record administration must grant a bachelor's degree or accept only candidates who already have a bachelor's degree. The curriculum includes courses in medical sciences, management sciences, health care administration, health record management, computer applications in health care, and health information management. Supervised clinical experience in health information departments is also included. Upon successful completion of a medical record administration program, the graduate is eligible to take the national certification examination to become a registered record administrator (RRA).

MEDICAL RECORD TECHNICIAN

Because of the great shortage of trained medical record administrators, it became evident by 1951 that there was a need for trained ancillary workers who would be qualified to work under the supervision of the medical staff in a small hospital, or under the supervision of a registered record administrator in a large hospital. Accordingly a curriculum was developed, and prerequisites for entrance (high school graduation) established for schools to train health information technicians.

In 1953 the first schools for the education of health information technicians were approved. Although initially hospital-based programs, at the present time all programs are offered in colleges and universities which grant an associate degree, except the Independent Study Program offered by AHIMA. The curriculum for the health information technician program includes courses in medical sciences; computer technology for health information systems; health information science; health information processing, retention, and retrieval; and personnel supervision. Supervised clinical experience in health information departments is also required. Upon successful completion of a health information technician program, the graduate is eligible to take the national certification examination to become an accredited record technician (ART).

Independent Study Program

While the medical record profession underwent its growing pains, the demand for qualified medical record personnel far exceeded the supply. In order to provide some measure of balance, the 1957 AHIMA House of Delegates approved the development of the Correspondence Course for Medical Record Personnel. Enrollment began in 1962, and by 1979 over 15,000 students had availed themselves of this educational opportunity.

In 1979 the AHIMA introduced a new, more comprehensive home study program entitled "Independent Study Program in Medical Record Technology" (ISP/MRT) to replace the Correspondence Course. Seventeen modules must be completed in the enrollment period of thirty-six months. Course content includes such subjects as medical terminology, medical record science, health care delivery trends, supervisory concepts, and directed clinical practice. In order to enroll in the ISP/MRT, a candidate must have completed prerequisite College coursework.

To be eligible to write the certification examination to become an accredited record technician, ISP/MRT graduates must also have 30 semester hours of college credit in anatomy and physiology; English composition; introductory computer course, College mathematics and electives.

In 1993, an Independent Study Program in Coding (ISP/Coding) was established to provide an alternative educational opportunity for students interested in becoming coding specialists. The program covers an introduction to the health record, medical terminology, basic pathology, basic and advanced ICD-9-CM and CPT coding principles, as well as DRG coding for reimbursement. Students are required to complete a college anatomy and physiology course.

CERTIFICATION

As medical record work began to take on a professional status, it was felt that a yardstick for measuring the ability of the workers was needed. In 1932 the AHIMA set up qualifications, including a written examination, to establish recognition of highly qualified health information practitioners as professionals. These standards for initial certification have been raised over time, as have standards for all allied health professions.

Currently an individual receives a Certificate of Registration, and is entitled to use the letters RRA (Registered Record Administrator) upon successful completion of the certification examination for health information administrators. A Certificate of Accreditation and the use of the letters ART (Accredited Record Technician) are provided candidates who successfully complete the certification examination for health information technicians.

CERTIFIED CODING SPECIALIST

In 1992, AHIMA began offering certification in coding to interested persons. The examination focuses on intermediate coding skills, and persons who pass the examination and follow AHIMA's continuing education requirements are allowed to use the term "certified coding specialist" or CCS after their names.

CONTINUI.NG EDUCATION

Just because a medical record professional receives a credential does not mean the educational process has ended. AHIMA, recognizing that the true professional is never finished with learning, initiated a continuing education (CE) program in 1975. At present, RRAs are required to earn 30 CE clock hours in two years and ARTs are required to earn 20 CE clock hours in two years. Failure to complete the required CE hours results in revocation of the individual's registration or accreditation status, and the person is no longer eligible to use the designated credentials. Appropriate completion of the requirements at a later date may result in the individual's certification being reinstated.

ROLES AND TITLES

Health information practitioners have traditionally been employed in hospitals. In recent years, however, many professionals have chosen careers within a variety of health care facilities. Some manage medical information in physicians' group practices, managed care groups, home health agencies, hospices, industrial and college health facilities, specialized hospitals, long-term care facilities, and ambulatory surgery centers.

Within health care facilities, the titles of information management professionals and their departments vary. Some may still be called medical record managers in medical record departments, while others are called medical or health information managers in health information services. This book refers to both titles, because both are in use in facilities.

Careers in health information management go beyond health care facilities, however. Professionals work in insurance companies, PROs, accounting firms, consulting companies, law firms, computer equipment companies, contracted service agencies, and virtually any business organization where data storage and retrieval is of great importance. Because of the intense need for health information services, some professionals start their own businesses to provide educational and consulting services.

Many health information professionals have obtained advanced degrees in information management, business administration, education, or public administration so they can pursue higher level jobs in special settings.

Many people predict that opportunities for health information professionals will be healthy in the next ten years, particularly as more non-acute facilities hire professionals and as the information needs in the health care industry continue to grow.

INTERNATIONAL FEDERATION OF HEALTH RECORD ORGANIZATIONS

AHIMA was the first national medical record association. While the original membership included many Canadian medical record librarians, the Canadians soon realized the advantages of having their own organization with common national goals; and in 1942 they organized the Canadian Association of Medical Record Librarians.

Prior to World War II, the medical record personnel of Great Britain were preparing for organization but had to delay until after the war. They organized in 1948 as the Association of Medical Records Officers of Great Britain.

By 1949 the Australian Hospital Association recognized the value of trained medical record personnel and sparked the impetus that brought about the organization of two state groups, the New South Wales and Victorian Associations of Medical Record Librarians. In 1952 the Australian Federation of Medical Record Librarians was organized. These additions brought about added interest in research in medical records and improvement in the quality of the medical record. Channels of communication were soon established between the members of the organized associations as well as with isolated workers in other countries around the world. It was believed that worldwide participation of medical record personnel would bring about advances in the establishment of international standards, the compilation of statistics for international comparisons, as well as disease classifications that could be adopted on an international basis. Therefore, the First International Congress on Medical Records was held in London in

1952 with representatives from nine countries participating. Additional Congresses were held every few years until the Fifth International Congress in Stockholm, where the International Federation of Health Record Organizations was established. The Sixth Congress, and first meeting of the Federation, was held in 1972 in Sydney, Australia. It is evident that international interest in medical records has spread rapidly and that the enthusiasm of the original sponsoring group, including AHIMA has been amply rewarded.

The International Federation of Health Record Organizations meets every four years at various locations around the world. The purposes of the Federation are similar to those adopted by the national organizations. The Federation attempts to serve as a means of communication among medical record practitioners in various countries and thus advance the standards of medical record science worldwide. The Federation promotes the development of techniques to improve the quality of medical record services. This is done partly by educational programs and other media developed for the exchange of ideas and experiences by medical record personnel on an international level.

SUMMARY

This chapter offers a brief look at the history and growth of health care facilities and professionals. Health care today is complex, as patients are treated in a variety of settings by a variety of professionals.

A key component in today's health care environment is patient information, and its management is the subject of this book. Individual patient records are invaluable for ongoing care, for research, for quality review, and for legal needs. Data that comes from individual patient records, too, is invaluable as facilities compete, grow and change.

The health information management professional is a key member of the health care team, combining knowledge of business, information management, and patient records with a professional and ethical commitment.

STUDY QUESTIONS

1. Describe the historical development of medical care in the US.

2. Summarize the reasons for the development of the Hospital Standardization Program by the American College of Surgeons.

3. Define the major types of health care facilities and the types of care they offer.

4. Describe the method accrediting agencies use to survey facilities.

5. Detail ten reasons why medical records are valuable to patient care.

6. Explain the control and ownership of medical records.

7. Identify another allied health profession and research its origins.

8. Define the roles of the medical staff in a health care facility.

9. Draw or describe a typical page from a medical record of the 1800s and the 1900s.

REFERENCES

American Osteopathic Association, *Accreditation Requirements of the American Osteopathic Association*, (Chicago: AOA, 1988).

Buckland, Ann, "Chief Information Officer—Try it on for Size," *Journal of the American Medical Record Association*, (August, 1988), p. 34-39.

Burda, David, "More Positions Available than Wanted in Medical Record Job Market," *Journal of the American Medical Record Association*, (October 1984).

Classification of Health Care Institutions, (American Hospital Association, 1974).

Editorial on Hospital Standardization, *Hospital Management,* (May 1919).

French, Ruth M., *Dynamics of Health Care*, 3rd Ed., (McGraw Hill, 1979).

Joint Commission on Accreditation of Healthcare Organizations, *Accreditation Manual for Hospitals*, (Chicago: Joint Commission, 1994).

Martin, Franklin H., "Hospital Standardization - Its Inception, Development and Progress in Five Years," *Surgery, Gynecology and Obstetrics*, (1922), 34:135-160.

chapter 2

DEVELOPMENT AND CONTENT OF THE HOSPITAL MEDICAL RECORD

The medical record is the who, what, where, when, and how of patient care. Medical records are the visible evidence of what the hospital is accomplishing. It is imperative that accurate, timely documentation be provided for each patient on each contact with a health care provider.

Reinforcing the importance of documentation in hospital medical records, the Department of Health and Human Services (DHHS) in the document Conditions of Participation for Hospitals and the Joint Commission on Accreditation of Healthcare Organizations in its Accreditation Manual for Hospitals state that an adequate medical record shall be maintained for every individual who is evaluated or treated at the hospital through inpatient, ambulatory (outpatient), home health, or emergency services. The health information practitioner should consult the most current editions of the aforementioned documents and also the licensure requirements of the applicable state to ensure an understanding of what comprises an "adequate medical record."

FLOW OF THE MEDICAL RECORD

When a person is admitted to a hospital, the person is considered an "inpatient." The medical record for the inpatient originates in the admitting department of the hospital, and sometimes begins even before admission in the form of preadmission testing or other data. Here, the patient or representative provides identifying and financial data and signs consent forms for treatment and release of information. A medical record number which is used on all medical record forms for the patient is assigned. Generally, this is a permanent identification number assigned by the hospital and used whenever the patient receives care at the hospital. A patient account number may also be assigned. This is a unique number that differentiates each hospitalization or other episode of care for billing purposes. The admitting department sends relevant portions of the information collected on admission to other departments in the hospital to inform them the patient is being admitted. The departments usually receiving data are the business office, data processing, medical records, nursing service, housekeeping, and dietary.

The next department to generate data on the patient is the nursing station to which the patient is assigned. Here a medical record of basic forms is compiled for the patient. When orders for various tests, treatments, and consultations are provided by the patient's physician, nursing service generates and routes or transmits via computer the requests to the appropriate departments. Nursing service is responsible for filing test results and making entries regarding nursing care on certain forms within the record. Many aspects of medical record documentation are computerized, with printouts becoming part of the medical record.

The attending physician who admits the patient is primarily responsible for the patient's care. The attending physician generates data by compiling a history of the patient, performing a physical examination, and recording the results. The physician also generates data regarding the patient when orders for diagnostic and therapeutic services are made, when the patient's condition and response to treatment are assessed through progress notes, and when the patient's course at the end of the episode of care is summarized. During hospitalization, data may be generated by other physicians who give care to the patient, such as in providing consultation, surgery, or other specialized evaluations or treatments. Data dictated by various physicians may be transcribed and entered in the medical record. The health information department employs transcriptionists who type patient histories, physical exams, consultations, operative reports, and discharge summaries. Usually pathology and radiology departments employ transcriptionists who type these reports. The physician who generates each of these reports should review and authenticate them.

Ancillary services provide additional support in the care of the patient. Departments most frequently referred to as ancillary are dietary, medical laboratory, physical therapy, occupational therapy, respiratory therapy, and social service. These departments receive requests for services, evaluations, and/or treatments for individual patients. The data thus generated

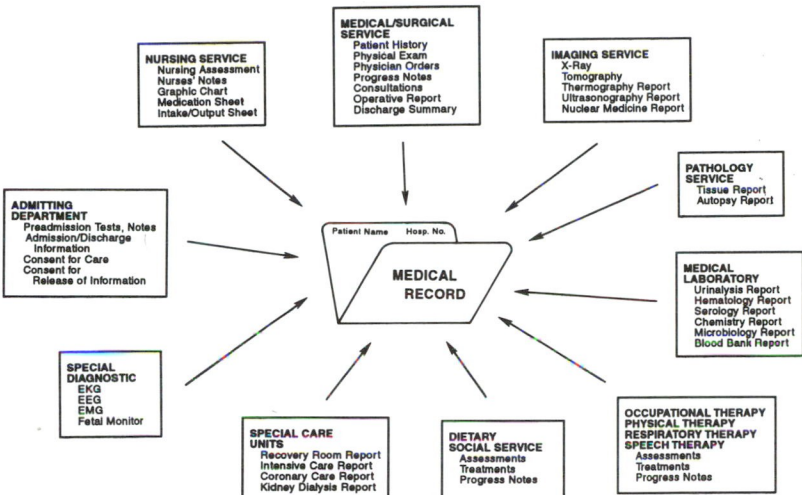

FIGURE 1. FLOW OF MEDICAL RECORD DATA

become part of the medical record, either by being placed in the record at the nursing station or, in the case of a patient who has been discharged, by the health information department. (See Figure 1.)

When a person goes to a hospital for ambulatory care, the patient is considered an "outpatient." Creation of ambulatory care records, in hospitals and other health care facilities, is covered in Chapter 3.

CONTENT OF THE MEDICAL RECORD

This section discusses the content of the acute general hospital medical record. The discussion is organized by describing the basic forms found in the majority of hospital medical records. While computerization of some position of the medical record exists in many hospitals, the data to be collected via the computer are often the same as the data contained in the forms described here. Many computer generate forms with the needed content at the end of a shift, day, or upon discharge.

Unless specified by requirements of approving agencies, the organization of data within and among the individual forms is determined by each hospital. A variety of sample forms are included in this chapter to demonstrate arrangements of data. As a result of the variety, the forms taken as a whole are not consistent in format. Inclusion of a form in this chapter is not to be construed as meaning the form is required or approved by licensing, certifying, or accrediting agencies. Individual hospitals should organize data to allow for efficient gathering and dispersing within its data system. Before adopting any form, it is imperative that a hospital critique the form to be certain it meets the individual needs of that hospital.

Because of the reduced size of the forms in this book, most have been left blank so the data items can be more easily read. In actual practice each item should have an entry. Items not pertinent to a particular patient are indicated by some type of entry, such as "not applicable" (NA). This indicates the item was not accidentally overlooked, which might be inferred from the presence of a blank item.

There are two broad classifications of hospital medical record data: administrative and clinical (reflecting the patient's illness(s) and treatment(s). Clinical data are usually subdivided into medical, nursing, and ancillary data. There are specific considerations for clinical data present in "special" types of hospital records such as obstetric, newborn, and short-stay records.

ADMINISTRATIVE DATA

Admission/Discharge Record

Basic identification and financial data are routinely collected on every patient except where not available. The data are collected at admission or prior to admission if pre-admission processing is done. These data are contained on a form referred to as the identification sheet, admission/discharge record, summary sheet, or face sheet. It is commonly computerized.

Sufficient information is contained in the sociological section to positively identify the patient including at a minimum the patient's name, address, date of birth, and next of kin. Basic clinical data are also supplied on this form. This data is described more fully in the section on clinical data.

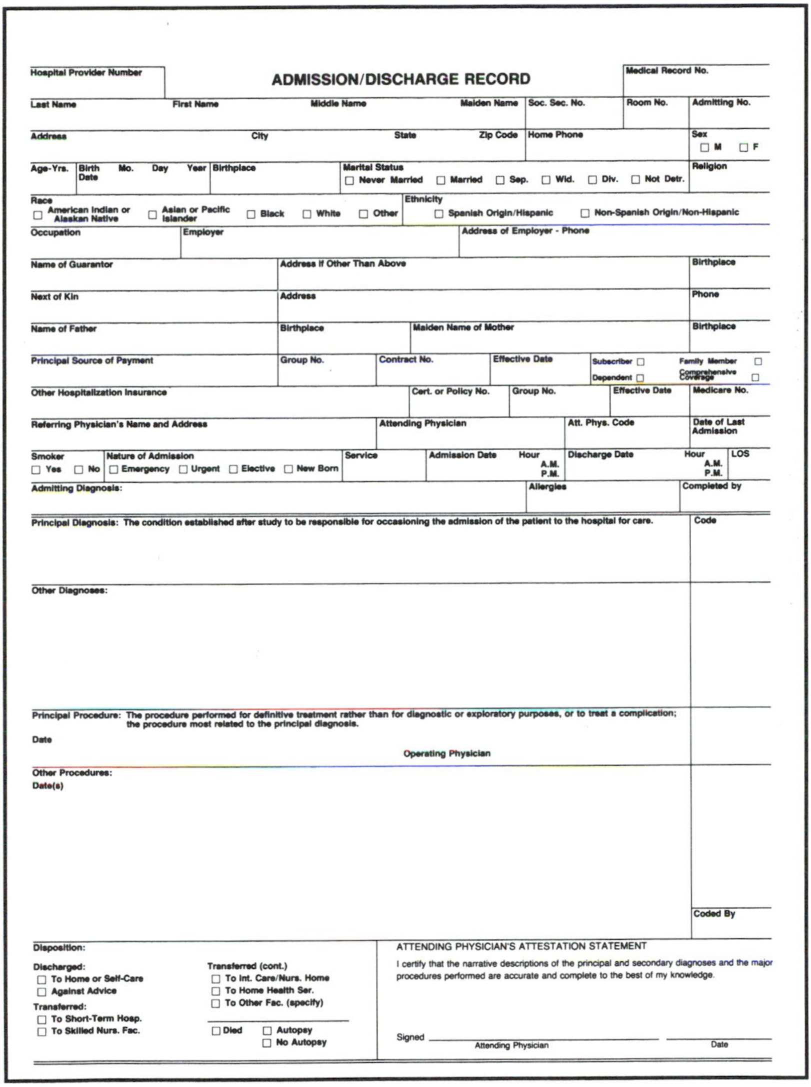

Hospital Provider Number

ADMISSION/DISCHARGE RECORD

Medical Record No.

Last Name | First Name | Middle Name | Maiden Name | Soc. Sec. No. | Room No. | Admitting No.

Address | City | State | Zip Code | Home Phone | Sex ☐ M ☐ F

Age-Yrs. | Birth Date Mo. Day Year | Birthplace | Marital Status ☐ Never Married ☐ Married ☐ Sep. ☐ Wid. ☐ Div. ☐ Not Detr. | Religion

Race ☐ American Indian or Alaskan Native ☐ Asian or Pacific Islander ☐ Black ☐ White ☐ Other | Ethnicity ☐ Spanish Origin/Hispanic ☐ Non-Spanish Origin/Non-Hispanic

Occupation | Employer | Address of Employer - Phone

Name of Guarantor | Address If Other Than Above | Birthplace

Next of Kin | Address | Phone

Name of Father | Birthplace | Maiden Name of Mother | Birthplace

Principal Source of Payment | Group No. | Contract No. | Effective Date | Subscriber ☐ Dependent ☐ | Family Member ☐ Comprehensive Coverage ☐

Other Hospitalization Insurance | Cert. or Policy No. | Group No. | Effective Date | Medicare No.

Referring Physician's Name and Address | Attending Physician | Att. Phys. Code | Date of Last Admission

Smoker ☐ Yes ☐ No | Nature of Admission ☐ Emergency ☐ Urgent ☐ Elective ☐ New Born | Service | Admission Date | Hour A.M. P.M. | Discharge Date | Hour A.M. P.M. | LOS

Admitting Diagnosis: | Allergies | Completed by

Principal Diagnosis: The condition established after study to be responsible for occasioning the admission of the patient to the hospital for care. | Code

Other Diagnoses:

Principal Procedure: The procedure performed for definitive treatment rather than for diagnostic or exploratory purposes, or to treat a complication; the procedure most related to the principal diagnosis.

Date

Operating Physician

Other Procedures:

Date(s)

Coded By

Disposition:

Discharged:
☐ To Home or Self-Care
☐ Against Advice

Transferred:
☐ To Short-Term Hosp.
☐ To Skilled Nurs. Fac.

Transferred (cont.)
☐ To Int. Care/Nurs. Home
☐ To Home Health Ser.
☐ To Other Fac. (specify)

☐ Died ☐ Autopsy ☐ No Autopsy

ATTENDING PHYSICIAN'S ATTESTATION STATEMENT

I certify that the narrative descriptions of the principal and secondary diagnoses and the major procedures performed are accurate and complete to the best of my knowledge.

Signed ____________ Attending Physician ____________ Date

Form courtesy of Physicians' Record Company

FIGURE 2. ADMISSION/DISCHARGE RECORD

Figure 2 is an example of an admission/discharge record. This example also contains the attestation statement required by Medicare, which some admission/discharge records may not include.

Attestation Statement

The attestation statement is a requirement of the Medicare prospective payment system. Via this statement the physician certifies that the principal and secondary diagnoses and the major procedures performed are accurately and completely

---

ATTESTATION STATEMENT

SAMPLE HOSPITAL, DRG ASSIGNMENT

PATIENT NAME: Doe, John   MEDICAL RECORD NO. 123456
ADMIT DATE: 01/01/89   DISCHARGE DATE: 01/10/89   BIRTH DATE: 09/01/1916
ATTENDING PHYSICIAN: Peter Adams, M.D.
PATIENT ACCOUNT NO. 890002

AGE: 73   SEX: Male   DISCHARGE DISPOSITION: 1 Home

MDC: 4   Diseases and disorders of the respiratory system

DRG: 87   Pulmonary edema and respiratory failure

ADMITTING DIAGNOSIS: 514   Pulmonary congestion/hypostasis

PRINCIPAL DIAGNOSIS: 514   Pulmonary congestion/hypostasis

SECONDARY DIAGNOSES:

276.5 Hypovolemia   (CC)

585   Chornic renal failure   (CC)

276.9 Electrolyte/fluid dis NEC   (CC)

403.9 Hypertensive renal dis NOS   More specific dx might be CC

PROCEDURES:

39.95 Hemodialysis

PRIMARY PAY SOURCE: 1 Medicare

ACTUAL LOS: 9	AVERAGE LOS: 7.0
	OUTLIER LOS THRESHOLD: 24
	NO. OF OUTLIER DAYS: 0
TOTAL CHARGES: $6,115	DRG PAYMENT: $4,467
	OUTLIER PAYMENT: $ 0
COST WEIGHT: 1.8078	TOTAL PAYMENT: $4,467

PHYSICIAN CERTIFICATION:

I certify that the narrative description of the principal and secondary diagnosis and the major procedures performed are accurate and complete to the best of my knowledge.

PHYSICIAN SIGNATURE: _____DATE: _____

FIGURE 3. ATTESTATION STATEMENT

documented in the medical record. The attestation statement may appear on the admission/discharge record (see Figure 2), or may be on a separate form. Frequently a hospital will use a computer to generate, via coded diagnostic and procedural data, an attestation statement which also contains Medicare reimbursement information (total charges and the Medicare "DRG Payment"). (Figure 3.)

CONDITIONS OF ADMISSION

TO

1. **General Duty Nursing:** The hospital provides only general duty nursing care. Under this system nurses are called to the bedside of the patient by a signal system. If the patient is in such condition as to need continuous or special-duty nursing care, it is agreed that such must be arranged by the patient, or his legal representative, or his physicians, and the hospital shall in no way be responsible for failure to provide the same and is hereby released from any and all liability arising from the fact that said patient is not provided with such additional care.

2. **Medical and Surgical Consent:** The patient is under the control of his attending physicians and the hospital is not liable for any act or omission in following the instructions of said physicians, and the undersigned consents to any x-ray examination, laboratory procedures, anesthesia, medical or surgical treatment or hospital services rendered the patient under the general and special instructions of the physician. The undersigned recognizes that all doctors of medicine furnishing services to the patient, including the radiologist, pathologist, anesthetist and the like, are independent contractors and are not employees or agents of the hospital.

3. **Release of Information:** The hospital may disclose all or any part of the patient's record to any person or corporation which is or may be liable under a contract to the hospital or to the patient or to a family member or employer of the patient for all or part of the hospital's charge, including, but not limited to, hospital or medical service companies, insurance companies, workmen's compensation carriers, welfare funds, or the patient's employer.

4. **Personal Valuables:** It is understood and agreed that the hospital maintains a safe for the safekeeping of money and valuables and the hospital shall not be liable for the loss of or damage to any money, jewelry, glasses, dentures, documents, furs, fur coats and fur garments, or other articles of unusual value and small compass, unless placed therein, and shall not be liable for loss of or damage to any other personal property, unless deposited with the hospital for safekeeping.

5. **Financial Agreement:** The undersigned agrees, whether he signs as agent or as patient, that in consideration of the services to be rendered to the patient, he hereby individually obligates himself to pay the account of the hospital in accordance with the regular rates and terms of the hospital. Should the account be referred to an attorney for collection, the undersigned shall pay reasonable attorney's fees and collection expense. All delinquent accounts bear interest at the legal rate.

The undersigned certifies that he has read the foregoing, receiving a copy thereof, and is the patient, or is duly authorized by the patient as patient's general agent to execute the above and accept its terms.

_____
PATIENT

_____
PATIENT'S AGENT OR REPRESENTATIVE

_____
RELATIONSHIP TO PATIENT

A copy of this Document is to be delivered to the patient.

Time of signing_____ 19____, Hour _____.M.

Witness: _____

| FORM A-144 | PHYSICIANS' RECORD CO., BERWYN, ILLINOIS - PRINTED IN U.S.A. | CONDITIONS OF ADMISSION |

Form courtesy of Physicians' Record Company

FIGURE 4. CONDITIONS OF ADMISSION

Conditions of Admission

The back of the admission/discharge form or a separate form is used for the conditions of admission (admission consent or authorization for admission form). The form provides a statement indicating that the patient agrees to receive basic, routine care. There usually is a statement to the effect that the hospital cannot guarantee the outcome. This form (Figure 4), when signed by the patient or guardian at admission, provides a record of consent to routine services, diagnostic procedures, and medical treatment. It is the responsibility of the admitting clerk to explain to the patient the contents of this form and its purpose.

Consent for Release of Information

A consent or authorization for release of information (Figure 5) allows the hospital to send copies of the patient's medical record to specifically named organizations. This form may also be found on the back of the admission/discharge form. The

AUTHORIZATION FOR RELEASE OF INFORMATION

To ______________ (NAME OF HOSPITAL) Hospital Number ______________

You are hereby authorized to furnish such professional information, in accordance with the policy of your hospital, as may be necessary for the completion of my hospitalization claims by ______________ (NAME OF THIRD PARTY)

______________ (NAME OF THIRD PARTY) from the medical records compiled during my hospitalization from ______________ 19____ to ______________ 19____ and are hereby released from all legal liability that may arise from the release of the information requested.

Date ______________ Signed ______________ (PATIENT OR NEAREST OF KIN)

Signed ______________ (PARTY INSPECTING RECORD) ______________ (RELATIONSHIP IF SIGNED BY OTHER THAN PATIENT)

Date of inspection of record ______________ 19____ Signed ______________ (ATTENDING PHYSICIAN)

Authorization must be signed by the patient, or by the nearest relative in the case of a minor or when patient is physically or mentally incompetent.

FORM C-409 PHYSICIANS' RECORD CO., BERWYN, ILLINOIS PRINTED IN U.S.A.

Form courtesy of Physicians' Record Company

FIGURE 5. AUTHORIZATION FOR RELEASE OF INFORMATION

patient's signature on this form authorizes the hospital to release medical information compiled during the current episode of care. The organizations which may receive this information are those which provide hospitalization insurance coverage including Medicare/Medicaid, workers' compensation, Blue Cross-Blue Shield, and private carriers. The American Health Information Management Association's position on confidentiality should be checked to ensure that release of information forms contain adequate information for an informed consent. Again, it is the responsibility of the admitting staff to explain to the patient the content of the consent and its purpose.

Advance directives, also known as living wills or durable power of attorney directives, are written instructions about the care a patient does or does not want. The Patient Self Determination Act, a federal law passed in 1990, requires health care facilities to ask patients whether they have advance directives and to document the response in the medical record. In addition, if there are state laws on advance directives, living wills, right to die, or death with dignity, hospitals must follow them as well.

The federal Patient Self Determination Act governs hospitals, skilled nursing facilities, home health agencies, and hospices that treat Medicare or Medicaid patients. Its major provisions require the following:

- Health care organizations must have policies about patients' rights to accept or refuse medical treatment, including the right to formulate advance directives. The policies must follow state laws, if applicable.
- At Admission, the institution must give the individual written information about what treatment decisions patients can make, along with the hospital's own treatment policies.
- The institution is required to document in the medical record whether the patient has an advance directive.

Special Consents

A special consent or authorization form (Figure 6) is required for any non-routine diagnostic or therapeutic procedures performed on the patient. This form provides written evidence that the patient agrees to the procedure(s) listed on the form. For the consent to be valid, the physician must discuss the procedures named, the risks, alternative procedures, and likely outcomes with the patient and/or guardian.

The *Conditions of Participation* require that the medical staff bylaws and rules and regulations state that a surgical operation may be performed only on consent of the patient or legal representative, except in emergencies. Also they require (in the section on the Surgery department) that a properly executed consent form for operation be in the patient's medical record prior to surgery.

AUTHORIZATION
AND
CONSENT TO OPERATION PROCEDURE

I, _____ authorize and consent to the performance upon myself (or) (name of patient) _____ of the following operation/procedure_____ _____ to be performed by or under direction of Dr.____ _____ at Community Hospital on_____.

I further consent to the performance of any additional procedures during the course of my operation/procedure which the physician or associates judge necessary or desireable to correct the existing condition or any other unhealthy condition which they may discover.

I realize that an operation/procedure requires numerous assistants, technicians, nurses, and other personnel, and I give my consent to such medical procedures and care by such personnel and Community Hospital befor, during, and after the operation/procedure to be performed.

I also consent to the disposal by Community Hospital of any tissue or parts which may be removed during my operation.

I have been advised by my physician about alternatives to the operation/procedure suggested, but I believe that the treatment suggested is the treatment or operation I should have.

My physician has advised me fully about the nature of the operation/procedure and the risks involved. I realize that neither the physician nor Community Hospital can guarantee any result.

I have read this authorization and understand it.

NOTE TO PATIENT: YOUR SIGNATURE BELOW INDICATES THAT YOU HAVE READ AND AGREED TO THE ABOVE, THAT THE OPERATIONS/PROCEDURES HAVE BEEN ADEQUATELY EXPLAINED TO YOU BY YOUR ATTENDING PHYSICIANS OR SURGEONS, THAT YOU HAVE ALL THE INFORMATION YOU DESIRE, AND THAT YOU AUTHORIZE AND CONSENT TO THE PERFORMANCE OF THE OPERATIONS/PROCEDURES MENTIONED ABOVE.

DATE:_____   SIGNATURE:_____ _____ _____

RELATIONSHIP (IF OTHER THAN PATIENT):_____

WITNESS' SIGNATURE:_____ _____

Signature of physician by which it is affirmed that the informed consent of the patient, or duly authorized agent, has been obtained to the outlined above.

DATE:_____   SIGNATURE:_____

FIGURE 6. SPECIAL CONSENT

The Joint Commission requires that there be evidence of informed consent for procedures and treatments for which consent is required according to the policy developed by the medical staff, governing body, and law. When consent is not obtainable, the reason is to be documented in the record. See Chapter 15 for further discussion of consents/authorizations.

CLINICAL DATA

Clinical data are the second broad category of medical record information.

Admission/Discharge Record

The medical information which is part of the admission/discharge record (Figure 2) usually includes the statement of diagnoses and procedures. The attending physician is responsible for supplying and authenticating this information. There is no requirement that the admitting diagnosis must be on this form, however, its presence here is helpful for room assignment in those hospitals with specialized services. It also assists nursing service in beginning care for the patient. Because insurers expect patients with certain diagnoses to be cared for on an outpatient basis, it is important that the admitting diagnosis be provided at or before admission. All diagnoses and procedures are to be written in full, without symbols or abbreviations, in acceptable terminology. The admission/discharge record may also provide such information as consultations, autopsy performance, presence of institutional (nosocomial) infections, allergies or sensitivities, and disposition of patient.

Medical History

The medical history of the patient is data the physician uses to establish a tentative provisional diagnosis on which to base the treatment of the patient (Figures 7 and 8). In the event that a reliable history cannot be elicited from the patient, the history must be obtained from the person best able to relate the facts. It is helpful to record the source of the history, i.e., the patient, parent, or friend. The history is to be completed within 24 hours of admission.

If the history and physical examination are performed by an unlicensed physician, intern, or medical student they should be countersigned by the resident and/or attending physician. If the attending physician does not agree with the data recorded, the attending physician's findings and pertinent observations should be recorded before signing.

To promote uniformity and completeness in the medical record, each facility should adopt a standard outline for the history, which may be printed on the history form. In a computerized system, the components of the history appear on the

HISTORY

Family Name	First Name	Attending Physician	Room No.	Hosp. No.

CHIEF COMPLAINT

Concise statement of complaints with date of onset and duration of each. Record in order of importance.

PAST HISTORY

Measles	Influenza
Whooping cough	Pleurisy
Mumps	Tuberculosis
Chickenpox	Asthma
Tonsillitis	Arthritis
Scarlet fever	Amebiasis
Diphtheria	Lues
Rheumatic fever	Gonorrhea
Typhoid fever	Injuries
Malaria	Operations
Pneumonia	Other

FAMILY HISTORY

If living health of, and if deceased cause of death of father, mother, siblings, children. Any familial:

Cancer	Heart disease
Tuberculosis	Allergy
Diabetes	Arthritis
Hemophilia	Other
Kidney disease	

INVENTORY BY SYSTEMS

GENERAL

Nutrition	Tremor
Fever	Weight gain
Night sweats	Weight loss
Falling hair	Other

SKIN

Eruptions	Jaundice
Cyanosis	Other

HEAD

Headache	Syncope
Trauma	Other

EYES

Eyestrain	Lacrimation
Diplopia	Glasses Date Last Checked
Photophobia	Blurring
Inflammation	Other

(over)

FORM D-219 — PHYSICIANS RECORD CO. · BERWYN, ILLINOIS · PRINTED IN U.S.A. — HISTORY (OVER)

Form courtesy of Physicians' Record Company

FIGURE 7. MEDICAL HISTORY (front)

display screen for the physician to use. Positive (the presence of a symptom) and negative data should be recorded. It is recommended that the terms "negative" or "normal" not be used except in summarizing stated facts. The data should reflect what the patient states. The physician's point of view may be expressed in the physical examination and subsequent notes. The following information is suggested content for the history.

HISTORY (Continued)

INVENTORY BY SYSTEMS
(continued)

EARS
Deafness   Dizziness
Discharge   Pain
Tinnitus   Other

NOSE
Colds   Obstruction
Epistaxis   Postnasal drip
Sinus's   Other

THROAT
Soreness   Dysphagia
Redness   Other
Hoarseness

RESPIRATORY
Chest pain   Dyspnea
Hemoptysis
Sputum   Other

NEUROMUSCULAR
Weakness   Varicosities
Joint pain   Deformities
Paresthesia   Other

CARDIOVASCULAR
Pain   Faintness
Asthma   Vertigo
Palpitation   Edema
Tachycardia   Other

GASTROINTESTINAL
Appetite   Stool
Distress   Shape
Pain   Color
Nausea   Mucous
Vomiting   Blood
Belching   Hemorrhoids
Flatulence   Hernia
Constipation   Other
Diarrhea

GENITOURINARY
Discharge   Pyuria
Sores   Hematuria
Frequency   Pain
Nocturia   Other
Incontinence

FEMALE - REPRODUCTIVE
Periods   Pregnancies, type
Frequency   and complications
Type   Labors, type and
Duration   complications
Abortions   Other

PSYCHOLOGICAL STATUS
Personality type Convulsions
Emotional state   Paralysis
Headaches   Nervous breakdown
Stress   Insomnia
Memory Loss   Suicidal behavior
Nightmares   Other

Taken by:_____
                        (Signature of physician taking history)

Date_____ Attending Physician_____M.D.

(D-219 BACK)

Form courtesy of Physicians' Record Company

FIGURE 8. MEDICAL HISTORY (back)

1. Chief complaint: nature and duration of the symptoms that caused the patient to seek medical attention, as stated in the patient's own words.

2. Present illness: detailed chronological description of the development of the patient's illness from the appearance of the first symptom to the present time.

3. Past medical history: a summary of childhood and adult illnesses or medical treatment, such as infectious diseases, pregnancies, allergies and drug sensitivities, accidents, operations, hospitalizations, and current medications.

4. Psychosocial or personal history: marital status; dietary, sleeping, exercise patterns; use of coffee, alcohol, other drugs, and tobacco; occupation; environment; daily routine; religious beliefs; and outlook on life.

5. Family history: diseases among relatives in which heredity or contact may play a role, such as allergies; infectious diseases; mental, metabolic, endocrine, cardiovascular, renal diseases; or neoplasms. The health of immediate relatives, ages at death, and causes of death should be recorded.

6. Review of systems: a systemic inventory to reveal subjective symptoms which the patient either forgot to describe or which at the time seemed relatively unimportant. Generally an analysis of the subjective findings will indicate the nature and extent of the physical examination required. The following data are examples of items which the physician is to include.

   a. General: usual weight, recent weight changes, fever, weakness, fatigue.

   b. Skin: rashes, eruptions, dryness, cyanosis, jaundice, changes in skin, hair or nails

   c. Head: headache (duration, severity, character, location).

   d. Eyes: glasses or contact lenses, last eye examination, vision, glaucoma, cataracts, eyestrain, pain, diplopia, redness, lacrimation, inflammation, blurring

   e. Ears: hearing, discharge, tinnitus, dizziness, pain.

   f. Nose: head colds, epistaxis, discharges, obstruction, postnasal drip, sinus pain.

g. Mouth and throat: condition of teeth and gums, last dental examination, soreness, redness, hoarseness, difficulty in swallowing.

h. Respiratory: chest pain, wheezing, cough, dyspnea, sputum (color and quantity), hemoptysis, asthma, bronchitis, emphysema, pneumonia, tuberculosis, pleurisy, last chest x-ray.

i. Neurological: fainting, blackouts, seizures, paralysis, tingling, tremors, memory loss.

j. Musculo-skeletal: joint pain or stiffness, arthritis, gout, backache, muscle pain, cramps, swelling, redness, limitation in motor activity.

k. Cardiovascular: chest pain, rheumatic fever, tachycardia, palpitation, high blood pressure, edema, vertigo, faintness, varicose veins, thrombophlebitis.

l. Gastrointestinal: appetite, thirst, nausea, vomiting, hematemesis, rectal bleeding, change in bowel habits, diarrhea, constipation, indigestion, food intolerance, flatus, hemorrhoids, jaundice.

m. Urinary: frequent or painful urination, nocturia, pyuria, hematuria, incontinence, urinary infections.

n. Genito-reproductive: Male-venereal disease, sores, discharge from penis, hernias, testicular pain or masses. Female-age at menarche; menstruation: frequency, type, duration, dysmenorrhea, menorrhagia; symptoms of menopause; contraception; pregnancies; deliveries; abortions; last Pap smear.

o. Endocrine: thyroid trouble, heat or cold intolerance, excessive sweating, thirst, hunger or urination

p. Hematologic: anemia, easy bruising or bleeding, past transfusions.

q. Psychological: personality type, nervousness, mood, insomnia, headache, nightmares, depression.

Qualified oral surgeons, who have been granted such privileges by the medical staff, may perform a complete history (and physical examination) on their patients. Dentists and podiatrists are responsible for documenting the patient's history pertaining to their area of expertise. If a complete history has been recorded within 30 days prior to admission, such as in the office of a physician or a qualified oral surgeon, a legible copy of this report may be placed in the hospital medical record, provided there have been no changes since the original was recorded; or if changes have occurred, these changes were documented at the time of admission.

Physical Examination

The physical examination (Figure 9) provides baseline data about the patient to assist the physician in determining a

FORM D-302 PHYSICIANS RECORD CO., BERWYN, ILLINOIS . PRINTED IN U.S.A.

HOSPITAL REGULATION: All Positive and Important Negative Findings Shall be Recorded.

Date_____ Hour_____ a.m. p.m. Age_____ Sex_____ Weight_____

Temp._____ Pulse_____ Resp._____ Blood Pressure_____

ORDER OF RECORDING

1. General
2. Skin
3. Eyes
4. Ears
5. Nose
6. Mouth
7. Throat
8. Neck
9. Chest
10. Heart
11. Abdomen
12. Genitalia
13. Lymphatic
14. Blood Vessels
15. Locomotor
16. Extremities
17. Neurological
18. Rectal
19. Vaginal
20. Diagnosis
21. Signature

Name Last	First	Middle	Hospital No.

Location in Hospital	Clinic or Service	Attending Physician

PHYSICAL EXAMINATION

Form courtesy of Physicians' Record Company

FIGURE 9. PHYSICAL EXAMINATION

diagnosis. The examination should include all body systems. The degree of detail depends upon the age and sex of the patient, the patient's symptoms, other physical findings or laboratory data.

The diagnosis portion of the physical examination may be a statement of a provisional (tentative) diagnosis. The physician records his impression based on the subjective statements of the patient in the history and his objective findings in the physical examination. The physician may have several diagnoses which he considers possible for the patient. The stating of several different diagnoses is referred to as the "differential" diagnosis.

Suggested content of the physical examination follows. Words in parentheses indicate sections which the physician may be likely to omit when the exam is entirely negative.

1. General survey: apparent state of health, signs of distress, posture, weight, height, skin color, dress and personal hygiene, facial expression, manner, mood, state of awareness, speech.

2. Vital signs: pulse, respiration, blood pressure, temperature.

3. Skin: color, its vascularity, any lesions, edema, moisture, temperature, texture, thickness, mobility and turgor, nails.

4. Head: hair, scalp, skull (face).

5. Eyes: visual acuity and fields, position and alignment of the eyes, eyebrows, eyelids; lacrimal apparatus; conjunctivae; sclerae; corneas, irises; pupils: size, shape, equality, reaction to light and accommodation; extraocular movements; ophthalmoscopic exam.

6. Ears: auricles, canals, tympanic membranes, hearing, discharge.

7. Nose and sinuses: airways, mucosa, septum, sinus tenderness, discharge, bleeding, smell.

8. Mouth: breath, lips, teeth, gums, tongue, salivary ducts.

9. Throat: tonsils, pharynx, palate, uvula, postnasal drip.

10. Neck: stiffness, thyroid, trachea, vessels, lymph nodes, salivary glands.

11. Thorax, anterior and posterior: shape, symmetry, respiration.
12. Breasts: masses, tenderness, discharge nipples.
13. Lungs: fremitus, breath sounds, adventitious sounds, friction, spoken voice, whispered voice.
14. Heart: location and quality of apical impulse, thrill, pulsation, rhythm, sounds, murmurs, friction rub, jugular venous pressure and pulse, carotid artery pulse.
15. Abdomen: contour, peristalsis, scars, rigidity, tenderness, spasm, masses, fluid, hernia, bowel sounds and bruits, palpable organs.
16. Genitourinary: scars, lesions, discharge, penis, scrotum, epididymis, varicocele, hydrocele.
17. Vaginal: external genitalia, Skene's and Bartholin's glands, vagina, cervix, uterus, adnexa.
18. Rectal: fissure, fistula, hemorrhoids, sphincter tone, masses, prostate, seminal vesicles, feces.
19. Musculoskeletal: spine and extremities, deformities, swelling, redness, tenderness, range of motion.
20. Lymphatics: palpable cervical, axillary, inguinal nodes; location; size; consistency; mobility and tenderness.
21. Blood vessels: pulses, color, temperature, vessel walls, veins.
22. Neurological: cranial nerves, coordination, reflexes, biceps, triceps, patellar, Achilles, abdominal, cremasteric, Babinski, Romberg, gait, sensory, vibratory.
23. Diagnosis.

The Joint Commission requires a report of a comprehensive current physical assessment. If one has been performed within 30 days prior to admission, such as in the office of a physician staff member, then a durable, legible copy of this report may be used in the patient's medical record if there have been no changes in the patient or if the changes are documented at the time of admission. When the patient is readmitted within 30 days for the same or a related problem, an "interval" physical exam reflecting any changes may be used, provided the original physical exam is readily available. Prior to surgery the medical record must contain a history, physical exam, and preoperative diagnosis. The recorded physical exam is to be authenticated by a physician or, when given the privilege, a qualified oral surgeon. The physical exam is to be completed within 24 hours of admission.

In conjunction with the history and physical examination, the Joint Commission further requires that there be a statement of impressions or conclusions drawn from the aforementioned data and a statement of the course of action planned for the patient while in the hospital.

Physician's Orders

The written or verbal orders constitute the attending physician's direction to nursing and ancillary services and house staff, regarding all medications and treatments for the patient. An example of a form for recording physician's orders is provided in Figure 10. Physician's orders are to be dated and authenticated by the physician giving the order. Routine or "standing" orders are a set of orders designed for routine care of patients with a certain diagnosis or procedure. When these are used as either a separate sheet or incorporated on the physician's order form, they are also to be signed by the physician. Most hospitals discourage the use of standing orders because the specified services may not be medically necessary for some patients. A discharge order should be written on every patient when the physician determines the patient may be released from the facility. Absence of a discharge order may indicate the patient left the hospital against medical advice (AMA), a fact which should be noted in the progress notes or discharge summary. Verbal orders of authorized practitioners may be allowed with certain limitations. Medical staff rules and regulations should state who may receive verbal orders and the time limits for affixing a signature to these orders. Medical staff rules and regulations may prohibit the use of such orders.

The Joint Commission specifies that the medical staff rules and regulations should define any category of verbal orders associated with any potential hazard to the patient, and require the responsible practitioner to sign such orders within. The time frame defined in the Medical Staff rules and regulations.

```
┌────────────────────────────────────────────────────────────────────────┐
│                                        ┌ USE NAME PLATE OR PRINT PATIENT ID HERE ┐ │
│                                          ↓   ↓   ↓   ↓   ↓   ↓   ↓   ↓   ↓       │
│            PHYSICIAN'S ORDERS                                             │
│                                                                          │
│  DRUG ALLERGIES                                                          │
│  ANOTHER BRAND OF DRUG IDENTICAL IN FORM AND        ☐                     │
│  CONTENT MAY BE DISPENSED UNLESS CHECKED                                 │
├──────────┬──────────────────────────────────────┬───────────────────────┤
│ Date & Time │       ORDERS AND SIGNATURE         │    Signature of       │
│  Ordered  │                                      │  Physician and Nurse  │
│           │                                      │   attending to order  │
```

FORM D-625 REVISED 7/83   PHYSICIAN'S ORDERS   PRINTED IN U.S.A.
PHYSICIANS RECORD CO BERWYN ILLINOIS

Form courtesy of Physicians' Record Company

FIGURE 10. PHYSICIAN'S ORDERS

Progress Notes

Progress notes are specific statements related to the course of the patient's illness, response to treatment, and status at discharge. The attending physician is responsible for recording continuing observations of the patient's progress. In integrated progress notes ancillary professionals, such as occupational, physical and respiratory therapists, also document the care they provide and the patient's response to treatment. Nurses' notes may or may not be included. When integrated progress notes are used, the progress notes form often allows for distinction between physician and other notes through the use of margins or columns (Figure 11 provides examples of two styles of progress notes).

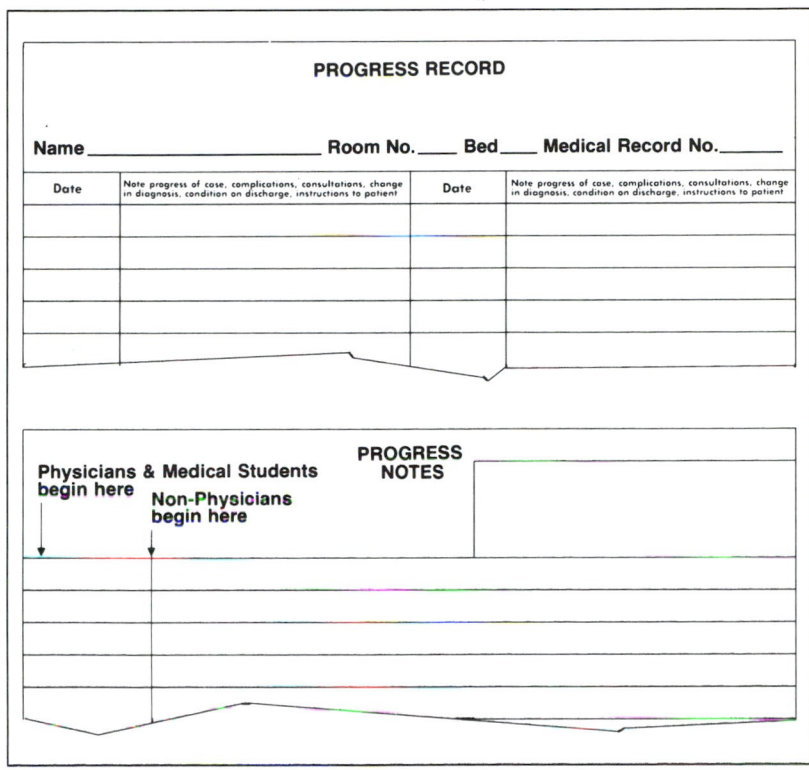

FIGURE 11. PROGRESS NOTES FORMS

Physician progress notes should include an admission note, follow-up progress notes, and a final note. The admission note summarizes the general condition of the patient at the time of admission. Pertinent information about the patient not recorded in the history or physical examination should be recorded here. Subsequent progress notes are written as frequently as required by the patient's condition and medical staff rules and regulations. All treatments provided and the patient's response to each are to be included in the progress notes. Any complications which the patient develops should also be documented in the progress notes. If the hospital has house officers, an end-of-service note is to be written as one house officer relinquishes the care of the patient to another. This note summarizes the patient's course of illness and treatment. The final note is a statement of the patient's general condition on discharge, discharge instructions including patient activity, diet, medications, and time for follow-up visit to a physician. If the patient expires while in the hospital, the final note describes the circumstances regarding the patient's death, the findings, whether an autopsy was performed, and the cause of death.

Pathology Reports

Pathology reports (Figure 12) consist of a microscopic and/or macroscopic (gross) description of tissue expelled (as in an abortion), removed from a patient during surgery, or during a specialized procedure (biopsy) to provide tissue for pathological analysis, or after death when an autopsy (or necropsy) is performed. A request for tissue examination identifying the clinical diagnosis is sent with the tissue specimen to the pathologist. The pathologist examines the tissue and writes a report which includes as a minimum a descriptive diagnostic report of gross specimens received. The pathologist and the medical staff jointly decide which categories of specimens require only a gross description and diagnosis and must follow any state laws on the subject. When a microscopic evaluation is performed, any tissue diagnosis is to be based on the microscopic findings. The pathologist is responsible for signing the pathology report. Hospitals which contract with an outside agency for pathology services are to obtain the original pathology report for inclusion in the record.

In the autopsy report the pathologist documents a summary of the history of the patient's illness and treatment, a detailed report of gross findings, microscopic findings, and anatomic diagnosis at autopsy. The pathologist is responsible for authenticating the autopsy report.

TISSUE REPORT

Clinical Diagnosis: Date:

Pathological Diagnosis:

Macroscopic Examination:

Microscopic Examination:

_____M.D.
SIGNATURE OF PATHOLOGIST

FORM D-1203   PHYSICIANS RECORD CO., BERWYN, ILLINOIS · PRINTED IN U.S.A.   TISSUE REPORT

Form courtesy of Physicians' Record Company

FIGURE 12. PATHOLOGY - TISSUE REPORT

Imaging Reports

Imaging reports are descriptions of diagnostic or therapeutic imaging services. Diagnostic procedures can include: x-ray, radioactive scanning, thermography, magnetic resonnance, computerized tomography, xerography, and ultrasonography. A physician, usually a radiologist, writes or dictates a description of what is seen and the implications for the patient. This interpretation, which the radiologist authenticates, becomes the report. For therapeutic purposes, x-ray and radioactive materials may be administered. The amount of the dose, the date, and time are documented. At the end of the treatment, a

X-RAY REPORT

Family Name	First Name	Home Phone	Room No.	Hosp. No.
Address	Occupation	Sex M F	Age—Years	X-Ray No.
Attending Physician		Date		O.P.D. No.

Submitted for (Please check) X-ray film ☐ Stereo ☐ Fluoroscopic exam. ☐ Complete exam. ☐ Discretion of Radiologist ☐ Treatment ☐

Dressings may ☐ may not ☐ be removed Previously rayed ____________

Clinical Summary ____________

Suspected pathology ____________

Attending Physician ____________ M.D.

Findings ____________

____________ M.D.
Signature of Roentgenologist

FORM D-1904 PHYSICIANS' RECORD CO., BERWYN, ILLINOIS - PRINTED IN U.S.A. X-RAY REPORT

Form courtesy of Physicians' Record Company

FIGURE 13. IMAGING- X-RAY REPORT

summary of the treatment is provided and is authenticated by the radiologist and becomes part of the medical record.

The most common form of imaging report found in the record is the x-ray (Figure 13). Some hospitals combine the request and report for radiologic services on one form. Often the upper portion contains the request. This portion contains the patient's name, hospital number and other identifying information, the part or region to be examined (which the attending physician documents), and the authentication of the attending physician. The bottom portion usually provides space for the interpretation and the radiologist's authentication.

Electrocardiograph Report

The electrocardiogram (ECG, EKG) is a graphic tracing which represents the electrical changes in heart muscle as the heart beats. The electrocardiograph report consists of the cardiologist's authenticated interpretation of an electrocardiogram. The actual graphic tracing may be filed in the medical record or in the EKG laboratory, available for reference if necessary.

Electromyographic Reports

The electromyograph report consists of the neurologist's or orthopedist's interpretation of an electromyogram (EMG). The EMG measures electrical activity in skeletal muscles at the motor unit level. The interpretation of these measurements is the responsibility of the neurologist or orthopedist.

Consultation Report

Consultation reports (Figure 14) contain an opinion about a patient's condition by a physician other than the attending physician. This opinion, requested by the attending physician, is based on a review of the patient's medical record, an examination of the patient, and a conference with the attending physician. Some hospitals use a form which combines a request for consultation with the consultation report. The consultant records findings, makes recommendations for the patient, and authenticates the report.

The *Conditions of Participation* require that the medical staff have established policies regarding the status of consultants. They further specify that a consultant must be well qualified by training, experience, and competence to give an opinion in the specialty in which his advice is sought. They also state that routine procedures, such as x-ray examinations, electrocardiogram determinations, tissue examinations, and

proctoscopic and cystoscopic procedures are not normally considered to be consultations. The categories of patients for
which consultations are required are (1) patients who are not
good medical or surgical risks, (2) patients whose diagnoses
are obscure, (3) patients whose physicians have doubts as to

CONSULTATION REPORT

CONSULTING PHYSICIAN REQUESTED (Please Print)   SERVICE   DATE REQUESTED

FROM:

NAME OF REQUESTING PHYSICIAN (Please Print)   SERVICE

BRIEF REASON FOR CONSULTATION (Including lab., X-ray results)

Signature of requesting M.D.

FINDINGS, OPINIONS, & RECOMMENDATIONS:

NAME OF CONSULTANT (Please Print)   SERVICE

DATE   TIME   SIGNATURE   M.D.

CONSULTATION REPORT   **CHART COPY**

FIGURE 14. CONSULTATION REPORT

the best therapeutic measures to be taken, and (4) instances
where there is a question of criminal activity. When the admission is an emergency, there may be exception to these require-

ments. The attending physician is responsible for requesting consultation.

Operative Data

Some hospitals group all the information pertaining to each surgical procedure. This collection of information is referred to as an operative set or section. The information usually contained in an operative section is: consent for surgery; pre-anesthesia, anesthesia, and post-anesthesia reports; the operative report; and if applicable, pathology report.

Anesthesia Report

When a patient undergoes a procedure which requires an anesthetic other than a local, an anesthesia report (Figures 15 and 16) is required. This form documents the preoperative medication, the amount of concentration, time given, and effect. Additionally this form lists the anesthetic agent, the amount, the technique used to administer it, the effect and duration of the anesthetic, the temperature, pulse, respiration and blood pressure, blood loss, blood transfusions and intravenous fluids given, and notations of the patient's condition throughout the procedure.

Any treatments given which are not documented elsewhere and surgical manipulation which may affect the conduct of anesthesia and complications arising during administration of the anesthetic are documented on the form. The practitioner providing the anesthetic (nurse anesthetist or anesthesiologist) is responsible for recording the information and authenticating the anesthesia report.

In conjunction with the administration of anesthesia there must be recorded in the medical record a pre-anesthesia and a post-anesthesia note. The pre-anesthesia note is often found in the progress notes and includes information on the choice of anesthesia, the medical procedure anticipated, the patient's previous drug history, past anesthetic problems and any potential anesthetic problems, a physical examination of the patient, summary of laboratory data, and pre-anesthesia medications.

The postanesthesia note may be in the progress notes, the recovery room report, or the anesthesia report. The postanesthesia report documents the patient's condition after anesthe-

sia, specifying the nature and extent of any anesthesia-related
complications. It is documented and authenticated within 24
hours after surgery by the practitioner who administered the
anesthetic.

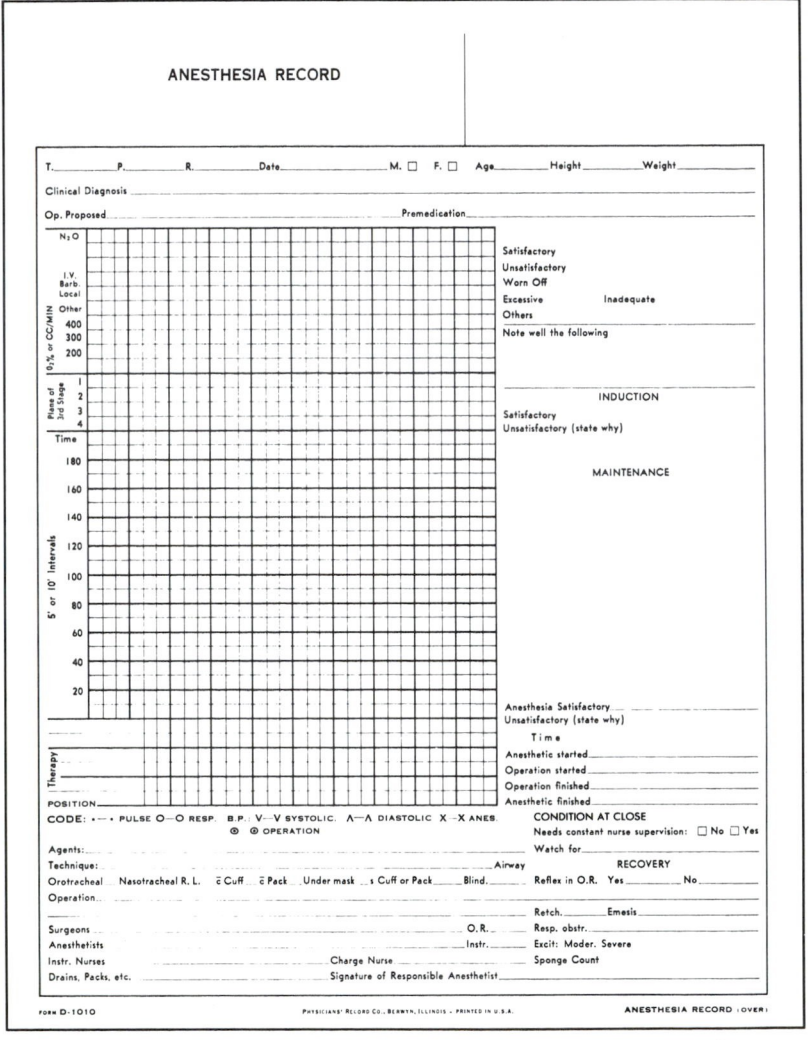

Form courtesy of Physicians' Record Company

FIGURE 15. ANESTHESIA REPORT (front)

Documentation of at least one postanesthetic visit which
describes the presence or absence of anesthesia-related complications is required by the Joint Commission. A note made in

the surgical or obstetrical suite or in the postanesthesia care unit does not ordinarily constitute a visit. The number of visits will be determined by the status of the patient. A visit should be made early in the postoperative period and again after

ANESTHESIA STUDY

PREOPERATIVE

Check negative conditions only. Record positive details below.

Resp._____Urol.___

Circ._____Neurol.___

G.I._____Obst.___

Gyn._____Metab.___

Positive:___

Anes. History

Urine_____B.P.___

Hb._____RBC_____WBC___

Other Lab. data___

POSTOPERATIVE

COMPLICATIONS	R.O.in	Op. Day		DAYS POSTOPERATIVE															Wks. P.O.	
		D	N	1	2	3	4	5	6	7	8	9	10	11	12	13	14	3	4
Nausea & Vomiting																			
Headache																			
Urinary retention																			
Backache																			
Laryngitis																			
Pulmonary																			
Shock																			

Remarks:___

(D-1010 BACK)

Courtesy of Physicians' Record Company

FIGURE 16. ANESTHESIA REPORT (back of Fig. 15)

complete recovery from anesthesia. Each note must specify the date and time. It is recommended that the postanesthesia note be made by a physician or qualified oral surgeon. All anesthesia personnel are encouraged to record postanesthesia notes for patients to whom they have administered anesthesia. It is acceptable for the physician or dentist who discharges the patient to make the documentation required if it is not feasible for anesthesia personnel to do so. It is recommended that the anesthesia records be completed promptly and filed in the medical record within 24 hours of completion.

Recovery Room Record

Patients are taken to the recovery room for immediate post-operative or post-anesthesia care. Pertinent data regarding the patient's condition on arrival and transfer from the recovery room, as well as information regarding the patient's condition and treatment while there, must be documented. This provides a complete record from the time the patient leaves the operating room until he arrives on the nursing unit. A form specifically designed for recording recovery room care is often used. This allows quick comparison of all required information, including vital signs, treatment, and progress. The post-anesthesia note may be documented on this form. Depending on the content of a particular form, it may be authenticated by either the nurse or physician, or both.

The Joint Commission states that when there is a post-anesthesia care unit, the medical record must contain the patient's level of consciousness on entering and leaving the unit, the vital signs, status reports of infusions, surgical dressings, tubes, catheters, and drains. If there is no special care unit, similar information is to be documented in the medical record.

Operative Report

The medical records of all patients who had surgical procedures performed must include an operative report (Figure 17). A preoperative diagnosis should be recorded in the medical record prior to surgery. It is helpful, though not required, to have the preoperative diagnosis included on the operative report. This allows quick comparison of the preoperative diagnosis with the postoperative diagnosis, which is to be documented on this form. The operative report also includes a full description of the findings, both normal and abnormal, the organs explored, procedures, ligatures, sutures, number of packs, drains and sponges used, and names of surgeons and assistants. The date and duration of surgery and the condition of the patient at the completion of surgery should also be stated. The operative report should be written or dictated immediately after surgery, authenticated by the surgeon, and filed in the medical record as soon as possible after surgery.

NAME

ROOM NO

(ADDRESS)

HOSP. NO

PHYSICIAN

OPERATIVE RECORD

DATE

Name of Procedure:			Began:	AM PM	Ended:	AM PM
Surgeon:		Assistant Surgeon:				
Instrument Nurse:	Circulating Nurse:		Sponge Nurse:			
Anesthetist:	Anesthesia:		Began:	AM PM	Ended:	AM PM

Pre-operative Diagnosis

Post-operative Diagnosis

Tissue Removed: To Pathologist: Yes / /   No / /

Sponge-Count: Gross Findings:

Drains:

Description of Procedure:

Signature of Surgeon Dr.

FORM 08-114   MOORE BUSINESS FORMS, INC.   **OPERATIVE RECORD**

Form courtesy of Moore Business Forms, Inc.

FIGURE 17. OPERATIVE REPORT

When there is a transcription and/or filing delay, a comprehensive operative progress note should be entered in the medical record immediately after surgery to provide continuity of care.

Discharge Summary

The discharge summary (or clinical resume-Figure 18) is a concise recapitulation of the patient's course in the hospital: the reason(s) for hospitalization; significant findings from ex-

DISCHARGE SUMMARY

Family Name | Room No. | Hosp. No.

Attending Physician | Date of Admission | Date of Discharge

Provisional Diagnosis:

Principal Diagnoses:

Additional Diagnoses:

Operative Procedures:

Brief History and Essential Physical Findings:

Significant Laboratory, X-ray and Consultation Findings:

Course in Hospital with Complications, if Any:

Condition, Treatment, Final Disposition on Discharge and Prognosis:

Special Instructions to Patient: (Diet, Medications, Follow-up Care, Physical Activity)

Date _____ Signed _____ M.D.

FORM D-103 (REV. 3/81) | PHYSICIANS RECORD CO., BERWYN, ILLINOIS - PRINTED IN U.S.A. | DISCHARGE SUMMARY

Form courtesy of Physicians' Record Company

FIGURE 18. DISCHARGE SUMMARY

aminations/tests; procedures; therapies provided and the response to these; condition at discharge; and instructions given regarding medications, physical activity, diet, and follow-up care. The description of the patient's condition upon discharge should be stated in a manner that allows comparison with the condition upon admission. Vague terms such as "improved" should be avoided. When pre-printed instructions are given to the patient, this fact should be documented in the record; and a sample instruction sheet should be on file in the health information department. All relevant diagnoses established by the time of discharge and all operative procedures should be recorded in acceptable terminology. When the discharge summary and the admission/discharge form both contain listings of final diagnoses and procedures, care must be exercised to insure that both listings are the same. A final progress note may substitute for a discharge summary in the following cases: patients who are hospitalized less than 48 hours with problems of a minor nature, normal newborns, and uncomplicated obstetrical deliveries. The JCAHO's 1994 standards also allow a transfer summary to be substituted for the discharge summary in the case of the transfer of the patient to a different level of hospitalization or residential care within the organization. The discharge summary should be written or dictated immediately after the discharge of the patient.

Nursing Data

The second type of clinical data found in the medical record is nursing data generated by the registered nurse, licensed practical nurse, and the nurse's aide. Some forms, such as the recovery room record discussed earlier, contain data documented by both nurses and physicians. There are, however, a number of forms in the medical record which are the sole responsibility of nursing personnel. A nursing assessment or nursing care plan for each patient is required. This document includes nursing diagnoses and statements of the nursing measures to be taken which will facilitate the medical care provided. Although traditionally nursing care plans were not filed in the medical record, today most hospitals include nursing assessments with the permanent medical record.

Nurses' Notes

The nurses' notes are narrative entries made by nursing personnel regarding their observations of the patient, care and treatment given the patient, and the patient's response to the therapy. Nurses' notes may be written on integrated progress note forms or on separate nurses' notes, which are similar in appearance to progress notes. Historically nurses' notes were written in different colors of ink to indicate the nursing shift on which the entry was made. This is no longer advisable as colors do not photocopy or microfilm well. The nurses' notes should describe the patient's needs, problems, capabilities and

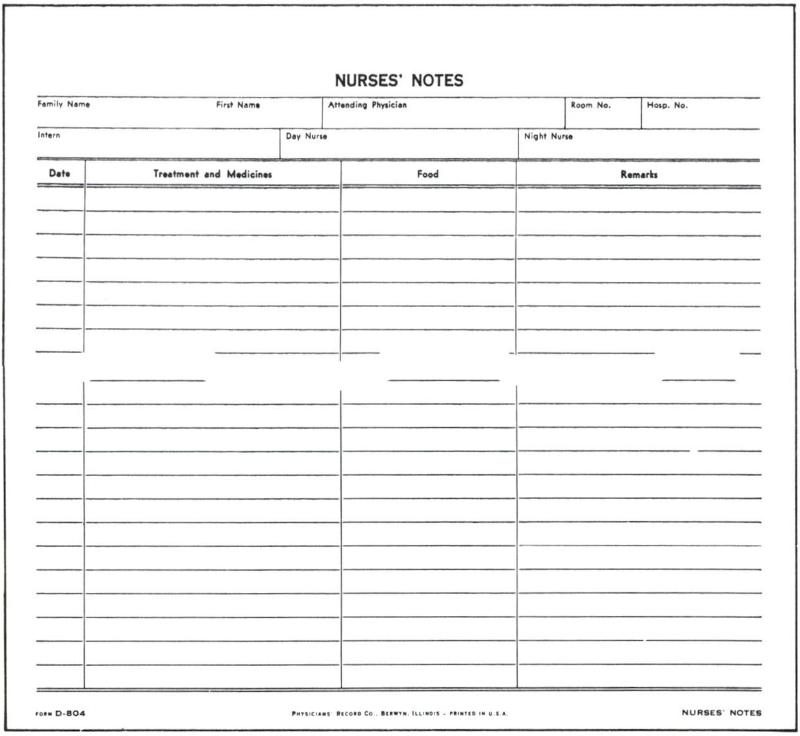

NURSES' NOTES

Family Name First Name | Attending Physician | Room No. | Hosp. No.

Intern | Day Nurse | Night Nurse

Date	Treatment and Medicines	Food	Remarks

FORM D-804 PHYSICIANS' RECORD CO., BERWYN, ILLINOIS - PRINTED IN U.S.A. NURSES' NOTES

Form courtesy of Physicians' Record Company

FIGURE 19. NURSES' NOTES

limitations in terms of the patient's actual behavior. Nursing intervention and patient response must be noted.

As much as possible, nurses' entries should contain objective data, such as stating the milliliters of fluids taken rather than subjective terms such as intake "poor" or "good." Any subjective data should be in the form of statements made by the patient, such as complaints of pain or emotional problems.

The nurses' notes usually consist of an admission note, subsequent notes as required by the patient's condition and hospital regulations, and a discharge note. The admission note includes the time of admission, how the patient arrived (wheelchair, stretcher, or walking), symptoms, signs, treat-

---

01/19/88 18:09 Page 1

SHIFT REPORT - CHRONOLOGICAL

W ,JOAN
Adm. Date: 01/13/88
Birth Date: 03/08/1949 age 38

Room 102   Bed 1   01/13/88 13:00 - 01/13/88 22:56
Hosp. Days: 1   Post Op: --
Height: 66.0 inches

Mr# 121212   Acc# 123
Doctor: DELTORO

OUTPUT - Stool
    01/13/88 22:27   JDD   RN   BOWEL MOVEMENT, small brown semi-formed stool guaiac negative
OUTPUT - Chest tube(s)
    01/13/88 22:26   JDD   RN   Volume 50 cc Suction 20 cmH2O drsg. dry & intact
OUTPUT - Other catheter
    01/13/88 22:25   JDD   RN   Volume 900 cc
INTAKE

    Lipids
    01/13/88 22:18   JDD   RN   Volume consumed 50 cc Left in bottle 100 cc
INTAKE

    TPN (Hyperal) 84 cc/hr Central line L. subclavian
    01/13/88 22:16   JDD   RN   Volume consumed 150 cc Left in bottle 850 cc IV site patent dressing
    intact no signs/symptoms of infiltration infusion pump monitoring
INTAKE

    D5W 42 cc/hr Central line L. subclavian
    01/13/88 22:14   JDD   RN   Volume consumed 300 cc Left in bottle 600 cc IV site patent
    no signs/symptoms of infiltration
ASSESSMENT - General
    01/13/88 20:37   JDD   RN   family visiting
INTAKE - P.O.
    01/13/88 18:31   JDD   RN   Volume 660 cc broth jello tea
ASSESSMENT - Diabetic
    01/13/88 17:36   JDD   RN   Blood Glucose 93 mg finger stick
WOUND SITES - Surgical
    left flank nephrostomy tube
    01/13/88 17:07   JDD   RN
    DR. J. SMITH NOTIFIED OF NEPHROSTOMY TUBE DRAINAGE
HYGIENE - Skin care
    01/13/88 17:05   JDD   RN   complete:bed:bath:back:care:given:bed:linen:changed:::::::::::::
    01/19/88 18:07   CB   RN   Record deleted: CHARTED ON WRONG PATIENT
OUTPUT - Chest tube(s)
    01/13/88 17:04   JDD   RN   Suction 20 cmH2O left chest tube to pleuro-vac inserted by MD
RESPIRATORY CARE - Nursing Interventions
    01/13/88 17:00   JDD   RN   oxygen therapy face mask ordered no c/o
RESPIRATORY CARE - Oxygen Administration
    01/13/88 17:00   JDD   RN

    NASALPRG   FM-% L/M   FT-% L/M   PED1%   VENT%
    40 0.4

    PART.RBTHR%   NON.RBTHR%   TRACH%   CPAP%   cmH2O

VITAL SIGNS

    TEMP PULSE RESP SYST DIAS MAP CVP WEIGHT
    01/13/88 16:42   JDD   RN   130.0

JDD : D   JOANN   RN
CB : B   CINDY   RN

W ,JOAN
Adm. Date: 01/13/88
Birth Date: 03/08/1949 age 38
Mr# 121212   Acc# 123
Doctor: DELTORO

FIGURE 20. COMPUTER GENERATED NURSES' NOTES

---

ment instituted, time and type of specimen sent to the laboratory, and the time the attending physician was notified of patient's admission. The discharge note would contain time of discharge, how the patient left and with whom, discharge instructions, and if transferred to another facility, the name of the facility. If the patient leaves without a discharge order and against the advice of the physician, this should be noted and

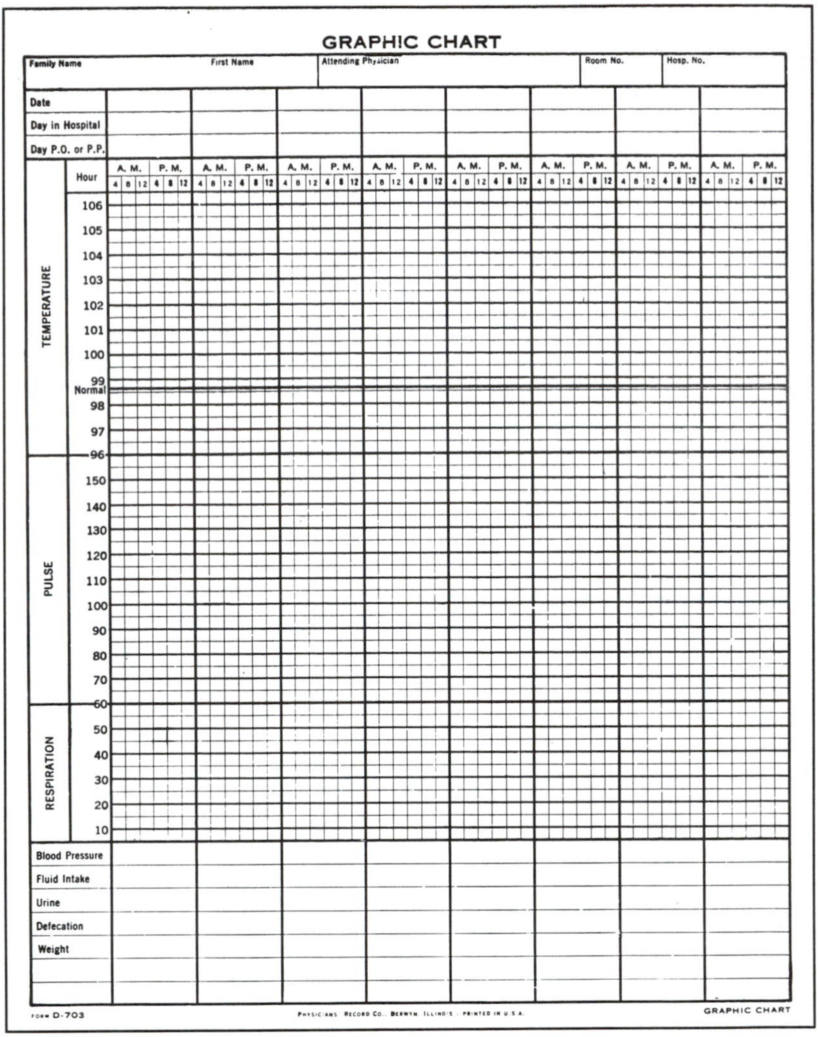

Form courtesy of Physicians' Record Company

FIGURE 21. GRAPHIC CHART

the reason. If the patient dies, the note should describe when life functions apparently ceased, the time the physician was notified, and the time a physician pronounced the patient dead.

Bedside terminal systems have greatly enhanced the ability to record progress notes and other nursing data. A sample of computer-generated nurses' notes is provided in Figure 20.

Graphic Sheet

The graphic sheet (vital sign or TPR sheet-Figure 21) is used to record several different parameters regarding the patient. Most commonly, the temperature, pulse, respiration, and blood pressure measurements are charted on this form. Other information which may be included is intake and output of fluids (and solids). One form usually provides space for charting and parameters, six times a day for several days. The patient's condition may require more frequent measuring of the vital signs. An additional form may be needed to allow for frequent documentation. Signatures of the individuals making these observations are usually not required.

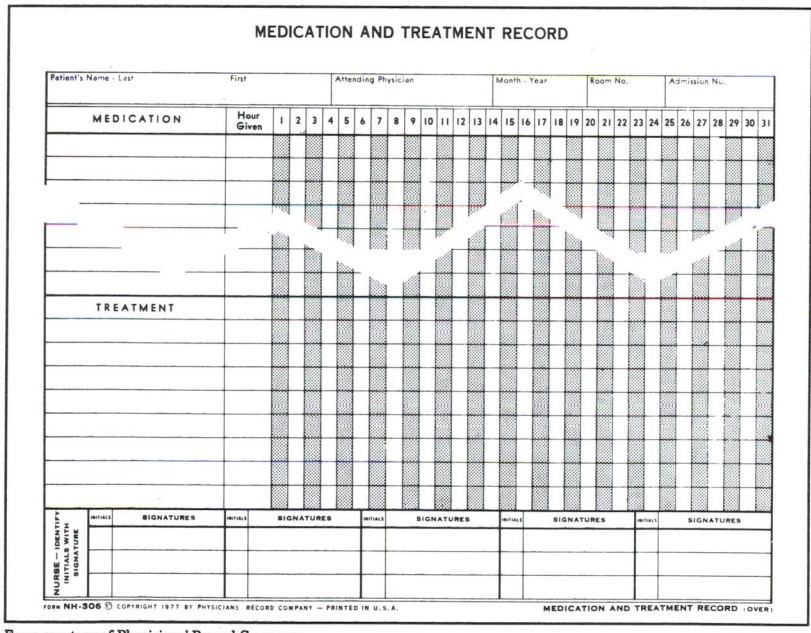

Form courtesy of Physicians' Record Company

FIGURE 22. MEDICATION SHEET

Medication Sheet

The medication sheet (Figure 22) provides documentation of the medicines given orally, topically, by injection, inhalation, and infusion. The date, time, name of drug, dose, and route by which it was given are documented after the drug has been administered. Intentional omission of medication is also documented in the medical record; and the reason for such is noted in the nurses' notes, such as in preparation for surgery. The professional giving the drug initials the entry.

Miscellaneous Reports

Nursing service personnel in specialized care units of the hospital, such as the intensive care unit (ICU), coronary care unit (CCU), or post-anesthesia room (recovery room) may be responsible for documenting observations about the patient on specialized forms. These forms allow for more frequent recording of observations and may be used in addition to or in place of routine forms.

Ancillary Data

The ancillary data contained in the medical record refer to are generated by health professionals other than physicians and nurses. The most common ancillary forms are medical laboratory, physical therapy, respiratory therapy, and social service reports.

Medical Laboratory Reports

The medical laboratory reports consist of various types of analyses or examinations of body substances such as blood, urine, and stool. The medical laboratory usually provides: blood bank, blood chemistry, hematology, microbiology, serology, and urinalysis tests and reports. The laboratory tests are performed only upon the orders of a physician. The clinical laboratory scientist or technician performs the test and prepares an original report of the results for the medical record. The reports must contain patient identification, name and date of examination, authentication of person performing the test, results, time in and time out of the laboratory, and the name of the laboratory when the test is performed outside the hospital. Reports should also be designed to facilitate comparison of each determination with pertinent reference values and sequential and related analyses. Reports must be completed promptly and filed in the medical record within 24 hours of completion. Hospitals with manual systems for documenting laboratory results commonly use small slips of paper which are placed on a collection sheet in the medical record, as shown in Figure 23.

LABORATORY REPORTS

MISCELLANEOUS LABORATORY

☐ Routine
☐ Preop.; Date Needed
☐ Not Emergency But Needed By Time
☐ Emergency Only Ordered By Physician. Report to Go Directly to M.D.

IF IMPRINT PLATE NOT USED PRINT HERE

DATE
PAT. NAME
HOSP. NO.
ROOM NO. (ADDRESS)

A123456

DATE REQUIRED	SPECIMEN DRAWN BY
REQUESTING PHYSICIAN	DATE
NURSE	TIME

ORDER ONLY ONE TEST ON THIS SLIP

☐ OUTPATIENT

Specimen _____

Examination Desired _____

REPORT:

REPORTED BY   DATE REPORTED

MISCELLANEOUS LABORATORY

☐ OUTPATIENT

CROSSMATCH RECORD		UNIT NUMBER					BLOOD BANK PRODUCTS SPECIFY UNIT		
PATIENT		DONOR		SALINE COMPATIBLE	ALBUMIN COMPATIBLE	COOMBS COMPATIBLE	ANTIBODY SCREEN	FRESH FRO-ZEN PLASMA	PLATELET CONCENTRATE	FIBRINOGEN
GROUP	TYPE	GROUP	TYPE					SALT-POOR ALBUMIN		CRYOPRECIPITATE
								PLASMA PROTEIN FRACTION (5%) 250 cc.		
		STARTED BY			STOPPED BY			RhoGAM		
Dᴴ								LOT OR UNIT NO.		
DATE GIVEN		TIME STARTED		TIME FINISHED		cc. ADMIN-ISTERED		REPORTED BY		
REACTION TO TRANSFUSION	☐ YES ☐ NO	IF YES, USE SEPARATE REPORT FORM						DATE REPORTED		

BLOOD TRANS. — BLOOD BANK PROD.

FORM D-408 PHYSICIANS RECORD CO. BERWYN ILLINOIS

LABORATORY REPORTS

Form courtesy of Physicians' Record Company

FIGURE 23. MEDICAL LABORATORY REPORTS

Laboratory computer systems generate a summary of all laboratory work performed on a patient. Often computers generate daily reports as well as weekly or other cumulative reports. To eliminate excessive paper, daily reports should be destroyed when cumulative reports are available. Figure 24 provides an example of a cumulative report. Some computer-generated results are very sophisticated in their appearance.

The medical record should contain complete and accurate information about blood transfusions. The American Associa-

```
                        COMMUNITY HOSPITAL


   PATIENT:Doe, Jane                           ROOM NUMBER:   3W/319-1
   UNIT NUMBER:16 19 12                         DATE PRINTED:08/30/88
   PHYSICIAN:Wilson, A. J.



                    NORMALS   07/10/88  08/23/88  08/27/88  08/29/88
                              R:0732HR  R:1915HR  R:1710HR  C:2255HR

   *****ROUTINE URINALYSIS*****

   RT. URINALYSIS
   COLOR                      YELLOW    YELLOW    YELLOW    YELLOW
   APPEARANCE                 CLOUDY    CLEAR     CLEAR     CLEAR
   SPECIFIC GRAVITY           1.015     1.020     1.010     1.020
   PH              5.0-8.0    8.0       6.0       6.0       6.0
   PROTEIN         0-10       TR        NEG       NEG       NEG
   GLUCOSE URINE   NEG -      NEG       NEG       2+*       NEG
   KETONES         NEG -      NEG       NEG       NEG       TR*
   BILE            NEG -      NEG       NEG       NEG       NEG
   OCCULT BLOOD    NEG -      TR*       NEG       NEG       NEG
   NITRITE         NEG -      NEG       NEG       NEG       NEG
   UROBILINOGEN    .1-1.0     0.1       0.1       0.1       0.1
   WBC/HPF         0-5        75*       5         5         2
   RBC/HPF         0-5        4         1         1         0
   EPITH. CELLS    NEG -      MOD*      FEW*      NEG       FEW*
   CAST            NEG -      NEG       NEG       NEG       NEG
   CAST            NEG -      NEG       NEG       NEG       NEG
   BACTERIA        NEG -      MANY*     MOD*      FEW*      NEG
   CRYSTALS        NEG -      AMPHO*    NEG       NEG       NEG
                              MANY
   MUCUS           NEG -      FEW*      FEW*      NEG       NEG
   MED TECH ID                DT/201    BR/211    TRIC      KC/214
                                                  FEW
                                                  BR/211


        MOD   =  MODERATE
        AMPHO =  MORPHOUS PHOSPHATE
        NEG   =  NEGATIVE
        TR    =  TRACE
        TRIC  =  TRICOMONAS

              FINAL LAB RESULTS
```

Form courtesy of Physicians' Record Company

FIGURE 24. CUMULATIVE LABORATORY RESULTS

tion of Blood Banks (AABB) in its *Technical Manual*, specifies that the transfusion form, which becomes part of the patient's record, should have the name and identification number of the intended recipient and the donor identification number. Notation of ABO and Rh groups of the patient and donor should be the same on the label of the blood lab as on the transfusion form. The perfusionist who administers the blood, checks identification information at the patient's bedside and documents on the transfusion form that this information has been checked. In addition, the perfusionist notes on the transfusion form whether the compatibility tag identifies the person performing the test and the interpretation of results. After the perfusionist checks the identifying information, the transfusion form must be signed to indicate that the identification was correct and to identify the person who started the transfusion. Notation of the date and time of transfusion, the nature of the transfusion product, its identification number, and the patient's condition at the start of transfusion should be recorded in the patient's medical record. After transfusion of each unit of blood, the patient care personnel (nurse) records the time, the volume and type of component given, the patient's condition, and the identity of the person who stops the transfusion and observes the patient.

Physical rehabilitation services

Physical rehabilitation services promote the restoration of the functional abilities of individuals with physical, cognitive, and/or sensoriperceptual impairment. These services include audiology, creative arts, occupational therapy, rehabilitation medicine, and speech-language pathology.

The JCAHO's requirements for medical record documentation include the reason for referral, a summary of the patient's clinical condition, and a treatment plan that assesses the functional ability of the patient and sets measurable goals. The patient's progress and results of treatment must be assessed at least monthly for outpatients and every two weeks for inpatients.

One common physical rehabilitative service, physical therapy, is described below.

Physical Therapy

Physical therapy reports (Figures 25 and 26) describe assessments and treatments including the use of exercise, heat, cold, water, electricity, ultrasound, and other physical means to restore the patient to useful activity. The assessment or treatment is ordered by the physician on the physician's order sheet or on a requisition which is sent to the physical therapy department by the nursing service. The therapist providing

PHYSICAL THERAPY EVALUATION	Date_____

PHYSICAL THERAPY EVALUATION

Date_____
Initial_____
Interim_____
Final_____

PATIENT NAME _____ | Patient Number _____ | Age: _____

DIAGNOSIS: _____

TO: _____

Physical Therapy Plan of Treatment has been reviewed with
_____patient
_____family
_____other agency personnel involved with patient's care

GOALS

Short Term:
1.
2.
3.

Long Term:
1.
2.
3.

PHYSICAL THERAPY PLAN OF TREATMENT:
1.
2.
3.
4.
5.

The PT Plan of Treatment is recommended pending physician's approval

_____, R.P.T.

The PT Plan of Treatment is amended and or approved by:

_____ Date _____
Physician

KEY: I: Independent   A: Needs Assist   S: Needs Supervision for Safety   U: Unable   NA: Not Applicable

Comments: If applicable remark on frequency, speed, assistive devices.

FUNCTIONAL ASSESSMENT

BED ACTIVITIES:
1. Rolls, turns in bed
2. Moves sideways in bed
3. Comes to sitting position
4. Sitting balance

TRANSFERS:
1. Wheelchair to and from bed
2. Toilet
3. Tub
4. Car

AMBULATION:
1. Wheelchair mobility
2. Comes to standing position
3. Standing balance
4. Initiates steps
5. Textures (carpets, outside)
6. Dynamic balance (movement)
7. Stairs
8. Uses elevators

ACTIVITIES OF DAILY LIVING:
1. Feeds self
2. Uses toilet
3. Dresses self
4. Bathes self

BEHAVIOR (Items below rated + or −)
1. Alert
2. Oriented to time, place, direction
3. Disoriented
4. Cooperative
5. Confused
6. Safety awareness

(OVER)

FIGURE 25. PHYSICAL THERAPY REPORTS (front)

the service documents the treatment given and the patient's response, dates and signs the report.

The initial report contains objective data regarding: behavior; joint evaluation; muscle/motor evaluation; respiratory evaluation; functional evaluation; and other evaluations, such as posture, skin, reflexes, prosthetics, orthotics, sensation, and edema, as necessary. Goals and recommended procedures to achieve these goals should be included.

EXERCISE TOLERANCE

a) Pulse Rate: b) Respiration   c) Blood Pressure

    Before Exercise_____   Rate_____   Before Exercise_____

    After Exercise_____   Quality_____   After Exercise_____

Endurance   General Posture

SPEECH IMPAIRMENT   AUDITORY IMPAIRMENT   VISUAL IMPAIRMENT
☐ Yes   ☐ No   ☐ Yes   ☐ No   ☐ Yes   ☐ No

SKIN CONDITION   SENSATION

GAIT ANALYSIS

MOBILITY   ASSISTIVE DEVICE

STRENGTH   RANGE OF MOTION

A. TRUNK   A. TRUNK

B. EXTREMITIES   B. EXTREMITIES

COMMENTS/RECOMMENDATIONS:

Frequency_____ Duration_____

Therapist_____

FIGURE 26. PHYSICAL THERAPY REPORTS (back of Fig. 25)

The progress notes or reports also are stated objectively to allow comparison to the initial findings and demonstrate progress toward the goals. Continual reassessment and adjustment of the treatment program should be performed in consultation with the physician and documented. Education of the patient and/or patient's family also should be documented. A discharge note or summary is recorded when service is discontinued to explain therapies provided and the patient's response to these.

PLEASE USE BALL POINT PEN AND BEAR DOWN

| DATE | PHYSICIAN'S ORDERS |

BE SURE TO IMPRINT PATIENT'S NAME BELOW

1. OXYGEN CONCENTRATION   (CIRCLE ONE)
   ROOM AIR ,   AIR DILUTION ,   100%

2. LENGTH OF RX.   (CIRCLE ONE)
   5 MIN. ,   10 MIN. ,   15 MIN.
   OTHER_____

3. CM H20 PRESSURE   (CIRCLE ONE)
   10 CM ,   15 CM ,   20 CM,
   OTHER_____

4. MEDICATION   (CHECK ONE)
   _____   3cc N/S
   _____   2.5cc N/S, .5cc BRONKOSOL
   _____   1.5cc N/S, .5cc BRONKOSOL
                 1cc MUCOMYST
   _____   2.5cc N/S, .3cc ALUPENT
   _____   1.5cc N/S, .3cc ALUPENT
                 1cc MUCOMYST
   _____   4cc ETHYL ALCOHOL
   _____   OTHER (SPECIFY)

   (I PPB-HAND HELD · INCENTIVE SPIROMETRY)

5. FREQUENCY   (CIRCLE ONE)
   OD.,   BID.,   TID.,   QID., _____ QHR.

6. COUGH,   DEEP BREATHE Pt. X 3

7. D/C Rx. IF PULSE >120, UNLESS
   SPECIFIED._____

8. CHARTS WILL BE FLAGGED AFTER 3 DAYS.
   IF NOT REORDERED, Rx. D/C'D.

THERAPEUTIC OBJECTIVES OF RESPIRATORY THERAPY

DATE: _____

PATIENT:_____ ROOM:_____

DIAGNOSIS:_____

( ) IMPROVE DISTRIBUTION OF VENTILATION
( ) DELIVERY OF AEROSOL MEDICATION
( ) PREVENT OR TREAT ATELECTASIS
( ) IMPROVE ARTERIAL OXYGENATION
( ) IMPROVE OR PROMOTE COUGH
( ) MOBILIZE SECRETIONS
( ) OTHER:_____

_____

PHYSICIAN_____ DATE_____

OTHER RESPIRATORY ORDERS:_____
_____
_____
_____
_____

FORM N01   SPEEDIPLY• PAT D MCP• PAT D MBF 28

Form courtesy of Moore Business Forms, Inc.

FIGURE 27. RESPIRATORY THERAPY REPORT

Respiratory Therapy Report

The respiratory therapy report (Figure 27) documents the assessments and treatments of the patient and the patient's response to these. The treatments provided by respiratory therapy include administration of oxygen, therapeutic gases, aerosols and humidity, mechanical ventilation, and emergency resuscitation. Evaluations and examinations provided by respiratory therapy include various pulmonary function tests such as spirometry, lung volume measurements, and arterial blood analysis. The Joint Commission states that respiratory therapy services shall be ordered by a physician and should state the type, frequency and duration of treatment, and as appropriate, the type and dose of medication, the type of dilutent, and oxygen concentration. This report and any related respiratory consultation should be placed in the medical record. All respiratory therapy services should be documented in the record including the type of therapy, date and time of administration, effects of therapy, and any adverse reactions. Upon discharge, the physician should document a timely, pertinent summary of the overall results of respiratory therapy and the need for long term oxygen therapy.

Social Service Record

Social service reports are developed by the social worker working with the patient. The social worker has access to and knowledge of a wealth of information about the patient, some of which is sensitive, personal data not recorded in the social service report for the medical record. The social service record should contain background, social information, and problems identified by the patient, his family, and the social worker. A plan of action, progress reports, and a discharge note should be documented in the medical record.

SPECIAL RECORDS

Special care units established in the hospital give specialized care to certain groups of patients such as those in the coronary care unit, intensive care, kidney dialysis, psychiatric unit, or rehabilitation unit. Wherever possible, regular medical record forms are used, but in some instances special forms must be developed to document the needed data.

Special medical record forms are often used for specific categories of patients such as obstetric, and newborn patients.

OBSTETRIC DATA

A complete hospital obstetric record includes several special forms: antepartum (prenatal) record, labor and delivery record, and postpartum record. The American College of Obstetrics and Gynecology identifies recommended content for these forms in its *Standards for Obstetric-Gynecologic Services.*

Antepartum Record

The antepartum or prenatal data (Figures 28-30) are started in the obstetrician's office or obstetric clinic, preferably very early in the pregnancy. The antepartum record should contain the following data:

Health history - including menstrual history, past pregnancies, number of full-term pregnancies, premature pregnancies, spontaneous and induced abortions, number of living children, spacing of previous pregnancies, length of gestation, route of delivery, sex and weight of newborn and any complications, drug sensitivities, blood transfusions, blood group and Rh type, diabetes and other metabolic disorders, vascular disease, sexually transmitted diseases, convulsive disorders, gynecologic abnormalities, and serious injuries. The previous administration of Rh immune globulin should be specifically noted.

Family history - presence or absence of metabolic disorders, cardiovascular diseases, malignancy, congenital abnormalities, mental retardation, and multiple births in immediate relatives

Social history - patient's occupation and work environment, ethnic origin, educational and religious background.

Physical examination - neck, breasts, heart, lungs, abdomen, pelvis, size of uterus, configuration and capacity of bony pelvis, rectum, and extremities.

Laboratory tests performed in the pregnancy - hemoglobin or hematocrit, urinalysis, blood group and Rh type, irregular antibody screen, rubella antibody titer, cervical cytology, and syphilis screen.

Risk assessment - including a problem list and recommendations for management, with special attention to such high risk factors as cesarean section, operation on the uterus or cervix, diabetes, hypertension, medical indication for termination of pregnancy, premature onset of labor, history of prolonged labor suggesting dystocia, multiple gestation, two or more abortions, use of drugs, alcohol and tobacco, and congenital abnormalities.

Health History Summary Date:

HOLLISTER
maternal/newborn
RECORD SYSTEM

PATIENT IDENTIFICATION

Patient's name _____

Age_____ Race_____ Religion _____ Marital status _____ Years married _____ Education _____ Occupation _____

Home address _____ Home tel. _____ Work tel. _____

Nearest relative _____ Relative's employer _____ Work tel. _____

Referring physician _____ Attending physician _____

Medical History	Patient	Family	Check and detail positive findings including date and place of treatment. Precede findings by reference number.
1. Congenital anomalies			
2. Genetic diseases			
3. Multiple births			
4. Diabetes mellitus			
5. Malignancies			
6. Hypertension			
7. Heart disease			
8. Rheumatic fever			
9. Pulmonary disease			
10. GI problems			
11. Renal disease			
12. Other urinary tract problems			
13. Genitourinary anomalies			
14. Abnormal uterine bleeding			
15. Infertility			
16. Venereal disease			
17. Phlebitis, varicosities			
18. Nervous/mental disorders			
19. Convulsive disorders			
20. Metabol./endocrine disorders			
21. Anemia/hemoglobinopathy			
22. Blood dyscrasias			
23. Drug addiction			
24. Smoking/alcohol			
25. Infectious diseases			
26. Operations/accidents			
27. Blood transfusions			
28. Other hospitalizations			
29. **No known disease**			

Menstrual History Onset ___ age Cycle ___ q ___ days Length ___ days Amount ___ L.M.P. ___ mo/day/yr ___ quality

Pregnancy History Grav ___ Term ___ Pret ___ Abort ___ Live ___ E.D.C. ___ mo/day/yr

No.	Month/year	Sex	Weight at birth	Wks gest	Hrs in labor	Type of delivery	Details of delivery. Include anesthesia and maternal or newborn complications. Use Risk Guide numbers where applicable
1							
2							
3							
4							
5							
6							
7							
8							

Sensitivities (detail positive findings)
30.☐ **None known**
31.☐ Antibiotics
32.☐ Analgesics
33.☐ Sedatives
34.☐ Anesthesia
35.☐ Other

Preexisting Risk Guide
Indicates pregnancy/outcome at risk
36.☐ Age < 15 or > 35
37.☐ < 8th grade education
38.☐ Cardiac disease (class I or II)
39.☐ Tuberculosis, active
40.☐ Chronic pulmonary disease
41.☐ Thrombophlebitis
42.☐ Endocrinopathy
43.☐ Epilepsy (on medication)
44.☐ Infertility (treated)
45.☐ 2 abortions (spontaneous/induced)
46.☐ ≥ 7 deliveries
47.☐ Previous preterm or SGA infants
48.☐ Infants ≥ 4,000 gms
49.☐ Isoimmunization (ABO, etc.)
50.☐ Hemorrhage during previous preg.
51.☐ Previous preeclampsia
52.☐ Surgically scarred uterus
53.☐ _____

Indicates pregnancy/outcome at **high** risk
54.☐ Age ≥ 40
55.☐ Diabetes mellitus
56.☐ Hypertension
57.☐ Cardiac disease (class III or IV)
58.☐ Chronic renal disease
59.☐ Congenital/chromosomal anomalies
60.☐ Hemoglobinopathies
61.☐ Isoimmunization (Rh)
62.☐ Drug addiction/alcoholism
63.☐ Habitual abortions
64.☐ Incompetent cervix
65.☐ Prior fetal or neonatal death
66.☐ Prior neurologically damaged infant
67.☐

Initial Risk Assessment
68.☐ No risk factors noted
69.☐ At risk
70.☐ At **high** risk

Signature

FIGURE 28. ANTEPARTUM RECORD

It is recommended that a copy or satisfactory abstract of the current prenatal information be available in the labor and delivery area by the estimated 36th week of pregnancy and arrangements made to obtain it as soon as possible if admission is necessary prior to this time.

This record is copyrighted by Miller Communications, Inc., and may not be reproduced without permission of Hollister Incorporated, the exclusive licensee under said copyright.

FIGURE 29. ANTEPARTUM RECORD

Labor and Delivery Record

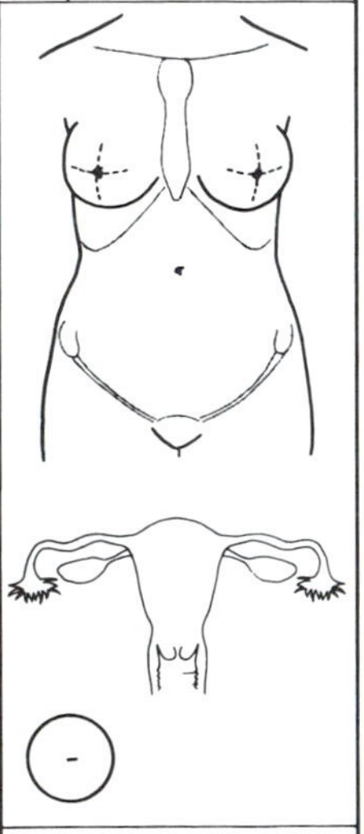

Specialized forms are used to document the patient's progress from the time of admission through labor and delivery to the postpartum period. These may be called Labor and Delivery Record or Labor and Delivery Summary and may consist of several forms depending on the arrangement of data (Figures 31 and 32). The antepartum record should be reviewed as soon as possible after admission and notations made regarding: parity, estimated date of delivery, blood group, Rh type, serologic tests for syphilis, rubella titer, and other important laboratory data. There should be an evaluation performed and documented by the admitting physician. If the patient has not had prenatal care, the evaluation should include a complete history, or an updated history if she has had prenatal care.

The updated history should include: time of onset of contractions, status of membranes, presence of any significant bleeding, time and content of last ingestions, drug intake, known allergies, use of contact lenses or eyeglasses, and presence of dentures. Notation should be made of attendance in childbirth classes, use and choice of analgesia or anesthesia, and plans for breast or bottle feeding. The extent of the admitting physical examination will depend on the condition of the patient. It should include the patient's blood pressure, pulse, temperature, frequency, quality and duration of uterine contractions, notation of leaking of amniotic fluid or unusual bleeding, pelvic examination, degree of cervical dilatation, effacement, fetal position, presentation, station of the presenting part, and heart rate. When there are no complications, trained nursing personnel may perform the initial pelvic examination.

During normal labor, the assessment of the quality of uterine contractions, fetal heart tones, and examination of the pelvis are done frequently to detect evidence of abnormality and to assess progress of labor. The patient's blood pressure, temperature, pulse, intake and output, and the fetal heart rate are also assessed frequently. Any significant sign or symptom, such as bleeding or meconium staining, should be evaluated by the physician.

Delivery data are recorded, such as: type of delivery, type of forceps used, blood loss, description of placenta and cord, episiotomy, laceration, anesthesia and other medications, and chronology of the labor and delivery. Data about the infant are also documented: apgar scores (which rate the infant at one minute and five minutes after birth), sex, weight, length, onset of respiration, abnormalities, and treatment to eyes.

Electronic fetal heart rate monitoring may be done prior to and during delivery. The tracings are part of the medical record and should include patient name, hospital number, and

Prenatal Flow Record

HOLLISTER® maternal/newborn RECORD SYSTEM

PATIENT IDENTIFICATION

Patient's name

Risk Guide for Pregnancy and Outcome

Preliminary Risk Assessment (detail risk factors from the HHS below)

☐ (0) No risk factors noted
☐ (1) At risk
☐ (2) **High risk**

Continuing Risk Guide (enter dates first noted and revise RISK STATUS)

Mo/day	Potential risk factors	Mo/day	**High** risk factors
/	3. Preg. without familial support	/	18. Diabetes mellitus
/	4. Second pregnancy in 12 months	/	19. Hypertension
/	5. Smoking (≥ 1 pack per day)	/	20. Thrombophlebitis
/	6. Rh negative (nonsensitized)	/	21. Herpes (type 2)
/	7. Uterine/cervical malformation	/	22. Rh sensitization
/	8. Inadequate pelvis	/	23. Uterine bleeding
/	9. Venereal disease	/	24. Hydramnios
/	10. Anemia (Hct < 30%:Hgb < 10%)	/	25. Severe preeclampsia
/	11. Acute pyelonephritis	/	26. Fetal growth retardation
/	12. Failure to gain weight	/	27. Premature rupt. membranes
/	13. Multiple pregnancy (term)	/	28. Multiple pregnancy (preterm)
/	14. Abnormal presentation	/	29. Low/falling estriols
/	15. Postterm pregnancy	/	30. Significant social problems
/	16.	/	31. Alcohol and drug abuse
/	17.	/	32.

Initial Prenatal Screen			Additional Lab Findings		
Mo day	Test	Result	Mo/day	Test	Result
/	Hct/Hgb		/	Hct/Hgb	
/	Patient's Blood type and Rh		/	Hct/Hgb	
/	Father's Blood type and Rh		/		
/	Antibody		/	Blood sugar	
/	Serology		/	Bacteriuria	
/	Rubella titer		/		
/	Urinalysis micro		/		
/	Pap test		/		
/	G.C.		/		
			/		

G T P A L | LMP mo/day/yr | EDC mo/day/yr

☐ Initial prenatal instruction
☐ Attends prenatal classes
☐ Cesarean section
☐ For sterilization
☐ Breast ☐ Bottle Feeding
☐ Circumcision

Quickening date mo/day/yr

Anesthesia

Baby's physician

See Add Prog Note

Flow Chart

Date	Weight this visit (Year / Pre-gravid)	Blood pressure	Protein	Sugar	Urine	Est. weeks gestation (dates/size)	Fundal height	Fetal heart rate	Edema			RISK STATUS (0,1,2)	
		/			/								
		/			/								
		/			/								
		/			/								
		/			/								
		/			/								
		/			/								
		/			/								
		/			/								
		/			/								
		/			/								
		/			/								
		/			/								
		/			/							Physician's signature	

FIGURE 30. ANTEPARTUM RECORD

date and time of admission and delivery. Relevant data such as examinations, changes in position of the patient, medications, and the corresponding times should be recorded on the tracings.

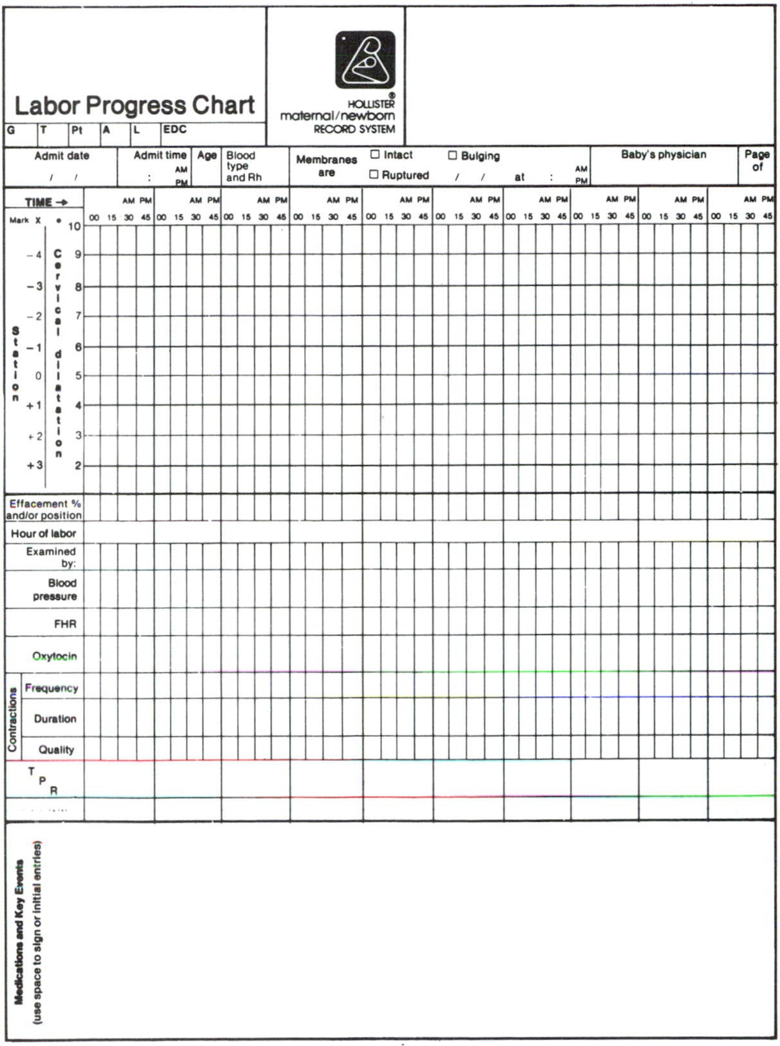

Labor Progress Chart

HOLLISTER® maternal/newborn RECORD SYSTEM

G | T | Pt | A | L | EDC

Admit date / / | Admit time : AM PM | Age | Blood type and Rh | Membranes are ☐ Intact ☐ Ruptured ☐ Bulging / / at : AM PM | Baby's physician | Page of

TIME → AM PM 00 15 30 45

Mark X •

Station: −4, −3, −2, −1, 0, +1, +2, +3

Cervical dilatation: 10, 9, 8, 7, 6, 5, 4, 3, 2

Effacement % and/or position

Hour of labor

Examined by:

Blood pressure

FHR

Oxytocin

Contractions: Frequency, Duration, Quality

T P R

Medications and Key Events (use space to sign or initial entries)

FIGURE 31. LABOR AND DELIVERY RECORD

Postpartum Record

The postpartum record (postpartum progress notes) contains information about the condition of the mother after delivery. It usually starts immediately after the patient is moved from the delivery room. Hospitals may use a regular progress note form, nurses' notes, or a special postpartum record to record this data. The information recorded is specific to post-delivery

Labor and Delivery Summary

HOLLISTER®
maternal/newborn
RECORD SYSTEM

Labor Summary

G	T	Pt	A	L	Type and Rh

Presentation — Position
- ☐ Vertex
- ☐ Face or brow
- ☐ Breech _____
- ☐ Transverse lie ☐ Compound
- ☐ Unknown

Complications ☐ None
- ☐ No prenatal care
- ☐ Preterm labor (≤ 37 wks.)
- ☐ Postterm (≥42 wks.)
- ☐ Febrile (≥ 100.4°) when admitted
- ☐ PROM (≥12 hrs. preadmit)
- ☐ Meconium
- ☐ Foul smelling fluid
- ☐ Hydramnios
- ☐ Abruption
- ☐ Placenta previa
- ☐ Bleeding-site undetermined
- ☐ Toxemia (mild) (severe)
- ☐ Seizure activity
- ☐ Precipitous labor (< 3 hrs.)
- ☐ Prolonged labor (≥ 20 hrs.)
- ☐ Prolonged latent phase
- ☐ Prolonged active phase
- ☐ Prolonged 2nd stage (> 2.5 hrs.)
- ☐ Secondary arrest of dilatation
- ☐ Cephalopelvic disproportion
- ☐ Cord prolapse
- ☐ Decreased FHT variability
- ☐ Extended fetal bradycardia
- ☐ Extended fetal tachycardia
- ☐ Multiple late decelerations
- ☐ Multiple variable decelerations
- ☐ Acidosis (pH < 7.2)
- ☐ Anesthetic complications
- ☐ _____
- ☐ _____

Induction ☐ None
- ☐ ARM ☐ Oxytoc. ☐ _____

Augmentation ☐ None
- ☐ ARM ☐ Oxytoc. ☐ _____

Monitor ☐ None

	FHT	UC
External	☐	☐
Internal	☐	☐

Medications — Total dosage

Time of last narcotic : A / P

Delivery Data

Method of Delivery
Cephalic
- ☐ Spontaneous — Type
- ☐ Low forceps
- ☐ Mid forceps
- ☐ Rotation _____ to _____
- ☐ Vacuum extraction

Breech
- ☐ Spontaneous
- ☐ Partial extraction (assisted)
- ☐ Total extraction
- ☐ Forceps to A.C. head

Cesarean (details in operative notes)
- ☐ Low cervical: transverse
- ☐ Low cervical: vertical
- ☐ Classical
- ☐ Cesarean hysterectomy

Placenta
- ☐ Spontaneous
- ☐ Expressed
- ☐ Manual
- ☐ Adherent
- ☐ Ut. exploration

Blood loss
- ☐ < 500 ml
- ☐ ≥ 500 ml
- Specify amount detail in Remarks _____ ml

Configuration
- ☐ Normal
- ☐ Abn. _____
Weighed (no) (yes) _____ gms.

Cord
- ☐ Nuchal cord x _____
- ☐ True knot
- ☐ ② ③ Umbilical vessels
Cord blood to (lab) (refrig.) (discard)

Episiotomy
- ☐ None — Suture
- ☐ Median _____
- ☐ Mediolateral
- ☐ Other _____

Laceration
- ☐ None
- ☐ ① ② ③ ④ Degree perineal
- ☐ Vaginal
- ☐ Cervical
- ☐ Uterine rupture
- ☐ Other _____

Surgical Procedures ☐ None
- ☐ Tubal ligation ☐ Curettage
- ☐ Other _____

Remarks: _____

Assisting _____

Delivery Data (cont.)

Delivery Anesthesia ☐ None
1 = Local 2 = Pudendal 3 = Paracervical
4 = Epidural 5 = Spinal 6 = General

Delivery Room Meds. ☐ None

Chronology — Date

		Time
EDC	/ /	
ADMIT TO HOSPITAL	/ /	A P
MEMBRANES RUPTURED	/	A P
ONSET OF LABOR	/	A P
COMPLETE CERVICAL DIL		A P
DELIVERY OF INFANT	/	A P
DELIVERY OF PLACENTA	/	A P

Infant Data

Apgar Scores

	Heart rate	Respiration	Muscle tone	Reflex irritation	Skin color	Totals
1 min						
5 min						

Resuscitation ☐ None — spontaneous respiration
- ☐ Oxygen
- ☐ Bag and mask
- ☐ Intubation
- ☐ Ext. cardiac massage
- ☐ Other _____
_____ mins. to sustained respiration

Nurse _____

Attending _____

Infant Data (cont.)

Medications
- ☐ None
- ☐ Volume expander
- ☐ Sodium bicarbonate
- ☐ Drug antagonists
- ☐ Umbilical catheter
- ☐ Other _____

Initial Newborn Exam
- ☐ No observed abnormalities
- ☐ Gross congenital anomalies
- ☐ Mec. staining ☐ Trauma
- ☐ Petechiae ☐ Other

Describe _____

Basic Data
ID bracelet no _____
Hospital record no _____
- ☐ Male ☐ Female
Birth order: _____ of ① ② ③ ④

Record procedures whether done in the delivery room or nursery

Weight _____ Length _____
- ☐ Vitamin K
- ☐ AgNo₃ 1% or _____
by: _____

Output
- ☐ Urine
- ☐ Meconium
- ☐ Gastric _____ (ml)
- ☐ Living at transfer to:

Deceased — Date
- ☐ Antepartum / /
- ☐ Intrapartum — Time A
- ☐ Neonatal (in deliv. room) _____ P

Date completed / /

FIGURE 32. LABOR AND DELIVERY SUMMARY

cases, such as: lochia, condition of breasts, fundus, perineum, medications, treatment, intake and output, and other pertinent information regarding progress. The observations and

documentation are completed by nursing personnel as frequently as the patient's condition requires. Each entry is dated
and timed.

NEWBORN DATA

A healthy newborn record contains a few routine forms such
as the admission and discharge form, and specialized forms
such as birth history, newborn identification form, and newborn physical examination and nursing record. The newborn's
condition such as prematurity or anomalies may require more
detailed observations and specialized forms.

Birth History

The birth history (history of newborn delivery) may be a
form (or forms) which is also used in the mother's medical
record, as shown in Figures 32 and 33, or may be a separate
form. The maternal information to be recorded is: previous
obstetric history; medical history; diseases during this pregnancy; mother's blood group and Rh type; tests for syphilis,
gonorrhea, herpes, and dates performed; drugs taken during
pregnancy, labor and delivery; duration of ruptured membranes and labor, including length of the second stage; method
of delivery and indications for such; placental abnormalities;
and estimated amount and description of amniotic fluid. The
newborn data recorded include: results of measurements of
fetal maturity and well-being, apgar scores at one and five
minutes, description of resuscitation, description of abnormalities, and problems occurring from birth until transfer to
the admission/observation area of the nursery.

This information may be compiled by the nurse and physician, with each authenticating his or her own entries.

Newborn Identification

While the newborn is still in the delivery room, two identical
bands indicating the mother's admission number, the newborn's sex, and the date and time of birth are placed on the
wrist or ankle. An identification form with information about
the mother and infant and an identification band number are
prepared. The birth records and identification bands should be
checked by both the nurse and responsible physician before the
newborn leaves the resuscitation area of the delivery room.

Footprinting and fingerprinting may also be used for newborn identification. Techniques such as sophisticated blood typing are now available and appear to be more reliable. Specific

Initial Newborn Profile

HOLLISTER
maternal/newborn
RECORD SYSTEM

1. Basic Data (entered by nursing personnel)

G T P A L

Mother's name _____

EDC ___ mo / day / yr   Delivery date ___ mo / day / yr   LMP ___ mo / day / yr

Time of birth ___ AM PM

Apgar at: 1 min ___ 5 min ___   Sex: ☐ Male ☐ Female ☐ Ambiguous

2. Physical Examination

Date of exam _____   Time of exam ___ AM PM   Baby's age at exam ___ hrs

Temperature _____   Respiration rate _____   Pulse rate _____

Femoral pulse ___ ☐ Normal   ☐ Absent/weak   ☐ Delayed

(Code ☑ = No abnormalities ☐ = Abnormalities present)

1 ☐ Reflexes   6 ☐ Thorax   11 ☐ Genitals
2 ☐ Skin color, lesions   7 ☐ Lungs   12 ☐ Anus
3 ☐ Head/Neck   8 ☐ Heart   13 ☐ Trunk/Spine
4 ☐ Eyes   9 ☐ Abdomen   14 ☐ Extremities/Joints
5 ☐ ENT   10 ☐ Umbilicus   15 ☐ Tone/Appearance

Description of abnormal findings — Please describe your findings objectively. Reserve your impressions or diagnoses for part 3 below. Please begin your findings with the reference number preceding each category

_____
_____
_____
_____
_____
_____
_____
_____

3. Impressions and Diagnosis

Initial Risk Estimate ☐ No risk factors noted   ☐ Low risk   ☐ Medium risk   ☐ High risk

_____
_____
_____
_____
_____
_____
_____
_____
_____

Newborn Risk Indicators —Please review these along with the prior risk information available to you, in order to arrive at your Initial Risk Estimate in part 3.

Observable at birth	Within 24 hrs. postpartum
☐ No risk factors noted	☐ No risk factors noted
☐ Abnormal presentation	☐ Abdominal distension
☐ Multiple birth	☐ Vomiting
☐ Low birth weight	☐ Failure to pass meconium (if
☐ Resuscitation at birth	skin not stained)
☐ 1 min. Apgar ≤5	☐ Melena
☐ 5 min. Apgar ≤7	☐ Apneic episodes
☐ Placental abnormalities	☐ Tachypnea (transient)
☐ Two cord vessels	☐ See-saw breathing
☐ Difficult catheterization	☐ Cyanosis
☐ >20ml. of gastric aspirate	☐ Petechiae/Ecchymoses
☐ Small mandible with cleft palate	☐ Jaundice
☐ Grunting	☐ Pallor
☐ Deep retractions	☐ Plethora
☐ Imperforate anus	☐ Fever
☐ Pallor	☐ Hypothermia
☐ Jaundice	☐ Arrhythmias
☐ Plethora	☐ Murmur
☐ Convulsions	☐ Lethargy
☐ Decreased tone	☐ Tremors (jitters)
☐ Congenital malformations	☐ Convulsions

4. Maturity Evaluation

Gest. age by dates ___ wks   Weight ___ lbs ___ ozs gms   Chest circ ___ cm

Gest. age by exam ___ wks   Length ___ cm   Head circ ___ cm

This infant is: ☐ Pre-term (<37 weeks)   ☐ SGA

classified as: ☐ Term (37-42 weeks)   ☐ AGA

☐ Post-term (>42 weeks)   ☐ LGA

5. Plans: diagnostic and therapeutic

_____
_____
_____
_____
_____
_____
_____
_____
_____
_____
_____
_____

Signature _____

FIGURE 33. NEWBORN PHYSICAL EXAMINATION

forms are required for each of these methods. Usually the nurse in charge of the delivery room is responsible for preparing and securing the identification bands and may prepare the identification sheet. Usually both the physician and nurse sign the identification form.

This record is copyrighted by Miller Communications, Inc., and may not be reproduced without permission of Hollister Incorporated, the exclusive licensee under said copyright.

FIGURE 34. NEWBORN PROGRESS NOTES

Newborn Physical Examination

The newborn's condition is assessed as soon as possible after birth. The initial physical examination (Figure 33) should include: date and time of birth; date, time and age at examination; sex; racial origin; birth weight, length, and head and chest circumferences; temperature; general appearance (e.g., activity, tone, cry); skin (e.g., pallor, cyanosis); head (size and shape of skull, molding, caput, hematoma, sutures, fontanels, size and position of jaw); facies; eyes;nose; mouth and pharynx; neck; thorax; lungs (respiratory rate and pattern, quality and distribution of breath sounds); heart murmur; circulation and peripheral pulses; abdomen; genitalia; anus; extremities; spine; neurological (posture, movements, state of consciousness, reflexes, symmetry, active and passive tone); and estimate of maturity.

The attending physician should examine the apparently normal infant no longer than 12 hours after birth. A newborn is also examined at least every three days if hospitalization continues and within 24 hours prior to the infant's discharge from the hospital. The results of these examinations are recorded in the infant's chart and signed by the physician.

Newborn Progress Notes

The newborn progress notes refer to information compiled by the nurses in the newborn nursery. This information may be written in narrative progress notes or may be entered on a flow chart, such as the newborn flow record (Figure 34), which is designed to allow for easier comparison of data. The American Academy of Pediatrics recommends that until the newborn's vital signs are stable (usually the first 6-12 hours after birth) there must be frequent recording of: temperature, heart, and respiratory rates; notations of color (cyanosis, jaundice); adequacy of peripheral circulation; type of respiration; state of consciousness; and presence of irritability, or twitching. Time of voiding and meconium stool should be noted. Weight should be measured and documented daily.

Other data usually recorded include: amount and type of intake and output, condition of the umbilical stump, any treatments or medications given, and any other pertinent observations.

Observations for the healthy newborn are made and recorded every eight hours until discharge. The specific time of observation is documented, and the entries are signed by the nurse making the observations.

FORMAT TYPES

Medical record format refers to the organization of the forms and/or their content within the medical record. There are three types of format: source-oriented, problem-oriented, and integrated.

Source-Oriented Medical Record

Traditionally, the hospital medical record is organized in sections according to the patient care departments which provide the care and the data; thus the term "source-oriented" medical record. Within each section the forms are arranged according to date. Usually the record is arranged in "reverse" chronological order at the nurses' station, so the most recent information is at the front and the oldest information is at the back of each section. Upon discharge of the patient, the record is often rearranged in chronological order from admission to discharge.

The major advantage to the source-oriented format is that it organizes reports from each source together, thus making it easy to determine the assessment, treatments, and observations a particular department has provided. Critics of the source-oriented medical record state it is not possible to quickly determine all of the patient's problems and treatments being provided for the patient at a given time, since the data from the various departments are organized in sections and not according to the problems of the patient or integrated in time sequence.

Problem-Oriented Medical Record

The problem-oriented medical record, commonly referred to as POMR, was introduced by Lawrence L. Weed, MD, in the 1960s. The POMR provides a systemic method of documentation to reflect logical thinking on the part of the physician directing the care of the patient. The physician defines and follows each clinical problem individually and organizes them for solution. The POMR has four basic parts: (1) database, (2) problem list, (3) initial plans, and (4) progress notes.

The database is a minimum set of data to be obtained on every patient, including chief complaint, present illness(es) patient profile (the patient's typical day) and related social data, past history and review of systems, physical examinations of defined content, and baseline laboratory data.

The problem list is contained on a form placed in the front of the record. "Problems" are anything that require management or diagnostic workup, including medical, social, economic, and demographic problems, past and present. The list should state the problems at the level of the physician's understanding of a particular problem. Thus, the problem list may contain a statement of a symptom, an abnormal finding, a physiologic finding, or a specific diagnosis. Conditions suspected or to be ruled out are not listed as problems but are noted in the initial plan. Additions or changes are made in the list as new problems are identified and active problems resolved. Problems are not erased; they are marked "dropped" or "resolved" and the date of the change recorded. Problems are titled and numbered and serve as a table of contents to the record.

The initial plans describe what will be done to learn more about the patient's condition, treat the condition, and educate the patient about the condition. Specific plans for each problem are delineated and fall into three categories: more information for diagnosis ("rule out" statements may be made here) and management; therapy (including statements of drugs, procedures, goals, and contingency plans); and patient education. The plans are numbered corresponding to the problem which they address.

Progress notes are the follow-up for each problem. Each note is preceded by the number and title of the appropriate problem and may consist of any or all of the following elements: subjective (symptomatic); objective (measurable, observable); assessment (interpretation or impression of the current condition); and plan statements. The acronym for this process is SOAP, and the writing of progress notes in the POMR format is often referred to as "soaping." The emphasis is on unresolved problems. In addition to the narrative notes to describe the patient's progress, flow sheets may be used in situations in which there are several factors being monitored or when the patient's condition is changing rapidly. The discharge summary and transfer note are also included in the "progress note" category. These should address all the numbered problems on the patient's list.

Dr. Weed recommended that certain other forms, such as physicians' orders, consultant reports, and nurses' notes, be in the problem-oriented style, with reference to titled and numbered problems.

Proponents of the POMR identify many advantages to this format: the physician is required to consider all the patient's problems in total context; the record clearly indicates the goals and methods of the physician in treating the patient; medical eduction is facilitated by the documentation of logical thought processes of the attending physician; and the quality assurance process is easier because the data are organized.

The major disadvantage of POMR is that the format usually requires additional training and commitment of the medical and professional staffs. Few acute care facilities maintain medical records that are fully problem-oriented. Many allied health professionals use the SOAP form of progress notes.

Integrated Medical Records

In the integrated format, all forms are organized in strict chronological order. On the nursing station the most current entries will be at the beginning of the record; on discharge the forms will be rearranged so that the entire medical record reads from admission to discharge. The key element is that forms from various sources are intermingled. Thus a record of a discharged patient may have the history and physical examination followed by a progress note, then a nurse's note, x-ray report, additional progress notes, consultation report, and so on. The forms for each episode of care are organized in separate sections of the record.

The advantage of the integrated format is that all information on a particular episode of care is together, thus providing a clear picture of the patient's illness and response to treatment.

The disadvantage of the integrated format is that it is difficult to compare similar information, for example, fasting blood sugar levels, over time because all reports of one type are not together in the record.

There may be varying degrees of integration of information. The most common variation allows for integrated progress notes, with all providers recording on the same form(s), in sequence. All other reports are maintained in source-oriented fashion.

Advantages to using integrated progress notes are: a patient's progress can be determined quickly because the current notes of all disciplines are together; the number of specialized forms is reduced, thus reducing the bulk of the record; and the team concept of health care is encouraged.

Disadvantages of integrated progress notes in a manual medical record system are: only one individual can document at a time; it may be difficult to identify the profession of the individual making a particular entry unless notes are always followed by the title of the recorder; and physicians often feel their documentation requires highlighting in some manner to differentiate it from that of other professionals caring for the patient.

The decision regarding the format of the medical record is usually made by the medical staff with recommendations from the medical record committee.

REQUIRED CHARACTERISTICS OF ENTRIES IN MEDICAL RECORDS

It has often been said that an adequate medical record indicates adequate care, and conversely, a poor medical record indicates poor care. It may be possible for a complete and thorough record to exist for a patient who received poor care, but the reverse is more likely to be true. A patient may have received adequate care which is poorly documented.

Appropriate Documentation

The quality of the medical record depends on information entered by those professionals authorized to provide care and responsible for documenting that care. Hospital and medical staff policies should determine who has this right and responsibility. The *Conditions of Participation* require that the medical staff have bylaws, rules, and regulations which include a provision for the medical staff to keep accurate and complete clinical records. It is further required that the record contain the originals of all reports.

The Joint Commission makes approximately the same statement adding that the record must contain information to identify the patient. The Joint Commission specifically states that entries may be made only by individuals given that right in hospital and medical staff policies. They describe the content of the record by stating that it must incorporate all significant clinical information pertaining to a given patient.

Authentication

Those professionals providing care to a patient and authorized to make entries in the record must document the care they provide and date the entry. They also verify that this care was given by authenticating the entry. The Joint Commission defines authentication as proof of authorship. The Joint Commission requires that medical records be dated and authenticated, and that there be a method established for identifying the authors of entries. The identification may be a written signature, identifiable initials, or computer key. When rubber stamps of signatures are allowed as a means of authentication (most commonly for pathologists and radiologists), the individual whose signature is represented by the stamp must place in the hospital's administrative offices a signed statement that he has the stamp and is the only one who will use it. No delegation of the use of the stamp is permitted by the Joint Commission

The *Conditions of Participation* specify that authentication may include signatures, written initials, or computer entry.

Every physician is to sign entries made, and a single signature by the physician on the admission/discharge record, where diagnosis(es) and procedure(s) are listed, is not sufficient to authenticate the entire record. In hospitals with house staff, the attending physician must countersign at least the history, physical examination, and discharge summary written by the house staff.

The parts of the record that are the responsibility of the attending physician are to be authenticated by the attending physician. If, for example, a physician assistant conducts and records the medical history and physical examination, the attending physician is required to sign these reports. Any entry which requires countersignature of the attending physician must be defined in the medical staff rules and regulations.

Abbreviations

Abbreviations and symbols are to be used only when they have been approved by the medical staff and when there is an explanatory legend available to those authorized to make entries in the record and to those who must interpret them. Each abbreviation and symbol should have only one meaning.

Timeliness

Because human memory can easily fail, it is imperative that entries regarding patient care be made as close as possible to the time of occurrence of the event(s) being documented. The Conditions of Participation address this issue by requiring that current and discharged patient records be completed promptly. Current records (the history, physical examination, and pertinent laboratory and x-ray data) are those which are completed within 24-48 hours after admission. Upon discharge of the patient, the record is to be completed within 30 days.

The Joint Commission requires that each clinical event shall be documented as soon as possible after its occurrence. Records of discharged patients are to be completed within a period of time specified in the medical staff rules and regulations which may not exceed 30 days. Completeness implies that the required forms are assembled and authenticated; all final diagnoses are recorded without use of abbreviations; and transcription of any dictated information is completed and inserted in the record.

Legibility

The usefulness of the record depends in part on the legibility of the entries. When it is economically feasible and appropriate, medical entries should be dictated and transcribed. When the transcribing and filing of reports cannot be accomplished in a timely fashion, entries providing sufficient information for continuity of care are to be made in the record.

Correction of Errors or Omissions

Errors are properly corrected by drawing a single line through the mistake, writing an explanatory statement, such as "wrong record," near it, and recording the correct information. The individual who notes the error corrects, dates, and signs the entry. The error should not be erased or painted out with correction fluid. If an entry is accidentally omitted, the entry is made after the last entry with an explanation of the omission and the reason for it being out of sequence.

RESPONSIBILITY FOR MEDICAL RECORD QUALITY

Medical Record Committee

The medical staff has responsibility for the overall quality of the medical record. In many facilities, quality review of medical records is performed by a separate medical staff committee, generally titled the medical record committee. In other facilities the ongoing evaluation of medical records may be designated as a responsibility of the entire staff, or of the executive committee. Regardless of the mechanism used, the medical staff is responsible for the maintenance of medical records that meet required standards for promptness, completeness, and clinical pertinence.

The following functions and responsibilities are usually assigned to the committee responsible for medical record review:

- Review of records for timely completion, clinical pertinence, overall adequacy for use in quality assessment activities, and, when necessary, as medicolegal documents.
- Review of records, including the results of all tests and therapies given, to assure they reflect the condition and progress of the patients.
- Determination of the format of the complete medical record, the forms used in the record, and the use of electronic data processing and storage systems for medical record purposes.

The health information practitioner must take an active role in helping the medical staff with medical record review. The health information practitioner will work closely with the committee chairman to prepare agendas for interesting committee meetings which must be held at least quarterly. For each meeting, summary information regarding the timely completion of medical records should be prepared. Health information personnel may also screen medical records to present those which do not meet documentation criteria for committee review. These selected cases would vary from month to month so that all types are eventually scrutinized. The committee then analyzes them carefully, and, in addition, checks a representative sample of those which the health information practitioner has accepted as adequate. These may be records chosen at random from the discharges, or they may be specific types of cases. In addition to reviewing the records of discharged patients, this committee should periodically perform an on-the-spot scanning of current inpatient records for completeness. This review is done on the patient units with the findings reported at medical record committee meetings.

The medical staff responsibility for medical record review goes beyond the inpatient record. Outpatient care medical records must also be reviewed, to determine that they are complete and sufficiently detailed to facilitate continuity of care. If the hospital administers a nursing facility, home health care program, or other health care delivery services records from these should also receive routine scrutiny.

Special review of emergency service records should be performed regularly by the Medical Record Committee to evaluate documentation of emergency patient care. Records of deaths occurring within 24 hours after admission to the emergency service should receive particular attention. Review of emergency records in disaster or riot situations is also indicated.

The medical staff bylaws must provide sufficient authority for the Medical Record Committee to reject substandard records, pass judgment on the quality of clinical entries, enforce staff rules regarding delinquent records, and in every way promote and encourage the maintenance of high standards. All physicians have signed an agreement to abide by the bylaws when they join the staff. Authority for disciplinary action of an individual physician is usually delegated by the governing body to the Executive Committee of the medical staff. Disciplinary action may take the form of suspension of admitting or surgical privileges or withholding other benefits.

Some hospitals find, however, that suspending physicians' privileges because of delinquent records is counter-productive. It is costly to the hospital to refuse patients. Suspending privileges may cause conflict between physicians and the hospital, even though records completion requirements are stated in medical staff bylaws. What's more, the suspension process requires a time-consuming effort on the part of the health information department to check the age of incomplete records and issue letters to physicians delinquent in their record keeping.

As a result, hospitals are using more innovative methods to encourage record completion. Some use incentives rather than penalties, such as recognition for good documentation habits or even sending unsigned reports to physicians' offices, as long as this practice does not conflict with either the hospital's policies or accrediting or regulatory agencies' requirements on confidentiality and integrity of records.

Technology offers records completion solutions too. Dictation systems are more user-friendly, so physicians in many hospitals can dictate from any touch-tone telephone. And signing reports—even the Medicare attestation statement—electronically is acceptable to JCAHO and to Medicare if certain controls are in place.

Some hospitals are coming to the decision that physicians must be accountable for their records without intense policing by the hospital. An increasing number of health information departments check only for the presence of signed major documents, such as the operative report and discharge summary.

Health Information Practitioner/Medical Staff Interface

In addition to working with medical record committee members in carrying out the committee's responsibilities, the health information practitioner interfaces with the medical staff individually and collectively in many other ways with respect to medical record functions:

- Assisting the medical staff in drawing up policies for medical record content/completion.
- Orienting house staff and new members of the attending staff to the hospital's medical record content and completion policies; manuals may be prepared for this purpose.
- Developing procedures to facilitate completion of incomplete records.
- Keeping physicians informed of the number of record requiring completion.
- Administering policies uniformly for completion of records.

- Providing timely transcription of reports for the medical record.
- Supplying data and assisting physicians in conducting research studies.
- Presenting educational programs for physicians on documentation requirements which impact on reimbursement.
- Making medical records available for ongoing care of patients.
- Developing or revising medical record forms.
- Providing statistics on individual physician's performance, such as the number of admissions or procedures.

SUMMARY

A medical record must be maintained on every person who receives hospital services. The preadmission or admissions office begins the medical record, and all departments which provide care to the patient add forms to the record to document the services given. The health information department processes the medical record and determines when it is complete. The completed medical record is retained in the health information department for future reference and safekeeping.

The medical record may be organized in one of several ways: source-oriented, problem-oriented, or integrated. Certain data must be documented in the medical record and in the manner required by licensing, certifying, and accrediting agencies. Some of the requirements for medical record content are very specific regarding the data to be included on particular forms; other requirements state that the data are to be documented in the medical record. Except where specifically stated in the requirements of the approving agencies, the content and layout of medical record forms is an individual determination made by each hospital.

The health information administrator with a knowledge of medical record content requirements can provide significant assistance to the hospital in providing quality care and meeting the requirements of licensing, certification, and accreditation agencies.

STUDY QUESTIONS

1. Describe the flow of information into the medical record.
2. Describe briefly the processing of the medical record within the health information department.
3. Define: source-oriented, problem-oriented, and integrated medical record formats.
4. Describe the proper method for correcting errors in the medical record.
5. Name three medical record forms which are usually the sole responsibility of nursing service.
6. State the four categories of patients for whom a consultation should be provided.
7. Name four types of special records maintained by hospitals.

REFERENCES

American Association of Blood Banks, *Technical Manual*, (Philadelphia: J.B. Lippincott Co., 1981).

Bates, Barbara, *A Guide to Physical Examination*, (Philadelphia: J.B. Lippincott Co., 1983).

Conditions of Participation-Hospitals, U.S. Dept. of Health and Human Services, (Washington, DC: Social Security Administration, June 17, 1986).

Dripps, Robert D., James E. Eckenhoff and Leroy D. Vandam, *Introduction to Anesthesia,* (Philadelphia: W.B. Saunders Co., 1982).

Egan, Donald F., *Fundamentals of Respiratory Therapy*, (St. Louis: C.W. Mosby Co., 1977).

"Even with law, hospitals write their own policies on advance directives," *Medical Records Briefing,* September 1991. pp 11-12.

"From faxes to computers, medical records managers find creative ways to get reports signed." *Medical Records Briefing*, September 1993, pp 7-9.

Glondys, Barbara A., *Documentation Requirements for the Acute Care Record,* (Chicago: AHIMA, 1994)

Guidelines for Perinatal Care, (Evanston: American Academy of Pediatrics and American College of Obstetrics and Gynecologists, 1983).

Herbert, Lauren A., "Basics of Medicare Documentation for Physical Therapy," *Clinical Management in Physical Therapy*, Vol. 1, No. 3, (1981): 13-14.

Hospital Care of Newborn Infants, (Evanston: American Academy of Pediatrics, 1977).

Joint Commission on Accreditation of Healthcare Organizations, *Accreditation Manual for Hospitals*, (Chicago: Joint Commission, 1994).

Lewis, LuVerne Wolfe, *Fundamental Skills in Patient Care*, (Philadelphia: J.B. Lippincott Co., 1984).

Mahoney, Elizabeth Anne et al., *How to Collect and Record a Health History*, (Philadelphia: J.B. Lippincott Co., 1976).

Managing Medical Record Completion, Opus Communications (Marblehead, MA, 1990).

Manning, Susan C., "Correcting the Health Care Record," *JAMRA* 53, (August, 1982): 76-78.

Rambo, Beverly and Lucile A. Wood, *Nursing Skills for Clinical Practice*, (Philadelphia: W.B. Saunders Co., 1982).

Sherman, Jacques L., and Sylvia K. Fields, *Guide to Patient Evaluation*, Garden City: Medical Examination Publishing Co., Inc., 1978).

Skurka, Margaret F., *Organization of Medical Record Departments in Hospitals*, 2nd Ed., (American Hospital Association, 1988).

Stoelting, Robert K. and Ronald D. Miller, *Basics of Anesthesia*, (Livingston, NY: Churchill, 1984).

Weed, Lawrence L., *Medical Education, and Patient Care*, (Cleveland: The Press of Case Western Reserve University, 1970.

chapter **3**

MEDICAL RECORDS IN AMBULATORY CARE

The provision of health care in the United States is changing. Care is no longer exclusively provided in a hospital (inpatient) setting or in a physician's office. Care is increasingly provided in a variety of ambulatory care settings. Health care consumers have many choices. Increasingly, ambulatory care through a health maintenance organization, urgent care center, hospital outpatient department, etc., is chosen as an alternative to an office visit to a private physician.

FACTORS INFLUENCING USE OF AMBULATORY CARE

There are several factors that influence the increased utilization of ambulatory care. A primary factor is the effort by the government, third-party payers, and the business community to contain or reduce health care costs. Medicare reimburses hospitals for inpatient services through a prospective payment system. This system provides hospitals with a financial incentive to discharge patients earlier, thus increasing their need for more intensive ambulatory care follow-up. Pressures to reduce costs have also resulted in increased reimbursement coverage for ambulatory services, and in some cases, insurance policies actually demand certain treatment be provided on an ambulatory basis.

Integral to cost-containment is the concern over the effect of the tremendous growth in the elderly population. The U.S. Census Bureau has projected a doubling in the age group 65 and over between 1980 and 2020 with an even more rapid increase in the 85 years and older age group. In order to meet the health care needs of this elderly population without massive increases in health care expenditures, cost-containment measures must be implemented and, therefore, utilization of alternatives to expensive inpatient care will continue to increase. In the future, however, the cost of these alternatives will be more closely scrutinized.

Two other factors that will continue to influence increased utilization of ambulatory care services are consumerism and scientific and technological advances. There is a trend toward alternative health care by the consumer. Patients are demanding more in terms of information and convenience; and for many, ambulatory care is preferred to inpatient care. Scientific and technological advances have allowed care previously performed in the hospital (e.g., dialysis, cancer chemotherapy, hyperalimentation, etc.) to be provided in an ambulatory setting. These advances, therefore, have made alternatives to inpatient care feasible.

AMBULATORY CARE

Ambulatory health care comprises services provided to patients who are neither hospitalized nor institutionalized as inpatients in a health care facility which is the site of the encounter. The National Committee on Vital and Health Statistics recently adopted this definition to describe care rendered in a multitude of ambulatory settings.

HOSPITAL-BASED AMBULATORY CARE

The provision of ambulatory care by hospitals has increased. In its publication called *Hospital Statistics,* the American Hospital Association cites the following growth statistics:

- Almost 81% of hospitals had organized ambulatory care programs in 1991.
- In 1991, visits to hospitals' ambulatory care services numbered over 323 million.

- Revenue growth as a percent of total growth was 24% in 1991.

Hospitals offer four types of services to ambulatory patients.

- Ancillary Services - When a patient is referred by a private physician to a hospital laboratory, radiology, and other services, the hospital is said to be providing ancillary services. In this ambulatory care situation, the physician gives the patient a requisition to obtain diagnostic or therapeutic services such as x-rays, laboratory tests, or physical therapy. The patient presents the requisition at the hospital. Hospital staff members provide the requested service, and submit a report on the services rendered to the physician's office. The patient returns to the physician's office for follow-up of the test results, physical therapy treatment, etc.

- Organized Outpatient Department or Primary Care Center - In this situation the patient utilizes the hospital's facilities to obtain ancillary services as well as on-going care. The patient is registered in the outpatient department or primary care center and is usually seen by physicians salaried by the hospital, although in some settings the patient may be seen by a private physician. Primary care generally refers to basic health services consisting of family medicine, general internal medicine, and/or pediatrics. It is often an initial point of care from which referrals are made for other more intensive, specialized services. The outpatient department generally refers to a broader range of services, including all the clinical specialties represented on the hospital's medical staff.

- Emergency Department - Most hospitals see a large number of patients in their emergency department for a wide variety of complaints. Simple procedures are often performed as are laboratory tests and x-rays in larger emergency departments.

- Ambulatory Surgery Facilities - An ambulatory surgery facility is defined by the AHA as a "free-standing or hospital-based facility, with an organized professional staff, that provides surgical services to patients who do not require an inpatient bed." Hospital-based facilities may be located at the hospital or may be satellite facilities located physically separate from the hospital. Free-standing ambulatory surgery centers (ASC), are often operated for profit and owned by physicians or investor-owned companies.

Ambulatory surgery is a fast-growing area within outpatient care. Consider these 1992 statistics (provided by SMG Marketing Group, Chicago, IL):

- Total surgeries performed in hospitals was 22,869,000. Of those, more than half—12,321,000—were outpatient surgeries.
- Non-hospital based surgeries, or operations performed in free-standing outpatient surgery facilities numbered 4.5 million.
- Operations performed in surgi-centers numbered almost three million, and another 1.7 million operations were performed in physicians' offices and other ambulatory settings.

Satellite Ambulatory Care Units

Some hospitals operate part of their organized outpatient department as a physically separate unit from the hospital, and may provide primary care only, comprehensive care, or services for special populations or for special needs (e.g., family planning, sports medicine, maternal and child care, preventive care, etc.). These satellite ambulatory care units medical record requirements are the same for these satellite units as for other hospital outpatient units. Of special concern in satellite units, however, is the flow of information between the satellite and the hospital. A system must be implemented to assure the indexing of a patient's ambulatory and inpatient care encounters, and records of these encounters must be readily accessible. Some health care facilities transmit medical records to satellite facilities by facsimile (FAX).

FREE-STANDING AMBULATORY CARE FACILITIES

There are many types of free-standing ambulatory care facilities. The physician's office provides a large percentage of free-standing ambulatory care. This office may be a solo practice, a private group practice, or a health maintenance organization. Public health departments often provide ambulatory care through neighborhood health centers. Increasingly, free-standing facilities are emerging that are for profit and operated by investor-owned companies.

Group Practice

The AHA defines a group practice as a "combined practice of three or more physicians and/or dentists who share office space, equipment, records, office personnel, expenses, and income." A group practice may be single specialty (i.e., all dentists, all gynecologists, etc.), or it may be multi-specialty and provide comprehensive care.

Health Maintenance Organizations

Health maintenance organizations (HMOs) emerged as an attempt to control health care costs. Federal legislation in 1973 provided financial support to HMOs that met federal regulations and this furthered the growth of HMOs. The AHA defines the HMO as an "organization that has management responsibility for providing comprehensive health care services on a prepayment basis to voluntarily enrolled persons within a designated population." A fixed premium is paid by members in return for the availability of all services included under the plan. Most plan options are comprehensive in nature. HMO plans include coverage of inpatient services, emergency services, and ambulatory care services. In addition, there are provisions for regular medical checkups, immunizations, and other preventive measures aimed at retaining good health. Eyeglasses, hearing aides, dental care, and prosthetic devices may also be covered.

There are three kinds of HMOs, and their information keeping practices vary:

- In staff model HMOs, physicians work only for the HMO in its facilities. Because staff model HMOs are discrete facilities, they often have medical records departments for the HMO.
- Group model or closed HMOs contract with physicians who continue to work in their private offices, usually treating only HMO patients. The physicians keep their own medical records, but must feed practice data into the HMO so it can monitor utilization, quality, and costs.
- Independent practice associations (IPAs) are similar to group model HMOs because physicians practice in their own office settings, keeping their own medical records

while giving practice data to the HMO for monitoring. Unlike most group model HMOs, however, physicians in IPAs treat HMO patients in addition to patients with other kinds of insurance.

Preferred Provider Organizations

Preferred provider organizations (PPOs) are also a response to escalating health care costs. PPOs are established by a panel consisting of health care providers or insurers. PPOs are similar to HMOs because a benefit package is offered to subscribers. The benefit package offered may include physician and hospital services as well as other services. The PPO panel contracts with providers to offer care to PPO subscribers at a negotiated cost that is usually discounted. Subscribers are free to use providers not affiliated with the PPO, but there is a financial incentive to use the contracted provider.

Unlike HMOs, PPOs utilize a fee-for-service system; so, there is a potential for cost increases even with a lower cost per individual service. For this reason, utilization review of both inpatient and ambulatory care is essential if costs are to be reduced or contained. There is no central location to store a patient's record or to coordinate care. Each provider has a separate record of patient care provided. The PPO obtains information regarding each provider's services and charges through claims submitted and, in some cases, through abstracts completed by the provider.

Neighborhood Health Centers

Neighborhood health centers (also known as community health centers) are specifically designed to bring health care to the economically disadvantaged. They are often operated by the local or state public health department. Residents in poverty areas often do not seek necessary medical services due to either lack of money, unavailability of primary care physicians, or other accessibility problem (such as a language or cultural barrier). Neighborhood health centers attempt to employ residents of the neighborhood to ease accessibility barriers and to keep costs low.

Treatment in the neighborhood health center is generally family centered. Indirectly, illnesses may result from crowded living conditions, unsanitary facilities, and other social and economic factors. Family care teams are used by the center to provide continuity of care to families encountering these types of problems. In such a system, the health care team usually includes an internist, pediatrician, nurse, and social worker. Continued emphasis is placed on preventive medicine procedures and education. Patients must understand the relationship between illness and living conditions.

Urgent, or Convenience, Care Centers

Urgent care centers, which may also be called convenience care centers, are often open 12 to 16 hours a day, seven days a week and offer convenient care for routine or minor emergency problems such as sprains, sore throats, etc. Most are for-profit companies. Unlike the HMO and PPO, these centers have no insurance component. Payment for care is strictly on a fee-for-service basis. Some will bill the patients' insurance plan if the plan covers ambulatory care, but many require direct payment (many accept credit cards) for which the patient must seek reimbursement from the insurance plan after the care has been rendered.

Additional information on the insurance aspects of ambulatory care, especially HMOs and PPOs, is included in Chapter 12.

ON-SITE AMBULATORY CARE

On-site ambulatory care is care provided in a nonhospital setting such as a business, educational institution, or prison. Industrial health clinics emphasize maintenance of employee health and safety. Student university health centers treat students and, sometimes, faculty within the university. Treatment may range from first aid to general medical care; in the case of industrial health clinics, it may include preemployment physicals and other programs such as stress management. The Joint Commission's ambulatory health standards as well as standards from the Accreditation Association for Ambulatory Health Care, Inc., are applicable to most on-site ambulatory care settings. In addition, the National Commission on Correctional Health Care, located in Chicago publishes three sets of standards, titled—*Standards for Health Services in Jails, Standards for Health Services in Prisons,* and *Standards for Health Services in Juvenile Confinement Facilities.* Health information management professionals should also refer to any applicable federal regulations for correctional medical information.

MEDICAL RECORD PROFESSIONALS IN AMBULATORY CARE

Many ambulatory care facilities do not have any professional medical record support. Increasingly, however, health information professionals are providing consultation services or working full or part time in ambulatory care facilities including physician's offices.

Health information professionals can provide valuable assistance in the development of integrated systems that improve the continuity of patient care and eliminate the need for unnecessary duplication of tests or examinations. When patient care data are readily available, care can be less costly and of higher quality.

Health information professionals can provide input and/or develop policies for providers regarding appropriate record content and format; exchange of patient data between providers; confidentiality of data; and the collection of comprehensive, uniform data and statistics.

AMBULATORY CARE RECORDS

Ambulatory care records and the standards applicable to them vary with the type of ambulatory care setting.

HOSPITAL-BASED AMBULATORY CARE RECORDS

Records for ancillary service outpatients may only include the results of the tests or services received. Complete medical and health information is not necessary as the patient returns to the private physician for further care. Often a formal medical record is not created. Reports of the ancillary services may be kept in the ancillary service departments, with a copy sent to the patient's private physician. If the ancillary service outpatient has been either an inpatient or outpatient on a previous occasion, the reports of the ancillary services should be filed with existing hospital medical records.

Because of the nature of emergency medical treatment, record systems must be developed to capture and integrate critical medical information from various sources in a concise and comprehensive manner.

There are two important elements in emergency medical documentation: Adequate information about the patient for dealing with life and death situations must be readily available. Information about the care provided in the emergency situation must be easily and accurately documented.

Adequate information for emergency care should be a concern long before emergency care is needed. The hospital should have medical record systems which allow for quick retrieval of previous inpatient and outpatient records. Often medical record department file areas are located near the emergency department. In hospitals with very active emergency departments, the file area may be staffed 24 hours a day. In other hospitals, procedures should be specified on who may have access to the file area and how records may be removed. Adequate controls should also be in place to ensure that records are available when needed. Hospitals with advanced computer systems may have recent records "online" (i.e., immediately accessible via a terminal), but frequently have older records archived "offline" and/or in paper or microfilm form that require human retrieval. The medical staff will determine the policy for routine record retrieval for emergency care, but the individual physician determines additional record retrieval requirements for each specific case.

The medical record itself should be organized in such a manner that critical information about a patient is immediately accessible. A unit medical record comprised of all inpatient, outpatient, and emergency care records provides maximum accessibility to information. Some hospitals use self-adhesive labels on the outside cover of the medical record to warn of allergies so that the patient is not administered drugs or other substances which may cause an adverse reaction. A single, up-to-date problem list compiling all active conditions both from inpatient and outpatient care is ideal. In the absence of such a comprehensive list, the face sheet of each inpatient admission should clearly document the diagnoses and procedures pertaining to that admission. Discharge summaries should reflect content that not only describes the inpatient event but provides information for subsequent care. In addition to the medical record itself, some hospitals or physicians encourage their patients to wear bracelets or neck tags with critical medical information about themselves, such as the fact that they are diabetic or have a cardiac pacemaker. Patient-carried computerized cards the size of credit cards are available on which to store limited medical information. The emergency department must have a microcomputer with a card reader to access the data.

Emergency medical information gathering and recording must be easy to do while focusing maximum attention on the patient. Often documentation begins with the ambulance service at the patient's home, workplace, accident site, or virtually any other place. This record must capture the patient's vital signs, ongoing condition, nature of illness or injury, and procedures performed. Upon arrival at the emergency department, a copy of the ambulance record may be appended to the hospital's emergency service report, or data may be abstracted from the ambulance record for the emergency service report. If the patient has been an inpatient or outpatient at the hospital, previous records must be made available for emergency care.

The Medicare *Conditions of Participation: Hospitals* specify items considered essential for treating emergency department patients. Included are patient identification; history of disease or injury; physical findings; laboratory and x-ray reports, if any; and diagnosis, treatment, and disposition of the case. The physician in charge of the case must sign the emergency outpatient record to validate its contents.

The Joint Commission requires that a medical record be kept each time a patient receives treatment from the emergency department. The physician responsible for the emergency service provided should authenticate the medical record. Items that should be documented include:

- Pertinent history of the present illness or injury, physical findings, and vital signs.
- Emergency care given to the patient prior to arrival.
- Diagnostic and therapeutic orders.
- Clinical observations including results of treatment.
- Reports of procedures, tests, and results.
- Diagnostic impressions
- Conclusion at the termination of treatment, including final disposition, patient's condition on discharge, and any

instructions given to the patient or family for follow-up care.

- A patient leaving against medical advice.

In addition, the Joint Commission expects hospital emergency services to keep a continuous register of information for every person seeking care. The register should include at least the name, age, date, time, means of arrival, nature of complaint, disposition, and time of departure of each patient.

A copy of the emergency department treatment form is usually sent to the patient's physician for use in providing follow-up care. A complete record of all the care given to the patient ensures the hospital of adequate legal protection. An emergency record similar to the one shown in Figure 1 can assure this complete documentation.

The content of emergency department records is often mentioned in state regulations. These requirements should be reviewed by health information professionals when developing emergency department medical records and record-retrieval procedures.

The hospital outpatient department or primary care center has recently been the focus of attention as non-emergency ambulatory care has been increasing and as the federal government begins to impose a prospective payment system for Medicare reimbursement of outpatient care. In the past, the content and organization of the outpatient medical record was left somewhat to chance. The hospital medical record department rarely assembled outpatient record contents in any specified order or analyzed the documentation for completeness. Diagnoses identified in the outpatient setting and procedures performed were generally not coded and indexed. (Coding is a procedure which assigns a numeric code to diagnostic and procedural databased on a medical classification system; indexing is the arrangement of the codes to allow for retrieval of records by specific diagnostic and/or procedural data.) If physicians wanted to study certain outpatient records, outpatient department staff may have been assigned to keep track of the patients identified by the physician for a brief period of time. Physicians may even have kept separate notes for themselves on interesting or special cases - transferring only minimal data on these patients to their hospital outpatient records.

While outpatient medical records have not changed drastically overnight, improvement is taking place. The increased intensity of outpatient services has necessitated improved documentation for continuity of patient care data. Patients often receive

EMERGENCY ROOM RECORD

Family Name | First Name | Middle Name | Home Phone | Arrival Date | Time A.M. P.M. | Hosp. No.

Address | City | State | Zip | Age | Date of Birth / / | Sex M F | Civil Status M S W D Sep | Religion

Employer | Address | Compensation Yes No

Relative or Friend; Parent or Guardian if a Minor | Address | Phone

Insurance Carrier | Contract No. | Effective Date | Subscriber Dependent | Family Member Comprehensive

Cert. or Policy No. | Group No. | Effective Date

Family Doctor | Notified Yes No | Brought By Relative Self Police Fire Other | Type of Service: Lab XR PH PT Other | S.S. No.

☐ Medicare Patient | Medicare No. and Other Information

BRIEF HISTORY

If accident state where, when and how injured; if illness describe; note care prior to admission:

NOTIFIED: Relative ☐ Coroner ☐ Police ☐ By Whom:

Allergies: | Last Tetanus: | Current Rx:

Nurse's Signature R.N. | Officer's Signature | Star | District | Time A.M. P.M.

PHYSICIAN'S REPORT

CONDITION ON ARRIVAL ☐ Good ☐ Fair ☐ Poor ☐ Shock ☐ Hemorrhage ☐ Coma ☐ Critical ☐ D.O.A. | TIME | TEMP. Oral Rectal | P. | R. | B/P

Treatment: Tetanus Toxoid ______ cc. Tetanus Antitoxin Test ______ Tetanus Antitoxin ______ units

Physical Findings:

Diagnosis:

Disposition of Case: ☐ TREATED & DISCHARGED ☐ ADMITTED Room/Bed ______ ☐ TRANSFERRED To ______ Via ______ | Time A.M. P.M.

CONDITION ON DISCHARGE
Good ☐ Satisfactory ☐ Serious ☐ Critical ☐ Expired ☐

INSTRUCTIONS TO PATIENT: See Dr. ______ ☐ in ______ days ☐ if further problems. Instruction ☐ Sheet Given ______

ADDITIONAL INSTRUCTIONS

PATIENT OR AUTHORIZED SIGNATURE | DATE | TIME .M. | ATTENDING PHYSICIAN M.D.

EMERGENCY ROOM CHARGES (Does Not Include Fee of Attending Physician)						OTHER SERVICES RENDERED
ITEM	CHARGE	ITEM	CHARGE	ITEM	CHARGE	
Emergency Room		Drugs		Cast Room		X-ray
Anesthetic		Oxygen		Examining Room		Laboratory
Antiseptics		Sutures				Physical Therapy
Dressings		Tetanus Antitoxin				

FORM D-2311 PHYSICIANS' RECORD CO., BERWYN, ILLINOIS - PRINTED IN U.S.A.

Form courtesy of Physicians' Record Company

FIGURE 1. EMERGENCY RECORD

outpatient care services over an extended period of time. Entries which document the care provided must be made each time an outpatient returns for care or treatment. For this reason it is very important that the patient's medical record be available at all times. The Joint Commission on Accreditation of Health-care Organizations states a system must be established either to consolidate a patient's records at the time of scheduled outpatient visit, or to incorporate pertinent medical information

Name											
Name_____ Clinic_____ DOB_____ Allergies:_____											
#	Entry Date	Chronic Problems	Rev. Res.	#	Entry Date	Temporary Problems	Recurrence Date				
							1	2	3	4	5

FIGURE 2. PATIENT PROBLEM LIST

(e.g., discharge summaries, operative reports, and pathology reports) in the ambulatory care record. A complete health picture of the patient must be available to everyone contributing to the patient's continuing care.

Medicare billing requirements for data in coded form have involved the medical record department in review of outpatient medical records and should further improve the organization and documentation in the record. Outpatient record entries should be arranged so that preceding remarks can be quickly

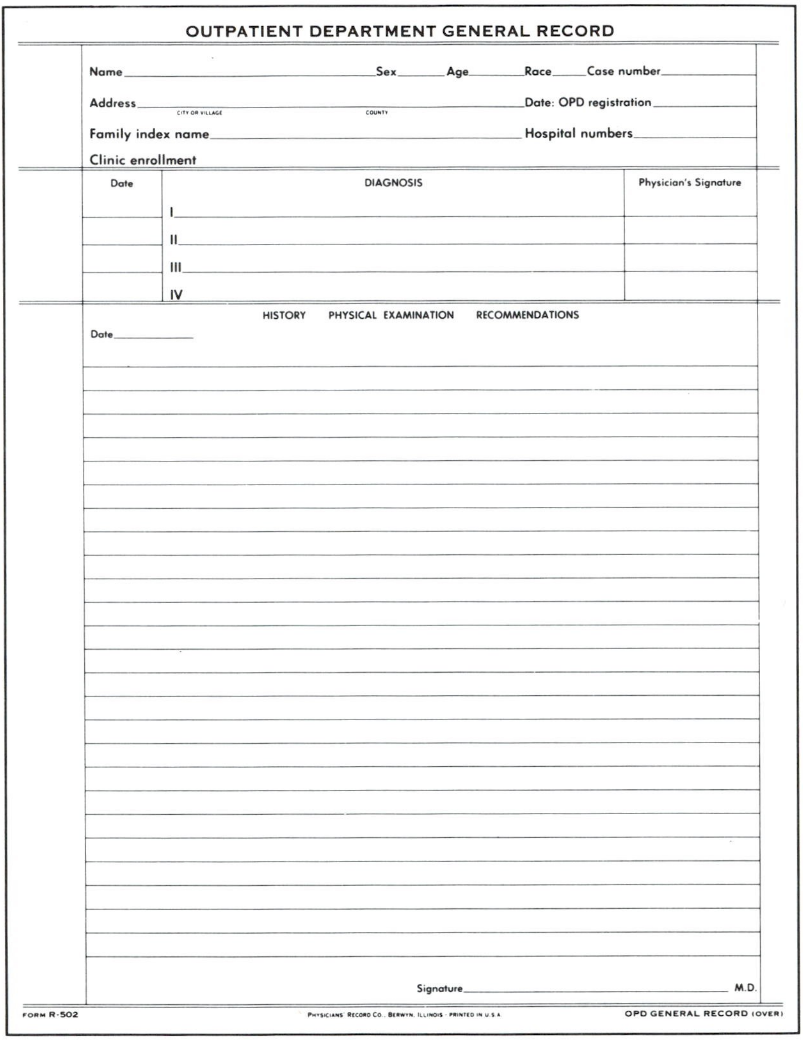
OUTPATIENT DEPARTMENT GENERAL RECORD

Name ______ Sex ______ Age ______ Race ______ Case number ______

Address ______ (CITY OR VILLAGE) ______ (COUNTY) ______ Date: OPD registration ______

Family index name ______ Hospital numbers ______

Clinic enrollment

Date	DIAGNOSIS	Physician's Signature
	I	
	II	
	III	
	IV	

HISTORY PHYSICAL EXAMINATION RECOMMENDATIONS

Date ______

Signature ______ M.D.

FORM R-502 Physicians' Record Co., Berwyn, Illinois · Printed in U.S.A. OPD GENERAL RECORD (OVER)

Form courtesy of Physicians' Record Company

FIGURE 3. AMBULATORY CARE RECORD (front)

scanned for the necessary medical data. Progress notes are usually arranged in chronological order. Referencing may be made to individual problems or conditions by use of the problem-oriented method of recording discussed in Chapter 2. Thus, data particular to one injury, such as a hip fracture, can be readily scanned by problem number and name. The Joint Commission requires hospital-based ambulatory service records

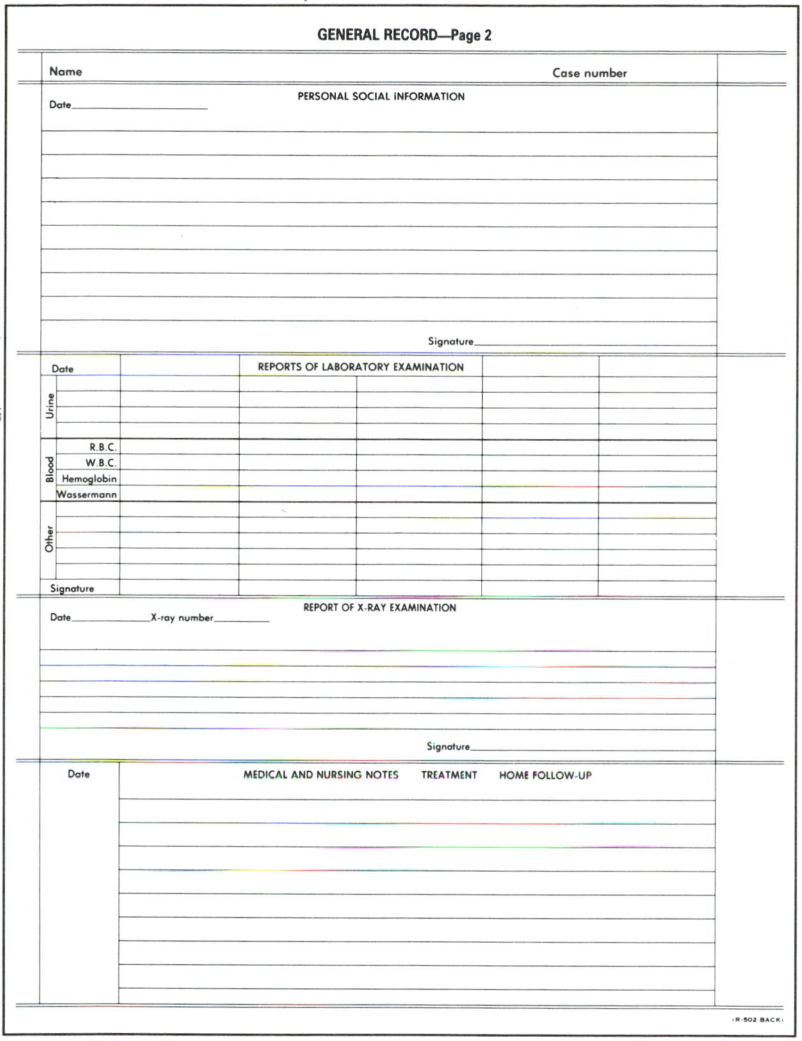

GENERAL RECORD—Page 2

Name   Case number

PERSONAL SOCIAL INFORMATION
Date

Signature

REPORTS OF LABORATORY EXAMINATION
Date

Urine

Blood — R.B.C. / W.B.C. / Hemoglobin / Wassermann

Other

Signature

REPORT OF X-RAY EXAMINATION
Date_____X-ray number_____

Signature

Date   MEDICAL AND NURSING NOTES   TREATMENT   HOME FOLLOW-UP

(R-502 BACK)

Form courtesy of Physicians' Record Company

FIGURE 4. AMBULATORY CARE RECORD (back of fig.3)

to include a list of known significant diagnoses, conditions, procedures, drug allergies, and medications. The list must be initiated and maintained for each patient by the third visit (Figure 2).

Both the federal government and the Joint Commission list a number of specific data items essential to a good outpatient record. The *Medicare Conditions of Participation: Hospitals* states that at least enough information must be included to ensure continuity of care, including the patient's medical history, physical findings, laboratory and diagnostic test results, diagnosis, and treatment record.

Individual states may also have regulations related to ambulatory care records. The health information practitioner should be thoroughly familiar with all applicable regulations at the state level. Other specific items of medical data included on medical record forms relate to the type of outpatient services rendered. An outpatient department record form which can be used to document required visit information is shown in Figures 3 and 4.

MEDICAL RECORDS IN FREE-STANDING FACILITIES

Medical record standards for free-standing facilities are found in the Joint Commission's *Accreditation Manual For Ambulatory Health Care* and in the Accreditation Association for Ambulatory Health Care's *Accreditation Handbook for Ambulatory Health Care*. Both groups accredit free-standing ambulatory care facilities such as private group practices, neighborhood health centers, health maintenance organizations, urgent care centers, ambulatory surgery centers, etc.

Contents

To assure the ongoing provision of effective medical care, the Joint Commission requires free-standing ambulatory care medical records to contain a summary list of significant past surgical procedures and past and current diagnoses or problems. The list should be conspicuously documented in each patient's record. The list should not repeat recurring problems or diagnoses and must include any significant surgical conditions, significant medical conditions, any allergies and untoward reactions to drugs, and currently or recently used medications.

In addition, all entries in the patient's record (for each visit) should be identified with the patient's name and number (when applicable) and should include:

- Date, department, and provider name and profession.
- Chief complaint or purpose of visit.
- Objective findings.
- Diagnosis or medical impression.
- Studies ordered, such as laboratory or x-ray studies.
- Therapies administered.
- Disposition, recommendations, and instructions to patient.
- Signature or initials of practitioner.

Many states have regulations applicable to some free-standing ambulatory settings, and health information professionals should be familiar with these as well as with any applicable federal regulations.

Format of Ambulatory Care Records

The arrangement of information in the patient's ambulatory care record should be convenient for those who must refer to it on a daily basis. The ambulatory care record should provide a ready means of communication among all providers. As discussed in Chapter 2, either the source-oriented, integrated, or problem-oriented method of recording may be used. In the source-oriented method, forms are filed in chronological order and placed in separate sections of the record by the type of form or service rendered. In an integrated record, progress notes are entered in strict chronological order by all providers of care, regardless of service. Problem-oriented progress notes are useful when a patient is seen for multiple problems at one time, and reference must be made to the treatment course of each.

Each ambulatory care facility should decide on a suitable format based on individual needs and preferences. The health information professional can assist the facility in choosing a suitable format and recommending necessary changes in the arrangement of health records.

Computerized Ambulatory Care Records

Computerized ambulatory care medical records have been in existence for a number of years. The COSTAR (Computer Stored Ambulatory Record) system was developed by the Laboratory of Computer Science at Massachusetts General Hospital in collaboration with the Harvard Community Health Plan in the

1960s. It has been operational since 1969. The COSTAR system is a comprehensive medical information system for ambulatory care which allows for the capture and storage of narrative medical information. Use of the system can result in a paperless record although printed record copies may be generated. The system is directory-based and thus allows for coded/standardized data. Data can be collected by clinical staff on encounter forms and later entered into the computer by clerical staff, or data can be entered directly by clinical staff. To ensure the quality of the database direct entry is preferable. Implementation of the COSTAR system requires a major personnel and financial commitment.

Several computer systems are also available for management of the ambulatory care facility. Such systems allow the physician to schedule patients; store, track, and analyze medical records; follow-up patients; manage business applications; conduct quality assurance studies; and link with a hospital.

The health information professional should be familiar with the various ambulatory care computer record systems available and should be actively involved in planning and implementing any such system. Key considerations when implementing a computerized record system are: (1) Who is the system for - the provider, the administrator, or the researcher? (2) How should the data be structured for ease of access? and (3) What type of patients will be included in the system - cardiac patients, pediatric patients, etc.?

ANALYSIS OF AMBULATORY CARE RECORDS

The accuracy and completeness of ambulatory care records are important to the patient, physician, other health care providers, and facility. Health information personnel may be delegated the task of quantitative review of the records after each patient visit or episode of care. A careful review of entries should be made to ensure that all required data are present and signed by the appropriate persons. If a hospital's ambulatory care record is not filed in the health information department, responsibility for quantitative analysis may be delegated to employees supervising records in the ambulatory care area itself.

A review of the quality of data entered in ambulatory care records should be performed by the medical staff on an ongoing basis. The health information department may be asked to assist in performance of this function, or it may be delegated to a medical staff committee. Record review requirements for ambulatory care records can be found in the applicable accreditation standards cited earlier in this chapter and in applicable government regulations.

AMBULATORY CARE DATA

In 1989 the National Committee on Vital and Health Statistics approved the Uniform Ambulatory Care Data Set developed by its Subcommittee on Ambulatory Care Statistics and the Department of Health and Human Services (DHHS) Interagency Task Force. The Interagency Task Force was charged with ascertaining the data needs of agencies within DHHS; and whereas the Subcommittee reviewed the data set from the broader perspective of other government agencies, the research community, and the private sector.

The purpose of the Uniform Ambulatory Case Data Set is to improve the comparability of ambulatory care data by defining a common core of standard data items with uniform definitions. The items in their data set are recommended for inclusion in the records of all ambulatory health care but do not, themselves, define a complete patient record. Although desirable, all items do not need to be recorded in the individual patient's medical record. Some items may be included in billing records. In such instances, however, the capability should exist to link data from the various data sources.

The data items delineate information which characterizes the patient, the provider, and the encounter. A few items are designed as optional.

Patient Data Items

  1. Personal Identification

    a. Name: Surname, first name, and middle name or initial.

    b. Numeric: A unique number for the individual that links personal characteristics of the person to all services received by the person within a health care system and across systems when services are covered under a third-party (government or private) reimbursement or funding arrangement.

  2. Residence (usual residence, full address, and zip code)

3. Date of Birth (month, day, year)

A minimum of three digits are required for year. If birth date is not known, interpolate year of birth from age.

4. Sex

   a. Male

   b. Female

5. Race and Ethnic Background

   a. Race:

      (1) American Indian/Eskimo/Aleut

      (2) Asian or Pacific Islander

      (3) Black

      (4) White

      (5) Other Race

   b. Ethnicity

      (1) Hispanic Origin

      (2) Not of Hispanic origin

6. Living arrangement and marital status (optional)

The Subcommittee and Interagency Task Force recognize that a person's social support system can be an important determinant of health status, access to health care services, and use of services. Frequently, marital status and/or living arrangement are used as surrogates for the social support system available to a patient. It is recommended that, when this information is needed for program design, targeting of services, utilization and outcome studies, or other research and development purposes, the following definitions should be used for living arrangement and marital status. In terms of measurement of social support the item on living arrangement will have greater utility than the item on marital status. However, the ultimate selection of items needs to be made on the basis of the context and purpose of the data collection.

Living Arrangement

   a. Alone

   b. With spouse (alternate: with spouse or unrelated partner)

   c. With children

d. With parent or guardian

e. With relatives other than spouse, children, or parents

f. With nonrelatives

g. Unknown

Multiple responses can be made to this item because of living arrangements that are a combination of spouse, children, parents, and nonrelatives.

In those data systems which choose to collect marital status in lieu of or in addition to living arrangement, the following categories should be used:

Marital Status:

a. Married—A person currently married. Classify Common Law marriage as "married."

b. Never married—A person who has never been married or whose only marriages have been annulled.

c. Widowed—A person widowed and not remarried.

d. Divorced—A person divorced and not remarried.

e. Separated—A person legally separated or otherwise absent from spouse.

f. Unknown.

These categories are mutually exclusive. Cohabitation should be grouped with married unless the purpose of data collection is specifically for health insurance benefit determination.

Longitudinal studies will have the opportunity to study transitions from one type of living arrangement or marital status to another.

Provider Data Item

An individual provider has been defined as a health professional who delivers services or is professionally responsible for services delivered to a patient, who is exercising independent judgment in the care of the patient, and who is not under the immediate supervision of another health care professional. An encounter is defined as a professional contact between a patient and a provider during which services are delivered.

The following characteristics should be collected for the provider of record for each encounter. If a user decides to collect the additional provider data element, discussed above under definitions, for the provider who initiated the encounter if different from the provider who delivered or was responsible for the services delivered, consideration also will have to be given to the necessary identification elements required for this item.

7. Provider Identification

a. Name: Surname, first name, and middle name or initial.

b. Numeric: A unique number that distinguishes the provider from all other providers and is the same for the provider in all settings where he may be in practice.

8. Location or Address

Full address and zip code for the location of the office or facility that is the usual or principal place of practice.

9. Profession (the one in which the provider is currently engaged)

a. Physician (M.D. or DO.) or Dentist (DDS or DM)
List specialty and or subspecialty (limit up to three)

b. Other Licensed or Certified Health Care Professional
List field of practice or specialty

c. Other Health Care Provider
List self-designated field of practice or specialty

Encounter Data Items

10. Date, Place or Site and Address of Encounter, if different from item 8.

a. Date of Encounter: Month, day, and year

b. Place or Site of Encounter (A list of 29 places of encounter is provided in the full description of the data set; examples include office, home, hospital outpatient, hospice, independent laboratory, and ambulance.)

c. Address of Facility where Services Rendered, when different from item 8.

11. Patient's reason for encounter (optional)

Includes the patient's stated reason at the time of the encounter for seeking attention or care. This item attempts to define what actually motivated the patient to seek care.

12. Problem, Diagnosis, or Assessment

Describes all conditions requiring evaluation, or treatment or management at the time of the encounter as designated by the provider. It is recommended that the standard coding convention for this purpose should be the widely-used *International Classification of Diseases* and, if existent, its clinical modification (currently ICD-9-CM), with all codes available for use. This approach should accommodate the coding of symptoms, ill-defined conditions, and problems when a firm diagnosis has not been established.

The condition which should be listed first is the diagnosis, problem, symptom or the reason for encounter shown in the patient's health care record to be chiefly responsible for the ambulatory medical care services provided during the encounter. List additional codes that describe any co-existing conditions. Do not code diagnoses documented as "probable," "suspected," "questionable," or "rule out" as if they are established. Rather, code the condition(s) or symptom(s) to the highest degree of certainty for that encounter.

13. Services

Describe all diagnostic services of any type including history, physical examination, laboratory, x-ray or radiograph, and others that are performed pertinent to the patient's reasons for the encounter; all therapeutic services performed at the time of the encounter; and all preventive services and procedures performed at the time of the encounter. Also, describe, to the extent possible, the provision to the patient of drugs and biologicals, supplies, appliances and equipment.

The diagnostics, therapeutic and preventive services should be captured in connection with the encounter where they are provided. The *HCFA Common Procedure Coding System* (HCPCS), which is based on CPT-4 for physician services and has been augmented for nonphysician services, currently is the most inclusive coding system for fostering uniformity in reporting these services.

14. Disposition

The provider's statement of the next step(s) in the care of the patient. As many categories as apply should be reported. At a minimum, the following classification is suggested.

a. No follow-up planned

b. Follow-up planned

   (1) Return anticipated as necessary but not scheduled

   (2) Return to the current provider at a specific date

   (3) Telephone follow-up

   (4) Returned to referring provider

   (5) Referred to other individual provider

   (6) Referred to other provider for consultation

   (7) Referred to an adjunctive provider agency

   (8) Transferred to other individual provider

   (9) Admit to acute-care hospital

  (10) Admit to residential health care facility

  (11) Other

15. Patient's Expected Sources of Payment

a. Primary Source

The primary source that is expected to be responsible for the largest percentage of the patient's current bill.

b. Secondary source

The secondary source, if any, which will be responsible for the next largest percentage of the patient's current bill.

c. Other source(s)

The categories for both primary, secondary, and other sources are as follows:

   1) Blue Cross/Blue Shield

   2) Other health insurance companies

   3) Other liability insurance

   4) Medicare

   5) Medicaid

   6) Workers compensation

   7) Self-insured employer plan

   8) Health Maintenance Organization (HMO)

   9) CHAMPUS

10) CHAMP VA

11) Other

   d. Payment mechanism (related to this service)

      1) Fee-for-service

      2) HMO/pre-paid plan

      3) Unknown or unidentified

16. Total Charges

All charges for procedures and services rendered to the patient during this encounter. This includes a technical component or facility fee when billed separately from the professional component.

COLLECTION OF AMBULATORY CARE DATA

Routine collection of patient information assists the hospital or the ambulatory care facility in analyzing its patterns of care and the demographics of its patient population. Through the implementation of an appropriate coding and indexing system, the information contained in the patient's health record can be compiled not only for payment purposes, but for administrative, research, and educational uses.

Commonly used units of measure in ambulatory health care include:

Encounter - a face-to-face contact between a patient and a provider who has primary responsibility for assessing and treating the patient at a given contact, exercising independent judgment.

Professional contact - professional contact occurs between a patient and a provider when the patient is physically present or when the provider is analyzing a specimen or interpreting an image, etc., of the patient for the referring physician.

Thus, an encounter occurs when a patient receives x-ray, laboratory, physical therapy services., etc., through a separate provider when those services are not completed at the time of the original encounter with the provider ordering the services. A professional contact also can occur between a patient and provider on the telephone and by other communication mechanisms for remote sites. Receiving services from a pharmacist or a supplier does not constitute an encounter.

Outpatient visit - the visit of an outpatient to one or more units or facilities located in or directed by the entity maintaining the outpatient health care services (clinic, physician's office, hospital/medical center).

Occasion of service - a specific identifiable instance of an act of service involved in the care of patients.

The differences noted in the above definitions point out some of the difficulties in collecting ambulatory care statistics. An outpatient visit may involve one or more outpatient occasions of service to the individual, depending on how many tests are done or outpatient units visited. Encounters may be with professional personnel responsible for the patient's care or with ancillary personnel, such as social workers, who assist in the care of the patient. Patients may have several encounters during one visit, and an ambulatory care facility needs to maintain data on the number and types of these encounters. Because of the differences expressed in each of these units of measure, many ambulatory care facilities find it useful to record data on outpatient visits, encounters, and occasions of service, in order that accurate patterns of care are documented and readily available

QUALITY MANAGEMENT

For many reasons, quality assurance methods for ambulatory care may differ from those used for inpatient care as ambulatory care is different in scope, provision, and documentation. Ambulatory care medical records of some providers may not be good data sources for quality studies since they may be brief; poorly organized; and illegible or incomplete, often containing no mention of relevant care by other providers. In addition, retrieval of records by diagnoses, problems, or by reasons for visits may not be possible since coding and indexing may not be performed. Quality activities are also limited by staffing and funding. Staff members available to conduct quality studies may have little formal training in medical terminology, anatomy and physiology, medical records, etc.

Quality management methods established must utilize available data and must be easily understood by the persons involved. Health information professionals should be active in helping to establish ambulatory care quality assurance programs as well as procedures for coding, indexing, and data collection.

The Joint Commission requires accredited ambulatory care facilities to have appropriate quality control mechanisms. These include:

- The coordination of a scheduling and staffing plan that facilitates accessibility and continuity of care and minimizes patient waiting time.
- A system for follow-up on broken appointments. A timely review, interpretation, and reporting, as appropriate, of diagnostic radiographic studies, laboratory tests, and electrocardiograms, to be available to the practitioner requesting such services in the provision of ambulatory care.
- A systematic review and evaluation of surgical patients who require hospitalization following ambulatory surgery.
- When authorized and appropriate, the provision, to the private practitioner or medical facility responsible for follow-up care, of a copy of the record or summary of ambulatory care services.
- The maintenance and evaluation of patient drug profiles, whenever possible. Inclusion, in the medical staff's review functions, of drug usage evaluation of ambulatory care patients who receive medications.
- Inclusion, in the medical staff's review functions, of blood usage review of ambulatory care patients who receive blood transfusions.
- Compliance with the requirements for radiation therapy, when provided.
- A means of communicating in the language of the predominant population groups served.

Also required is an ongoing quality assurance program designed to objectively and systematically monitor and evaluate the quality and appropriateness of patient care, pursue opportunities to improve patient care, and resolve identified problems. The scope of the quality assurance program should include the evaluation of the quality and appropriateness of diagnostic and treatment procedures; the quality, content, and completeness of medical record entries; clinical performance; the use of medications; patient satisfaction; the quality and appropriateness of surgical and anesthesia services, when provided; and the quality and appropriateness of emergency services, when provided. There must be quality control in pathology and laboratory services, and in radiology services, when provided.

SUMMARY

Ambulatory care is an integral component of the health care delivery system in the United States, and in recent years utilization of ambulatory care has increased markedly. Medical records maintained for ambulatory care assume a vital role in ensuring the continuity of patient care. The more diversified the health care delivery system becomes, the more important the role the information plays in the provision of continuous patient care. Health information professionals must take an active role in the development of quality records and information management procedures in ambulatory care facilities.

STUDY QUESTIONS

1. What factors influence increase utilization of ambulatory care and other alternatives to inpatient care?

2. List the four types of hospital-based ambulatory care.

3. Define "ambulatory surgery facility" and describe its present rate of growth.

4. What data elements should be recorded in emergency records according to the Medicare *Conditions of Participation*? According to the Joint Commission?

5. According to the Joint Commission, what data elements should be recorded at the time of each ambulatory care visit?

6. List various types of free-standing ambulatory care facilities and describe the medical record requirements according to the Joint Commission and the Accreditation Association for Ambulatory Health Care.

7. Describe the Joint Commission requirements for ambulatory care quality assurance.

REFERENCES

Benson, Dale S., William Van Osdol, and Peyton Townes, "Quality Ambulatory Care: The Role of the Diagnostic and Medication Summary Lists," *Quality Review Bulletin*, (June 1988).

Cook, Michael J., "Computerized financial systems in the ambulatory care marketplace," *Journal of Ambulatory Care Management*, Vol. 8, No. 2, (May 1985).

Department of Health and Human Services, "The Uniform Ambulatory Care Date Set," *Report of the National Committee on Vital and Health Statistics and its Interagency Task Force in the Uniform Ambulatory Care Data Set*, 1989.

Farley, Pamela J., "Hospital and Ambulatory Services for Selected Illnesses,"*Health Services Research*, Vol. 21, (December 1986).

Feste, Laura, *Ambulatory Care Documentation*, (Chicago American Medical Record Association, 1989)

Glossary of Health Care Terms, American Health Information Management Association, 1994, Chicago, IL.

Henderson, John A., "Surgery center growth slows; more procedures done," *Modern Healthcare*, (June 6, 1986).

Horn, Susan D., June D. Buckle, and Christopher M. Carver, "Ambulatory severity index: Development of an ambulatory case mix system," *Journal of Ambulatory Care Management*, (November 1988):53-62.

Hospital Statistics, American Hospital Association, 1993, Chicago, Il.

Joint Commission on Accreditation of Healthcare Organizations, *Accreditation Manual for Hospitals*, (Chicago: Joint Commission, 1994).

Joint Commission on Accreditation of Healthcare Organizations, *Ambulatory Health Care Standards Manual*, (Chicago: Joint Commission, 1994).

Kelly, William, Herbert Fillmore, and Paul Tenan, "Case Mix Classification and Ambulatory Care," *Business and Health*, U.S. No. 7, (May 1988): 41-44.

Kraft, David P., "Quality of Care and the Accreditation of Health Services; What Is the Relationship?"*Journal of American College Health*, Vol. 37, (November 1988).

Miller, Laird L., and Joanne E. Miller, "Using supply and demand economics to purchase health care," *Journal of Ambulatory Care Management,* Vol. 10, No. 4, (November 1987).

Nelson, Robert A., "Planning for an ambulatory care computer system," *Journal of Ambulatory Care Management*, Vol. 8, No. 2, (May 1985).

Palmer, R. Heather, "The Challenges and Prospects for Quality Assessment and Assurance in Ambulatory Care," *Inquiry 25*, Vol. 25, No. 1, (Blue Cross and Blue Shield Association, Spring 1988): 119-131.

Ross, Donna J., and Kathleen E. Hughes, "A new attitude: Contracting for success with alternative delivery systems," *Journal of Ambulatory Care Management*, (February 1987).

Sabin, Margaret, and Debra Fox-Filiessman, "The Exploding Demand for Ambulatory Data," *Computers in Healthcare*, Vol. 9, No. 6, (June 1988).

Schneider, Karen C., et al., "Ambulatory visit groups: An outpatient classification system," *Journal of Ambulatory Care Management*, (August 1988).

Wakefield, Douglas S., and Robert L. Ludke, "Developing an ambulatory care risk management (ACRM) program," *Journal of Ambulatory Care Management*, (November 1988).

chapter *4*

CLINICAL RECORDS IN LONG TERM CARE AND REHABILITATION FACILITIES

Providing clinical records is an important goal in the management and operation of long term care and rehabilitation facilities. The content of clinical records is different, but the procedures for their maintenance in these type of facilities may be similar to those in acute care. However, because of differences in the recording of data, the clinical record system in a long term care facility should not duplicate the system used in an acute care setting. The individual needs of the institution must be considered when organizing the record system. This chapter summarizes guidelines for record content, data collection activities, quality assurance and improvement, utilization review, and record management principles applicable to long term care and rehabilitation facilities.Although long term care and rehabilitation are often directed at two different populations there are enough similarities in the populations that their clinical record requirements are also similar. Most significant is that both populations require care over a long period of time. Changes in physical status are not as dramatic as they are in an acute care setting. Both long term care residents and rehabilitation patients have chronic conditions, although the long term care resident generally has chronic diseases, whereas rehabilitation care patients often have disabilities resulting from congenital factors, accidents or injuries. The long term care resident is generally elderly, whereas the rehabilitation patient may be of any age. In both settings, residents and patients require assistance with and training in the activities of daily living. The generally younger rehabilitation patients, however, may receive more extensive training beyond activities of daily living including basic education and alternate career training. Long term care is generally provided as inpatient care. Rehabilitation care may be both inpatient and outpatient.

LONG TERM CARE FACILITIES

Long term care facilities are an integral part of the health care delivery system. The focus of long term care changed in 1987 with the passage of the Omnibus Budget Reconciliation Act (OBRA). After numerous delays, federal regulations were issued in 1991 to implement OBRA in long term care facilities. The regulation revised and consolidated the requirements that facilities furnishing LTC must meet to participate in either or both the Medicare and Medicaid programs. These regulations replaced the former *Conditions of Participation* that were developed under the Medicare program. These long term care requirements and related state regulations should be carefully reviewed when developing policies and procedures for the maintenance of clinical records.

Nursing home is a generic term used to denote a health care facility for the elderly. Often, designations indicating level of care for a specific facility are specified in licensure regulations. Skilled care is the most comprehensive level, with patients needing continuous nursing service and a variety of support services on a routine basis. Intermediate or nursing facility care is not as complex. These residents may require a limited degree of support and nursing services.

Facilities may be licensed to provide more than one level of care, so patients may move from one level of care to another according to their needs.

Generally, state regulatory agencies have different systems for assessing the appropriate level of care and determining reimbursement. Clinical record personnel will find it useful to acquaint themselves with the specific systems used in their states. Level of care may also be defined by a classification system such as the Resource Utilization Groups used in some states. There are other methods of case-mix based reimbursement systems used by Medicaid programs funding nursing facility residents in other states. The term "nursing facility" is now being applied to facilities participating in the Medicaid program that were previously called intermediate care facilities. Many different types of LTC facilities are now available providing many options to the elderly and disabled, such as assisted living, rest homes, independent living, respite care, and hospice facilities.

Given such a variety of options, the resident and patient population and thus documentation requirements will vary from one long term care institution to another. At one end of the spectrum are the frail and/or ill elderly persons who no longer are able to live independently. They have generalized chronic physical deterioration needing a variety of supportive services to maintain the normal activities of daily living, and have a variety of chronic disease conditions requiring regular physician, nursing, and other professional health care services. Medical record documentation is, therefore, characterized by ongoing, repeated documentation of chronic care, interspersed with major medical episodes.

At the other extreme are patients who come to a facility for comparatively shorter stays, many often with more specific and time-limited diagnostic situations which totally or partially resolve during the convalescent or rehabilitative stay.

LEGAL, REGULATORY, AND ACCREDITING STANDARDS

Fundamental to the operation of a long term care facility is licensure by the state agency empowered to regulate such facilities. The agency issues regulations which include specific areas of medical record content and practice. During licensure renewal, significant aspects of the medical record content and system may be reviewed. If an area is not in compliance, the facility must file its plan of correction, specifying the manner and time frame in which it will bring the practices into compliance. A properly developed medical record system should assist facilities in maintaining compliance with state, federal, and local requirements. Ongoing medical record review and related monitoring will help reduce noncompliance with respect to documentation by all personnel who provide care to residents.

The federal LTC regulations apply to all facilities that participate in the Medicare/Medicaid programs. As with state regulations, a facility must correct deficiencies identified through periodic surveys.

The third set of standards flows from voluntary participation in the Joint Commission on Accreditation of Healthcare Organization's program of accreditation. This accreditation body has developed standards for long term care facilities. Facilities that wish to have accreditation status apply to the Joint Commission, participate in the site visit survey, and, if found in compliance, are issued the accreditation certificate appropriate to the facility's level of care. Unlike the state and federal regulations, compliance with the Joint Commission standards is voluntary.

Although a particular facility may not seek Joint Commission status, clinical record personnel may find it useful to obtain such standards as a reference. A particular facility's policies may be more stringent than the state and federal regulations. The Joint Commission's guidelines provide a basis for such policy development, as do professional practice standards for LTC published by the American Health Information Management Association.

NURSING FACILITIES

THE PROFESSIONAL AND ADMINISTRATIVE STAFF

Ownership of nursing facilities reflects the same variety as hospitals although a higher percentage of facilities are for-profit entities. Under any form of ownership there will be an administrator designated as the chief executive officer responsible for the day-to-day running of the facility. Most state regulations require that the administrator of a nursing facility be licensed by the state.

A medical director will coordinate the work of the medical staff and provide oversight for the medical and professional care rendered. Each resident has an attending physician responsible for his care.

The director of nursing service plays a key role in long term care. Because of the nature of care delivered in many facilities, physician presence is more limited than in the acute care setting.The role of the director of nursing service is that of primary agent for day-to-day supervision of care and coordination with physician services. Clinical record personnel interact frequently with the director of nursing services in matters of resident care and documentation. Nursing personnel include a mix of registered nurses, licensed practical nurses, and aides. A variety of other professional health care providers render services in the nursing facility, including the activities director, occupational therapist, physical therapist, podiatrist, dentist, dietician, pharmacist, and social worker. When the facility is relatively small, some of these practitioners provide services on a contractual basis. The designation of professional credentials in documentation is important.

Clinical record personnel should include a credentialed practitioner, either as an employee of the facility or as a consultant. Responsibility for the day-to-day operations of the clinical record service must be assigned to an employee of the facility. Normally clinical record personnel report to the chief executive officer, but in some facilities, they report to the director of nursing service.

CLINICAL RECORDS IN NURSING FACILITIES

Each resident in a nursing facility must have an individual record. Clinical records should be simple, realistic, and flexible but should also be detailed enough to contribute to care and treatment. A clinical record should contain complete information about the resident's illness and treatment. Events should be recorded in the order in which they occur. This complete chronological recording justifies the diagnosis and proves that the condition warrants the treatment and the end result. Documentation must be sufficiently detailed to provide a basis for reimbursement by the various private and public funding agencies.

The following section describes the items typically included in a clinical record for nursing facilities which participate in the Medicare/Medicaid programs, comply with state licensure regulations, and participate in Joint Commission accreditation.

Identification Data

Information in the identification section of the record should include enough data to positively identify each resident. Examples of entries which may be collected are listed below. Items which may change should be kept current with the changes posted in the resident's clinical record in a highly visible place, e.g., the identification sheet. These items are preceded by an asterisk.

- Resident's name, including aliases and nicknames
- Marital status
- Facility number
- *Address
- *Telephone number
- *Age
- Date of birth
- Place of birth
- Citizenship
- Social Security number
- Religious preference
- Clergyman and address
- Mortuary preference
- Military service
- Insurance

- Medicare number
- Medicaid number
- Sex
- Next of kin or responsible agent
- Address and telephone number of nearest of kin or responsible agent
- Usual occupation
- Date of admission
- Time of admission
- Admitted from
- Referred by
- Attending physician
- Dentist
- Other information needed to satisy state requirements

A combined identification and summary sheet is displayed in Figure 1. When this type of form is used, the physician is responsible for writing the final diagnosis and condition of the resident or prognosis at discharge. The attending physician's signature may be requested if the facility desires verification of physician entries directly on the identification and summary

Reprinted with permission of Briggs Corporation, Des Moines, Iowa 50306

FIGURE 1. RECORD OF ADMISSION

sheet. It should be noted that such a summary sheet does not replace the formal discharge summary which constitutes a separate document. The date and time of discharge as well as the place to which the resident was discharged should be filled in by appropriate personnel.

RESIDENT TRANSFER FORM
(INTER-AGENCY REFERRAL)
(Reference tags: F200-A, F205-F208)

RESIDENT'S LAST NAME | FIRST NAME | MI | SEX ☐M ☐F | SOCIAL SECURITY NUMBER

RESIDENT'S ADDRESS (Street, City, State, Zip) | DATE OF BIRTH | RELIGION

DATE OF THIS TRANSFER | FACILITY NAME AND ADDRESS TRANSFERRING TO | PHYSICIAN IN CHARGE AT TIME OF TRANSFER

Will this physician care for resident after admission to new facility? ☐YES ☐NO

DATES OF STAY AT FACILITY TRANSFERRING FROM: ADMISSION | DISCHARGE

PAYMENT SOURCE FOR CHARGES TO RESIDENT
A. ☐ SELF OR FAMILY
B. ☐ PRIVATE INSURANCE
C. ☐ BLUE CROSS BLUE SHIELD
D. ☐ EMPLOYER OR UNION
E. ☐ PUBLIC AGENCY (Give name)
F. ☐ OTHER (Explain)

NAME AND ADDRESS OF FACILITY TRANSFERRING FROM | NAME AND ADDRESSES OF ALL HOSPITALS AND EXTENDED CARE FACILITIES FROM WHICH RESIDENT WAS DISCHARGED IN PAST 60 DAYS.

CLINIC APPOINTMENT SCHEDULED | DATE | TIME | ☐CLINIC APPOINTMENT CARD ATTACHED | DATE OF LAST PHYSICAL EXAMINATION | DATE OF LAST BOWEL MOVEMENT

RELATIVE OR GUARDIAN (Name, Address, Phone Number, Relationship to Resident) | WAS THIS PERSON NOTIFIED REGARDING THIS TRANSFER? ☐ YES ☐ NO | WAS THIS PERSON (OR WAS THE RESIDENT) GIVEN INFORMATION ON HOW TO CONTACT THE STATE OMBUDSMAN? ☐ YES ☐ NO

DIAGNOSES AT TIME OF TRANSFER — EMPLOYMENT RELATED: ☐YES ☐NO
(a) PRIMARY
(b) SECONDARY

VITALS AT TIME OF TRANSFER: Ht. ______ Wt. ______
T ______ P ______ R ______ B/P ______

REASON FOR TRANSFER

CHECK ALL THAT APPLY

DISABILITIES: ☐Amputation ☐Paralysis ☐Contracture(s) ☐Pressure Ulcer

INCONTINENCE: ☐Bladder ☐Bowel ☐Saliva

IMPAIRMENTS: ☐Mental ☐Speech ☐Hearing ☐Vision ☐Sensation

ACTIVITY TOLERANCE LIMITATIONS: ☐None ☐Moderate ☐Severe

RESIDENT KNOWS DIAGNOSIS? ☐Yes ☐No

POTENTIAL FOR REHABILITATION: ☐Good ☐Fair ☐Poor

DIET, DRUGS, AND OTHER THERAPY
at Time of Discharge

Diet Order:
Therapy:

Current Medications	Strength & Frequency	Time Last Dose	Amt. Sent

☐May NOT use generic substitutes
*(Physician or nurse must sign below - See verification of meds.)

IMPORTANT MEDICAL INFORMATION
(State allergies if any)

ADVANCE DIRECTIVES: ☐Yes ☐Attached ☐None

BED HOLD POLICY
Given to resident ☐ Yes ☐ No
Attached ☐ Yes ☐ No, reason: ______

Chest X-Ray Date ______ Result ______
C.B.C. Date ______ Result ______
Biochem Date ______ Result ______
Urinalysis Date ______ Result ______

SUGGESTIONS FOR ACTIVE CARE

BED
Position in good body alignment and change position every ______ hrs.
Avoid ______ position.
Prone position ______ times/day as tolerated.

SITTING
______ hr(s.) ______ times/day.

WEIGHT BEARING
☐Full ☐Partial ☐None
on ______ leg.

EXERCISES
Range of motion ______ times/day
to ______ by
☐resident ☐nurse ☐family.
Stand ______ minutes ______ times/day.

LOCOMOTION
Walk ______ (distance) ______ (no.) times/day.

SOCIAL ACTIVITIES
Encourage: (☐group ☐individual) activities
(☐within ☐outside) home.

Transportation: ☐Ambulance ☐Car ☐Car for handicapped ☐Bus

VERIFICATION OF MEDS
*Signature of Physician or Nurse X ______ Date ___/___/___

CFS 2-4/2P © 1992 Briggs Corporation, Des Moines, IA 50306 (800) 247-2343 Printed in U.S.A.

RESIDENT TRANSFER FORM
☐Continued on Reverse

Reprinted with permission of Briggs Corporation, Des Moines, Iowa 50306

FIGURE 2. RESIDENT TRANSFER FORM (front)

Transfer or Referral Statement

Nursing facilities need basic facts about each resident in order to provide appropriate care. These facts may be obtained from the transfer or referral form (Figures 2 and 3). When a resident is admitted to the facility, this form should accompany the resident; if it is not immediately available, this form should be requested immediately from the referring hospital, physi-

RESIDENT TRANSFER FORM (continued)

SELF CARE STATUS
(Check level of ability. Write S in space if needs supervision only. Draw line across if inapplicable.)

		Independent	Needs Assistance	Unable To Do
Bed Activity	Turns			
	Sits			
Personal Hygiene	Face, Hair, Arms			
	Trunk & Perineum			
	Lower Extremities			
	Bladder Program			
	Bowel Program			
Dressing	Upper Extremities			
	Trunk			
	Lower Extremities			
	Appliance, Splint			
Feeding				
Transfer	Sitting			
	Standing			
	Tub			
	Toilet			
Loco-motion	Wheelchair			
	Walking			
	Stairs			

BED ☐ Low   Mattress: ☐ Firm ☐ Reg.
Other ___
Side Rails: ☐ Yes ☐ No

BEHAVIOR ☐ Cooperative ☐ Oriented X ___
☐ Disruptive ☐ Belligerent ☐ Combative
☐ Senile ☐ Suspicious ☐ Withdrawn

MENTAL STATUS
☐ Alert ☐ Forgetful ☐ Confused

COMMUNICATION ABILITY	Yes	No
Able to make needs known		
Can speak		
Can hear		
Can write		
Understands speaking		
Understands writing		
Understands gestures		
Understands English		

If no, state language spoken or understood: ___

DIET
☐ Regular ☐ Low Salt ☐ Diabetic ☐ Bland
☐ Low Residue ☐ Other ___
☐ Feeds Self ☐ Needs Help
☐ Partial Assist ☐ Total Assist

RESIDENT USES
☐ Appliance
☐ Catheter (date of last change ___/___/___
☐ Colostomy ☐ Cane ☐ Crutches ☐ Prosthesis
☐ Walker ☐ Chair ☐ Hearing Aid
☐ Dentures (Specify ___)

OTHER EQUIPMENT

ADDITIONAL PERTINENT INFORMATION
(Explain necessary details of care, diagnosis, medications, treatments, prognosis, teaching, habits, preferences, etc. Therapists and social workers add signature and title to notes.)

SOCIAL INFORMATION
(Adjustment to disability, emotional support from family, motivation for self-care, socializing ability, financial plan, family health problem, etc.)

PERSON COMPLETING THIS FORM: Signature/Title ___ Date ___/___/___
RESIDENT TRANSFER FORM

FIGURE 3. RESIDENT TRANSFER FORM (back of Fig. 2)

cian, or other facility. The transfer or referral form should state the reason for admission, the diagnosis, current medical information, and the rehabilitative potential. The physician should also certify the level of care required and for what time period such care is anticipated.

Additional items that this statement should contain are:

— Identification data from the summary sheet of the record

—Name of transferring institution

—Name of receiving institution

—Date of transfer

—Hospital diagnoses/hospital number if transferred from a hospital

—Nurse's report including patient attitudes, behavior, interests, functional abilities (activities of daily living), unusual treatments, nursing care problems, nutrition, current medications and when last given, condition on transfer, and chest x-ray data and findings.

—Physicians' report including the reason for admission, order of medications, treatment, diet and activities, significant laboratory and x-ray findings, diagnoses, prognosis, and a brief summary of treatment.

Automatic transfer of information from a hospital to a nursing facility is often achieved by a transfer agreement signed by both the hospital and the nursing facility. Once in effect, the referring institution sends pertinent clinical information directly to the facility receiving the resident. The transfer or referral form, copies of the hospital discharge summary, history and physical examination, and other relevant reports accompany the resident to the nursing facility.

Residents may also be transferred from the nursing facility to other health facilities for other levels of care. Depending on the type of care required, residents may be transferred to an acute care hospital, another long term care facility, an ambulatory care center, or to a home care agency. The type of facility receiving the resident will determine the amount and type of information required. A copy of the transfer form is retained in the facility's record for the resident; the original accompanies the resident.

Admitting Evaluation or Assessment

An admitting evaluation or assessment is performed on every patient upon admission to the nursing facility. The attending physician examines the resident and records an admission history and physical examination in the clinical record. Nursing service, dietary, activities, and social service visit the resident, make their assessments and enter their initial evaluation of the resident's condition. If therapy orders are received on admission, the appropriate therapists will also begin evaluating the resident's needs.

Included in the attending physician's admitting evaluation are the medical and social history, physical examination, and treatment plan. The physician should date and sign the entire report. Some items that have an orientation specific to nursing facility care are discussed here.

Reason for Admission - A concise statement of those conditions or circumstances which resulted in the resident's placement in the nursing facility. It will become the basis for the development of further statements which determine the level of care needed.

Social History - A description of the social environment of the resident, including where the resident lives, his friends, his occupation, and his family relationships and dependence on those relationships. This segment of the record is typically compiled by social service staff and is often the basis for the discharge plan.

History and Physical Examination - To be performed and recorded by the physician within 48 hours after admission or as required by state regulations. A hospital or private physician examination completed within five days prior to admission may be used if signed and dated notations of changes in the resident's condition as entered in the record by the attending physician.

According to facility policy and certain standards, an annual physical examination by the physician may be completed. This annual examination should include all items listed in the original examination, including significant changes in the resident's condition and any change in treatment plan. A tickler file can be maintained to help ensure the timely scheduling of annual physical exams. This file is organized by date to remind personnel of examinations or treatment updates which are due. It is useful to correlate this tickler file with that maintained by the nursing service which usually schedules the examinations.

Comprehensive Care Plan

An interdisciplinary care plan emphasizes the interrelationship of each aspect of resident care. The care plan is initiated when a resident is admitted to the facility, and it is the working tool that provides a comprehensive care plan with input from each discipline involved in the care. It flows from the Minimum Data Set (MDS) assessment, and Resident Assessment Protocol Summary (RAPS), as well as the physician's care plan. Each health care professional also contributes his or her unique skills toward fostering resident progress.

The plan of care includes an assessment, statement of goals, identification of specific activities or strategies to achieve the goals, periodic assessment of goal attainment, and periodic updates. It also includes input from the resident and/or the resident's sponsor or surrogate. It is reviewed and revised as often as regulatory agencies dictate, as the goals are reached, or as the resident's status changes.

Many forms are on the market for care plans and computerized versions are available.

Changes in the care plan may be easily summarized at the time of resident discharge to provide a substantial portion of the discharge summary, showing either attainment of the goals established at admission, or changes in resident status which required modification of those goals. The plan of care provides a basis for later evaluation of the quality of care and the general pattern of care given in the institution.

Discharge Plan

A discharge plan is begun at the time of admission giving a general assessment of expectations for discharge, e.g., return to family care after a period of convalescence. The discharge plan focuses on after-care for the resident or on the needs of the resident which must be met to advance to a more independent lifestyle. Frequently this assessment and detailed planning are done through contract with a community agency such as a home health agency or similar social service group. Items to be included on the discharge plan include the living arrangements of the resident after discharge, the services required to keep the resident in the community, and the agency used in the discharge planning process.

Orders

At the time each resident is admitted, the facility must have physician orders for the resident's immediate care. At a minimum, this includes dietary, drugs if needed, and routine care to maintain or improve the resident's functional abilities. All orders must be signed and dated.

Because physicians do not visit residents in a nursing facility frequently, telephone orders are common. State licensure regulations should be reviewed for the specifics concerning who may record a telephone order and the time frame within which such an order must be signed.

With all verbal orders, the entry should be immediately recorded in the clinical record by the person who received the order. This individual should provide the date and time of the order and sign the entry. The professional designation of the receiver should be indicated, e.g., RN, RPT, etc.

Automatic stop orders for restricted medications are a routine procedure and should be delineated in the facility's policy manual. Under an automatic stop system, medications such as narcotics, sedatives, stimulants, antibiotics, tranquilizers, and anticoagulants are discontinued after a time specified by the facility, unless ordered specifically for a longer time. When the stop order goes into effect, the staff should notify the physician that the drugs are being discontinued. No prescription can be refilled or ordered without an order from the attending physician.

Specialized rehabilitative services such as physical therapy, occupational therapy, and speech therapy are provided only after a physician's order is received.

At the time of temporary or permanent discharge from the facility, a specific order must be written and signed prior to the discharge, leave, or transfer of the resident.

Drug Regimen Review

The drug regimen of each resident must be reviewed at least once a month by a licensed pharmacist. The findings of this review are documented in the record and reported to the attending physician and the director of nursing, and these reports must be acted upon.

Progress Notes

Progress notes consist of statements about each resident's progress as noted by various professional staff members. They give a chronological report of the resident's situation and include statements about reactions to treatment, general attitudes affecting treatment, and notations of any change in condition. They may be written by the physician, nurse, physician assistant, or any health professional providing care to the resident. All progress notes should be dated and signed. The provider of care, in signing the note, should also indicate his professional specialty.

Progress notes should be written by the physician any time the resident is seen.

Nurses' notes must be documented throughout the course of treatment. (The time frame for these entries will be dependent upon the requirements established by the facility's regulatory agency). These notes address the general condition of the resident. Items typically addressed include vital signs, skin conditions, mental status, appetite, ability to perform activities of daily living, and other specific signs and symptoms potentially requiring treatment. Nurses' notes should also be written when any non-routine event occurs, such as an incident. All notes are dated and signed with the nurse's name and professional designation.

All medicines and treatments given should be recorded on the resident's record. These are often recorded on a separate medication administration form. Drug reactions, any apparent change in the condition of the resident, any accident, and the date and time of these occurrences should be noted and signed. Drugs to be administered "as needed" (PRN medications) should be charted as to time and date given, the reason for administration, and the result. After a drug has been discontinued or the resident has been discharged, the remaining portion of the drug should be accounted for in the clinical record. A notation should be made in the nurses' progress notes that the medication has been destroyed, given to the resident if authorized in physician's orders, or returned to the pharmacy. If the medication has been destroyed, the means of destruction should be noted along with the nurse's signature and the signature of another nurse as a witness. Both entries should be dated. If the medication was given to the resident, instructions should be given to the patient in layman's terms. Entries should state that the medications went with the patient, the name of the medications, and a statement that instructions were provided to the resident regarding the usage of the medications. The nurses notes and transfer forms are the two places where this information is most commonly found. Such inclusions provide clarity of information and protect the resident as well as the facility.

Special forms may be used for recording vital signs (temperature, pulse, and respiration), blood pressure readings, intake and output, weight and height, medication and treatments, activities of daily living, and use of I.V.'s or other special services.

Social Service Reports

The psychosocial aspect of resident care is assessed through regular interaction by the social service staff. Social service assessment begins in some instances before admission through a preadmission assessment to determine proper placement of the resident. If the preadmission assessment leads to formal admission to the facility, these preadmission notes become part of the clinical record. For those applicants who are processed through the preadmission stage but are not admitted, the preadmission documentation is maintained for the length of time any business record is kept. The reason for nonadmission to a facility should be clearly stated in such preadmission assessments.

The social service staff participates in the development of the interdisciplinary care plan for each resident, makes periodic updates, records any contacts with the resident or family, and summarizes such findings as required by the resident's condition.

During discharge planning, the social service staff may coordinate community services and/or alternate placement of the resident. Such activities are documented in the discharge plan.

Special Reports

Laboratory, radiographic, and other diagnostic services are provided to residents upon written order of the physician. Reports of tests done during the resident's stay should be dated, signed, and filed in the record. The physician should be notified of test results as they are received. Such services are often provided through contacts with outside providers. Per federal regulations, reports from outside labs must include the name and address of the issuing laboratory.

Diagnoses

Admitting diagnoses should be recorded in the resident's clinical record at the time of admission, usually on the identification and summary sheet. Any diagnosis made during the stay in the facility should be added to the record and dated by the physician. If space is provided on the identification and summary sheet, subsequent diagnoses may be recorded here, or a separate diagnosis list may be maintained. Final diagnoses should be entered in the clinical record by the attending physician at the time of discharge, death, or transfer.

Discharge Summary

When a facility anticipates discharging a resident, a resident must have a discharge summary that includes a recapitulation of the resident's stay, a final summary of the resident's status to include the items required by federal regulations (found in paragraph (b) (2) of 483.20). The summary must be available at the time of the discharge for release to authorized persons and agencies with the consent of the resident or legal representative. The summary must include a postdischarge plan of care that is developed with the participation of the resident and his or her family, which will assist the resident to adjust to his or her new living environment.

A discharge summary is also necessary in each clinical record regardless of whether the discharge was anticipated. Facilities may use the same format as the discharge summary for anticipated discharges or may have a second one for all others.

Miscellaneous Reports

Forms containing information of an administrative nature are often filed at the end of the record or may be in an administrative file. The following items must be kept in the clinical record:

- The admission agreement between the facility and the resident or his responsible agent. In some states it may be necessary to have a consent to care form signed by the resident before certain treatments can be implemented. This is a legal protection for the facility.

- A property and valuables list should enumerate articles retained by the resident in the room and those held for safekeeping by administration. Such items as eyeglasses, dentures, and prostheses should be noted.

- Releases - Release from responsibility for leave of absence should be signed by the resident or the person legally responsible for him. This protects the facility in case of accident and helps to prevent possible false claims. Release from responsibility for discharge should be signed when the resident wishes to leave against medical advice. Consent for autopsy as well as release of the body to the mortician should be signed by the nearest of kin. These consents legally protect the facility. A written authorization for the release of information should be signed by the patient or his legal representative before the facility gives information to an insurance company, attorney, or anyone asking for data about the resident. This written authorization should be filed with the record with an indication of material released under its provisions.

- In case of death, a copy of the death certificate may be kept as part of the clinical record if it is available. When an autopsy is performed, a copy of this report should become a part of the record.

- Resident's rights acknowledgment enumerates the resident's rights during his stay. A resident must be informed of his rights prior to or at the time of admission and periodically thereafter, and there should be written evidence of this. A printed form containing the rights may be signed by the resident and placed in the record as proof of his being informed of these rights. If there are any changes in these rights, an updated copy should be signed and dated by the resident and added to the clinical record.

Accident/Incident Reports

Unusual incidents or occurrences involving residents, employees, or visitors should be recorded on an incident report form. Complete information on findings and treatment should be recorded. Anything out of the ordinary, such as a fall from bed, administration of a wrong drug, or an accident involving a visitor should be reported on special accident or incident report forms (Figure 4).

Such reports are used for administrative purposes only and should not be filed in the clinical record. They are most often

INCIDENT AND ACCIDENT REPORT

"An Incident is any happening which is not consistent with the routine operation of the hospital or the routine care of a particular patient. It may be an accident or a situation which might result in an accident."

Person Involved (Last Name, First Name, Middle Initial) | MALE ☐ FEMALE ☐ | Nursing Unit ______ | Name of First Person to See Incident or Accident

Date of Incident | Time of Incident A.M. P.M. | Exact Location of Incident: Patient's Room ☐ Corridor ☐ Bathroom ☐ Dining Room ☐ Other (Specify)

PATIENT ☐ | Patient's Condition Before Incident: Ambulatory ☐ Assistive Device ☐ Wheelchair ☐ Safety Belt: Yes ☐ No ☐ Bedfast ☐ Alert ☐ Confused ☐ Disoriented ☐ Sedated ☐ Agitated ☐ Other (Specify)

Were Bed Rails Present YES ☐ NO ☐ UP ☐ DOWN ☐ | Was Height of Bed Adjustable YES ☐ NO ☐ UP ☐ DOWN ☐

EMPLOYEE ☐ | Department | Job Title

Remained on Duty: YES ☐ NO ☐ | Assigned Shift: FIRST ☐ SECOND ☐ THIRD ☐

VISITOR ☐ | Home Address | Home Phone

OTHER (Specify) ☐ | Occupation | Reason for Presence at This Facility

Property Involved ☐ Equipment Involved ☐ Describe: | Repairs Requested YES ☐ NO ☐ | Was person authorized to be at location of incident: YES ☐ NO ☐

Describe Exactly What Happened: Why it Happened: What Causes Were. If any Injury, State Part of Body Injured. If Property or Equipment Damaged, Describe Damage.

Was Person Involved Seen by a Physician YES ☐ NO ☐	When	Where	Physician's Name
Was First Aid Administered and/or Examination Given: YES ☐ NO ☐	When	Place Administered	By Whom
Was Person Involved Taken to Hospital YES ☐ NO ☐	When	Where Taken	By Whom

Indicate on Diagram Location of Injury

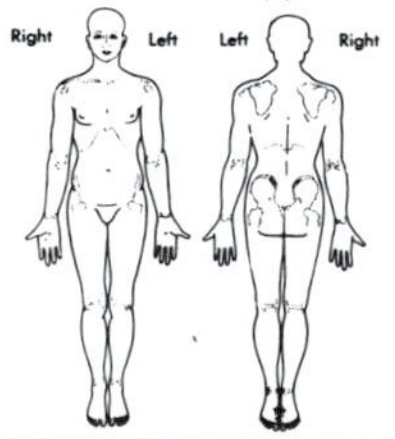

TYPE OF INJURY

1. Laceration ☐
2. Hematoma ☐
3. Abrasion ☐
4. Contusion ☐
5. Strain ☐
6. Puncture ☐
7. Scratch ☐
8. Illness ☐
9. Other (Specify) ☐
10. None Apparent ☐

PHYSICIAN STATEMENT, TREATMENT, RECOMMENDATIONS:

PHYSICIAN SIGNATURE DATE

Name, Address & Phone No. of Witness(es)

Corrective Action:

Date of Report | Signature and Title of Person Preparing Report | Department Head Signature | Administrative Signature

Prepare in Duplicate (No Carbon Paper Necessary)

FIGURE 4. INCIDENT REPORT

kept in a separate file in the chief executive officer's office. Although the report is not filed in the resident's clinical record, the information contained on it should correlate with the information recorded on the nurses' note, the physician's progress note (if any), or any other practitioner's entry.

A facility must immediately inform the resident, consult with the resident's physician, and if known, notify the resident's legal representative or an interested family member when there is an accident involving the resident which results in injury and has the potential for requiring physician intervention.

ARRANGEMENT OF THE MEDICAL RECORD

The arrangement of the record should meet the needs of the nursing facility Most facilities arrange records in reverse chronological order while the resident remains in the facility. When records are thinned or residents discharged, the record is rearranged into straight chronological sequence.

While the resident is in the facility, the record should be arranged for the convenience of the physicians, nurses, and other health care personnel. The sequence of documents should be spelled out so consistency of practice is maintained. If the order of the record during the resident's stay is different from the final arrangement for permanent filing, the sequence may be rearranged at the time of final review. If the record retention schedule indicates record destruction after an approved time limit when there is no activity associated with the records of discharged residents, it may be useful to arrange the record at discharge in the order that permits easy retrieval of information to be kept permanently, followed by all material which will be destroyed. This eliminates a detailed purging of the chart at the time of record destruction. Figure 5 and 6 are examples of a sequence of both open and closed records.

CLINICAL RECORD PROCESSING AND DATA COLLECTION

Review of Clinical Record Content

Procedures for the quantitative review of records while residents are in the facility should be developed by the health information practitioner. This consists of checking that the required reports and signatures have been included in each record according to the prescribed time frames. Because the length of stay for nursing facility residents often extends to

SAMPLE ORDER FOR INHOUSE (OPEN)CLINICAL RECORDS*

TAB	CONTENT
ADMISSION RECORD	ADMISSION/DISCHARGE RECORD
	ADMISSION AGREEMENT/RE-AGREEMENT
	AUTHORIZATION
	TRANSFER FORMS
	MISCELLANEOUS COPIES OF RECORDS FROM TRANSFERRING FACILITY
	MDS/COMPREHENSIVE ASSESSMENT
	TRIGGER LEGEND
	RAP SUMMARY
	QUARTERLY REVIEWS
HISTORY & PHYSICAL	HISTORY AND PHYSICAL
PHYSICIAN ORDERS	MONTHLY ORDERS
	TELEPHONE ORDERS
	STANDING ORDERS
	WEIGHT RECORD
PROGRESS NOTES	PHYSICIAN'S PROGRESS NOTES
NURSES' NOTES	NURSES' NOTES
	NURSES' ADMISSION ASSESSMENTS
MEDICATION & TREATMENT	MEDICATION RECORDS
	TREATMENT RECORDS
	FLOW SHEET
	SKIN GRIDS
	BLADDER/BOWEL TRAINING SCHEDULE
	TOILETING SCHEDULE
	TURN SCHEDULE
	BEHAVIOR GRID
LAB & SPECIAL REPORTS	LAB REPORTS
	X-RAY REPORTS
	EKG REPORTS
	DENTAL EXAM SHEETS
REHAB & THERAPY	PHYSICAL THERAPY PROGRESS NOTES
	PHYSICAL THERAPY MONTHLY MODALITY SHEET
	PHYSICAL THERAPY ASSESSMENT
	OCCUPATIONAL THERAPY PROGRESS NOTE
	OCCUPATIONAL THERAPY MODALITY SHEET
	OCCUPATIONAL THERAPY ASSESSMENT
	SPEECH THERAPY PROGRESS NOTE
	SPEECH THERAPY MODALITY SHEETS
	SPEECH THERAPY ASSESSMENT
SOCIAL SERVICE	SOCIAL SERVICE PROGRESS NOTES
	SOCIAL HISTORY AND EVALUATION
ACTIVITIES	ACTIVITY PROGRESS NOTES
	ACTIVITY ASSESSMENT
DIETARY	DIETARY PROGRESS NOTES
	DIETARY NUTRITIONAL ASSESSMENT
MISCELLANEOUS	PERSONAL INVENTORY SHEET
	COPY OF GUARDIANSHIP OR POA PAPER

* ALL INFORMATION IN THE INHOUSE RECORDS SHALL BE MAINTAINED IN REVERSE CHRONOLOGICAL ORDER WITH THE MOST RECENT BEING FIRST.

FIGURE 5. SAMPLE ORDER FOR INHOUSE (OPEN) CLINICAL RECORD

SAMPLE ORDER FOR CLINICAL RECORDS
OF DISCHARGED RESIDENTS

* ADMISSION RECORD
* ADMISSION AGREEMENT
* ACKNOWLEDGMENT OF RECEIPT OF RESIDENT RIGHTS
* AUTHORIZATIONS
* CERTIFICATION/RECERTIFICATION (MEDICARE)
* TRANSFER FORM
* COPIES OF RECORDS FROM TRANSFERRING FACILITIES
* HISTORY AND PHYSICAL EXAMINATION
* CONSULTATION REPORTS
* PHYSICIAN ORDERS
    STANDING
    MONTHLY
    TELEPHONE
* PHYSICIAN PROGRESS NOTES
* DISCHARGE SUMMARY
* REHABILITATIVE INFORMATION
    PT EVALUATION/NOTES
    OT EVALUATION/NOTES
    SPEECH EVALUATION/NOTES
* SOCIAL HISTORY/ASSESSMENT/NOTES
* DISCHARGE PLAN
* ACTIVITY ASSESSMENT/NOTES
* NUTRITIONAL ASSESSMENT/NOTES
* TRIGGER LEGEND SHEET
* RAP SUMMARY
* QUARTERLY REVIEWS
* COMPREHENSIVE ASSESSMENT/MDS
* NURSING ASSESSMENT WEIGHT RECORD
* NURSING NOTES/MONTHLY SUMMARIES
* MEDICATION RECORDS
* TREATMENT RECORDS
* RESIDENT CARE FLOW SHEET
* DECUBITUS RECORD
* INTAKE AND OUTPUT RECORD
* RESIDENT CARE PLAN (NURSING, ACTIVITIES, DIETARY, AND
    SOCIAL SERVICE)
* INDIVIDUAL HABILITATION PLAN
* PERSONAL INVENTORY EFFECTS SHEET
* MISCELLANEOUS

* THESE ITEMS SHOULD BE FOUND IN EVERY RECORD.
SPECIAL NOTE: INFORMATION IN THE DISCHARGED RECORD SHOULD
BE MAINTAINED IN CHRONOLOGICAL ORDER.

FIGURE 6. SAMPLE ORDER FOR CLINICAL RECORDS OF DISCHARGED RESIDENTS

years, the system for review of records should focus on each stage of care so timely documentation is fostered. Time frames for such review are as follows; admission period, monthly review, quarterly review, annual review, special analysis at time of temporary transfer and return, and discharge review. Figures 7 and 8 are forms which reflect this continuous chart analysis.

If information or a signature is missing, reminders should be given to the staff member who is responsible for entering the documentation or signing the information in the record. Members of the clinical staff are responsible for review of records for quality of care. Professional record personnel can assist the physicians in this qualitative review by summarizing periodically the patterns of chart deficiencies and by making available summaries of the documentation requirements of various legal and accrediting agencies.

Data Collection

The resident's physician and the staff of the nursing facility record information needed for care and information required by standard-setting and licensing agencies. Clinical record personnel should routinely abstract data from medical records of discharged and deceased residents and, as needed, from the inpatient records.

The following statistics have been found useful for meeting the needs of the nursing facility management: inpatient census, percentage of occupancy, length of stay, and death rate. The length of stay may be further refined in order to reflect those relatively short stays (a few months) as compared to the more typical length of stay which involves years. Where there is a pattern of transfer to and from acute care facilities for medical episodes, these patient movements may also be part of the statistical profile needed by management.

Statistics should be gathered in a uniform way using standard definitions. A minimum data set for use in long term care facilities is mandated for all certified facilities. The federal requirements which address this document are found under CFR 483.20. A nursing facility should use standard definitions where they exist or agree in advance on definitions to use within the facility to foster consistency and comparability. Data collection should be reviewed from time to time to ensure data needs are met. Definitions for terminology used in many health care facilities are also found in the *Glossary of Health Care Terms* published by the American Health Informtion Manage-

Inhouse Audit / Analysis Sheet

KEY CODE:

I = Incomplete   C = Complete   M = Missing   N = Non-Applicable   S = Signature Needed

Resident Last Name	First Name		Init.		Station	Room	Bed		Physician	
Item				**Dates of Audit**						
1 H&P										
2 TB Test										
3 Rehab Potential										
4 Recertification										
5 Physician Orders										
6 Telephone Orders										
7 Standing Orders										
8 Physician Visits										
9 Physician Progress Notes										
10 Nurses Assessments										
11 Nurses Notes										
12 Nurses Monthly Summary										
13 Monthly Weights										
14 Intake/Output										
15 Lab/X-ray Reports (per orders)										
16 PT/OT/Speech Reports (")										
17 Social History										
18 Social Assessment										
19 Discharge Plan										
20 Social Service P.N.'s										
21 Activity Assessment										
22 Activity Progress Notes										
23 Nutritional Assessment										
24 Nutritional Progress Notes										
25 Resident Care Plan										
26 Nursing										
27 Dietary										
28 Activity										
29 Social Service										
30 PT/OT/Speech										
31 Personal Inventory Sheet										
32 MDS/RAP Summary										

FIGURE 7. INHOUSE AUDIT / ANALYSIS SHEET

ment Association. This text also provides additional discussion of basic statistics and manner of compilation.

All events such as admissions, discharges, temporary hospital transfers, temporary leaves, including absences against medical advice, and deaths should be reported on the daily census report. Statistics on resident movements should be detailed for each care unit of the facility. Each day the resident

DISCHARGE CHART ANALYSIS	
C = Completed M = Missing S = Signature Needed N = Not Applicable I = Incomplete	
ADMISSION RECORD	
ADMISSION AGREEMENT	
ACKNOWLEDGMENT OF RECEIPT OF RESIDENT RIGHTS	
AUTHORIZATIONS/CONSENTS	
TRANSFER FORMS	
HISTORY AND PHYSICAL/T.B. TEST	
LAB, X-RAY AND EKG REPORTS	
STANDING ORDERS	
PHYSICIAN ORDERS	
TELEPHONE ORDERS	
PROGRESS NOTES	
DISCHARGE SUMMARY	
NURSING ADMISSION ASSESSMENT/MDS/TRIGGER LEGEND/RAP SUMMARY	
SKIN ASSESSMENT SHEETS	
NURSING NOTES	
DISCHARGE NURSING NOTE	
MONTHLY SUMMARIES	
MEDICATION RECORDS/TREATMENT SHEETS	
INTAKE-OUTPUT RECORDS	
MONTHLY VITALS/WEIGHTS	
SOCIAL HISTORY/ASSESSMENT/PROGRESS NOTES	
DISCHARGE PLANNING	
ACTIVITY ASSESSMENT/PROGRESS NOTES	
NUTRITIONAL ASSESSMENT/PROGRESS NOTES	
PHYSICAL THERAPY EVALUATION/PROGRESS NOTES	
SPEECH THERAPY EVALUATION/PROGRESS NOTES	
OCCUPATIONAL THERAPY EVALUATION/PROGRESS NOTES	
RESIDENT CARE FLOW SHEETS	
CARE PLAN/IHPs	
PERSONAL INVENTORY SHEET	
MISCELLANEOUS	

Reisdent Name: _____

Admitted: _____   Discharged: _____

FIGURE 8. DISCHARGE CHART ANAYLSIS

is on a leave for temporary hospital transfer, his name must appear on the report. This daily census report should also include the number of residents present each day. A monthly tabulation of these figures is compiled providing a basis for further statistical computations.

Quality Assessment and Assurance

A facility must maintain a quality assessment and assurance committee consisting of the director of nursing service, a physician designated by the facility, and at least three other members of the facility's staff. The committee must meet at least quarterly to identify issues with respect to which quality assessment and assurance activities are necessary and develop and implement appropriate plans of action to correct identified quality deficiencies.

Each discipline, department, or service providing care should be involved in identification of important aspects of care including high-risk, high-volume, and/or problem-prone clinical activities. Providers should also identify clinical indicators related to the quality and appropriateness of care for the important aspects and define the levels of performance related to each clinical indicator that represents the threshold at which a more intensive evaluation of the quality and appropriateness of care is initiated.

Utilization Review

Utilization review is the function of ensuring that resources are effectively and efficiently utilized. The appropriateness of the use of a nursing facility does not depend on the resident's potential for recovery or an improved outcome in the same manner as it does in an acute care hospital. Rather, utilization is considered to be medically appropriate if the resident requires daily nursing services to maintain present medical status or prevent deterioration of the medical condition. The process of utilization review is thus one that focuses on continuing stay review at regular intervals, as defined by regulatory and accrediting agencies.

HOME CARE

"Home care" describes services (medical and nonmedical) provided to patients and their families in their home or place of residence.

Home care is an integral component of the health care delivery system in the United States. Because of cost containment measures, the increasing elderly population, consumerism, and improved health care technology, the number of home care providers is rapidly increasing. In response to the Medicare prospective payment system, many hospitals are now vertically integrating by offering home care services to their patients. Hospital patients are being discharged faster. In response, home care services are becoming more clinical, such as I.V. infusion therapy.

LEGAL, REGULATORY, AND ACCREDITING STANDARDS

Medical record documentation in Medicare certified home health providers is now virtually dictated by the Medicare *Conditions of Participation for Home Health Agencies*. The *Conditions* require that home care agencies have record documentation policies that result in efficient completion of standard Health Care Financing Administration (HCFA) forms. These forms include:

- Home Health Certification and Plan of Treatment
- Plan of Treatment/Medical Update and Patient Information Addendum
- Home Health Agency Intermediary Medical Information Report

The National League for Nursing has an accreditation program for home care providers called the Community Health Accreditation Program (CHAP). Primarily voluntary nonprofit and government agencies participate in this program. The League's standards require that service records be maintained for each patient, and they outline what each record should contain. The League has an Administrator's Handbook for Community Health and Home Care Services which contains some home care record forms and some record management guidance.

The National Homecaring Council represents and accredits agencies providing homemaker/home health aide services. Its standards contain some record keeping guidance for these home care providers.

The Joint Commission on Accreditation of Healthcare Organizations has a specific set of standards for home care providers. It includes requirements for medical record documentation, and specifies that a patient's completed home care record must become part of the patient's hospital unit medical record.

The health information professional should also refer to Public Health Service guidelines and to any applicable state regulations. It must be emphasized that state regulation may be the only mandatory requirements that home care providers must meet if they are not accredited or Medicare certified.

In addition, many providers are not certified and may not even have regulations governing them or reimbursement from the federal government. Nevertheless, they exist to provide personal care and clinical services to patients and families in their homes.

PROVIDERS OF CARE

There are currently about 7,000 Medicare certified home health organizations, but it has been estimated by the National Association for Home Care that there are over 17,000 home care providers who may offer one or more home care services. These other providers may be non-certified home health agencies, home care staffing companies, or home care equipment companies. Equipment companies often furnish durable medical equipment directly to patients and are, therefore, often responsible for patient education regarding the equipment's use. A home care staffing company may furnish selected services such as the services of home health aides, companions, or homemakers. These companies may provide some services at a patient's request or may provide services in conjunction with a home health agency and/or in response to doctors' orders.

Home health agencies provide a broader range of services; and to be Medicare certified, a home health agency must provide skilled nursing care and at least one of the following therapeutic services - physical, speech, or occupational therapy; medical social services; or home health aide services. HCFA defines five major Medicare provider home health agency categories: (1) hospital or provider-based, (2) proprietary, (3) private nonprofit, (4) government (state or local health and welfare departments), and (5) voluntary nonprofit (visiting nurse associations).

THE HOME CARE MEDICAL RECORD

The smooth flow of information about a patient, often referred to as a "client" of home care, is particularly important to home care because the providers of care perform their services in the patient's home and are physically removed from other health care providers. Information from all providers regarding their visits must be efficiently incorporated in the patient's medical record.

Medicare certified agencies must submit the HCFA standard forms to their fiscal intermediary. Regardless of an agency's certification status, general documentation guidelines should be followed.

In 1986, the Foundation of Record Educatiojn of the American Medical Record Association completed a W. K. Kellogg Foundation-funded home care project. Through its advisory committee, forms and guidelines for documentation were developed. The following section describes these guidelines.

Initial Database

An initial database should include admission/referral/general information, initial clinical information, transfer information from transferring facility, initial nursing assessment, relevant reports of diagnostic and therapeutic procedures, and a problem list. The physician having primary responsibility for the patient's care must be designated. The composition of the patient's household and the name of a person who will assume responsibility for care if required must be included, as well as the suitability or adaptability of the patient's residence for the provision of the required health care services.

Plan of Treatment

All care provided must be based on a written plan of treatment. The plan must be established by the attending physician in conjunction with agency staff, and it must be reviewed by agency personnel and the attending physician at least once every 60 days and as often as the severity of the patient's condition requires. The physician's signature is required on all initial and on all subsequent plans of treatment.

The plan of treatment must document all pertinent diagnoses, including mental status, types of services and equipment required, frequency and duration of visits, prognosis, rehabilitation potential, functional limitations, activities permitted, nutritional requirements, medications and treatments, any safety measures to protect against injury, instructions for timely discharge or referral, and any other appropriate items.

Ongoing Documentation

Procedures and documentation must assure that the medical record at all times reflects an accurate, current picture of the patient's status and the services being provided. For each home visit there should be clinical progress notes. Adequate documentation of home health aide services, dietary/nutritional information, and other services such as those of therapists or social workers must be included. All drugs and treatments administered must be ordered in writing by a physician. In particular, "do not resuscitate" orders, when discussed with the patient and next of kin, must be documented. "Routine care only" orders are not adequate. Medications administered by the agency staff must be documented and any beneficial and adverse drug effects delineated.

Patient Summaries

At least every 61 days a patient summary must be documented and forwarded to the patient's attending physician and to the referral source. This is a part of the review of the treatment plan. Upon a patient's discharge, a summary must be documented which includes the agency admission and discharge dates, discharge reason and status, and a synopsis of care provided. When a patient is discharged by a specific service of the agency prior to agency discharge, a summary should be written and either incorporated into or filed with the final discharge summary.

Consent for Care

An informed consent for care must be signed by the patient and filed in the medical record. Often a copy is provided the patient as well.

Service Agreement

Patients should also sign a service agreement which outlines the services to be provided, the times services will be provided, the charges, and the parties responsible for payment.

Record in the Home

Many agencies maintain some written information in the patient's home. This often includes the agency name and telephone number, staff names and visit schedule, emergency plans, patient/family instructions, and a listing of a patient's medications with potential side effects and instructions recorded. When this is done a form or progress note reflecting the care should be included in the agency's medical record.

HOME CARE RECORD PROCESSING AND DATA COLLECTION

Review of Medical Record Content

Home care records should be reviewed throughout a patient's care episode, not just at discharge from home care. Some items that should be monitored are (1) the presence of initial assessments and care plans, (2) the prompt return of care plans and orders sent to the attending physician for signature and review, (3) the documentation of care plan reviews at, as a minimum, 60-day intervals, and (4) the documentation of all visits. If visits are not documented or not documented properly (i.e., do not reflect skilled nursing care), agencies may lose Medicare reimbursement. Many agencies, therefore, monitor visit documentation very closely.

To assure that established policies are followed in providing services, check the latest state and federal regulations as well as standards from the Joint Commission and other accrediting organizations.

Collection of Home Care Data

To assure availability of standard data for program evaluation, quality management activities, research, and administrative functions, each individual home care program must document standard, uniform data for each of its patients.

Uniform data must also be recorded if meaningful comparisons are to be made between home care providers and if data are to be available for health care planning. Medicare-certified providers document the standard data required by Medicare.

The Joint Commission's 1993 standards address various levels of home care. For any home care patient, JCAHO requires that home care providers document at least the following data:

- identification data
- name and phone number of family member or significant other

- description of any safety measures needed to protect the patient
- notes on the adaptability of the home for home care
- notes for each service provided, including the data, staff person, and care provided
- identity of other individuals and organizations known to be involved in the patient's care
- any instructions given to the patient on discharge by the home care organization, and
- transfer forms, summaries or copies of records from transferring organization

For patients receiving home health, clinical respiratory, or personal care and support services, Joint Commission requires the following to also be documented in addition to the above requirements for any patient.

- a description of any functional limitations, activity restrictions, and
- a statement of any change in the patient's condition

For patients receiving home health or clinical respiratory services, JCAHO requires the following documentation in addition to the above requirements:

- name of the patient's physician
- principal and secondary diagnoses on admission
- any surgical procedures relating to the admission
- patient history as it relates to home health services
- current medication profile
- information on any allergies or diet restrictions
- initial and ongoing assessments
- signed and dated progress notes describing physical and psychosocial signs and symptoms, treatment provided, and response to treatment
- test results and procedure findings
- orders authenticated by the patient's physician, and
- any advance directives for care or any such discussions with patients

When patients are discharged from home health or home clinical respiratory service, JCAHO requires a discharge summary to be added to the record. It should include the following:

- date of discharge

- reason for discharge, including names of any organizations to which the patient is transferred
- overall status as well as the status of problems identified through the course of care, and
- a summary of the care provided

Diagnostic classification systems used by a home care provider should meet the needs of the provider as well as the requirements of its reimbursement source(s). The use and documentation of nursing diagnoses varies by home health agency. (See Chapter 9.) ICD-9-CM coding may also be performed. Whatever system is used, coding should be complete and performed according to the particular system's coding instructions. Coding must reflect the requirements of the reimbursement source and must include indexing of assigned codes so data and medical records are easily retrievable for quality assurance studies, research, and so forth.

For Medicare reimbursement purposes, a visit is defined as each time a health worker furnishes home health services to the beneficiary. Therefore, if two different care givers see a patient on the same day it would be two visits; but if a nurse provides several services during the same visit, charges may be submitted for only one visit.

Quality Management

Quality Management in home care presently focuses largely on program evaluation rather than on the quality assessment of patient care. Both types of evaluations are important and should be reflected in a home care program's quality assurance plan.

The Joint Commission requires the monitoring and evaluation of the quality and appropriateness of patient care services as well as the resolution of any identified problems. Objective criteria, developed by a home care program's staff, must be used to perform the required monitoring and evaluation. This should include ongoing identification of important aspects of care that focus on high-risk, high-volume, and/or problem-prone activities. Measurable indicators of the quality and appropriateness of each important aspect of care, which specify activities, events, occurrences, and/or outcomes should be defined. One indicator should be patient satisfaction. The identification of the level of performance related to each indicator should also be specified. Level of performance represents the extent to which care is effective, adequate in quantity, and provided in the setting best suited to the patient's needs and represents the threshold at which further evaluation of the quality and appropriateness of care is initiated.

Medicare requires an annual review of a home health agency's total program but does not require an evaluation of patient care. The National League for Nursing has standards for evaluation which address program evaluation, the quality of care delivered by each discipline, and utilization review.

Utilization Review

Initially felt to be a supportive service provided primarily for Medicare recipients, providing care in the home has been extended to pediatric, obstetric, respiratory, and other medical and surgical specialties, with private insurance now viewing the practice as cost-effective. There are two key issues in reviewing the utilization of home health, the first is the appropriateness and medical necessity for the level of care provided, and the second is the appropriateness of the care giver utilized.

Assessing the appropriateness and medical necessity for home health is a complex issue as services have been extended to "high-tech" areas such as chemotherapy and even ventilator care. It is necessary to determine that the patient's primary medical condition lends itself to the types of therapies that can be provided, that there are no secondary conditions which would be compromised by not being in an acute or nursing care environment, that the patient has support persons available to assist when necessary and monitor response when home health personnel are not available, that the living environment is conducive to supporting home health services without causing complications, and that the service provided is staffed and managed in a manner immediately responsive to the patient's medical condition, therapies, supplies, and support services.

The appropriate level-of-care giver should be assessed on a regular basis. Usually available are the companion/homemaker, home health aide, and nurse. Various ancillary clinical therapists also assist in the care process. Cost over-utilization can occur when a caregiver is used beyond the level of medical necessity, such as a registered nurse who is used to bathe and turn a patient. Under-utilization occurs when the caregiver is not trained to provide the level of care that is demanded, such as a licensed practical nurse administering chemotherapy.

As with all utilization management systems, appropriate documentation leading to a database is critical to the monitoring and review system. Although retrospective review of record documentation is a necessary part of the review system, due to the frequent extended use of home care, concurrent documentation, together with on-site assessment and observation should also be used.

THE HOSPICE

Hospice programs offer dying persons and their families or significant others an alternative to traditional care for terminal illness. A hospice provides palliative medical care to the terminal patient and psychosocial and spiritual support to the patient and his family. Hospice care and support are provided by an interdisciplinary team (which includes volunteers) in the patient's home or residence and in an inpatient setting. The care setting is dependent on the patient's condition and on the support available in the home. Most hospice patients have a primary care person assigned, and this is the person mainly responsible for looking after the patient in the home. This person may be the next of kin but need not be. Generally, patients receive inpatient care when acute symptom management is required or when the primary care person needs a respite. Most hospice patients spend the majority of their hospice stay at home, and many receive both home care and inpatient care during a hospice care episode. Sometimes care is not provided directly by a hospice but the hospice arranges or contracts for the care in a home health agency or an inpatient facility. Regardless, the patient still remains a hospice patient, and the hospice coordinates his care.

The family is provided support before and after the patient's death. Most hospice programs follow survivors for at least a year after a patient's death. The level of support provided to survivors is largely dependent on the assessed needs as well as on the survivors' desire for support. Support may be provided by professional staff but is often provided by volunteers.

MEDICAL RECORDS IN HOSPICE PROGRAMS

Hospice medical records document information on the patient and his family or significant other(s). Records must contain the patient's and the primary care person's identifying information. To assure well-coordinated, continuous hospice care, it is vital that records be well documented. The hospice record is the

---

A. FUNCTIONAL ASSESSMENT (Record Code For Each Function)

ASSESSMENT CODES I = Can Do Alone   2 = Can Do With Assistance   3 = Unable To Do   4 = Not Determined

FUNCTION	CODE	COMMENTS
1. BATHING OR SHOWERING		
2. SHAMPOOING		
3. NAIL CARE		
4. HAIR CARE		
5. DRESSING		
6. BOWEL AND BLADDER		
7. TRANSFERRING IN AND OUT OF BED OR CHAIR		
8. WALKING		
9. STAIRS		
10. MOBILITY OUT OF HOME		
11. DOES PATIENT HAVE A HISTORY OF FALLS?		

B. PATIENT CARE REQUIRMENTS

	YES	NO	COMMENTS
1. CATHETER			
2. COLOSTOMY/ILEOTOMY			
3. OXYGEN/RESPIRATORY EQUIPMENT			
4. WALKER			
5. WHEELCHAIR			
6. COMMODE			
7. HOSPITAL BED			
8.			
9.			

C. SUITABILITY OF PATIENT/FAMILY RESIDENCE

1. STAIRS   COMMENTS_____
       YES   NO

2. SAFETY HAZARDS   DESCRIBE_____
       YES   NO

3. SAFETY MEASURES NEEDED_____

4. ADEQUACY OF ENVIRONMENT_____

ACTIVITIES OF DAILY LIVING (Page 1 of 2)	Imprint Patient Identification or Write-In Information Below Patient's Name Medical Record No.

Hospice Project/FORE of AMRA 5/84 Form #4

FIGURE 9. HOSPICE CARE (page 1 of 2)

communication tool between the various interdisciplinary team members and between the hospice and the contracted inpatient facility or home health agency.

In 1984 the Foundation of Record Education of AHIMA completed a W.K. Kellogg Foundation-funded hospice project. The primary objective of this project was to develop a model hospice

---

D. ACTIVITIES

1. CURRENT ACTIVITIES (Describe)_____

_____

_____

2. LIMITATIONS IMPOSED BY ILLNESS (Describe)_____

_____

_____

E. REFERRAL(S) FOR HOME ASSISTANCE (e.g. home health aide, homemaker, etc.)

_____

_____

F. DIETARY

1. ROUTE OF FOOD INTAKE ☐ By Mouth   ☐ Feeding Tube   ☐ IV   ☐ Other_____

2. ALTERATIONS IN TASTE/SMELL_____

3. APPETITE_____

4. ALCOHOL INTAKE_____ 5. FOOD RESTRICTIONS_____

6. FOOD/FLUID LIKES/DISLIKES_____

7. MEAL PATTERNS_____

8. COMMENTS_____

_____

G. REST/SLEEP (Check yes or no for each)

SYMPTOM	YES	NO	COMMENTS/DESCRIPTION
1. SLEEP DISORDERS			
2. CHANGES IN SLEEP HABITS			
3. SLEEP AIDS			
4. NAPS			
5.			

H. WHAT DOES PATIENT ESPECIALLY WANT FROM HOSPICE?_____

_____

I. SOURCE(S) OF INFORMATION:_____

Date _____ Information Recorded By _____

                                                    Signature and Title

	Imprint Patient Identification or Write-In Information Below
ACTIVITIES OF DAILY LIVING (Page 2 of 2)	Patient's Name
	Medical Record No.

Hospice Project/FORE of AMRA 5/84 Form #4

FIGURE 10. HOSPICE CARE (page 2 of 2)

medical record. This model record is available in *A Medical Record Handbook for Hospice Programs*. The model record forms are not copyrighted and health information professionals are encouraged to copy and use the forms or to adapt the forms to a particular hospice's needs.

The hospice handbook contains many other guidelines, several of which will be referred to later in this section. The guidelines and the model record were developed by a Hospice Project Advisory Committee which consisted of professionals employed by hospice programs, as well as representatives from various organizations (Joint Commission, American Hospital Association, American Medical Association, and the National Hospice Organization). The documentation guidelines in the handbook were intended to provide guidelines to all hospices. Therefore, health information professionals should ensure hospices are documenting in accordance with these guidelines even if they are not required to meet Joint Commission or Medicare documentation requirements. The handbook also addresses several hospice record management concerns. For instance, it recommends that the hospice record become part of the patient's unit record when the hospice is based in a hospital or a home health agency; and that the patient index file contain information on the patients receiving hospice care as well as the survivors being followed through bereavement programs.

The Joint Commission includes accreditation standards for hospice programs in its standards for home care. For details, refer to the latest JCAHO standards.

Medicare regulations generally require the same documentation as Joint Commission standards. Differences primarily reflect signature and time requirements. The Medicare regulations prescribe a specific hospice organizational structure and state that a hospice must maintain control of a patient's care provided at a contracted inpatient facility. The contracted inpatient facility must follow the care plan established by the hospice, and the hospice record must at least include a summary of all inpatient services provided.

Medicare reimburses hospices at four different rates for the following care levels: routine home care, continuous home care, inpatient respite care, and general inpatient care. Continuous home care (8 hours or more of continuous, predominantly nursing care) and general inpatient care (care for acute symptom management that cannot be performed in the home) are the more intensive care levels, and when this care is provided, the medical record must justify that this care was needed.

The National Hospice Organization has hospice program standards but has no formal accreditation program. The program standards state that accurate and current records should be kept on all patients. State hospice regulations should also be referred to for record documentation requirements. The model hospice record should meet Joint Commission hospice standards and hospice Medicare regulations if documented per instructions and if standards and regulations are adhered to regarding frequency, signatures, and time requirements for documentation.

HOSPICE RECORD PROCESSING AND DATA COLLECTION

Review of Content

Each hospice should have a system to review medical records on a frequent, ongoing basis. It is recommended that records be reviewed shortly after admission (within five days of an inpatient admission and within ten days of a home care admission), on discharge, and on an ongoing basis (every 30-60 days). It is also recommended that volunteer documentation be filed in the medical record and that it be reviewed and initialed by the volunteer coordinator and the team nurse coordinator prior to filing.

Collection of Hospice Data

Hospices must collect data in a uniform manner if services are to be evaluated and comparisons made within and among hospice programs. Data on the care provided by hospice programs are needed for both internal and external planning. There are presently few computer systems that are specifically developed for hospice data collection. A hospice management information system was developed by the Hospice Foundation of Miami, Florida, through a project funded by the Arthur Vining Davis Foundation. The system is capable of collecting and processing patient demographic, diagnostic, and care information. A plan of care can be printed, and the system can be used to provide up-to-date patient care information to the on-call nurse.

The FORE of AHIMA hospice project reviewed several existing classification systems and recommended that hospice programs use the *International Classification of Diseases, Ninth Revision, Clinical Modification (ICD-9-CM)* to code a patient's and a survivor's diagnoses and problems (see Chapter 9). Hospices should also maintain diagnosis and problem indexes. In hospital-based programs, coding and indexing should be coordinated with the hospital's health information department.

There are two recognized hospice care episodes. The first episode begins with the patient's/family's admission to the hospice program and ends at the time a patient dies or is discharged from the hospice program. This episode includes all home care and inpatient care provided to the patient either directly or through contract with an inpatient facility or home health agency. The second care episode begins with the survivor's admission to bereavement follow-up (the day following a patient's death) and ends when the survivor is discharged from bereavement follow-up.

As previously mentioned, the recommended service data set items should be recorded by all hospices. From this data, the minimum statistics listed below should be calculated.

- —Average Daily Census, preferably by type of service provided (home care, bereavement, inpatient).
- —Average Length of Patient's Hospice Stay (the first hospice episode).
- —Average Number of Total Days of Inpatient Care and Home Care Received by Patients/Families.
- —Average Length of Bereavement Follow-up (the second hospice episode).

The hospice handbook contains formulas for the above statistics. Hospices that are Medicare certified should calculate a separate statistic that reflects the aggregate number of home care days and inpatient days received by Medicare patients. This is necessary because Medicare will not reimburse hospices at the inpatient care rate when, in a given year, the aggregate inpatient care days exceed 20 percent of the total care days.

Quality Assurance

The Joint Commission requires hospices to monitor and evaluate the quality and appropriateness of hospice program services. There should be routine collection of information pertaining to the delivery of interdisciplinary team services. This information should be assessed (using objective criteria), and important problems regarding care delivery or opportunities to improve patient/family services identified. Once problems or opportunities are identified, action must be taken and the effectiveness of this action evaluated. At least annually there should be documented evidence that quality assurance program findings resulted in action taken relating to patient/family services, administration or supervision, or in-service and/or continuing education. The quality assurance program's findings and conclusions should be coordinated, to the degree possible, with any inpatient facility or agency providing services (through contract or arrangements) to a hospice program's patients/families.

Utilization Review

Hospices monitor allocation of resources to run efficiently, and to resolve any identified problems. To do this a hospice must use objective criteria to review a randomly selected sample of medical records. This review should monitor concerns such as:

1. the appropriateness of the level of services and the team services provided,
2. the appropriateness of admission,
3. stays exceeding six months, and
4. delays in providing team service.

Utilization review should result in documented action being taken. The utilization review plan should be reviewed at least annually and revised as appropriate.

Medicare regulations require hospices to conduct ongoing assessments of the quality and appropriateness of the services provided. Services provided through arrangements or contracts must be assessed. There must be documentation of the mechanisms used to monitor care, the problems identified and resolved, and the suggestions made for improving care.

RESPITE CARE

Respite care is defined as care given by a provider to a person living in the community to provide a break to family members that normally provide the care. Respite care can be divided into two categories: services that are provided in home and services that are provided out of home. In home services include nursing care and home health aides provided through visiting nurse associations. Out of home services include nursing homes and adult day care centers. Adult day care centers provide an alternative to out of home services such as nursing homes that require the patient to stay overnight. These centers are usually open eight hours a day, five days a week, with the patient attending as many or as few sessions as desired. Regulatory agencies' requirements for medical records must be followed in all areas of respite care.

REHABILITATION FACILITIES

Rehabilitation facilities may be of many types, including comprehensive inpatient rehabilitation, outpatient medical rehabilitation, and programs for spinal cord injury, chronic pain management, brain injury, infant and early childhood developmental disabilities, vocational evaluation, work adjustment, occupational skill training, job placement, respite, community mental health, alcoholism and drug abuse treatment, and psychosocial care.

The range of services provided is also extensive. Some examples are: patient advocacy, audiology, dentistry, driver training, education, guardianship, independent living skills instruction, job placement, nursing, orthotics and prosthetics, recreational services, speech-language pathology, and 24-hour crisis intervention.

Every person served by a rehabilitation facility first undergoes an intake and orientation program. This program screens individuals for admission and provides referrals when the specific facility cannot accept a person. This process also includes obtaining diagnostic, treatment, and training data from cooperative programs and medical data from other health care facilities. The facility must establish and follow specific procedures for assessment to determine an individual's program of rehabilitation.

The individual's program should focus on reintegration of the individual into the community. This may be accomplished through maximizing independent functioning, the establishment and maintenance of relationships, etc. Where services are delivered primarily in the facility, the individuals served are usually concerned with their functioning in the community. In a work-oriented program, examples would include training the individual in how to use transportation to go to work, training the family, if applicable, in how to motivate the individual to keep a job, establishing procedures to stimulate the individual to take medications as prescribed, etc. Community integration in a residential program could be reflected in such activities as assisting the person served to interact appropriately with neighbors, use the local transportation system, utilize community resources for recreation, shopping, worship, etc. A psychosocial program might assist the person to deal with interpersonal relationships on a job.

The individual's program and its goals should constantly be reviewed and modified as the individual progresses in the treatment program. Referrals to other agencies may also be needed. Finally, procedures for discharge and follow-up should be established and implemented.

Follow-up is conducted to support the gains of the person served and for quality assurance. Follow-up of persons served should determine to what degree the person's program has been successful and whether the services offered are optimum. It is through information gathered during follow-up contacts that the staff is able to ascertain if further services are required and evaluate the effectiveness of services and programs. The need for the organization to be flexible and to modify its programs can be met best through awareness of the degree to which persons served achieve their goals.

REHABILITATION RECORDS

Facilities that provide rehabilitative care may be accredited by the Commission on Accreditation of Rehabilitation Facilities (CARF). CARF requires that a single case record be maintained for anyone admitted to the facility. The completed case record should include the following:

- Case identification data
- The name and address of the personal representative, conservator, guardian, and/or representative payee, if one has been appointed for the person served;
- Pertinent history, diagnosis of disability, rehabilitation problems(s), goals, and prognosis;

- Reports of assessment and individual program planning;
- Reports from referring sources;
- Reports of service referrals;
- Reports from outside consultation and from laboratory, radiology, orthotic and prosthetic services, etc.;
- Designation of the program manager for the individual. A written policy identifying who is responsible for the program management of given groups would remove the necessity for this information in the case record;
- Evidence of the individual's, and where appropriate, the family's participation in the decision making process of the individual's program;
- Evaluation reports from each service;
- Reports of staff conferences;
- The individual's total program plan;
- Plans from each service;
- Signed and dated service and progress reports from each service;
- Correspondence pertinent to the person being served;
- Release forms;
- A discharge report;
- Follow-up reports.

Rehabilitation and physical medicine case records are unique because although all essential data are located in the case record, duplicates of some worksheets are maintained by service units. The worksheets contain information which is valuable to that service unit such as raw scores and daily attendance. These worksheets do not substitute for the case record. CARF states that the main record should receive first priority when recording case information.

QUALITY ASSURANCE

CARF provides guidelines for assessment of program quality for individuals served in rehabilitation facilities. These include:
1. The organization should have an established written system which provides for an internal review of the program of services for individuals served.

2. The review should result in a determination as to whether:
   a. Application of each service began at the appropriate point during the individual's course of service.
   b. The appropriate services were provided for an adequate duration.
   c. The appropriate goals were stated for each service in the individual's program.
   d. The services produced the desired results in terms of the stated goals of the program and the needs of the individual.
3. The system should provide for designated staff review of cases no less than quarterly.
4. No person should review his/her own cases.
5. The review should involve at least a sampling of persons served, including persons discharged.
6. The review should occur, on an individual case basis, during the course of providing services between admission and discharge.
7. The review should be conducted irrespective of sources of funding for those served.
8. Results of the review should be documented and reviewed periodically by the organization's administration.
9. As a result of the review, a plan of corrective action should be initiated.

UTILIZATION REVIEW

The process of utilization management for rehabilitative medicine parallels that of acute care with the exception of four key differences: preadmission evaluation, establishment and ongoing evaluation of the treatment plan, assessment of the coordination of the rehabilitation team, and the mandatory inclusion of discharge planning for every case.

It is necessary to assess prior to all admissions whether rehabilitation is possible, the type of program that is necessary, and the existence of any social or environmental factors which might affect the outcome. After formal acceptance into a rehabilitative program, it is necessary to assure that goals have been established to guide the caregivers in their various disciplines and to assess the patient's progress. Continuing stay review focuses on the appropriate use of professional services to achieve these goals and the patient's continuous response.

Since coordination of various disciplines is vital to a successful outcome, assessment of the production efficiency of rehabilitation involves evaluating that team conferences are held on a regular basis, that goals and objectives are reviewed, and that documentation is provided on a concurrent basis to facilitate communication. A critical factor in the coordination of the rehabilitation process is the initiation of discharge planning in the early stages of goal development so that the level of self-sufficiency that is set as a physical objective may also be realized on a social and environmental level. Although the time frames involved in ilitative care are extended, the focus of review must be on the receipt of care that can be medically expected to improve the patient's condition and can only be rendered in the rehabilitation setting.

New initiatives in this area involve the use of ambulatory services whenever they are available and are possible for the patient to access on a regular basis. Also, employer sponsored private review programs are following a "case management" approach which coordinates the patient's rehabilitation potential, medical services, and ability to return to an appropriate productive employment situation.

GENERAL MEDICAL RECORD MANAGEMENT PRINCIPLES

CLINICAL AND MEDICAL RECORD FORMS

Chapter 7, "Forms Design and Control" gives principles of forms development for clinical record documentation. These principles are applicable to long term and ilitative care facilities. Because the patient population is relatively low, printing large quantities of forms at one time could result in waste should revision be necessary. A balance is needed between the cost savings gained by having a large quantity printed and the usage rate over a one or two-year period. Changes in the regulatory agencies' requirements will affect the forms' content. This should also be considered when determining the quantity and usage rate of forms.

FILING SYSTEMS

A filing system is necessary to protect records and to facilitate their location. An effective filing system for long term care and rehabilitation records should enable one to identify a resident's record, to locate it quickly, and to retrieve it from any location in the facility. Because of the long duration of care, clinical records may remain for weeks, months, and even years at the nurses' station or in a provider's possession until the time of discharge. Consequently, many basic principles of filing systems apply both to the inpatient records (e.g., charge-out system) as well as to the closed records which are processed for permanent filing upon discharge. The system should be that which does the job best; but whatever method is chosen, all parts of the record should be kept in one place as a unit.

This principle, filing all records in one place as a unit, has particular application in situations where a voluminous record is thinned out. When material is removed from the active portion of the record, the portion removed should be kept in a central location as the primary material. For example, in a nursing facility the active portion of the chart will remain in the active folder or chart holder; the thinned portion will be kept in a locked file in a central location, preferably the record department. At the time of discharge, both sections of the chart will be merged again. This same principle, one record in one location, applies to multiple charts for the same resident, as in the situation of a resident who has more than one admission to the facility.

ALPHABETIC VERSUS NUMERIC FILING

The records of residents who have been discharged may be filed either in alphabetic or numeric order. Alphabetic filing is suitable for a very small facility or one having a low resident turnover rate. In this system, the record is filed by last name, first name, and middle name in strict alphabetical order.

In large facilities or in those with short stay, numerical filing is recommended. In this system, the record is filed in strict numerical sequence by resident number.

Permanent storage of the records is facilitated through the use of file folders. Because activity levels for discharged records are relatively low, a lightweight folder is acceptable. See Chapter 8 for further discussion of numbering and filing.

RETENTION OF RECORDS

Clinical records should be kept by the facility as long as required under the statute of limitations or state record-retention regulations. Licensure regulations usually specify the re-

CLINICAL RECORD DESTRUCTION LOG

RESIDENT NAME	ADMISSION	DISCHARGE	DATE OF BIRTH	REC. NO.

The Records Listed Above Were Destroyed On_____.

The Method of Destruction Was_____.

_____   _____
Clinical Record Supervisor   Administrator

_____
Witness

FIGURE 11. CLINICAL RECORD DESTRUCTION LOG

tention period for a given state. The statute of limitations sets a time limit on initiating lawsuits involving residents and their treatment in the health facility. The time limit varies among states and for different types of lawsuits.

In the absence of a state or other regulation, the federal LTC regulations, and accrediting standards, coupled with a review of record usage after discharge, provide the chief executive officer and the clinical record practitioner a sound basis for the development of a record retention schedule specific to the facility. When records are destroyed after the required retention period, basic information is retained permanently, including resident name, date of birth, admission and discharge dates. A sample clinical record destruction log is shown in Figure 11. Such a log shows records have been destroyed according to facility policy.

RELEASE OF INFORMATION

The clinical record is a confidential document. All employees of the facility are responsible for assuring that no unauthorized person ever takes any of these records out of the file, reads, copies, or otherwise tampers with them. Some individuals are authorized to access this information, and health information personnel should be ready to make it available to them. Since legal requirements and restrictions about release of medical information vary from state to state, the facility should have a local attorney outline basic rules to follow. Many component state associations of the American Health Information Management Association have compiled handbooks for the release of information for their respective states; these resources are available from such professional groups. Using the pertinent legal advice and related professional association material, the administrative staff, including the clinical record practitioner, should develop a policy on the release of information for the facility. Chapter 15 of this text provides a detailed review of pertinent points, including record ownership, disclosure of information, court subpoena and/or deposition processes, and resident access.

Three areas in release of information in the long term care facility deserve particular attention. The first is the processing of information when a resident is being transferred from the facility for continuing care. In these instances, AHIMA's position statement on "Confidentiality of Patient Health Information" specifies that a release is not necessary since the information is being released to another health care provider currently involved in the care of the patient. The transfer form should be completed to go with the resident

The second point, also associated with the transfer of residents from one facility to another, involves specificity of authorization. When material is released from the present facility's record, the only material it is empowered to release is that generated during the course of treatment at the facility. There should be no re-release of information obtained from previous settings. The resident's authorization covers only the record as generated in the course of treatment at each specific facility. Should another facility need such prior information, it is its duty to obtain the necessary consent of the resident and to set in motion the necessary procedures for obtaining such material.

CONSULTING

Many facilities utilize the services of a credentialed health information practitioner to review their long term or rehabilitation care facility's clinical record department. While some facilities employ the practitioner full-time, others contract with the practitioner for consulting services. Consulting is one area of continued growth for the health information practitioner. It allows the practitioner to utilize technical, administrative, teaching, and writing skills.

The consultant makes visits to the facility to review clinical record department operations to ensure that the regulatory agencies' requirements are met. Frequency of visits will be dependent upon regulatory requirements and/or the agreement between the consultant and the facility. The consultant reviews the department to ensure that records are kept in accordance with professional standards and practices. The records should be complete, accurately documented, readily accessible, and systematically organized. Random audits of both active and closed medical records may be performed. The consultant also reviews the facility's policies and procedures for maintaining complete medical records. Special emphasis should be placed on reviewing the facility's policies and procedures regarding the confidentiality of the medical records to safeguard this information against unauthorized use, loss, or destruction. Usually within two weeks after a visit, the consultant provides the administrator with a written report of findings and recommendations.

The consultant may provide inservice training sessions to the staff. In these cases, the consultant needs to develop a program outline, handouts when necessary, and a test to see if the attendees learned from the session.

The consultant may also be called upon to help the health information designee in providing reports to administration. Such reports may include the compiling of statistics regarding bed occupancy and transfers to other facilities, the compiling of statistics for patient diagnoses and the appropriate ICD-9-CM codes for the diagnoses, and the compiling of statistics regarding problem areas found in the facility's medical records.

SUMMARY

Clinical records are an integral part of long term and rehabilitation care facilities. The basic content and minimum standards of the record should be considered when developing a record system. This chapter has defined these basic contents along with other pertinent areas related to the record in long term care and rehabilitation facilities. Those engaging in the maintenance of clinical records in these environments must carefully review the appropriate regulatory and accrediting agencies requirements.

STUDY QUESTIONS

1. Distinguish between the long term care patient and rehabilitation patient.
2. Identify the standards which pertain to the operation of a long term care facility. Which agencies standards are voluntary, which are mandatory?
3. Describe the purpose and content of the following:
   Transfer or referral statement
   Physician's admitting evaluation
   Patient care plan
   Progress notes
   Physician discharge summary
   Accident/incident report
4. Describe the appropriate arrangement of the medical record while the patient is in the nursing facility and upon discharge.

5. Define home health care.
6. List the forms which the Health Care Financing Administration requires of Medicare certified home health agencies.
7. Identify the components of home health record documentation.
8. Define hospice, identify agencies which establish standards for hospices, and describe medical record content appropriate for hospice programs.
9. Define respite care.
10. Identify the primary accrediting agency for rehabilitation facilities.
11. Describe the content of a completed case record describing rehabilitation services.
12. Explain the purpose of review of medical record content, data collection, quality assurance, and utilization review in long term care facilities.
13. Describe the role of the health information consultant in long term care.

REFERENCES

American Medical Record Association, *Consulting: Another Dimension, Part I - Principles of Consulting* (Chicago: AMRA, 1977).

American Medical Record Association, *Consulting: Another Dimension, Part II - Long Term Care* (Chicago: AMRA, 1979).

American Medical Record Association, *Professional Practice Standards for Long Term Care* (Chicago: AMRA, 1988).

American Health Care Association, *Quest for Quality: Self-Appraisal Guide for Long Term Care Facilities* (Washington, D.C.: AHCA, 1982).

American Hospital Association, *Medical Rehabilitation Services in Health Care Institutions* (Chicago: AHA, 1986).

Berger, Audrey, "The Medical Record Consultant in Long-Term Care," *Topics in Health Record Management: Records in Nontraditional Settings* (March, 1985): 39-45.

Cameron, James M., "Case-mix and Resource Use in Long-Term Care," *Medical Care* (April, 1985): 296-309.

Cofer, Jennifer and Hugh Greeley, *Quality Improvement Techniques for Long Term Care* (Opus Communications, Marblehead, MA, 1993).

Commission on Accreditation of Rehabilitation Facilities, *Program Evaluation in Inpatient Medical Rehabilitation Facilities* (Tucson: CARF).

Commission on Accreditation of Rehabilitation Facilities, *Standards Manual for Organizations Serving People with Disabilities* (Tucson: CARF, 1988).

"Conditions of Participation: Comprehensive Outpatient Rehabilitation Facilities," *Code of Federal Regulations,* Title 42, Part 485, Section 485.50-485.74 (Subpart B).

"Conditions of Participation: Hospice Care," *Code of Federal Regulations,* Title 42, Chapter IV, Part 418; Section 418.50-418.100 (Subpart C)

"Conditions of Participation - Skilled Nursing Facilities, *Code of Federal Regulations,* Title 42, Section 405.1101-1137 (Subpart K)

Curtis, Mary Role, "The Treatment Plan System: Management Tool for Multidisciplinary Patient Care," *Journal of the American Medical Record Association* (April, 1982)

Ellis, Jack A. N. and Susan Helbig, *The Health Care Consultant as a Change Agent* (Chicago: AMRA, 1981).

Federal Register, February 2, 1989, pp 5316-5318.

Federal Register, September 26, 1991, pp 48826-48829.

42 CFR, Part 431, et al., Medicare and Medicaid; *Requirements for Long Term Care Facilities and Nurse Aide Training and Competency Evaluation Programs;* Final rules.

Glondys, Barbara A., *Today's Challenge: Content of the Health Record - Documentation Requirements in the Medical Record* (Chicago: AMRA, 1985).

Goines, Brenda M., *Medical Record Policies and Procedures* (Englewood Cliffs, NJ: Brady Communications Company, Inc., 1985).

Hoyer, Robert, *"Highlights of the First National Home Care Agency & Hospice Inventory,"* CARING Magazine, July 1993, pp 54-58.

Joint Commission on Accreditation of Healthcare Organizations, *Accreditation Manual for Home Care* (Oakbrook Terrace, IL, 1993).

Joint Commission on Accreditation of Healthcare Organizations, *Accreditation Manual for Long Term Care Facilities* (Chicago: Joint Commission, 1994).

Joint Commission on Accreditation of Healthcare Organizations, *Quality Improvement in Home Care* (Oakbrook Terrace, IL, 1993).

Kay, Eleanor and Barbara S. Nodiff, *Quality Assurance Manual for Long-Term Care Facilities* (National Health Publishing, 1988).

Kitanik, Barbara, "Determining Software Needs in Long-Term Care," *Software in Healthcare* (Oct.-Nov., 1984): 80-82.

Kleffel, Dorothy, "Home Health Record Systems: A Challenge to the Medical Record Profession," *Topics in Health Record Management: Ambulatory Care* (March, 1981): 33-44.

"Long Term Health Care: Minimum Data Set," *Report of the National Committee on Vital and Health Statistics,* (Hyattsville, Maryland: National Center for Health Statistics, 1980): DHHS No. PHS 80-1158.

Marrelli, T. M., *Handbook of Home Health Standards and Documentation Guidelines for Reimbursement,* second edition (Mosby, 1994).

Mary Ann Lowe, *Patient Care Plans in Long Term Care Facilities* (Ypsilanti, Michigan: Nursing Home Publishing Associates, 1983).

Miller, Susan C., *Documentation for Home Health Care: A Record Management Handbook* (Chicago: AHIMA, 1986).

Miller, Susan C., *A Medical Record Handbook for Hospice Programs* (Chicago: AHIMA, 1984).

Stevens, Linda and Carolyn R. Kirk, "The Role of the Health Record Practitioner in Public Health Nursing and Home Health Care Agencies," *Topics in Health Record Management: Records in Nontraditional Setting* (March, 1985): 61-64.

Wilde, Donna J., "Home Health Agencies with Multiple Programs: Flexibility is Key for Clinical Records," *Topics in Health Record Management: Records in Nontraditional Settings* (March, 1985): 1-12.

chapter **5**

MENTAL HEALTH RECORDS

HISTORY OF MENTAL HEALTH CARE
IN THE UNITED STATES

Mental health care was almost nonexistent in the United States until the early 19th century. One of the earliest pioneers was Dorothea Dix, who worked hard to improve the lot of mental health patients and the facilities in which they were housed. It was due to her persistence that the government enacted federal legislation which granted states land upon which mental hospitals could be built. These institutions, many of which are still in existence, served the population for many decades.

Almost one hundred years later, in 1946, the National Institute of Mental Health (NIMH) was created as an agency of the Federal Government. Studies at that time and later pointed up the fact that existing facilities were used mostly for holding the mentally ill or treating individuals in crisis situations, and that the great majority of patients needed more active care.

A major study entitled "Action for Mental Health" was published in 1960 and resulted in the passage of the Community Mental Health Centers Act of 1963. Its goal was to establish multiservice programs which would meet different and multiple needs of mental health patients. Several hundred Community Mental Health Centers have been established to provide treatment for mental illness in all of its various forms. These centers can be free-standing, under one roof, under several roofs, connected with a hospital, or variations of these.

Public Law 94-63, passed July 29, 1975, is known as the "Special Health Revenue Sharing Act of 1975" and contains amendments to previous acts involving such areas as Health Revenue Sharing and Community Mental Health Centers. The amendments cover many items and relate specifically to services offered, comprehensive mental health services, and reimbursement.

Title XVIII of the Social Security Act provides payment for medical services in mental health facilities for persons over age 65 or under age 18. Title XIX provides assistance to states (at their discretion) for their mental health care programs. Both of these acts bring into focus reimbursement, utilization review, and the *Conditions of Participation for Hospitals.* Concern for the mentally ill and resulting legislation have placed emphasis on the need for better care of the mentally ill and documentation of that care.

The first set of Joint Commission on Accreditation of Healthcare Organization standards for psychiatric programs was published in 1972. Over the next several years, special standards were developed and published for child and adolescent psychiatric programs, for alcohol and drug abuse rehabilitation programs, and for programs treating the developmentally disabled.

With the movement in the late 1970s toward one set of standards for facilities providing multiprograms, standards for adult psychiatric, child and adolescent, and alcoholism and drug abuse programs were combined into one manual called the *Accreditation Manual for Mental Health, Chemical Dependency, and Mental Retardation / Developmental Disabilities Services* (MHM). The latest edition of this manual also includes standards for mentally retarded and developmentally disabled programs. Effective October, 1987, all facilities which provide psychiatric care and are licensed as a hospital are required to be surveyed under the *Accreditation Manual for Hospitals* (AMH). Standards for psychiatric programs have been incorporated into the AMH in those areas where the needs are different. Facilities which provide psychiatric care but are not licensed as a hospital such as free-standing alcoholism and drug abuse rehabilitation programs and community mental health centers are surveyed under the MHM.

Although there are certain characteristics unique to mental health records, general medical record documentation requirements and record-keeping practices are applicable. In the mental health care facility, the health information practitioner will be responsible for many of the same activities that take place in the acute care general hospital. The health information professional must be familiar with the Joint Commission standards and state licensing requirements. In addition, the health information practitioner should be prepared to provide appropriate service to the medical staff in its committee activities and to the clinical staff in its clinical charting activities.

In this chapter, emphasis will be placed on record-keeping practices that are of more significance in mental health facilities than in acute care facilities. Much of the information presented regarding documentation requirements is based on the Joint Commission's MHM. The health information practitioner should have access to these standards as well as the *Medicare Conditions of Participation*. The state mental health code should also be available for review of state documentation and record-keeping requirements.

CONTENT OF MENTAL HEALTH RECORDS

According to the American Psychiatric Association, the mental health record should document the evaluation, treatment, and course of the patient's illness. It provides a means of communication between the physician and other staff members contributing to the patient's care. The mental health record is also a basic source of information for study and evaluation of the care rendered and for reimbursement by third-party payers. The mental health record should contain all pertinent clinical information, which at a minimum should consist of:

- identification data
- source of referral
- reason for referral
- patient's legal status

- all appropriate consents for admission, treatment, evaluation, and aftercare
- admitting psychiatric diagnosis
- psychiatric history
- record of the complete assessment, including the complaints of others regarding the patient as well as the patient's comments
- medical history, report of physical examination, and record of all medications prescribed
- provisional diagnoses based upon assessment which includes intercurrent diseases as well as the psychiatric diagnoses
- written individualized treatment plan
- documentation of the course of treatment and all evaluations and examinations
- multidisciplinary progress notes related to the goals and objectives outlined in the treatment plan
- appropriate documentation related to special treatment procedures
- updates to the treatment plan as a result of the assessments detailed in the progress notes
- multidisciplinary case conferences and consultation notes which include date of conference or consultation, recommendations made, and actions taken
- information on any unusual occurrences such as: treatment complications, accidents or injuries to the patient, morbidity, death of a patient, procedures that place the patient at risk or cause unusual pain
- correspondence related to the patient, including all letters and dated notations of telephone conversations relevant to the patient's treatment
- discharge or termination summary
- plan for follow-up care and documentation of its implementation
- individualized aftercare or post treatment plan

PATIENT MANAGEMENT

INTAKE

Each mental health program should develop policies and procedures that specify the information to be obtained on all applicants or referrals for admission, the procedures for accepting referrals from outside agencies and organizations, the records to be kept on all applicants, the statistical data to be kept on the intake process, and the procedures to be followed including alternative referrals when an applicant is found ineligible for admission.

Every state defines categories of admission (such as voluntary and involuntary for specified durations) and requirements for reporting admissions.

ASSESSMENT OF THE PATIENT

Each program should conduct a complete assessment of each patient. Assessment is the process of gathering and ordering facts about a patient by means of interviewing the patient and significant others, observing the patient, performing physical and mental examinations of the patient, and conducting other diagnostic tests. The purpose of the assessment is to identify the patient's needs during the current course of treatment and to serve as a basis for development of the patient's individualized treatment plan. The assessment should include identification of physical, emotional, behavioral, social, recreational, legal, vocational, nutritional , and developmental needs.

Physical Assessment

The physical assessment should include a medical, alcohol, and drug history, and an appropriate laboratory workup. In inpatient programs, a physical examination must be completed within 24 hours of admission. In other types of programs, the need for a physical examination is determined by the physician; and the rationale for not conducting a complete examination should be documented. In programs serving children, adolescents, and mentally retarded/developmentally disabled patients, motor development and functioning; speech, language and hearing functioning; visual functioning; and the patient's immunization status must be assessed.

Emotional and Behavioral Assessment

An emotional or behavioral assessment should be completed and documented in the patient's record. The following items should be included:

- history and previous emotional, behavioral, and substance-abuse problems and treatment;
- the patient's current emotional, behavioral functioning;
- a direct psychiatric evaluation, when indicated;
- a mental status examination appropriate to the age of the patient, when indicated;
- psychological assessments, when indicated; and
- other functional evaluations of language, self-care, and social affective and visual-motor functioning, when indicated.

Social Assessment

The social assessment should include information related to the patient's environment and home, religion, childhood history, military service history, financial status, peer group, and the patient's family circumstances including the family constellation and current living situation.

Recreational Assessment

An activities assessment should include information relating to the patient's skills, talents, aptitudes, and interests.

Legal Assessment

A legal assessment is not always conducted, but when appropriate it should include a legal history and a discussion to determine if the patient's legal situation will affect the patient's progress in treatment. If it is determined that it will, it should be included in the patient's problems to be addressed.

Vocational Assessment

A vocational assessment is not always conducted, but when appropriate it should include a vocational history, educational history which includes academic and vocational training, and a discussion with the patient regarding past work experiences, attitudes toward work, and possibilities for future education, training, and employment.

Nutritional Assessment

A nutritional assessment is not always conducted, but when appropriate it should be documented. Patients being treated for eating disorders or patients having physical conditions which require special diets should have a nutritional assessment.

Other Assessments

In addition to the initial assessments just described, there are circumstances which arise during the course of the patient's treatment which require special assessment. Examples of these are:

- prior to the implementation of seclusion
- prior to the application of restraints
- prior to the use of electroconvulsive therapy
- after a therapeutic pass

Documentation requirements for these and other circumstances are discussed in the Special Therapies section of this chapter.

Results of all assessments conducted should be documented in the patient's mental health record. They should reflect the fundamental needs of the patient and should include appropriate multidisciplinary clinical input. Assessments serve as the foundation for the development of the patient's individualized treatment plan.

Treatment Plan

The Joint Commission requires that each patient have a documented plan of treatment. The MHM do not define the elements of the plan, however, the *Consolidated Standards Manual* standards describe in very specific terms the content of a treatment plan and the frequency of documentation. Medicare also requires an individualized treatment plan in its *Conditions of Participation for Psychiatric Facilities*.

Content of the Treatment Plan

Goals and Objectives: The treatment plan should contain specific goals which the patient must achieve and which are based upon the patient's need as derived from the initial assessments. The treatment plan should also contain specific objectives which relate to the goals and should include expected achievement dates. These should be written in measurable terms in order to assess the patient's progress in attaining them. Setting goals and objectives in measurable terms (1) assures that each patient has an individualized treatment plan; (2) requires specific action which leaves little room for guessing; (3) communicates the same goal expectation

---

INITIAL TREATMENT PLAN

PATIENT NAME: MEDICAL RECORD NO.:   DATE:

I. Briefly identify major problems, objectives, goals, and disposition planning:

      PROBLEMS:

      OBJECTIVES:

      GOALS:

      DISPOSITION PLANNING:

II. CURRENT DIAGNOSIS:

      AXIS   I.

      AXIS   II.

      AXIS   III.

      AXIS   IV.

      AXIS   V.

III. ESTIMATED LENGTH OF HOSPITALIZATION:

IV. TREATMENT: (specify therapist where applicable)

      A. MEDICATION LIST: DOSAGE:

FIGURE 1. INITIAL TREATMENT PLAN (front)

---

to all staff members who work with the patient; and (4) enables those involved in the ongoing treatment of the patient, or other qualified personnel, to determine what treatment is being carried out.

Treatment Modalities: The treatment plan should describe the services, activities, and programs planned for the patient; should specify the staff members assigned to carry out the planned treatment; and should specify the frequency of the treatment modalities.

B. ☐ MEDICAL WORKUP:
    ☐ PHYSICAL EXAM:
    ☐ LABORATORY/X-RAY:
    ☐ OTHER:

C. ☐ PSYCHOLOGICAL TESTING:

D. ☐ SPECIAL PROCEDURES AND/OR CONSULTATIONS:

E. ☐ SCHOOL OR EDUCATIONAL EVALUATION:

F. ☐ SOCIAL WORK: (i.e., special evaluation, disposition planning, etc.)
_____
_____
_____
_____

G. ☐ ACTIVITIES THERAPY: (include goals and objectives)
_____
_____
_____
_____

H. ☐ NURSING CARE: (include goals and objectives)
_____
_____
_____
_____

I. ☐ THERAPY:
    1. INDIVIDUAL: ☐ Brief ☐ Full Sessions____times per wk. with_____
    2. GROUP:_____times per wk. with_____
    3. FAMILY:_____times per wk. with_____

DATE:_____   SIGNATURE:_____

FIGURE 2. INITIAL TREATMENT PLAN (back of Fig.1)

FREQUENCY OF DOCUMENTATION

Inpatient, Residential, and Partial-Day Programs: A preliminary treatment plan should be developed upon admission based upon the intake assessment. An initial treatment plan should be developed within 72 hours of admission based upon the assessments conducted within that time frame. This plan is used to implement immediate treatment.

FIGURE 3. MASTER TREATMENT PLAN

As the patient is re-evaluated, the treatment plan is updated as well. In its 1993 MHM, the Joint Commission says the treatment plan should be reviewed at least at these key decision points:

- at the time of transfer or discharge,
- at any major change in the patient's condition,
- at the conclusion of the initial treatment and any subsequent estimated lengths of treatment,

---

REVISION OF MASTER TREATMENT PLAN

WEEK_____

PATIENT NAME:_____ DATE:_____

TREATMENT TEAM:
Psychiatrist: Primary Nurse:
Social Worker: Activities Therapist:
Educational Liaison: Dietary Consultant:
CD Counselor:

FORMULATION:

DIAGNOSIS: AXIS   I.
           AXIS II.
           AXIS III.
           AXIS IV.
           AXIS V.
NEEDS ASSESSMENT AND TREATMENT METHODS:

EXPECTED DATES OF ACHIEVEMENT (New)

I. GOAL:
        OBJECTIVES:

   STATUS IN ACHIEVING GOAL AND OBJECTIVES:
   TREATMENT METHODS — Frequency — Person or Discipline Responsible:

EXPECTED DATES OF ACHIEVEMENT (New)

II. GOAL:
        OBJECTIVES:

   STATUS IN ACHIEVING GOAL AND OBJECTIVES:
   TREATMENT METHODS — Frequency - Person or Discipline Responsible:
                    (Continue goals and objectives if applicable.)
DIAGNOSTIC QUESTIONS AND PROCEDURES: (Include specific unresolved diagnostic problems and techniques
to be utilized to refine these.)

DISCHARGE PLANNING: (Need for continued hospitalization, expected length of stay, aftercare planning.)
        METHOD:
PATIENT AND FAMILY PARTICIPATION IN AND RESPONSE TO THE TREATMENT PLAN:

                                    _____
                                         ATTENDING PSYCHIATRIST

FIGURE 4. REVISION OF MASTER TREATMENT PLAN

- every ten visits or every three months of outpatient care, which-ever comes first, and
- every three months of inpatient treatment.

Outpatient Programs: An initial treatment plan should be developed at intake based upon assessment of the patient's presenting problems, physical health, emotional status, and behavioral status. If the number of patient visits is more than 10, a master plan should be developed and should be based upon a comprehensive assessment of the patient's needs. This master plan should be reviewed and updated as needed every 10 visits or every three months, whichever comes first.

Programs Treating the Mentally Retarded/Developmentally Disabled: Requirements for preliminary, initial, and master treatment plans, and review and update of the master plan are identical to those for residential programs. In addition, when a patient has attained majority or is emancipated, there should be documentation that the treatment plan was reviewed by a multidisciplinary treatment team and that the following were considered:

- civil and legal rights; and
- the need for the patient to remain in the program.

OTHER REQUIREMENTS

The patient should be involved in the development of the treatment plan, and this involvement should be documented in the patient's record. The family or significant others should also be involved in the treatment plan, and this, too, should be documented.

In reviewing the patient's mental health record, one should be able to determine from the treatment plan (1) what is being treated; (2) what treatments are being used; (3) the goals of treatment; and (4) who is responsible for carrying out the various treatments. The treatment plan should also clearly state the criteria, written in measurable terms, for termination of treatment services. (See sample forms in Figures 1, 2, 3, and 4.)

PROGRESS NOTES

Documentation of the patient's progress should be contained in the patient's mental health record. The progress notes are considered to be part of the treatment plan. The progress notes should include documentation of implementation of the treatment plan, treatments provided, and the patient's response to that treatment. Revisions and updating of the treatment plan should also be documented in the progress notes.

Progress notes are used to review the progress of the patient. Such reviews are often conducted in multidisciplinary case conferences. Records of these conferences are documented in the progress notes or on special forms designed for that purpose. Documentation should identify persons in attendance. All entries should be properly dated and signed.

DISCHARGE SUMMARY AND PLANS
FOR AFTERCARE

The discharge summary and plans for aftercare are also included in the patient's record as part of the treatment plan. The discharge summary should be completed and filed in the patient's record within 15 days of discharge. The discharge summary should include a clinical resume that summarizes the following:

- results of the initial assessment and diagnosis
- significant findings
- course and progress of the patient with regard to each identified clinical problem
- clinical course of the patient's treatment
- final assessment including the general observations and understanding of the patient's condition initially, during treatment, and at discharge
- recommendations and arrangements for further treatment including prescribed medications and aftercare
- final diagnoses

When appropriate, a written aftercare plan for continuing treatment should be developed describing the responsibility of the organization for facilitating the transfer of the patient to another phase or modality of the program, to another program, an agency, to an individual, and /or to the patient's personal support system.

SPECIAL THERAPIES

Mental health care facilities sometimes utilize procedures not generally found in the acute care hospital setting. Examples of special procedures are use of restraints, seclusion, psychosurgery, electroconvulsive therapy, the use of unusual medications or experimental drugs, therapeutic passes, and behavior modification techniques.

When it becomes necessary or desirable to treat a patient utilizing special procedures, the rationale for their use and the clinical indications must be clearly stated in the patient's record. The record should also contain evidence that indications for the special procedure have been reviewed by the head of the professional staff, or other appropriate persons, prior to implementation.

Seclusion and Restraint

If a patient is to be placed in seclusion or in restraints, the physician must first conduct a clinical assessment of the patient. This must be documented in the patient's record and should include the clinical justifications for the use of seclusion and/or restraint and a summary of what less-restrictive intervention was tried without success necessitating seclusion and/or restraint. A written order must also be entered in the record prior to restraint or seclusion, and it shall be for a limited time not exceeding 24 hours. In an emergency, restraint or seclusion may be utilized by trained, clinically privileged staff. However, the assessment and order for the use of emergency restraint or seclusion, which must be documented in the record, may not exceed one hour. The physician's oral order shall be required if restraint or seclusion is to be continued. It is further required that staff members provide appropriate attention to these patients at 15-minute intervals. This should also be documented in the patient's mental health record. It is important to remember that restraint or seclusion requires clinical justification and should be used only to prevent a patient from self-injury, injuring others, or from causing serious damage to the facility. Seclusion might also be used to prevent serious disruption of the therapeutic environment. Seclusion and restraint should never be implemented as punishment or for the convenience of the staff. It is generally recommended that seclusion should be considered as a viable treatment procedure before restraints. Seclusion, without the use of restraints, is a less restrictive alternative to restraints, which also incorporates seclusion for the safety of the restrained patient. All use of seclusion and restraint for longer than 24 hours should be reported to the head of the professional staff who should review each case and investigate unusual or possibly unwarranted patterns of utilization.

ECT AND OTHER THERAPIES

Electroconvulsive therapy, psychosurgery, behavior modification procedures that use painful stimuli, and the use of experimental or unusual drugs require the written informed consent of the patient or appropriate legally responsible person before the procedure can be carried out. Such consents are to be made part of the patient's record. Consents for any of these procedures may be withdrawn, verbally or in writing, at any time.

Therapeutic passes are an important treatment modality for mental health patients. Therapeutic passes are used to assess the patient's ability to function outside of the safe and secure hospital environment, to assess the patient's ability to appropriately respond to daily activities and stimuli, to augment the patient's treatment plan by providing for enhancement of socialization and to foster a sense of freedom and self-determination. They are also used to allow the patient an opportunity at resuming role responsibility and to foster repair of ruptured or difficult family relationships. Therapeutic passes should be well documented in the patient's record, as third-party payment for the care may be difficult to obtain. Documentation should include the justification for the therapeutic pass and the patient's response to the therapeutic pass. The proper use of therapeutic passes in relation to the patient's treatment plan may prevent premature discharge and the necessity of a readmission to continue treatment.

Behavior modification programs based on point systems, token economies, and/or level systems are becoming popular in the treatment of adolescent patients. These programs are usually very specific in relation to the patient's behavior and progress in the program. The patient's record should document the patient's progress within the program and in relation to his illness.

Patient's rights are becoming an important issue in the treatment of mental health patients. It is extremely important that the patient's mental health record document any denials of patient's rights. Documentation should include the "good cause" for denial and the restoration of the right(s) when good cause no longer exists.

The health information practitioner needs to be aware of any state laws which may place further constraints on the use of these special procedures, and state requirements for consents and other documentation. The mental health code of a particular state is usually a good source for this type of information.

RECORD DOCUMENTATION

Problem-oriented, goal-oriented, source-oriented, or a combination of one or more of these documentation systems may

---

3-11 Shift: Patient attended all activities throughout shift. Behavior was appropriate and she appeared in good spirits. She appeared sullen and sat alone in the corner of the patient lounge following the multifamily group. She did not interact with the other patients in the discussion of the TV show being watched and appeared to be reading a magazine instead. At 11 P.M. the patient was observed scratching at right wrist with a staple. She refused to talk about it at first, but then admitted she was "angry with my mom because she didn't show up for family group—I hate her." Scratches are superficial, area cleansed and doctor notified. Patient is on close observation with 15-min. checks and staff is working with her on discussing feelings rather than acting them out.

FIGURE 5. SOURCE-ORIENTED (NARRATIVE) PROGRESS NOTE

be useful in mental health facilities. Source-oriented is probably the least favorable of the three. In the source-oriented record, information relevant to any one of a patient's problems, or goals, is scattered at random in admission notes, social histories, progress notes, nurses' notes, or in x-ray and laboratory reports. The record becomes bulky, is unorganized, and, as a result, retrieval of vital information is both difficult and frustrating. Communication among treatment team members is hampered, and ultimately patient care is negatively affected.

In a goal-oriented and problem-oriented approach, problems are identified and numbered. Treatment plans identify the problems by number, and specific goals are decided upon. Plans of action for each of the problems are established and related to the various disciplines. This allows members of the multidisciplinary team to document in relation to problems, goals, or both. In mental health, documentation related to the

---

Example B. Same as Example A but incorporating steps in treament plan.

3-12-85   Goal #2: Dealing with angry feelings.

Observations (O): Joe related in group how he used anger to distance himself from others. He said that he could never talk with his parents as they never listened to him, and this made him feel helpless. "Lashing out" then made him feel better. Joe stated he is willing to work this out in group therapy.

Plan (P): Joe will undergo the "insult-compliment" exercise in the next group psychotherapy session and will give group members feedback on this experience.

3-19-85   G: Dealing with angry feelings.

O: Joe has shared with the group members his historical and current pattern in dealing with anger. He is able to apply his insights in the group and appears to be trying out new behaviors regarding the expressions of his negative emotions. Group members gave him very supportive and insightful feedback. While somewhat defensive initially, Joe heard and responded well to feedback.

P: Joe will relate at least five negative emotions to various group members relative to group members' behavior by 3-26-85.

FIGURE 6. GOAL-ORIENTED PROGRESS NOTES

patient's strengths, program participation, and daily functioning are important in assessing the patient's need for continued treatment, the effectiveness of the treatment plan, and the progress of treatment. All members of the team participate in monitoring and documenting the patient's progress in treatment plans and progress notes. It is important for the record to document the patient's response to treatment in relation to the various disciplines involved. Patients may be responding in one area and not another. Examples of the various documentation systems are provided in Figures 5, 6, 7, and 8.

Example A: Simple Format

3-12-85   Goal #2: Will deal more effectively with angry feelings and upsettings emotions.

Movement Toward Goal (MTG): Joe related in group how he used anger to distance himself from others. He said that he could never talk to his parents as they never listened to him, and this made him feel helpless. "Lashing out" then made him feel better. Joe stated he is willing to work on this in group therapy.

3-18-89   Goal #2: Dealing with angry feelings

MTG: Joe has shared with the other group members his historical and current pattern in dealing with anger. He is able to apply his insights in the group and appears to be trying out new behaviors regarding the expressions of his negative emotions. Group members gave him very supportive and insightful feedback. While somewhat defensive initialy, Joe heard and responded well to the feedback.

FIGURE 7. GOAL-ORIENTED PROGRESS NOTES

REVIEW PROCESS

ONGOING QUANTITATIVE AND QUALITATIVE ANALYSIS

The health information practitioner should assume responsibility for review of patient records. In an inpatient acute care psychiatric facility, this review should be conducted at least weekly while the patient is hospitalized. In an outpatient or partial-day program, this review should be conducted at least monthly. In a residential or long term psychiatric setting, this review should be conducted monthly. A final review should take place within one working day of the patient's discharge. The focus of review is on quantity, timeliness, and quality of clinical documentation.

The health information practitioner should develop a form to assist in the review process. The form should list all items that are to be checked. When in the process of developing the list, refer to the facility's medical staff bylaws, rules, and regulations; the Joint Commission standards under which the facility is accredited; and the *Medicare Conditions of Participation* for mental health record documentation requirements. The state's mental health code should also be consulted.

Part of the patient record review process includes the coding of diagnoses and procedures and the maintenance of an indexing system for location of patient records by diagnosis and

---

Problem #1: Self-Mutilative Behavior

S: "I don't want to talk about it— leave me alone."

O: Observed to be scratching at R. wrist with staple from magazine at 11 P.M. Three superficial 1-inch scratches on inner aspect of R. wrist with little bleeding. Area cleansed with soap and water. Patient affect: angry and sullen and refused to discuss incident. After 15 minutes 1:1 was able to state anger that mother did not show up for multifamily group tonight. Talked about being let down by mother and was able to contract that she would notify staff if she felt upset again.

A: Angry and hurt at mother. Feels that she doesn't get enough attention from mother and that mother doesn't care about her. Acting out rage by hurting self. Does not appear to be actively suicidal at present. Continues to show poor impulse control and difficulty expressing self with words.

P: Avoid secondary gains for scratching behavior. Matter-of-fact approach. Focus her to discuss what she was feeling before incident. Reinforce self-disclosure. 15-min. checks. Watch for infection and keep scratches clean.

FIGURE 8. PROBLEM-ORIENTED PROGRESS NOTES

procedure. While the *Diagnostic and Statistical Manual of Mental Health Disorders (DSM-III-R)* is used extensively by mental health practitioners to describe mental health disorders, coding may also need to be done using the *International Classification of Diseases* (ICD-9-CM) for reimbursement. Chapter 12 provides a full description of DSM-III-R and its compatibility with ICD-9-CM.

QUALITY MANAGEMENT

Quality management is a process of monitoring and evaluating that focuses on quality of care issues in the health care facility. The Joint Commission's process involves:

- the identification of the most important aspects of the care the organization provides;
- the use of indicators to systematically monitor these aspects of care in an ongoing way;
- the evaluation of care when monitoring raises suspicions about its quality or appropriateness, in order to identify problems or opportunities to further improve care; and
- the taking of actions to resolve problems or improve care, and evaluation of their effectiveness.

In mental health care facilities several types of quality assurance reviews should be performed. The Joint Commission requires:

- evaluation of the use of special treatment procedures;
- review of the use of unusual or experimental drugs;
- medication usage review, including the review of medication records, adverse reactions, and medication errors;
- review of patient care incidents.

The quality and appropriateness of patient care provided in the anesthesia, dental, dietetic, emergency, nursing, pathology, pharmacy, radiology, and rehabilitation services should also be monitored and evaluated.

The clinical performance of all individuals both with and without clinical privileges should be monitored and evaluated through:

- meetings of clinical services, departments, units, or teams to consider findings from ongoing monitoring activities of the professional staff;
- clinical supervision aspects of patient care monitoring;
- patient care evaluation; and
- professional staff peer review.

Relevant findings from these quality assurance activities are considered as part of:

- the reappraisal/reappointment of professional staff members;
- the renewal or revision of individual clinical privileges; and

- the mechanisms used to appraise the competence of all those practitioners who do not have clinical privileges.

The Joint Commission also requires the following organization functions to be reviewed:

- infection control;
- utilization review; and
- maintenance of the quality and content of mental health records.

While the Joint Commission delineates the basic process of quality assurance (see Chapter 16 for greater detail), implementation in a mental health facility requires some special adaptations. Perhaps the most unique features are the fact that outcome indicators are generally behavioral and identifiable only in incremental steps over a long period of time. The American Psychiatric Association has developed behavioral indicators. These often must be applied differently in adult, adolescent, and child care. To obtain the full picture of behavioral care quality assurance often requires aftercare follow-up for a period of 18 months to two years.

Quality assurance, utilization review, and mental health record analysis are closely integrated. Concurrent analysis which reviews records against the multidisciplinary team's treatment plan ensures not only a complete record on discharge, but the opportunity for quality and utilization intervention.

UTILIZATION REVIEW

Utilization review in mental health is a challenge because of concerns about confidentiality. The tendency of mental health professionals to limit clinical information in mental health records related to privileged communications makes it difficult for payers and their agents to understand what "value" they and beneficiaries are receiving in mental health care. Additional problems in assessing psychologic necessity of care result from frequently significant variations in utilization patterns among providers for the treatment of similar conditions and from the difficulty payers frequently have in either understanding or believing clinical documents. Many of these problems can be attributed to poor documentation, lack of qualified mental-health personnel evaluating care for payers, and inherent difficulties in analyzing the benefit value from claims data. Nevertheless, problems in assessing mental health care for reimbursement purposes remain the single greatest dilemma for payers.

The Joint Commission requirements for utilization review in mental health facilities require the review or the use of the organization's resources to identify underutilization, overutilization, and inefficient use of the organization's resources.

In a mental health facility Joint Commission requires monitoring that includes consideration of:

- the appropriateness and clinical necessity of admissions;
- continued stays in and discharge from an inpatient or residential program;
- continued treatment and/or rehabilitation;
- the appropriateness, clinical necessity, and timeliness of supportive services; and
- the utilization of staff, space, and, as indicated, other organizationwide resources.

The facility's utilization review process including written plan, criteria, and length-of-stay norms should be reviewed and evaluated at least annually and revised as necessary to reflect the findings from utilization review activities. Chapter 16 also provides information on utilization review.

RELEASE OF INFORMATION

The health information practitioner is responsible for the development of policies and procedures which safeguard the patient's right to privacy. The policies and procedures developed should specify the conditions under which information may be disclosed, who may release information under various circumstances, and the procedures for releasing information from the patient's mental health record.

The policies and procedures for the release of confidential patient information must take into consideration the applicable state laws; Joint Commission requirements, and if applicable, the federal regulations related to alcohol and drug abuse patients. It is recommended that all policies and procedures be developed to meet the most stringent laws or regulations which might apply to patient information within the facility. Policies and procedures which differ for different types of patients may make it possible to breach patient confidentiality simply by notifying a requestor that a more stringent requirement exists for a particular patient.

Federal regulations pertaining to the confidentiality of alcohol and drug abuse records are found in Title 42, Part 2 of the Federal Regulations. The Federal Regulations are very specific and stringent in regard to the release of confidential patient information.

CONSENTS

All consents for release of information are to be made part of the patient's record. The date the information was actually released, and the person who released the information should also be included in the record.

When developing policies and procedures for release of information and consent forms for the mental health facility, the health information practitioner should consult the mental health code of the state in which he practices. State requirements and/or state mental health requirements are sometimes beyond the standards of the Joint Commission and regulations of the federal government. It is also important to be familiar with which laws, rules, and regulations pertaining to the release of confidential patient medical records exempt psychiatric and/or substance abuse records.

Many states have developed laws related to access to the mental health record by the patient or authorized representative. It is important that these laws be carefully reviewed to determine the extent to which they apply to psychiatric and/or substance abuse records. Specific policies and procedures should be developed for implementing patient access requirements to psychiatric and substance abuse records or portions of general acute records that include psychiatric or substance abuse information.

In addition to written procedures for release of information, the health information practitioner is responsible for the security of mental health records. Policies should be developed indicating who, within the facility, has access to records and under what conditions access is allowed. For example, there should be a policy which states that only those members of the treatment team involved in the care and treatment of the patient have access to the patient's mental health records.

Records should be stored in secured filing areas. When records are removed from the files, a referencing system should permit location of the mental health record at any time. Records removed from the files should be removed only to other secured areas or should be returned to the permanent file area at the end of each day.

The Joint Commission requires that mental health records be retained at least five years from the date the case is officially closed. However, the health information practitioner should also check the state mental health code for state record-retention requirements. For example, some states require that records be kept for a specified number of years after competency has been established, and most states require that the records of minors be kept at least one year after a minor has reached the age of majority.

In Chapter 15 the contents of a valid consent form for the release of medical information are delineated.

SUMMARY

There have been profound changes taking place in the care of the mentally ill, especially in the last two decades. New treatment methods require fresh approaches to clinical record documentation. Psychiatric hospitals face continued pressure to cut costs while continuing to provide quality care. More and more third-party payers, surveying agencies, and other patient care reviewers are demanding access to patient information.

Health information practitioners practicing in mental health facilities have the opportunity to apply their skills in meeting these new challenges and to develop more efficient ways of documenting mental health care.

STUDY QUESTIONS

1. What are the minimum data requirements for mental health records?
2. What elements are included in the complete assessment of the mental health patient?
3. What are the elements of an individualized treatment plan? How frequently is documentation required?

4. When a patient is placed in seclusion, what data must be recorded in the patient's record?

5. Explain the difference between source-oriented, problem-oriented, and goal-oriented documentation.

6. What is the focus of record review of mental health records? What is the frequency of review in the various settings?

7. What does the Joint Commission require for a consent to be valid in a mental health facility? How does this differ from the Federal Regulations for alcohol and drug abuse patients?

REFERENCES

Confidentiality for Alcohol and Drug Abuse Records, Title 42, Part 2 of the Federal Regulations.

Individual Treatment Planning for Psychiatric Patients, (National Institutes of Mental Health, 1978).

Joint Commission on Accreditation of Healthcare Organizations, *Accreditation Manual for Hospitals*, (Chicago: Joint Commission, 1993).

Joint Commission on Accreditation of Healthcare Organizations, *Accreditation Manual for Mental Health, Chemical Dependency, and Mental Retardation/Developmental Disabilities Services (MHM)*, (Chicago: Joint Commission, 1993).

Stricker, George and Alex R. Rodriguez, Ed., *Handbook of Quality Assurance in Mental Health*, (New York: Plenum Press, 1988).

Topics in Health Record Management: Mental Health Records, (Gaithersburg, MD: Aspen Systems Corporation, 1985).

chapter **6**

MANAGEMENT OF MEDICAL
RECORD CONTENT

The medical record is the permanent, legal document which must contain sufficient information to identify the patient, justify the diagnosis and treatment, and record the results. But because documentation in the medical record is performed by a variety of health care providers — physicians, nurses, therapists, and others — and because it is performed as a secondary activity following the rendering of patient care, documentation may not always be as accurate or complete as necessary and desirable. A busy physician may inadvertently record a progress note in the wrong patient's medical record; a nurse may get a call to assist a patient and forget to record a medication given. Regular analysis of the documentation in the medical record should be performed to manage the content of the medical record so it fulfills its purposes of communicating patient care information; of serving as evidence of the patient's course of illness and treatment for various legal, reimbursement, and peer evaluation reviews; and of furnishing clinical data for administrative, research, and educational activities.

A health care facility's medical staff relies on health information practitioners to analyze medical record documentation and notify them of omissions or inconsistencies which make the medical record incomplete or inaccurate. Different types of reviews may be done at different times relative to the patient's occasion of service. Each health care facility decides on the type or types of analyses to be done according to their documentation needs and medical staff policies.

TYPES OF MEDICAL RECORD DOCUMENTATION ANALYSES

There are three types of health information documentation analyses. They are quantitative analysis, qualitative analysis, and statistical analysis. Each is defined briefly in this overview. Quantitative and qualitative analyses are described in detail in the remainder of the chapter.

Quantitative analysis is performed by health information practitioners to identify areas of the medical record that are incomplete, such as a missing pathology report of tissue removed during surgery. In quantitative analysis a list of recording requirements is often used to identify deficiencies in medical record documentation. For example, the list could include "all entries must be dated and signed," and "all tissues removed during surgery must have a pathology report."

Qualitative analysis is the identification of inconsistent or inaccurate documentation. In qualitative analysis the health information staff applies knowledge of disease processes, the policies and standards established by the health care facility's administration and medical staff, and various licensing, accrediting, and certifying agency standards to review medical record documentation. For instance, during qualitative analysis it might be noted that a complication has not been recorded on the face sheet or that the terms left and right have been interchanged. The health care provider, however, makes the final decision that documentation is incomplete or inaccurate, and follows hospital policy to make the necessary additions or corrections. Qualitative analysis may also identify patterns in documentation where additions or corrections to specific medical records are not appropriate, but where improvements could be made through redesign of forms, educational activities, or other methods. Noting that one physician consistently fails to record a discharge progress note may be an example of such a pattern. This might be corrected by pointing out that the physician may be denied reimbursement for the visit to the patient on that day. Figure 1 summarizes the characteristics of quantitative and qualitative analyses.

CHARACTERISTICS OF MEDICAL RECORD DOCUMENTATION ANALYSES

QUANTITATIVE ANALYSIS

- Identifies obvious areas that are incomplete or inaccurate.
- Uses a prescribed list of recording requirements.
- Applies knowledge of medical record content to the analysis.
- Performed by a person trained on the job.
- Result is a list of deficiencies which can be completed by the health care provider in the normal course of facility procedures.

QUALITATIVE ANALYSIS

- Identifies inconsistencies and omissions that may potentially be incomplete or inaccurate.
- Performed by application of general principles of documentation and/or specific criteria.
- Applies knowledge of medical record content, disease process, and policies and standards established by the facility administration and medical staff, and various licensing, accrediting, and certifying agencies to the analysis.
- Performed by credentialed medical record practitioner.
- Results include:

  1. A list of deficiencies which can be completed by the health care provider in the normal course of facility procedures.

  2. Identification of patterns of poor documentation practices for which improvement should be sought through individual discussion, referral to quality assurance program, or by educational means.

  3. Identification of potentially compensable events to be reported to the facility's risk management, quality assurance program, or legal counsel, as applicable, for further review.

FIGURE 1. MEDICAL RECORD DOCUMENTATION ANALYSIS

Quantitative and qualitative analyses should be distinguished from clinical quality reviews. Quantitative and qualitative analyses are reviews of documentation in medical records designed to assist health care providers in improving their documentation. Quantitative and qualitative analyses result in completion of specific medical records by the health care provider and improved documentation practices. Clinical quality reviews, on the other hand, are performed by peer groups of health care providers to ensure the care delivered is of high quality. They use medical records as the documentation of the care, but their primary focus is on the care delivered, not on the way it was documented.

Statistical analysis entails abstracting data from medical records for administrative and clinical decision making. Diagnostic and procedural data are coded and can be used to retrieve specific medical records for research purposes or to define and evaluate the health care facility's case mix. A uniform set of data is also abstracted from the medical record and transmitted to the business office for billing purposes. Statistical analysis utilizes nomenclatures and classification systems, indexes and registers, and health care statistical methodology. These topics are discussed in greater detail in succeeding chapters.

The three types of analyses may be performed concurrently with the patient's occasion of service and/or retrospectively after the occasion of service has ended. In hospitals, analyses have traditionally been performed in the health information department retrospectively upon termination of the hospitalization. This affords an opportunity to review the medical record as a whole, although it delays the completion or correction of documentation. In order to ensure that quality care is provided within the hospital's resources, concurrent analysis, performed on the nurses' station to identify omissions or discrepancies quickly before they are compounded or misinterpreted, is used in some hospitals.

In order to implement concurrent analysis, the health care facility should evaluate the costs and benefits. Concurrent analysis may require additional personnel and materials. Additional space on the nursing units may be required.On the other hand, concurrent analysis which improves medical record completion rates and thus improves flow of information to the business office, can improve cash flow. Other benefits, such as improved utilization of resources, potentially improved patient care through timely and improved documentation, and decreased expenses in handling incomplete medical records, are less easy to quantify but are believed to accrue.

In long term care facilities, analyses have usually been performed during the patient's period of residency, although at monthly, semimonthly, and even quarterly intervals. Health information practitioners or other administrative staff are beginning to perform more frequent analyses with an eye toward improving care and utilization of the facility's resources.

Quantitative and qualitative analyses have rarely been performed by health information practitioners on ambulatory care records, although increased utilization of these services will increase the need for analyses of medical record documentation.

QUANTITATIVE ANALYSIS

Definition

Quantitative analysis is a review of prescribed areas of the medical record for identifying specific deficiencies. The prescribed areas are usually written in a procedure developed jointly by the facility's health information manager and health care providers in accordance with the facility's medical staff bylaws and administrative policies, and the standards of its licensing, accrediting, and certifying agencies. Each facility develops its own procedure, so there are many variations. For instance, in some facilities the procedure may describe a review of only physician documentation, because nurses, therapists, and other provider groups are rarely named as parties to malpractice suits and thus their deficiencies are not as significant as those of physicians Still other hospitals may look only for signatures and reports required by accrediting and licensing agencies. They may supplement that minimal review by regularly reviewing the documentation details of selected samples of records and presenting the data to appropriate medical staff groups.In facilities where nonphysician providers have been involved in malpractice suits, or where their documentation has been questioned in insurance audits or for other reasons, quantitative analysis may be performed on all documentation. Another common variation occurs in facilities with computerized medical information systems. Since access to a computer is by a personal identification method (code, key, or physical attribute), facilities with computer systems may not require a written signature for authentication; and, therefore, quantitative analysis would not include a check for signatures.

Purpose

The purpose of quantitative analysis is primarily to identify obvious and routine omissions that can be easily corrected in the normal course of the hospital's procedures. This procedure makes the medical record more complete for reference in continuing patient care; for protecting the legal interests of the patient, physician, and hospital; and for meeting licensing, accrediting, and certifying requirements.

Results

Quantitative analysis identifies specific deficiencies. These deficiencies should be completed by the health care provider within a short time of their identification. The medical staff bylaws specify a time frame for completion of medical records, in accordance with licensing, accrediting, and certifying agency requirements.

Components of Quantitative Analysis

The basic components of quantitative analysis include a review of the medical record for:

1. correct patient identification on every form,

2. presence of all necessary reports,

3. required authentication on all entries, and

4. good recording practices.

Review for Identification

Whether performed concurrently or retrospectively, quantitative analysis usually begins with the checking of each page of the medical record, for the patient's identification — at least the patient's name and medical record number. If a page is missing identification, the page should be reviewed to determine if it belongs to the patient whose medical record is being analyzed and identification recorded. An advantage of performing quantitative analysis concurrently is that pages with missing identification may be more easily identified.

Review for Necessary Reports

There are certain reports that are common to all medical records in a given facility. For example, in a hospital the reports of the medical history, physical examination, clinical observations (progress notes), and conclusions at termination of hospitalization (clinical resume and statement of final diagnoses and procedures) are common. Other reports are necessary depending on the patient's course in the hospital. If the patient had diagnostic tests, consultations, or surgery, reports of these procedures are required. The procedure for quantitative analysis should specify which reports to check for, at what times, and under what circumstances. For instance, if a history and physical examination have not been performed within 24 hours of admission, this deficiency should be identified on concurrent analysis. If a physician dictates operative reports, and the report for a particular surgery is missing upon retrospective analysis, this is identified as a deficiency. It should be noted, however, that if a report of an action is missing because the action was not done, the report cannot be considered a deficiency that the health provider can add to the medical record. For instance, if there is no physician progress note on a given day because the physician did not visit the patient on that day, the physician should not be asked to write a progress note.

Review for Authentication

Quantitative analysis also ensures that prescribed entries are authenticated. Authentication may be a signature, rubber stamp in sole possession of the owner, initials if identifiable within the medical record, or computer access code or key; and should include the professional title (MD, RN, etc.) of the author. An entry should not be signed by someone other than the author, although the facility may require countersignature of entries made by house staff and students to demonstrate supervision by qualified professionals. Where countersignature is required, both the signature of the author and supervising professional should be included, as well as a note regarding the review of the entry, such as "reviewed," "concur with," or "carry out orders as noted."

Review for Recording Practices

Entries should also follow good recording practices. While quantitative analysis cannot solve problems of illegibility or incomplete content, it can aid in noting where entries are not dated, where errors have not been appropriately corrected, where there are skipped spaces that should be lined through to prevent subsequent tampering - particularly in progress notes and physician orders and where abbreviations have been used in the statement of final diagnoses and procedures. Error correction is a particularly important aspect of documentation. Alterations can easily raise questions of authenticity and negligence. When it is necessary to correct an error (such as when the health care provider has written in the wrong patient's medical record), the health care provider should be advised to draw a single line through each line of the error, add a note explaining the error (such as "wrong patient's medical record"), date and initial it, and then make the correct entry in chronological order indicating which entry it is replacing. If there is any doubt as to the subsequent admissability of the entry, it is a good practice to have a professional colleague witness the correction process.

By ensuring that all forms are present in the correct arrangement and that all entries are authenticated and reflect minimum standards of good recording practices, quantitative analysis is an important part of improving the accuracy and completeness of medical records.

QUALITATIVE ANALYSIS

Definition

Qualitative analysis is a review of the content of medical record entries for inconsistencies and omissions which may signify that the medical record is inaccurate or incomplete. Such an analysis requires knowledge of medical terminology, anatomy and physiology, fundamentals of disease processes, medical record content, and the standards of licensing, accrediting, and certifying agencies. It is usually performed by a credentialed health information practitioner.

Purpose

As is true of quantitative analysis, qualitative analysis is performed to make the medical record complete for reference in patient care, protect legal interests, meet regulatory requirements, and for accurate data and statistical analysis. Because it is more in-depth than quantitative analysis, however, it serves these purposes more fully, and it also contributes background or supporting information for quality and risk management activities. Qualitative analysis also assists in diagnosis and procedure-coding specificity and sequencing which are important for ongoing medical research, administrative studies, and reimbursement.

Results

Qualitative analysis may result in the identification of correctable deficiencies, patterns of poor documentation, and potentially compensable events. Many of the findings of qualitative analysis are deficiencies in specific medical record entries which the health care provider can correct. For example, an ophthalmologist may identify a cataract and its extraction as the final diagnosis and operation on the face sheet of a medical record. Upon qualitative analysis the history and physical examination report and the progress notes may reveal that the patient is being treated for insulin-dependent diabetes. The physician should be requested to list this condition on the face sheet.

Some inconsistencies or omissions in documentation, however, cannot be verified after the fact, and, therefore, cannot be corrected. These represent poor documentation practices which hopefully, upon identification, can be improved in subsequent documentation. For instance, in performing a physical examination, a physician may actually examine every body system but may record information about only those systems which are abnormal. This practice may result in no direct harm to any patient. However, there may be a time when the medical record is used as evidence in court, and the physician may be questioned about the evaluation and normalcy of those body systems about which there is no documentation.

Inconsistencies or omissions in documentation may also reflect actual patient care practice problems which are potentially compensable events - an occurrence that has resulted in harm to the patient and that may possibly expose the facility and/or provider to professional or general liability claims and may require the facility and/or provider to pay damages to the person harmed. In a classic case, the physician ordered "watch condition of toes" of a young patient with a fractured tibia, omission of entries reflected lack of observation. A suit for negligence followed when irreversible ischemia required amputation.

Where qualitative analysis identifies patterns of poor documentation or potentially compensable events, neither of which can be corrected after the fact, the documenting health care provider should be made aware of the faulty documentation and offered assistance or suggestions for future improvement. It should never be suggested that the documentation be rewritten, as such entries are alterations and will not stand up under scrutiny. In all cases, raising the issue of improving documentation practices with a health care provider must be done with diplomacy. The effectiveness of constructive criticism frequently depends on the rapport the health information practitioner has with the health care provider. It may be necessary for the health care provider to perform a self-evaluation or to participate in a peer review of documentation so poor practices can be discovered by the offender or by peers. Providing educational reminders of good documentation practices or exhibiting classic instances of poor documentation and its results may also be helpful in improving documentation.

Components of Qualitative Analysis

Qualitative analysis may be performed "free-style" by applying the general principles of good documentation to the review of the medical record content, or a set of documentation criteria may be developed and applied. Using criteria is more objective and provides written backup, especially for detecting patterns of poor documentation. The components of qualitative analysis include a review of the medical record content (assuming the completion of quantitative analysis) for:

1. complete and consistent recording of diagnostic statements,

2. consistency in entries by all health care providers,

3. description and justification for the course of the patient's hospitalization,

4. recording of all necessary instances of informed consent,

5. application of good documentation practices, and

6. occurrence of a potentially compensable event.

Review for Complete and Consistent Diagnostic Statements

Diagnostic statements will be made throughout the medical record, each reflecting the level of understanding of the patient's medical condition at the time it is recorded. For example, upon admission to a hospital there should be an admitting diagnosis stating the reason for admission. The history and physical examination should document an impression or provisional diagnosis which generally must be confirmed through additional diagnostic studies. In certain cases, the impression or provisional diagnosis cannot be narrowed down to one diagnosis, but rather several possible diagnoses with similar symptoms must be further evaluated. This comparison is called a differential diagnosis, and frequently is stated as "rule out (one or more diagnoses)," or "(diagnosis 1) versus (diagnosis 2)." Prior to surgery, a preoperative diagnosis should be recorded in a preoperative progress note. This diagnosis is a statement of the reason for surgery or the expected findings upon surgery. A postoperative diagnosis, recorded in a postoperative progress note, states the clinical findings of the surgery. Both preoperative and postoperative diagnoses should be included in the operative report. A great difference in these diagnoses may be suggestive of inadequate diagnostic workup or other issues related to quality of care. A pathological diagnosis may be required to provide a definitive postoperative diagnosis. A pathological diagnosis is a description of the morphology, or cellular characteristics, of the tissue removed during surgery; whereas a clinical diagnosis describes the etiology (cause) and/or abnormal functioning of an organ or system, or the body as a whole.

Upon termination of the hospitalization, all final (clinical) diagnoses and procedures should be stated on the face sheet or in the discharge summary. The analyst should check this list to determine that it is complete, consistent with documentation, and in correct sequence. The final diagnoses will include the principal diagnosis, any complications, and those comorbidities affecting the hospitalization. The principal diagnosis must be carefully distinguished because of reimbursement reporting requirements. The *Uniform Hospital Discharge Data Set* (UHDDS), which establishes definitions for official hospital reporting, defines the principal diagnosis as "that condition established after study to be chiefly responsible for occasioning the admission of the patient to the hospital for care."

Secondary diagnoses are complications and/or comorbidities. A complication is a condition arising during the hospitalization that modifies the course of the patient's illness or the medical care required. Some complications include decubitus ulcer, post-operative hemorrhage, adverse reactions to medications, hospital acquired infections, neurological deficits, surgical emphysema, and injuries (perforations and punctures during surgery, falls, etc.). A comorbidity is a condition existing at the time of hospitalization which has potential for affecting the course of illness or medical care provided. Comorbidities are active conditions for which the patient is receiving treatment or being monitored, such as insulin-dependent diabetes mellitus or hypertension. Comorbidities may include personal history of illness or "status post" conditions when these factors influence the patient's condition. For example, if the patient previously had carcinoma of the breast, "history of carcinoma of the breast" may be listed as a comorbid condition, as the potential for recurrence must always be evaluated. "Status post cardiac bypass surgery" is an example of a condition that should also be listed.

The Uniform Hospital Discharge Data Set refers to secondary diagnoses as "other diagnoses." The UHDDS definition for other diagnoses is "all conditions that co-exist at the time of admission, that develop subsequently, or that affect the treatment received and/or length of stay. Diagnoses that relate to an earlier episode which have no bearing on the current hospital stay are to be excluded."

Procedures need to be listed completely. Each health care facility should specifically identify procedures which are to be recorded on the admission/discharge record and/or discharge summary. Some health care facilities require physicians to record only procedures performed in the operating room (OR). Other health care facilities require physicians to delineate, in addition, procedures such as bone marrow biopsies, cardiac catheterizations, blood transfusions, and CAT scans. As a minimum, most health care facilities require that all procedures influencing reimbursement be listed. For the Medicare prospective payment system, lists of "OR" and "non-OR" procedures have been issued.

When procedures are listed they should also be sequenced with the principal procedure first as clearly identified. The principal procedure is "one which is performed for definitive treatment rather than one performed for diagnostic or exploratory purposes, or was necessary to take care of a complication."

In the July 31, 1985, *Federal Register*, the federal government gave this additional advice on reporting procedures:

- All significant procedures are to be reported. A significant procedure is surgical in nature, or carries a procedural risk, or carries an anesthetic risk, or requires specialty training.

- When more than one procedure is reported, the principal procedure is to be designated. If there appear to be two procedures that are principal, then the one most related to the principal diagnosis should be selected.

Review for Entry Consistency

Qualitative analysis includes a review of medical record entries for consistency. Consistency refers to agreement or harmony of parts one to another and to a whole. As has already been mentioned, diagnostic statements in a hospital should be consistent from admission through discharge. Documentation should reflect progressively more information about the condition for which the patient was admitted. In an ambulatory care facility diagnostic statements should also be consistent across visits for a given problem. In an initial visit the physician may report only a symptom or abnormal result of a diagnostic study. After subsequent visits the diagnosis should emerge. Diagnostic statements should also demonstrate consistency among parts of the medical record. In a hospital or ambulatory surgery center the operative report, tissue report, results of diagnostic studies, and consent forms should be consistent. Differences here usually reflect poor documentation practices.

Other entries should also reflect consistency. Three common areas where inconsistencies can result in miscommunication of patient care information are progress notes written by different members of the health care team; orders, medication records, and progress notes not matching; and admitting and discharge information recorded by different health care personnel. For instance, a nurse's progress note may indicate that the patient spiked a fever, while the physician may indicate patient was afebrile. Such inconsistency leaves open to question whether or not the physician evaluated the condition and decided to take no action.

Review for Description and Justification of Course of Treatment

In addition to consistency, the medical record as a whole should also display specificity and thought processes. The medical record must describe and justify the course of the patient's hospitalization. The medical record, therefore, must document results of diagnostic studies, treatment, patient education, and patient location fully. "Test results normal," "patient doing well," and "patient given instructions" are examples of generalizations which describe nothing. The medical record should also display thought processes - the reasoning that leads to each decision, even if the decision is to take no action (as might have been the case in the previous example of the fever). This is especially important when there is a change in treatment plan. Not only should the alternate treatment be described, but the purpose for the new treatment, modification, or discontinuance should also be explained.

Review for Recording Informed Consent

Information regarding patient consent for treatment should be carefully delineated. The physician should carefully record the information provided to the patient to enable the patient to give an informed consent or to withhold consent. Each health care facility has a policy consistent with legal requirements on informed consent. The health information practitioner must know this policy and apply it when performing qualitative analysis. Physicians should be encouraged to not merely comply with the policy, but to take care in recording all instances of informed consent, such as describing of possible side effects from medication when its administration does not normally require completion of a special "consent form."

Review for Documentation Practices

Other characteristics of documentation which are qualitatively analyzed include evidence of timely recording of entries, legibility, use of approved abbreviations throughout the content, and avoidance of extraneous remarks. The medical record should contain no unexplained time gaps. This is especially important in emergency situations where not only is there a tendency to document less due to lack of time, but increased risk for error and subsequent scrutiny of entries for malpractice. Legibility refers to penmanship, use of ink for permanence of recording, and the careful completion of forms. Illegible entries and those with abbreviations not on the list of medical staff approved abbreviations are useless. Finally, while the medical record should reflect honest and candid statements, these should be recorded with caution. The medical record should never contain derogatory or critical comments. In the event such a comment is made, the author should either elect to let it stand, being aware of possible legal consequences, or treat it as an error (see previous discussion on error correction).

Review for Potentially Compensable Events

Finally, qualitative analysis should identify any potentially compensable events. Figure 2 displays a sample of some criteria which may be used in identifying potentially compensable events. The concept of identifying and analyzing "nonspecific clinical occurrences" originated with InterQual Incorporated, a consulting firm to health care providers, when consulting for the California Medical Insurance Feasibility Study (CMIF). The medical record should fully document an occurrence of harm to the patient.

INCOMPLETE MEDICAL RECORD CONTROL

The result of quantitative and qualitative analysis is the identification of specific deficiencies, patterns of poor documentation, and potentially compensable events.

Incomplete/Delinquent Medical Records

Medical records with specific deficiencies that can be completed by a health care provider are termed incomplete medical records. Health care providers are notified they have incomplete medical records and are expected to complete them within a time specified in the medical staff bylaws. When an incomplete medical record has remained incomplete after the defined time for completion has expired, the incomplete medical record is referred to as a delinquent medical record. Frequently, health care facilities determine and monitor their "incomplete medical

SAMPLE CRITERIA FOR IDENTIFYING POTENTIALLY COMPENSABLE EVENTS UPON QUALITATIVE ANALYSIS

Medical Record No.: _____   Analyst: _____   Page 3 of 4

	YES	NO	DEFICIENCY/PROBLEM DESCRIPTION
QUALITATIVE ANALYSIS — SCREENING CRITERIA, CONT.			
Does the medical record contain appropriately signed authorizations and consents?			
a. For routine treatment			
b. For surgical procedures/hazardous treatment			
QUALITATIVE ANALYSIS — POTENTIALLY COMPENSABLE EVENTS			
Is this admission for complication or incomplete management of problem on previous admission to this hospital?			
Was there an unexplained transfer from a general care unit to a special care unit during this admission?			
Is there an infection not present on admission?			
Is there a neurological deficit present at discharge which was not present on admission?			
Did the patient suffer cardiac or respiratory arrest during this admission?			
Was the patient transferred to another acute care facility except for administrative reasons?			
Was a procedure cancelled or repeated due to improper preparation of patient, technician error, or equipment failure?			

FIGURE 2. IDENTIFYING POTENTIALLY COMPENSABLE EVENTS

record rate" and their "delinquent medical record rate." The incomplete rate is the number of incomplete medical records over the number of discharges or other forms of patient care episodes during the required completion period. For example, if a hospital discharges 75 patients in the 30 days in which providers are given to complete their medical records, and 25 are incomplete, the incomplete rate for that period is 33 percent. The delinquent rate is calculated as the total number of delinquent medical records over the average number of discharges during a completion period. For example, if the hospital currently has 50 delinquent records in total, and it averages 75 discharges per period, its delinquent rate is 50 over 75 or 67 percent.

A delinquent rate of over 50 percent (representing more than a full period's discharges or episodes of patient care) is considered a serious problem. Of course, many factors influence how this rate is interpreted. If the incomplete rate is very high, one can expect a higher delinquent rate. The age of the delinquent medical records is also a factor. A 40 percent delinquent rate of medical records remaining incomplete for only two or three extra weeks may be more desirable than a delinquency rate of 20 percent representing medical records of several months delinquency. The type of delinquency is another factor. Delinquencies due to missing history and physical examination reports, operative reports, or signatures on attestation statements are more serious than delinquencies due to missing discharge summaries or signatures on progress notes. The completion period also affects the delinquency rate, especially when comparing rates across facilities.

Deficiency Notification

Health care providers need to know they have incomplete medical records and what deficiencies they contain. When concurrent analysis identifies deficiencies, they can be noted directly on the medical record commonly by a form inserted within the medical record, adhesive tape or rubber stamp placed on the cover, a removable sticker placed directly on the medical record form containing the deficiency, or a combination of these techniques. The next time the provider documents in the record, it is expected the deficiency will be corrected. When retrospective analysis is performed, or when deficiencies remain from concurrent analysis upon discharge, health care facilities have different ways of getting medical records completed. In some facilities health care providers are expected to routinely visit the health information department to attend to record deficiencies. In other facilities, providers may be notified in writing that they have incomplete medical records and asked to visit the health information department; or, in other facilities, providers may request the records be brought to a specified location within the facility. Such notification may be a copy of the deficiency form or may be a standard notification announcement. In still other facilities, incomplete medical records may be held on the nursing station until they are completed; or they may be routinely brought to the provider's office within the facility. Medical records should not be removed from the facility for completion, for they must be available for any emergency care required by the patient and for other purposes.

When performing retrospective analysis, specific deficiencies may be noted on the same type of form, tape, stamp, or sticker as described for concurrent identification of deficiencies. See Figure 3 for samples of such deficiency forms.

Filing of Incomplete Medical Records

When incomplete medical records are kept in the health information department, they may be filed in the permanent file, a separate incomplete file by provider name, or a separate incomplete file by medical record number. Each way has advantages and disadvantages. Filing incomplete medical records in permanent files makes them less accessible to providers but saves retrieval time if the medical records are very active. This arrangement may be most appropriate for hospitals with ambulatory care services to which patients return after discharge. The means of filing which is most accessible to providers is in a separate file by provider name. If multiple providers, such as the attending physician, surgeon, consultant, and respiratory therapist, have deficiencies on the same medical record, a cross-reference system must be established. Filing incomplete medical records in a separate file by number is a compromise between filing them in a permanent file and separately by provider name.

Computerized incomplete systems can be very helpful for controlling all aspects of incomplete medical records. Once specific deficiencies are input into the computer with the assis-

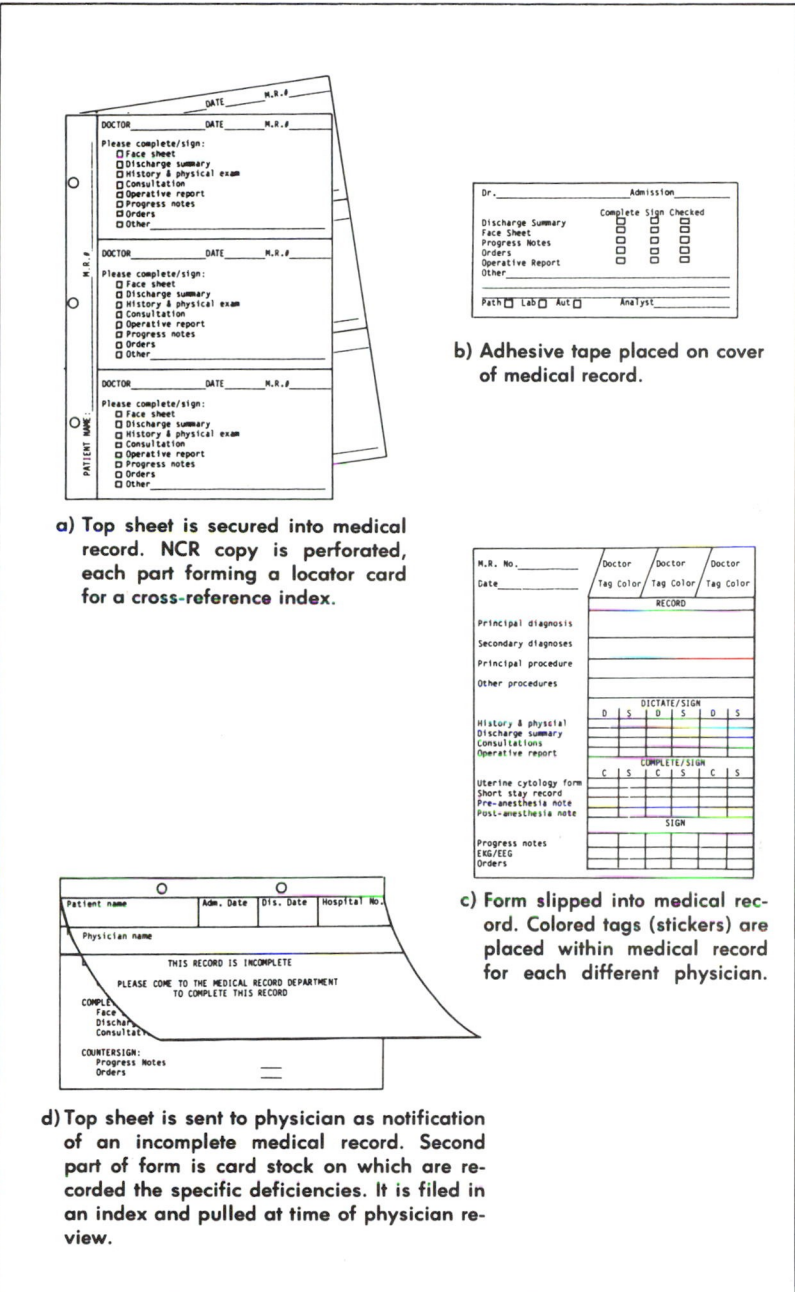

a) Top sheet is secured into medical record. NCR copy is perforated, each part forming a locator card for a cross-reference index.

b) Adhesive tape placed on cover of medical record.

c) Form slipped into medical record. Colored tags (stickers) are placed within medical record for each different physician.

d) Top sheet is sent to physician as notification of an incomplete medical record. Second part of form is card stock on which are recorded the specific deficiencies. It is filed in an index and pulled at time of physician review.

FIGURE 3. SAMPLE DEFICIENCY FORMS

tance of computer prompts, several outputs can be generated. For instance, a printed list of deficiencies can be generated. A series of notices of incomplete and delinquent medical records can be generated for the provider, as well as a composite list of provider's incomplete and delinquent records for department chairpersons. Statistics can also be computed, including not only the general incomplete and delinquent rates, but rates per provider, types of deficiencies, age of delinquent medical records, etc. The computer can also aid in medical record location, such as in situations where multiple providers have deficiencies on the same medical record.

Final Chart Check

When providers have worked on incomplete medical records, it is advisable to do a "final chart check," or "reanalysis" of these records to ensure that all deficiencies have been completed. It is extremely important that medical records be completed on a timely basis, for incomplete medical records affect the quality of patient care which can be rendered in a health care facility. Incomplete medical records also impact on the facility's licensure and accreditation status. For instance, the Joint Commission on Accreditation of Healthcare Organizations indicates that substantial, serious, or sustained medical record deficiencies or delinquencies may be the basis for a hospital receiving less than the maximum accreditation status. In the event that a medical record remains incomplete after a health care provider has terminated his or her association with the facility, the facility policy should be followed for filing the record as incomplete. Usually, the medical record committee will review the record and write a note to the effect that it could not be completed due to the resignation or death of the responsible provider.

HANDLING INFORMATION ON DOCUMENTATION PRACTICES AND POTENTIALLY COMPENSABLE EVENTS

When qualitative analysis identifies poor documentation which cannot be completed or corrected after the fact, the health information practitioner must be guided by the medical staff bylaws, hospital administration, and the AHIMA Code of

Ethics. Every situation may ultimately indicate a different action for solution. Frequently, patterns of poor documentation identify a need for more focused peer review by medical staff committees, including the medical record committee, tissue committee, quality management, etc. For instance, if it is noticed on qualitative analysis that a form for newborn physical exam reports routinely contains some omissions, it may be appropriate to advise the medical record committee to evaluate the form for possible revision. Another example occurs when it is noted that records completed by orthopedic and ophthalmology specialists rarely contain reports of gynecologic exams on female patients. Concerned that early signs of cancer may be going unnoticed, it could be recommended that the quality assurance program study this finding in more depth.

The provider may also be contacted directly about poor documentation practices. For instance, qualitative analysis may identify that one physician writes with an aqua-colored felt-tip pen which bleeds through the paper, obscuring the writing on the other side and not photocopying well. A sample may be shown to the provider and a request made to use another writing instrument.

General information about improving poor documentation practices may be distributed through a newsletter, bulletin board announcements, or in-service programs. For instance, information on sequencing of principal diagnoses and their impact on reimbursement may best be distributed by in-service programs. A newspaper clipping about a malpractice case in which poor documentation was a factor may be posted on a bulletin board or summarized in the facility's newsletter.

Finally, when a potentially compensable event has been identified, the facility's risk manager, quality assurance program, or legal counsel, as applicable, should be notified. Early identification and analyses of these events to determine whether there is liability potential can result in timely and prudent efforts to minimize potential losses.

In handling any information on poor documentation and potentially compensable events, it is extremely important to maintain the confidentiality of the information. This information is sensitive, and only those authorized to handle such information should be provided with the information. It may even be advisable to keep such records in a locked file, rather than in the general file area.

SUMMARY

The medical record contains pertinent information about each patient provided care at a health facility. The medical record must be written in a timely manner and contain sufficient information to identify the patient, support the diagnosis or reason for health care encounter, justify the treatment, and accurately document the results. Managing the content of the medical record through analysis of documentation is an important function of the health information department in all health care facilities. By reviewing all medical records during or following an occasion of service for completeness and accuracy, the health information practitioner makes a significant contribution to the health care facility. The nature of the analyses performed in a specific health care facility depends on the policies and needs of the facility's medical staff and administration and on the demands of the facility's licensing, accrediting, and certifying agencies. There are as many variations as there are facilities, for each adapts the general procedures outlined in this chapter to its own unique situation.

STUDY QUESTIONS

1. What is the major purpose of quantitative analysis, qualitative analysis, and statistical analysis?
2. What are the major differences between quantitative and qualitative analyses and quality assurance?
3. What are the advantages and disadvantages of concurrent and retrospective analyses?
4. How do analyses of medical record documentation differ among health care facilities?
5. What general characteristics of documentation does a person performing qualitative analysis look for in a medical record?
6. Distinguish between the following sets of terms:
    a. incomplete medical records/delinquent medical records

    b. deficiency/pattern of poor documentation/potentially compensable event.

7. Explain the various ways health care providers may be notified of incomplete medical records, be informed of deficiencies in specific medical records, and have access to incomplete medical records. Describe how computerization can aid the process.

REFERENCES

American Medical Record Association, *Glossary of Health Care Terms*, (Chicago, IL: AHIMA, 1994).

Berger, Elaine, et al., "Managing the Medical Record on a Concurrent Basis; Facts and Possibilities," *Journal of the American Medical Record Association*, (May, 1988 and June, 1988).

Care Communications, *The Record That Defends Its Friends*, (Chicago, IL: Care Communications, Inc., 1979).

Czecowski-Bruce, Jo Anne, *Privacy and Confidentiality of Health Care Information*, (Chicago, IL: American Hospital Publishing, Inc., 1984).

Federal Register, July 31, 1985, pages 31038-31040.

Flora, C. Rosalia, "Coordinating DRG Assignment Through Inpatient Record Analysis," *Journal of the American Medical Record Association*, (August, 1984).

Freeman, Tanya J., "Setting the Stage for Improved Record Content," *Journal of the American Medical Record Association*, (May, 1984).

InterQual, Inc., "Identifying and Analyzing Clinically-Related Occurrences," *InterQual, Inc.*, (Chicago, IL: InterQual, Inc., 1982).

Joint Commission on Accreditation of Healthcare Organizations, *Accreditation Manual for Hospitals*, (Chicago, IL: Joint Commission 1994).

Kessler, Paul, and Eric D. Joseph, *The Risk Management Primer*, (Chicago, IL: Care Communications, Inc., 1981).

Lee, Margaret P., "Concurrent Medical Record Analysis in a Community Hospital," *Journal of the American Medical Record Association*, (June, 1984).

Shlala, Thomas J., "Concurrent Chart Analysis and DRG Assignment in a Prospective Environment," *Journal of the American Medical Record Association*, (November, 1988).

"Seattle hospital streamlines record analysis with focused reviews for completeness," *Medical Records Briefing*, September 1992, pg 5-6.

chapter **7**

FORMS DESIGN AND CONTROL

Data are the lifeblood of health care facilities. Medical, financial, administrative, and operational data are essential. These data are frequently collected, processed, and/or presented to the user via forms. Inefficiencies in forms design, maintenance, and cost control may occur because of the large number of forms utilized by multiple users with differing needs. Poorly designed forms can result in inadequate data collection, laxity in documentation, erroneous information, duplication of effort, and mistakes. It has been estimated that an average 300-bed hospital spends as much as $700 annually per bed simply on the printing and storage of forms. Forms design and control systems are thus critical in ensuring that every form serves a desired purpose, only necessary forms are maintained, and all forms are readily available to users.

Every health care facility has the responsibility to provide forms to fit its needs. Neither the American Hospital Association nor the Joint Commission on Accreditation of Healthcare Organizations recommends any specific medical record or administrative forms. In some communities, several facilities have joined together and adopted basic medical record forms acceptable to the medical staffs of each facility. This is helpful to the physician who practices in more than one facility. The advent of computers has also made it easier for physicians and other health care providers as well as administrative staff to communicate data necessary to care for patients and carry out the business of the health care facility.

It is popularly believed that computers eliminate many paper forms. This is not necessarily the case, however. Paper forms are often used as an intermediary between the human communicator and the computer. These forms need to be carefully designed to ensure appropriate data collection and guidance for entering data into the computer. If users get the idea that paper forms are forbidden in an electronic environment, "home-grown" intermediate forms may be worse than no forms at all. Computers may also generate more paper than ever existed in the manual environment. Daily and cumulative reports of every conceivable type can result in a multiplicity of unused paper. Even where electronic information handling has created a near "paperless" environment, the environment is not "formless." Paper forms have only been replaced with touch-screens, "mouses," "windows," and other such technologies. In many cases this allows the user to become the forms designer. In such an environment, data element standardization programs, procedural guidelines, and input/output controls are required.

Many organizational patterns exist for forms management, especially as computerization has occurred. The health information practitioner may have full responsibility, or another individual designated as the forms manager may be responsible for managing the inventory, ordering, and stocking of paper forms, with an information systems manager responsible for computer input and output. Desktop publishing software for microcomputers allows virtually anyone to design professional appearing forms. Most health care facilities have a forms committee or subcommittee of the medical record committee which approves the design of forms for use in the medical record, and possibly for other uses. The health information practitioner assists this committee by making available the various requirements and statutes that may control the content of medical records. The health information practitioner is also familiar with the data requirements of various organizations and agencies. Understanding the flow of data and information throughout the health care facility ensures that forms or computer programs are designed to expedite communications. Knowledge of forms design and computer input/output techniques also makes the health information practitioner invaluable in this process.

Forms design and control, whether for paper construction or computer use, involves many factors. Forms design requires consideration of data elements, physical layout, user completion, paper, and printing. Forms control includes forms inventory, forms identification, ongoing review and revision, and purchasing.

FORMS DESIGN

A form should be designed to meet the purpose for which it is to be used. A primary consideration is whether the form is to be used to collect data or report information. Data are raw facts and figures. Information is data which have been processed in some meaningful and useful manner. Basic design rules include:

1. Study the purpose and use of the form and design it with the user in mind.

2. Design the form as simply as possible; omit unnecessary data or information.

3. Use standard terminology for all data elements, or provide definitions; label all information.

4. Include guidelines as necessary to ensure data collection or interpretation consistency.

5. Sequence data items logically, in relation to their source document or in the order of their capture; present information in a manner which captures the reader's attention.

Forms serve many purposes. Forms demand action. For example, they may require the obtaining of a signature, thumb print, or identification card imprint for authentication purposes. Data collection forms cause documentation to occur. Report forms demand a decision or identify a course of action. Forms also instruct the user what to do, what data must be gathered, where to obtain data, how to collect it, and what to do next. Forms fix responsibility and identify records for filing and future reference. Forms standardize, ensuring consistency in data collection and interpretation. Perhaps most importantly, forms communicate. For example, results of diagnostic studies are communicated from the laboratory to the physician, financial information is supplied to the chief executive officer from the finance office, and so forth. Because forms serve many purposes, each form must be designed to fulfill its purposes.

While forms ease work load by guiding and directing the user, forms can also add to work load. Forms that collect unnecessary data or are difficult to complete take time away from other activities. Forms that do not clearly and concisely present information take time to interpret or validate. Forms should be reviewed regularly to ensure that they are easy to use, serve to collect all data needed, eliminate collection of nonessential data, and present information in a meaningful manner.

Forms are often completed and used by many different people, so the terminology on the form should be known to all. Standard terminology should be used where it exists. For example, the Uniform Hospital Discharge Data Set (UHDDS) provides standard definitions for data commonly collected in hospitals. This data set is described in Chapter 11—Health Care Statistics. Other data sets exist as well. If a standard definition is not to be used or does not exist, the form should supply the definition. Even for commonly collected data it is important to provide guidance. For example, dates are commonly written in two-digit, month-day-year format in the U.S. In collecting birthdate information, however, it may be necessary to use four digits for the year. Abbreviations, codes, and contractions save space, but should be used only when their meaning is clear to all who must read the form. Since many forms in health care facilities have become "public," or open to inspection by licensing, accrediting and regulatory agencies, the courts, and patients or their representatives, abbreviations should be avoided.

Sequence of items on the form is another important consideration. Entry spaces in the body of a data collection form should be arranged so as to permit a continuous writing, typing or entry operation - from left to right and top to bottom. Numbering items makes reference easier and faster and also serves as a reference for detailed instructions. Data to be entered on the form should be grouped by related items whenever possible. If more than one person is responsible for completing a form, the data to be filled in by each individual should be grouped on the form according to the sequence of entries. Data on the form should also appear in the same order as similar items on other forms or records from which or to which data are transcribed, or in the same order as data are expected to be received, dictated, etc.

SPECIAL CONSIDERATIONS FOR PAPER FORMS DESIGN

Although design rules apply to both paper forms and computer data entry screens and reports, there are also differences to consider in the construction of forms for the two media. Five major components usually exist on paper forms. These are heading, introduction, instructions, body, and close.

1. Heading

The heading includes the title and information about the form. The title of a form may appear in one of several places. Standard positions are: top left, center, top right, left or right bottom. In a vertical card file, for example, the title should be placed at the bottom of the form to reserve the top portion for fill-in data. In a visible file, the title should be at the top so that pertinent control information can be seen at the bottom. A subtitle should be used when the main title needs further explanation or qualification. When forms are to be completed by or sent to persons outside the organization, the health care facility's name and address should be included in the title.

Other information about the form includes form identification, edition date, and page numbers. The lower-right margin is the best location for the form identification and edition date. In this location, tearing into or obliterating the information is avoided if the form is stapled in the upper left corner. Form identification is also visible if the forms are bound at the top or along the left side. Stocking of forms is also facilitated by having form identification at the bottom.

When a form consists of several separate pages or is back printed, the form identification should appear on each side and every page. In this way, if a photocopy of one side or one page is separated from the others, it can be easily identified. It also assists in the proper collation of forms with multiple pages.

The edition date or publication date should appear on each form. This assists the user in determining whether the current edition is being used and helps in the disposition of obsolete stock. The edition date usually appears next to the form number.

When there are multiple pages of a form, page numbers should be assigned. The page number can be in a numerical or alphabetical sequence. The page number can be placed in the upper-right corner or lower-right corner of the form. This will help the printer in assembling the materials for printing and in collating.

When designing a form which requires continuation sheets and the number of such pages is unknown to the user at the outset, each page should be provided with a space for page insertion, such as "Page_____of_____pages." The page number and total number of pages are entered in the blank spaces by the person completing the form.

2. Introduction

The introduction explains the purpose of the form. Sometimes the purpose is identified in the title. When further explanation is necessary, an explicit statement may be included on the form to explain its purpose.

3. Instructions

General instructions should be brief and placed at the top of the form. The user should be able to immediately determine how many copies are required; who should submit the form; and to whom copies should be sent. Instructions can be placed on the front of the form if there is enough space. If more detailed instructions are required, the reverse side of the form can be used; however, a reference to this should be included in the general instruction section. Lengthy instructions may also be placed on a separate sheet or in a separate booklet. Instructions may be provided as an administrative directive prescribed by the facility. Instructions should not be placed among entry spaces because that gives the form a cluttered appearance and hinders completion.

4. Body

The body is the part of the form that is devoted to the substantive work of the form. Careful consideration must be given to the arrangement of the data requested or information provided which includes proper grouping, sequencing, and aligning. Consideration must also be given to margins, spacing, rules, type styles, and recording method.

Margins - Margins add not only to a form's appearance and usefulness but to the ability to physically construct a form. Reproduction facilities require margins as working space for sprocket holes which permit the mechanical gripping of paper during the printing process, and for trimming the paper when several copies of a form are printed on large sheets. A minimum margin of 2/16 inch should be allowed at the top, 3/6 inch at the bottom, and 3/10 inch at the sides. If card stock is used, at least 1/8 inch should be allowed as margin on all sides. Obtain printer's specifications for margins when the image for a form is to extend to the edge of the paper or card. This process is called bleeding, and this style can result in increased handling costs.

Spacing - Spacing refers to the size of the data entry areas. When designing a form where the data will be entered with a typewriter, follow these guidelines:

Horizontal Spacing: Allow 1/12 inch for elite or 1/10 inch for pica type. 1/10 inch accommodates either elite or pica and allows for maximum entry space. Allow extra spacing, if desired, to prevent crowding.

Vertical Spacing: There are six vertical lines per inch on the standard typewriter, elite or pica. Allow 1/6 inch, or its multiple, for each line of typing. If an executive typewriter is used, allow 5.28 vertical lines per inch.

Follow these guidelines for handwritten spacing:

Horizontal Spacing: Provide 1/10 to 2/12 inch per character.

Vertical Spacing: Provide 1/4 inch to 1/3 inch. When a box design is used, 1/3 inch is required.

When a form can be filled in by hand or by typewriter, or a combination of both, determine the horizontal space by the hand fill-in requirements and the vertical space by the typewriter requirements. The 1/3 inch vertical spacing will accommodate either handwritten or typewritten entries.

Rules - A rule is a vertical and/or horizontal line. The line may be solid, dotted or in close parallel which serves several purposes. Rules divide the form into logical sections, direct the writer to enter data in the proper space, instruct the writer as to the desired length of data to be entered, guide the reader through the communication, and add to the physical attractiveness of the form (if arranged properly). Rules are often used to form boxes. The box design increases available space on a form as much as 25 percent.

Boxes are used in two principal design techniques, the "line" box and the "x" or "ballot" box. The line boxes are a series of rules of equal heights, arranged horizontally on a line, being just wide enough for fill-in data. When the designer can line the vertical rules from one line to another, it presents an orderly arrangement and reduces tab stops. Length and width of boxes should follow the guidelines for spacing of rules. Captions describing required entries should be in the upper left hand corner of the box or immediately above the box in which case the entire line box is available for data entry.

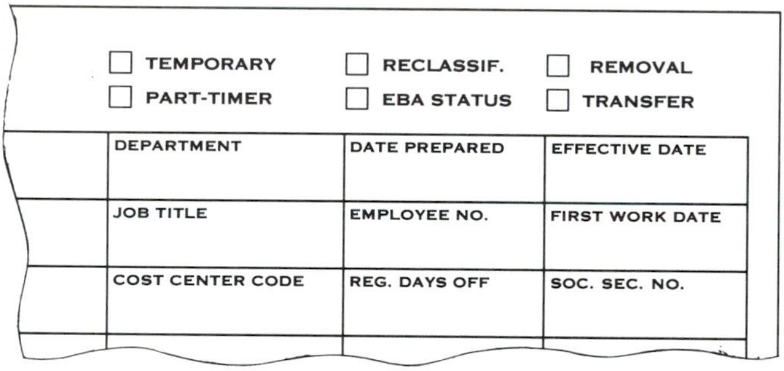

□ TEMPORARY	□ RECLASSIF.	□ REMOVAL
□ PART-TIMER	□ EBA STATUS	□ TRANSFER
DEPARTMENT	DATE PREPARED	EFFECTIVE DATE
JOB TITLE	EMPLOYEE NO.	FIRST WORK DATE
COST CENTER CODE	REG. DAYS OFF	SOC. SEC. NO.

FIGURE 1. BALLOT BOX AND LINE BOX EXAMPLES

The "x" or "ballot" box is a square ranging from 1/12" (for typewriters) or 1/4" (for handwriting or double spaced typewriter lines). Sufficient area should be allowed between each horizontal box with its applicable printed data and the next box. For vertical boxes the box should precede the data although the arrangement is clearer and more orderly if data length varies. Some space may be lost at the right.

Light or heavy rules or designs around a particular section of a form or around the entire form are called borders. A border can highlight a section. If it is around the entire form it makes it more attractive. Other functional considerations of forms design are blockouts and screening. Blockouts are a means of eliminating data from one or more parts of a multiple-part form by printing over the space to be eliminated or covered. Screening or shading is an effective way to emphasize or de-emphasize certain areas of a form. If done in the same color as the printing on the form, it gives the illusion of a second color. If done in a separate color, it becomes a bright signal.

Type Style - Type style is important in regards to readability and distinctiveness. For any one form, it is best to keep the number of different type sizes and styles to a minimum. Items of equal importance should be printed in the same type throughout the entire form. Normally, italic and boldface type should be used for emphasis but confined to words where special stress is required.

Recording Method - Most forms are produced by hand, typewritten or computer printed. Other methods of recording data include optical character recognition and bar code, which serves as direct input into a computer; and tracing performed by monitoring devices. In addition to the general principles of good forms design, special considerations of the OCR or bar code equipment and layout are important considerations.

5. Close

The last major component of a paper form is the close. This is the space for authenticating or approving signatures.

SPECIAL CONSIDERATIONS FOR PAPER FORMS CONSTRUCTION

In addition to the components which are unique to paper forms design, there are also construction considerations. These include: creating the master, physical building of the form, ink, paper, carbonizing, and duplicating method. Most construction characteristics of forms are rather technical in nature, and it may be desirable or necessary to consult a professional printer before a final decision about the form's construction is made. However, it is necessary for the health information practitioner to understand the underlying considerations in order to explain facility needs to a printer.

Creating the Master

Once the content of the form is decided upon, a master must be created from which copies of the form will be duplicated.

Forms may be simply typewritten or word processed, with rules drawn by hand. This should only be done for forms used exclusively in-house, and generally then only on a temporary basis.

Forms may be professionally typeset. Typesetting equipment costs from $50,000 to $500,000; thus printing companies or other professionals must perform this service. Typesetting permits proportional spacing and kerning (adjustment of spacing between lines), more than one type style and size on the form, integration of text and images (i.e., line drawings, photographs, etc.), and image scaling and halftoning (process of converting a continuous tone image to one comprised of dots in order to print gradations of tone). When a form is to be typeset, the health information practitioner or other forms manager must work closely with the typesetter to select characteristics of the design. A health care facility will often have a specification sheet it uses that defines standards for typesetting certain types of forms to ensure consistency.

Desktop publishing software allows a health care facility to either prepare text for typesetting or to produce a master on a high quality computer printer. Desktop publishing software is available for use on microcomputers. It allows the user to organize, directly on the computer, text and images in the same size and appearance as on final copy. In this way, the final arrangement is decided upon before submitting to typesetting. Desktop publishing software utilizes word processed text stored in computer files. It then adds codes which produce the various features desired. Images may be brought into desktop publishing software through a scanner and line drawings (such as rules) can be created directly in the desktop publishing program.

Output of desktop publishing depends on the quality of the copy desired. The difference between professional typesetting and computer printout is largely resolution (i.e., how many dots are used to form a character). Laser printers produce characters at 300 dots per inch, while typesetters produce output at 1270 to 2540 dots per inch. Output from laser printers can provide very satisfactory quality for certain types of forms or other documents. Problems with resolution (such as a jagged appearance - sometimes only noticeable through a magnifying glass) depend somewhat on the type of laser printer and the paper to which the document is printed. Other features of laser printers, which run in price from $650 or less to as much as $25,000 or more for a very high quality commercial printer, include size of memory and page description language availability. These features impact the ability to print a full page at a time, and the size of images which can be incorporated into text.

Physical Building of Form

Physical building of the form refers to its size and special properties. It is generally a good practice to utilize only standard size forms, especially if they are to be filed or photocopied. Decisions concerning factors such as the size of the form, the location of the data on the form, and the location of holes or other fastening devices on the form are affected by the kind of equipment used to process the form and the filing system employed. Printing on the reverse side of the form is yet another consideration which relates to photocopying and the physical consideration of paper weights.

The physical building of a form is particularly important where there is a need for making duplicate copies in one writing. The number of copies a form should contain depends on who requires a copy and when the copy is needed. Multi-copy forms afford a quick means of supplying copies, but usually not more than ten to twelve (and even less if handwritten) can be reproduced clearly. Multi-copy forms require only one writing, minimize mistakes, help attain uniformity, and save on photocopying time and cost. However, it is best to keep the number of copies at a minimum, for excess paper tends to contribute to inefficiency. When designing multi-copy forms, routing instructions should be placed at the bottom of the form.

Multiple copies may be reproduced as form sets or continuous or strip forms. A form set is several copies of a form, prefastened and precollated. A unit set is a form set held together by gluing (padding) one edge. A stub set or snapout set is a number of copies held together by a perforated stub, which may include interleaved carbon. After the stub set is completed, the stub is grasped in one hand, and the copies are snapped apart. The stub can be a corner or the entire top, bottom or side of the form. A fanfold set is one in which all parts are printed simultaneously on one sheet of paper then copies are folded back and forth into a set like an accordion. Continuous forms or strip forms are printed from a single roll of paper, each form being separated from the next by a horizontal perforation, Continuous forms are desirable for continuous processing through typewriters or computers, and often are punched on one or both margins for ease in machine feeding.

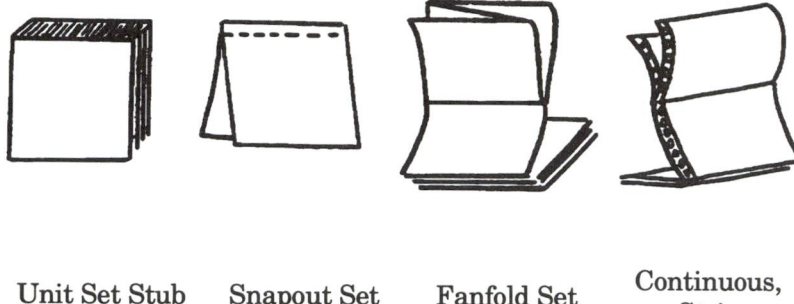

Unit Set Stub   Snapout Set   Fanfold Set   Continuous, Strip

FIGURE 2. TYPES OF FORMS SETS

Normally forms building solves most problems of fastening because the forms are held together by stubs or perforations until decollated. The most common fastening devices used are crimp, which is several small paper tongues die-cut through all copies forcing the tongues to protrude slightly into the succeeding copy or carbon; gluing one or both edges of the forms together; sewing with actual needle and thread; tongue-in-slot; and staples.

Ink

Although many forms are printed with standard black ink, consideration may be given to using special types of ink or colors. The ink selected should provide proper contrast to the paper and should give a clear, uniform, and smooth imprint. Certain printing processes require a certain type of ink. Use of more than one color of ink adds to the cost of the form and complicates photocopying, microfilming, and scanning into optical imaging systems.

Paper

There are five physical properties of paper which need to be considered in designing forms. These are weight, grade, grain, finish, and color. These properties relate to the form's permanency, durability, writing quality, readability, and microfilming. Permanency refers to how long the paper can be kept. Durability relates to one's ability to handle the paper many times. Paper quality also affects one's ability to write quickly and smoothly and the paper's ability to accept ink from printing devices. The ability to erase or apply opaquing fluid is also determined by the paper quality. Readability is affected primarily by the paper's interaction with light i.e., the amount of glare from a paper. Paper type also influences microfilming, as some colors, finishes, print types, and print sizes do not microfilm well.

Paper is usually sold by weight. Sometimes weight is referred to as substance or stock. A ream is the common measurement for quantity of paper and is approximately 500 sheets. Thus weight refers to how many pounds 500 sheets of a certain size of paper weigh. Paper weight influences permanency, durability, writing quality, and readability.

Names are frequently given to common weights of paper. Bond paper is a term applied to nearly all forms printing and reproduction papers of 11 to 24 pounds. They are relatively strong and clean, and have good erasing, printing, and permanence qualities. Manifold paper is a light 7 to 11 pound paper, usually referred to as "tissue." It is usually used for copies. The same weight paper but one with a transparent, "crinkled" finish is known as onion skin. Ledger paper is heavier than bond paper (24-36 pounds) and has a superb erasing quality, usually used for accounting and bookkeeping machine functions. Bristol, postcard, board, tag, duplicating, safety, and newsprint are other common paper types.

Grade of paper refers to the quality of the paper and is chiefly based on the kinds of materials used in the manufacturing process. Paper is made from rags, mechanical wood pulp, sulfite wood pulp, soda wood pulp, and sulfate wood pulp, which are used in varying amounts, depending upon the kind of paper desired. The grade selected for a form depends upon such things as the life of the form, the amount of handling, and the appearance. Generally, the more rag content, the longer the life of the paper:

100% rag	100 years life expectancy
75%	75 years

50%	50 years
25%	25 years
100% sulphite - Grade I	20 years
100% sulphite - Grade II - V	15 years
Newsprint	5 years

A watermark on paper is a transulent marking that is visible when a sheet of paper is held to the light. A watermark is applied to paper as it is being made and serves to identify the grade and manufacturer or the identification of the organization ultimately using the paper. Watermarks are generally only applied to high grade paper.

Grain of paper is the direction of the fibers making up the paper. The grain determines the paper's rigidity. This is a consideration if a form must feed through an office machine, such as a typewriter, printer, or photocopier.

Finish of paper refers to a chemical coating that may be applied to it. The condition of the paper surface can be rough (low finish), slick (high finish), or even glossy (very high finish). One of the major types of finishes is an electrostatic chemical applied to paper used in photocopiers and other electric or electronic equipment to keep the paper sheets from sticking to each other and feeding through the equipment smoothly.

Colored paper for forms frequently affords an effective medium for securing a strong appeal, a unique identification, and a simple means of facilitating the handling of forms. However, colored paper usually costs more than white. Contrast must also be considered for some colors are more difficult to read than others. Some colors will not photocopy, microfilm or scan into optical imaging systems effectively. A solution to this can be to use a colored or screened border.

Carbonizing

Carbonizing or producing copies is another consideration in paper forms construction. Carbon can be achieved in several ways: by inserting carbon paper by hand, one-use carbon interleaved into the form, carbon in a machine ("floating carbon"), and spots of wax carbon applied to the back of the form during manufacturing (ideal for selective copying). Carbonless paper (NCR = no carbon required) eliminates the dirtiness of carbon.

These forms are printed on paper chemically treated on one or both sides. Copies are obtained simultaneously with the original writing, the same as with carbon paper types. Though this is more costly than the use of carbon paper, the labor cost of inserting carbons, cleaning, etc. is often greater than the total cost of carbonless paper.

Duplicating Methods

A prime responsibility of the forms designer is to determine the most economical and/or practical way of producing a form in the quantity desired. Essentially, there are three major ways to reproduce forms: office duplication, commercial printing, and purchase of standard forms.

Office duplication requires two steps: preparation of a master copy and application of the master to a printing duplicator. Photocopying is probably the easiest of the duplicating methods, but is by far the most expensive. Unless only a trial of a form is being made, photocopying large quantities should not be considered. Spirit duplicating is the process of using an inked ditto paper for preparing the master and running it in a ditto machine that transfers ink to plain paper. This is an acceptable manner to reproduce a small number of forms (20-300) for intra-departmental, single sheet use. Dittoes are easy to prepare, economical, but are not very desirable in appearance. Stencil duplicating is more common, especially for forms which will change. The master is prepared on a special waxed-type of stencil paper and then run through an inking machine to produce copies on plain paper. As many as 300-2,000 copies of a single sheet from a master may be run at a very acceptable level. One limitation to stencil duplication is that the more rules there are, the fewer the number of good copies that can be made. Offset duplicating offers speed, versatility, and the capability to produce many clean, sharp copies. Offset equipment can often be found in the print shop of a large health care facility. This method can produce up to 100,000 copies. Paper masters can be prepared on a typewriter or word processor. Some brands can be reused, but not all. Metal masters must be prepared by a special machine. These may be reused and are especially suitable for complicated forms requiring unusual print sizes or type styles.

Commercial printing also involves two basic steps: preparation of a metal plate from original layouts and placement on a printing press. The printed result is extremely readable, high in quality, and permits extra color to be added to the form. In most cases, other operations such as punching, perforating, collating, carbon interleaving, and pre-numbering can be done simultaneously with the printing operation. Two basic commercial printing methods are used: letter press or raised type, and offset which is the same as offset duplicating except that the press is bigger and faster and can handle multiple operations.

Purchasing standard forms from a publishing company is a third option for obtaining forms. Purchase of such forms is generally cheaper than hiring a commercial printer, though more expensive than duplicating methods. While "crash imprinting" can customize the form to a certain extent, such as printing the name of the health care facility on the form, one generally sacrifices flexibility and uniqueness.

SPECIAL CONSIDERATIONS FOR COMPUTER FORMS DESIGN

There are two major considerations which are unique to data collection and information reporting via a computer: the screen format or layout, and the printout.

Screen Format

The computer has changed the conventional concept of the form because computers deal with data and document images on the screen, not printed forms. While it is true that prescribed formats for data entry, storage, and retrieval may be used in computerized information systems, discrete data elements, once captured, do not hold a fixed relationship with any parent document.

The focus on the data elements within a computer shifts design from forms to format. Instead of thinking in terms of a limited number of pre-printed forms with standardized blocks of prescribed data elements, virtually an infinite number of variable formats which can be tailored to specific information communication needs may be considered in a computer environment. Furthermore, the use of "windows," and unstructured imaging software allow users to design their own forms on a computer screen. Users can vary any element of design with the touch of a "mouse," a finger (touch-screen), or by use of functional keyboard keys.

Computer technology has come to the point where forms are not simply "automated." This was true of the technology in the 1960s and 1970s. Structured and hierarchical relationships appropriate to manual information processing environments are increasingly inappropriate in automated environments. Thus the focus of "format" design must be on ensuring that necessary data are captured. The logic of the computer program must prompt for data entry even though it may allow for data to be entered in any sequence at any time.

An example of the shift in "forms" design to "format" design for computerization may best be illustrated in the hospital admitting process. In a manual environment, the hospital required an admission officer to interview the patient or relative to obtain necessary demographic and insurance data which was typed on a form. Sometimes a worksheet was prepared in the physician's office or given to the patient; the data was then transferred to the permanent document in the hospital. The admission form was frequently multipart in order to distribute copies to the nursing station, business office, and others to alert them of the admission. Sometimes the form itself was initiated by the physician's office, or, with advance notice, the hospital may have obtained some information from the patient via telephone in advance of the admission and recorded on the form. The paper form was subject to loss, partial or total destruction, and illegible, incomplete, and untimely entries.

When the process was first automated, the computer screen basically became the form. Legibility was improved and the chance of loss or destruction was significantly reduced. Yet, the hospital still controlled data entry which essentially replicated manual form completion.

Computer technology now allows the physician's office, emergency department, or other location to electronically initiate the admission and supply data in a format preferred by that site. One day the patient may present to the hospital with a "smart card," which provides identification, insurance, and even medical information which results in direct entry of data into the admission processing as well as the clinical history taking. No form or screen entry may be required at all, or the admitting officer's screen may display only prompts specific to the data that are lacking on this particular patient. Once the patient is admitted, the physician may use a screen containing pull-down menus to select the type of data entry or retrieval desired; or a mouse may be used to point to text or graphic display for which data are to be input or output. While looking at one subset of data on a patient, the physician may also view a window containing data from another subset, or even data on another patient.

Such a system, however, requires the construction of data element controls and overrides. While the admitting department may be allowed to override a prompt requiring certain data, that missing data, if critical, must be captured later. An exception report of missing data may be generated at the end of the day, or discharge processing may not be permitted without entry of the missing data. The physician entering a history and physical exam may be required to respond to every element of a minimum data set before exiting the system. Thus forms design has shifted not only to computer screen format but computer logic design as well.

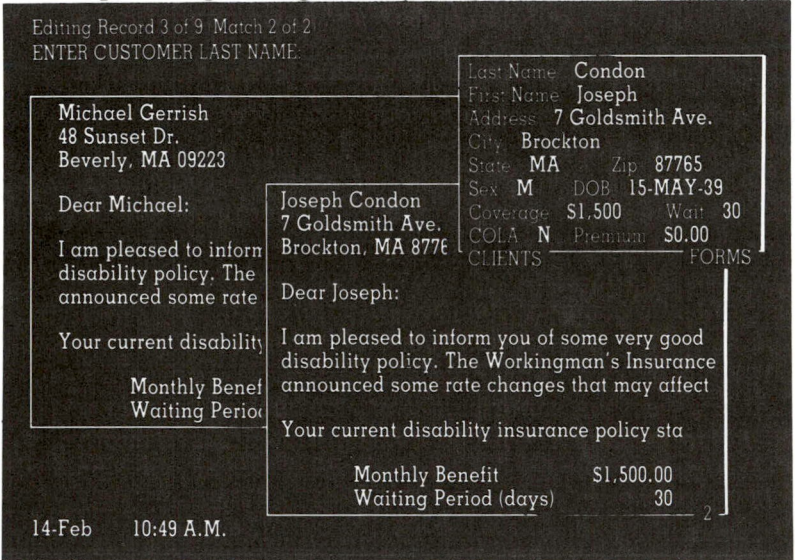

FIGURE 3. SAMPLE SCREEN WITH PULLDOWN MENUS

Printout

Printout refers to any paper product of a computer, which may be a copy of data entered, a "dump" of file or record contents, or a report displaying data that has been processed into useful information. Considerations with respect to printouts include distribution and thus confidentiality of copies, storage, and forms design.

Because there are still many cultural, legal, technical, and administrative barriers standing in the way of a completely paperless society, many more printouts than are probably necessary are generated. Health information management practitioners must take an active role in developing policies for the printing, distribution, storage, and destruction of printouts. Factors to consider include confidentiality of the information in the printout, the availability of terminals, the purpose of the printout, the retention of data in the computer system, alternate forms of storage, and the availability of shredders.

Design of printout forms is also an important factor. While computer screens can display data in many ways such as in tables, series of screens, and graphics, most printouts are not created to display data with such visual appeal. Not all printers can print graphics. Report generators which allow a user to produce tailored printouts, even from data in different databases, are somewhat time-consuming to use. Thus, much of what is printed out from a computer is not in a very desirable format. Without using a report generator, computers print data without margins, rules, headings, or other design characteristics. The health information practitioner may need to see that programs which generate information include at least a minimum of design characteristics if the users do not wish to use a report generator to create their own formats.

FORMS CONTROL

Just as forms design is not a random process, forms control should not be haphazardly performed either. Forms control encompasses the following objectives:

1. To insure the efficient design and construction of forms and their integration into all phases of the information processing system.
2. To develop and maintain proper specifications for the economical production and usage of needed forms.

3. To educate and assist operating personnel in designing their own forms when consistent with the aims and controls of the forms control program.

4. To stop the origination of useless forms, to combine forms which serve similar needs, to eliminate unneeded forms, and to create additional forms when such addition serves the information processing system better than combined forms.

5. To provide an effective brake on the natural inclination of personnel to change existing forms at whim.

In a paper environment, forms control includes: forms inventory, forms identification, ongoing review and revision (forms analysis), and purchasing. In a computerized system, data element inventory takes the place of forms inventory and programming logic takes the place of forms identification. Purchasing applies only to special forms of paper (e.g., OCR) input or output.

Forms Inventory

If a (paper) forms control program does not exist, the first step in implementing such a program is to obtain an inventory of all forms. This inventory should then be kept up to date at all times. A forms inventory includes a forms history file and subject/title file.

A forms history file provides a complete picture of each form in the organization from development to current status. It should be arranged according to the numbering system used to identify forms, which should be as simple as possible.

A forms history file can be set up by establishing a folder for each form and filing by form number. Each folder should eventually contain the following:

- A copy of the current edition of the form and any previous editions.
- Drafts showing significant stages of development and pertinent correspondence.
- A copy of the directive authorizing use of the form.
- The original request for approval of the form and any requests for revisions indicating the names of all units using the form and the rate of use.

- Evidence relating to the official final approval for the printing or reproduction and issuance of the form.
- A record of all actions taken on the form, including a cross-reference to the subject/title file.

The forms history file should be periodically reviewed and updated. Folders on discontinued or obsolete forms should be removed from the active file on a timely basis, appropriately annotated, and placed in a separate discontinued history file for such time as required by the organization's records retention schedule.

A forms subject/title file provides the mechanism by which forms dealing with related subject matter are brought together. One copy of each form is classified by purpose and placed in a subject/title folder.

The main purposes of the subject/title file are to:

- Avoid the creation of a new form when an existing form could be revised to serve the need.
- Detect those forms which might be eliminated or which might be consolidated with similar forms.
- Identify forms which should be analyzed and redesigned for simplification and uniformity of format, nomenclature, item sequence, spacing, size, and so forth.
- Generate studies of forms in relation to the systems and procedures used.

The subject/title file is not an easy file to develop because of the many possible subject headings that could be assigned to some forms. However, one subject heading can be selected and forms filed under that heading, producing as many cross-reference cards as necessary to tie the subjects together and facilitates location of the form. It is the best type of control file to use when making an analysis of the organization's forms. Maintenance of the forms subject/title file may be facilitated by using database software on a microcomputer.

Identification

Forms control requires that all forms be appropriately titled and identified, as previously described. Form identification is usually a number issued sequentially and prefixed or suffixed by a code for the originating department or section. As an example, the identifying line of the first form generated by the

Jewish Hospital of Michigan would appear as follows for a new form back printed; the front side numbered; the originating department Medical Records with a code number of 10; and the edition date January 1990:

0001a-10 01/90 MRD Copyright 1990 JHM

It is recommended that when a form is back printed (printed on both sides), or if the form comprises several pages, the primary form number (the sequential number) should have as its last character a lowercase alphabetic character, such as an "a" to represent the first page and a "b" to represent the reverse side of the form or the next page, and so forth.

For forms used in an automated environment, one may wish to identify each one by assigning the computer program number that will be receiving the data input. Facilities may wish to use computer-readable identification, such as bar coding, on forms that will be scanned into an optical imaging system. Computer readable identification allows the scanner to automatically index the type of form, thus speeding the process and eliminating the need for manual indexing of the form.

A Forms Control Register is essential for the proper control of form numbers issued, as well as for other identifying information. It can be maintained either manually or by computer. The register should include information on: form number, title, form size, edition date, revision date, and originating department.

Serial numbering of forms is another form of identification. It is advisable to number forms only when a high degree of control is required, such as admitting forms, purchase orders, etc. Much time can be wasted if the numbers are not used properly. A special forms control log is required to track the usage of serially numbered forms.

Forms Analysis

Ongoing review and revision of forms is the critical step in forms control. Forms analysis should begin by fact finding - a process which provides complete information about the form. Because (parts of) forms can become obsolete without the person preparing the form even being aware of it, it is important to regularly review forms, not just when the supply runs out or when a change is requested.

Some of the reasons which prompt an analysis of forms are: the existence of operational problems such as backlogs, bottlenecks, unusual time lags, repetition, or numerous errors; areas suggested by top management for potential savings and improvement; and suggestions made by the operating staff. Another reason why health information managers are taking fresh looks at the forms in use in their facilities is to prepare for computerization, especially optical imaging. Completely revising paper forms and controlling their numbers can be a multi-year process and is often a first step toward automation.

The forms analysis process may be aided by issuing a regular forms questionnaire to all users. A forms questionnaire in itself is a form which serves as a management tool: providing a written reference for cross-sectioning information (especially where there is more than one user of the form or where there are several related forms). The questionnaire may be completed by the users, or used by the forms analyst as an interview guide. Remember, as a form itself, the questionnaire needs to be reviewed periodically to insure that it is asking the questions relating to new requirements or new methods of handling forms.

In addition to the questionnaire, the following sources should be checked to obtain background information related to forms:

Manuals, regulations, or directives which describe functional responsibilities and procedures that relate to the forms under study.

- Forms History File and Forms Subject/Title File
- Completed forms which shows the types of errors made in com pleting the forms.
- Organizational charts which show the relationships of the department responsible for the form to other departments.

Fact confirmation is the second step in forms analysis where the facts about a form are summarized and presented to the users for their examination and verification. For example, one user may indicate that certain data being collected is no longer being used. However, another user, or the person initially filling out the form, may have need for the data.

Challenging the form by getting the user to think about each item in terms of its own merit and its cost is the next step.

Some questions to ask include: is the form necessary at all, does it really serve its stated purpose, are there forms already in the system that show the same data or at least enough of the data to serve the stated purpose, does the form produce

FORMS FLOWCHART

FORMS:　NAME_____ NUMBER_____ REVISION DATE_____

ORIGINATING DEPARTMENT:_____

DEPT.	OPERATION	Seg. No.	Worksheet A1	A2	HAR B1	B2	B3	B4	HAR Photocopy C1
			FORMS COPIES		Hospital Admission Record (HAR)				HAR
	Physician signs authorization for admission	0							
ADMITTING DEPARTMENT	Prepares	1	X	X					
	Sends Original to patient	2	X						
	Files Copy until	3		F					
	Original returned	4	X						
	If not returned on time, calls patient on phone	5		=					
	Prepares from Worksheet	6	X	X	O	O	O	O	
	Destroy	7	D	D					
	Has patient sign Authorization	8			X				
BILLING	Initiates Account	9				X	X	X	
	Add charges as occur	11				X	X	X	O
	Completes account	13				X	X	X	
	Send to Third Party Payors	16					X	X	D
	Files Original Bill	17				F			
M.R. ON NURSING STATION	Placed in Medical Record	10			X				
	M.D. adds diagnosis	12			X				
	Sends to Medical Records	14							
MEDICAL RECORD DEPARTMENT	Photocopies for Billing	15			X				
	Codes	18			X				
	Files	19			F				

KEY:

X　　the form is subject to an operation, specified in the left-hand column

O　　the form initiates the creation of a new document

X⌐▽　the form is sent to a department or employee already listed on a higher plan

=　　the form is used for checking purposes

V　　the form is verified　　　　　　　　　　　　　　　F　　the form is filed

X-O　the form is merged into another object　　　　　　D　　the form is destroyed

FIGURE 4. FORMS FLOWCHART

meaningful data for other aspects of the system, what would be the consequence if the form did not exist? If the form is necessary, a forms flowchart (Figure 4) can be used to analyze the distribution of the form and/or its copies. Are all the copies necessary, does each copy serve the stated purpose, does the recipient of each copy have any authority to take action based on data appearing on the copy — if not — why does that person get a copy, and if a copy is for information proposes, would it be cheaper to refer to a permanent copy in a central file? On the other hand, there may be too few copies which result in recipients making costly photocopies. If the form and all copies are necessary, is all data necessary? In addition to the overall merit of the form and its distribution, the content of the form should be analyzed. Does each item serve the stated purpose, what would be the consequence if individual data items were omitted, can they be reduced or eliminated?

Forms analysis also includes review of specifications and elements of design relating to paper, ink, punching, etc. A checklist is of great value here. Each health care facility should develop its own checklist of standard forms design considerations, spelling out hospital policy on titles, copies, hole punching, and so forth.

It is extremely rare that a form exists as an isolated document. Almost always it exists as one of several forms which are interdependent. So, item analysis or rearrangement of data may not fully result in cost reductions. A multiform analysis or data frequency chart (Figure 5), may be helpful in identifying forms which may be combined.

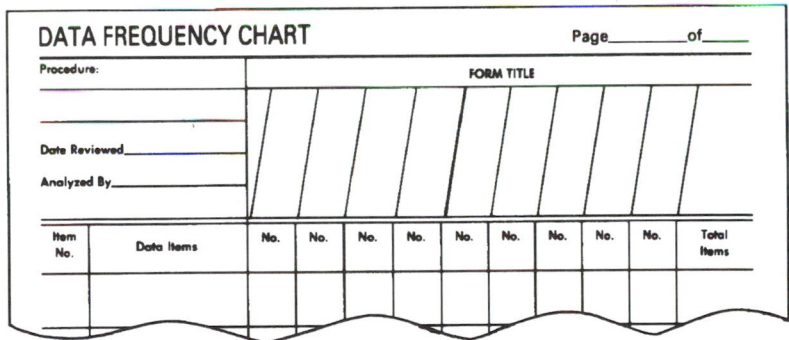

FIGURE 5. DATA FREQUENCY CHART

Purchasing

The purposes of forms control are the proper design of forms to insure the collection of needed information with maximum efficiency, elimination of obsolete forms, consolidation of forms to minimize duplication of effort, and minimization of printing costs. The essential ingredient in forms control is to have unbreakable rules backed by administration and medical staff. These rules should include a means of controlling the source of ordering and printing. The purchasing department and print shop should operate with an unequivocal statement that no form can be ordered, reordered, or changed without the approval of the appropriate forms committee chairperson or delegated representative (often the health information

REQUEST FOR NEW OR REVISED FORM

INSTRUCTIONS THIS FORM MUST BE COMPLETELY FILLED OUT AND FORWARDED TO FORMS CONTROL
ALL REQUESTS FOR NEW OR REVISED FORMS MUST HAVE A SAMPLE OR ROUGH DRAWING ATTACHED. | DATE

REQUEST FOR ☐ NEW FORM ☐ REVISED FORM | FORM TITLE | PRESENT FORM NO.

PURPOSE OF NEW OR REVISED FORM

WHAT PROMPTED THIS REQUEST?
☐ ORGANIZATION CHANGE ☐ PROCEDURE CHANGE ☐ TO IMPLEMENT ESTABLISHED PROCEDURE
☐ INTERNAL DEPT REQUIREMENT ☐ REQUEST OF ANOTHER DEPT ☐ MGMT ☐ GOVT, CUSTOMER OR OTHER REQMT

FORM PREPARED ☐ DAILY ☐ WEEKLY ☐ MONTHLY ☐ OTHER (EXPLAIN) ______

DATA ENTERED BY ☐ HAND ☐ TYPEWRITER ☐ OTHER (EXPLAIN) ______

FORM FILED BY ☐ DATE ☐ SUBJECT ☐ NUMBER | FORM FILED IN ☐ FOLDER ☐ BINDER ☐ OTHER (EXPLAIN) ______ | FORM USED INTERNALLY ONLY ☐ YES ☐ NO | FORMS OBSOLETED

DATA TO BE ENTERED ON (GIVE FORM NOS) | DATA TO BE ENTERED FROM (GIVE FORM NOS)

DISTRIBUTION OF FORM

PART	PERSON OR DEPT RECEIVING COPY	REASON COPY IS REQUIRED
1		
2		
3		
4		
5		
6		

FORM PRENUMBERED ☐ YES (Give Reason) ☐ NO

START UP QTY | MONTHLY USE THEREAFTER | ANNUAL QTY

NEW EQUIPMENT REQUIRED

EXPECTED BENEFITS TO BE DERIVED FROM NEW OR REVISED FORM

EXPECTED DOLLAR SAVING $______ PER YEAR | EFFECT ON CLERICAL WORKLOAD WORKLOAD WILL BE: ☐ INCREASED______ HRS PER MONTH ☐ DECREASED______ HRS PER MONTH

REQUESTED BY | PLT & DEPT | APPROVED (Dept Head)

Form courtesy of Association for Systems Management

FIGURE 6. REQUEST FOR NEW OR REVISED FORM

practitioner). Without strong control, mass confusion can result. The health care facility may wish to have a Request for New or Revised Form (Figure 6) to initiate the forms analysis necessary to create or change a form.

In order to lay out the proper form design, it is important to know the quantity of forms to be ordered, because the methods of reproduction govern the form design.

It is usually sufficient to order a six- to twelve-month supply of a form, depending on the discounts and the storage space available. If the form is subject to critical changes within a short period of time, one may wish to order a smaller supply. A standard form should be used for stocking, printing, and ordering forms.

Certain types of forms take longer to produce than others. Enough lead time (from the date the order is placed to the date of delivery) must be allowed to achieve the desired implementation date. Below are estimated time periods for the reproduction of just a few types of forms. These estimates can vary based on locality and the season in which the forms are to be reproduced:

Single-part forms (up to 11" x 17")	2 to 3 weeks
Single-part forms (over 11" x 17")	3 to 4 week
Tags and envelope	4 to 8 weeks
Carbon-interleaved snap-out forms	8 to 12 weeks
Continuous forms	10 to 15 weeks

Some printers will make arrangements to warehouse forms and make drop shipments as they are needed. This method enables one to take advantage of the lower cost per thousand that is available as the size of the order is increased. A good deal of foresight must be exercised to be assured that a heavily used form will be able to endure for a year or more without any changes in design or construction

SUMMARY

Forms analysis and control are the management tools of data communications. Whether a form is a specially designed piece of paper for a manual system, the format of a computer screen, the logical presentation of data elements in a computer environment, or a computer printout, forms design is important to ensure effective data collection and dissemination. Although forms control is needed primarily for paper forms, consideration must also be given to computer programming logic and printout management. Forms design and control require a defined purpose and coordinated effort. The health information practitioner lends forms expertise as well as knowledge of the information flow within a health care facility to the design of forms that will reduce direct costs as well as indirect costs of handling and processing. Well-designed forms are the key to efficient and effective data communication, which contributes directly to the productivity of all members of the health care team and ultimately to quality patient care.

STUDY QUESTIONS

1. Explain the statement that computer data communications are not "form-less."
2. Identify design rules for data collection forms.
3. Identify the five components of paper forms.
4. What construction considerations must be made for paper forms?
5. Describe the evolution of forms with respect to computerization.
6. What are the objectives of a forms control program?
7. What are the components of a forms control program?

REFERENCES

Amatayakul, Margret, "Forms Management," *Topics in Health Record Management* (June, 1984): 53-59.

Baker, Bob, "Creating and Managing the Business Form Electronically," *The Office* (November, 1986): 15, 19.

Christian, C.W., "Four Major Functions of a Forms-Management System," *The Office* (July, 1983): 77-78.

Clark, Jessie L., "On Developing An Effective Forms Management Program," *The Office* (December, 1980): 43.46.101.

Freidman, Selma, "Forms Management," Topics in Health Record Management (June, 1984): 53-59.

Garvey, Ed, "A Primer on Forms Productions, Design and Purchasing," *Topics in Health Record Management* (June, 1988): 26-35.

Horton, Forest Woody, "The Formless Form," *Records Management Quarterly* (July, 1984): 48-52.

Jacobs, Marvin, *Forms Design Clear and Simple* (Cleveland, OH: Formsman Inc., 1978).

Langer, Gary F., "Forms Management Programs: A How-To Approach For Controlling Healthcare Costs," *Healthcare Financial Management* (May, 1983): 10-20.

Meisner, Dwayne, "Taking Stock: A Guide to Business Papers," *Administrative Management* (November, 1974): 64-68.

Myers, Gibbs and Leslie H. Matthies, "Forms Order Quantities," *Journal of Systems Management* (November, 1984): 6-7.

Myers, Gibbs and Leslie H. Matthies, "New or Revised Forms," *Journal of Systems Management* (May, 1984): 20-21.

Myers, Gibbs and Leslie H. Matthies, "Pen and Pencil Forms," *Journal of Systems Management* (July, 1984): 40-41.

Myers, Gibbs and Leslie H. Matthies, "Self Instruction on Forms," *Journal of Systems Management* (September, 1984): 40-41.

"Well designed paper forms speed automation," *Medical Records Briefing* (June 1993): 1, 3-4.

chapter 8

FILING METHODS, STORAGE, AND RETENTION

Operations in many areas of a health care institution can be severely hampered by poor management of records; therefore, it is imperative that the health information practitioner establish systems and procedures for the efficient numbering, filing, distribution, storage, and retention of health informations throughout the facility. Efficiency in these functions is perhaps the most important single factor in establishing good rapport with other departments of the health care facility.

RECORD NUMBERING AND FILING SYSTEMS

Medical records in most health care facilities are filed numerically according to patients' medical record numbers. Alphabetical filing by patient names is cumbersome and subject to more error than numerical filing. There are several types of numbering and filing systems. Regardless of which of these systems is utilized, medical records requiring new numbers should have them assigned chronologically, and this number should be common to all departments of the facility.

SERIAL NUMBERING AND FILING

In serial numbering, the patient receives a new number for each occasion of treatment by a health care facility. If a patient is registered three times, three different numbers are assigned. For example, the patient Edward Brown is admitted to a hospital and receives the number 52783. When he returns for outpatient follow-up one week after discharge, he is registered under number 52829. If he is admitted to the hospital again the following year, he receives the third number - 64287. All numbers assigned to a patient are recorded in the master patient index.

Because a new number is issued for each occasion of service, a new medical records is also developed. This means the patient's medical records are filed in as many places in the file as the number of times the patient has received care at the facility and given another number.

UNIT NUMBERING AND FILING

In unit numbering, the patient is assigned a number on the first admission or visit which is retained for all subsequent admissions and treatments. For example, with unit numbering, each time Edward Brown arrives at the hospital for treatment, documentation on his care will be compiled under the first number he was assigned - 52783.

Unit numbering provides a single record which is a composite of all data gathered on a given patient, regardless of the number or types of services provided. The patient's entire medical record is thus filed as a unit in one folder under one number.

SERIAL-UNIT NUMBERING FILING

The serial-unit system is a synthesis of the serial numbering and unit filing systems. Each time the patient is registered, a new hospital number is assigned; but the previous records are continually brought forward and filed under the latest number issued. Thus, if patient Edward Brown returned for an outpatient visit following discharge, he would receive number 52829; but his inpatient admission data, filed under 52783, would be brought forward to be filed with the notes made during his most recent visit. A unit record is thus created. When the older records are brought forward, an outguide must be left in the file where the old record was pulled to indicate the new number under which the record is now filed. The empty chart folder marked with a referral to the new number is a satisfactory outguide.

OTHER ADAPTATIONS OF UNIT NUMBERING AND FILING SYSTEMS

The unit numbering and filing system is very popular with health care facilities due to the ease of retrieving patient information filed in one place under one number. Two adaptations of unit numbering are of particular note - social security numbering and family numbering.

Social Security Numbering - The use of social security numbers for patient identification is very controversial. They are used effectively in Veterans Administration hospitals which receive assistance from the Social Security Administration for location of unknown numbers. But other health care facilities have used the social security number as a patient identifier with varied success. The American Hospital Association recommends that social security numbers not be used as the medical record numbering system.

When considering using the social security number as the patient's medical record number, it should be understood that the social security number is not a national identifier. There is no legal requirement that every U.S. resident have a social security number. There are certain federal and state laws that require an individual to have a social security number; however, where use of the number is not required by law, the person may refuse to provide the number.

An advantage to using the social security number to identify a patient is that it is unique to the patient and distinguishes the patient from any other patient in the facility. However, individuals who do not have social security numbers must be issued "pseudo numbers."

"Pseudo" social security numbers may be issued from a special number series used only for those patients admitted without social security numbers. The Veterans Administration issues pseudo numbers in a special way. The assignment is based on numerical designations for the patient's initials and utilization of the birth date for the balance of the number. The code for numerical assignment to the alphabet is as follows:

1 abc	5 mno	9 yz
2 def	6 pqr	0 used when
3 ghi	7 stu	no middle
4 jkl	8 vwx	initial

Thus, John Brown, born January 1, 1946, would be issued the following number:

4	0	1	-	0	1	-	0	1	4	6
J	No	B		January			First		1946	
	Initial									

Other disadvantages to using this number include instances where patients have more than one social security number (in some cases patients have had five or more), and the fact that a nine-digit number is thought to be excessively long.

Planning for expansion of the medical records file area is difficult with the social security numbering system. Since patients arrive randomly at the facility, some areas of the file may fill up faster than other areas. This requires constant shifting of medical record folders to provide for an even distribution of the files.

Family numbering - Another adaptation of unit numbering is the family numbering system. Family numbering usually consists of placing extra pairs of digits signifying placement of the individual in the household. These digits are usually placed immediately before the regularly assigned number. Prefix number pairs have a definite sequence and meaning, so 01 is head of household (either mother or father), 02 is spouse, 03 is child or other family member, and so forth.

An illustration of this is shown below:

```
    01- 123456
    /        /
  head   family number (the same for all members of
   of                  that family)
household
    02- 123456
    /
  spouse
    03- 123456
    etc.
    /
  children or
other member
```

All patient information on one family is thus filed together by the family number. In the example above, the number 123456 provides a unit number for each family member and it groups the records of one family together for easy reference of related problems. This system is particularly helpful for neighborhood health centers and mental health centers utilizing family counseling techniques. The major disadvantage of family numbering is the frequent change and reassignment of numbers as family composition changes. Through divorce, a spouse may become head of another separate household. A child may become a spouse or head of a household through marriage. In these circumstances, a new household number must be assigned, resulting in an entirely new record.

ADVANTAGES AND DISADVANTAGES OF UNIT NUMBERING AND UNIT FILING

The Joint Commission on Accreditation of Healthcare Organizations suggests facilities use a unit record system or when not feasible, that a system be established to routinely assemble all divergently located inpatient, ambulatory care, and emergency record components when the patient is provided care. A unit record provides a complete picture of the patient's medical history and therapy, and it eliminates the task of gathering separate parts of a patient's record. To maintain a unit record, some form of binding all parts is necessary. A fastener with two prongs may be used with tabbing or indexing (Figure 1).

When a unit filing system is maintained, records documenting multiple occasions of treatment may become so thick that additional folders are needed to house one complete medical record. In order to alert filing personnel and health care professionals using the record that a medical record is contained in several folders, each folder should be marked with both the volume number and the total number of volumes. For example, the first folder is labeled "Volume 1 of 4," the second folder "Volume 2 of 4," etc. It is necessary to relabel all folders on one patient whenever another volume is added to the set.

When a unit record is utilized, it is essential that those responsible for assigning numbers determine whether or not the patient has been previously treated by the facility. With the unit numbering system, the patient is not assigned another number if previously registered. Occasionally a patient may mistakenly be assigned a new number. This error can be rectified by voiding the number on the most recent admission and filing the record under the first number issued to that patient.

In a manual system, the voided number is usually not reassigned to another new patient since it requires a great deal of clerical time to track the number and enter the new patient's name on the correct page in the number index. If numbers are

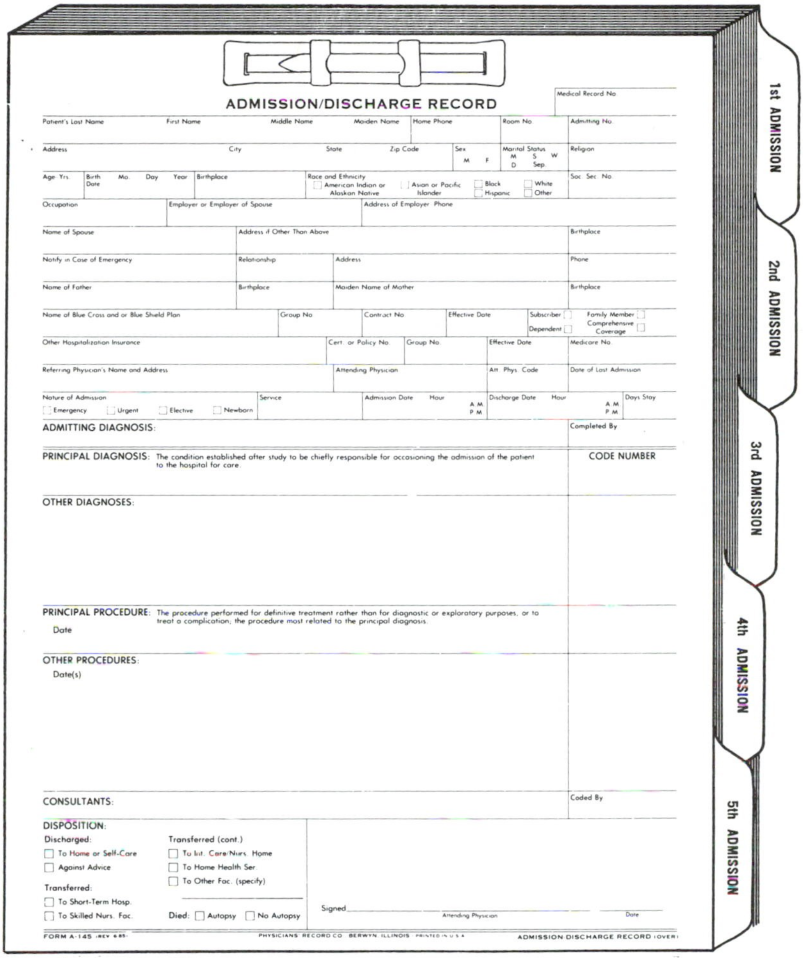

Courtesy of Physicians' Record Company

FIGURE 1. FILE FOLDER WITH TWO-PRONGED FASTENER AND CHART DIVIDERS

computer generated, the task of tracking unused numbers is not difficult if the computer program is designed to reuse such numbers.

FILE EXPANSION

Planning for file expansion is affected by the choice of a numbering system. When using the unit numbering and filing system, it is necessary to leave 25 percent of the shelves open because additional room is needed to allow for expansion of the individual medical records.

When using the serial-unit filing system which moves medical records forward, gaps may occur on the shelves as records are pulled. This is particularly apt to happen when readmission rates are high. With the serial numbering and filing system the shelves remain constant, expanding only at one end of the file as new numbers are assigned to patients.

PURGING OF FILES

Purging inactive records from the file is simple when using serial and serial-unit numbering and filing. The medical record number is an indicator of the age of the record: the lower the number, the older the record. With serial-unit numbering and filing, records of patients who are readmitted are always moved forward and filed under a higher number. Those records not moved forward within a prescribed time period are designated inactive. With the serial system, older records (those with the lowest numbers) are easily selected from the file shelves for inactive storage. In these systems, however, the remaining active records must be physically shifted back to allow room at the front of the file area for new records.

With the unit system, purging inactive records requires that the contents of each folder be individually inspected to determine the year of the last admission, ambulatory care visit, or emergency treatment; since the medical record number is not an indicator of record activity. Health care facilities that use unit numbering often mark the outside of each patient's folder with the year of most recent treatment activity to facilitate the purging process. This can also be accomplished by using pressure-sensitive color coded tabs with the year preprinted on the tab. Computer systems can sometimes generate listings of patient records with no activity since a specified date, which can then be used to assist in accurately identifying records to be purged.

NUMBER SOURCES

A health care facility usually creates its own bank of medical record numbers, arbitrarily deciding the highest number of digits it wishes to use before starting over again with the number 1. The number of digits used in the medical record number for both manual and automated systems should be adequate to cover anticipated growth based on hospital projections over a specified time period. For most facilities, a six-digit number, from 000001 to 999999, will supply numbers that are easy to remember and which will meet the need for many years. Starting a new number series for each year with a letter or number prefix (e.g., 90-456231 or A-456231) is not advisable, since an error in the prefix makes record retrieval extremely difficult.

Numbers which have not yet been assigned in a manual situation are usually held in a master control book by the health information department or patient registration area. The choice of where numbers are controlled depends on the needs of each facility and the procedures used to issue them. The responsibility for number allocation should be placed where the most accurate and trouble-free operation can be accomplished.

If a facility is automated, the computer program can control the issuance of numbers by automatically assigning the next sequential number to a new patient admission. The computer can also search the file to determine if the patient already has an assigned unit number.

If the health information department retains responsibility for number control, blocks of numbers (100, 200, or 500 consecutive numbers) are often issued to patient registration areas with a consistently high volume of new admissions. This practice reduces the amount of requests received by the health information department for number assignment.

CHANGING FROM SERIAL TO UNIT NUMBERING

Changing from serial or serial-unit to unit numbering and filing is easily accomplished by following the steps below.

1. Select a date to make the change, preferably the first day of the calendar or fiscal year.

2. Begin issuing unit numbers on the selected day. (The last unused serial number can be used to begin the unit system or an entirely new series, if desired.)

3. Assign readmitted patients a new unit number, bringing forward their previous records and filing them under the new number. Leave empty folders of the previous records

in their original places in the file. Make a cross-reference on the folder to the new unit number.

4. Leave in the file under their original numbers all records of patients not readmitted. After a specified time, all medical records remaining in the original file area may easily be purged from the active file area and taken to inactive storage.

TYPES OF FILING

Straight Numeric Filing

Straight numeric filing refers to the filing of records in exact chronological order according to medical record number. Thus, consecutively numbered records appear in sequence on the file shelves. For example, the following four medical records would be filed in consecutive order on a shelf: 465023, 465024, 465025, 465026. It is simple to pull any number of consecutively numbered records from the file for study purposes or for inactive storage. Probably the greatest advantage of this type of filing system is the ease with which personnel are trained to work with it.

This approach to filing has certain disadvantages. Because a clerk must consider all digits of the number at one time when filing a record, it is easy to misfile. The greater the number of digits that must be recalled when filing, the greater the chance for error. Transposition of numbers is common: Record 465426 can be misfiled as Record 464526. A more serious drawback to straight numerical filing is that the heaviest filing activity is concentrated in the area housing the medical records with the highest numbers (representing the newest records). Several clerks filing records at the same time in the same area are bound to get in each other's way. Finally, quality control of filing is difficult with this system. Since clerks are usually filing in the area of the most current records, it is not feasible to fix responsibility for a section of the file to one clerk.

Terminal Digit Filing

Terminal digit filing is a simple and accurate filing method which increases productivity of file clerks. Usually a six-digit number is used and divided with a hyphen into three parts, each part normally containing two digits. The primary digits are the last two digits on the right-hand side of the number. The secondary digits are the middle two, and the tertiary digits are the first two on the left side of the number (Figure 2). In a terminal digit file, there are 100 primary sections, ranging from

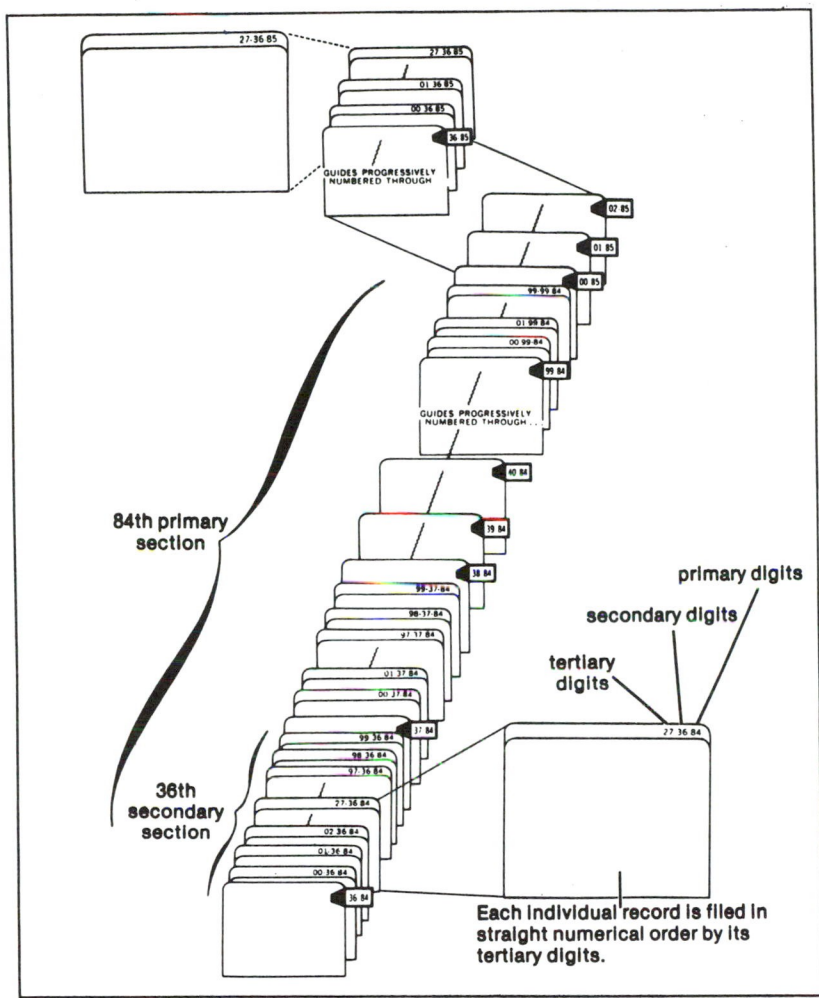

FIGURE 2. TERMINAL DIGIT FILING

00 to 99. When filing, a clerk considers the primary digits first, taking the record to the corresponding primary section. Within each primary section, groups of records are matched according to secondary digits. After locating the correct secondary digit

section, the clerk files in numerical order by the tertiary digits. In the file, the second tertiary digit changes with every record. Note the following sequences in a terminal digit file.

46-52-02	98-05-26	98-99-30
47-52-02	99-05-26	99-99-30
48-52-02	00-06-26	00-00-31
49-52-02	01-06-26	01-00-31

The terminal digit method of filing with six numbers has been described, but adaptations can be made to use five, seven, or even the nine digits found in the social security number. With a five-digit number, it can be broken into three sections, as follows:

0-23-45   1-23-45

With seven digits, the breakdown might be:

023-45-67   123-45-67

The nine digits in the social security number can be broken down in many ways, but it is common to break the last group of four numbers into two sections, calling the last two digits the primary digits and the second pair the secondary digits. Then the remaining five digits are used for sequential filing as follows:

243-09-5228 BECOMES	24309	-	52	-	28
	TERTIARY DIGITS		SECONDARY DIGITS		PRIMARY DIGITS

The family numbering system, as described earlier in this chapter, consists of a six-digit family number and a two-digit prefix to identify each individual family member. Since all parts of a family's record are placed together in the file, the terminal digit application of 01-623472 would require that the records be filed by the last six digits.

01	-	62	34	72
head of household		tertiary digits	secondary digits	primary digits

The advantages of terminal digit filing are numerous. As new records are added to the file, their terminal digit numbers are equally distributed throughout the 100 primary sections. Only every 100th new medical record will be filed in the same primary section of the file. This eliminates congestion that results when several clerks file active records in the same area of the file. Clerks may be assigned responsibility for certain sections of the file. As medical record numbers are assigned in straight numerical order, the work is evenly distributed with each clerk having approximately the same number of active records in each section. Inactive records may be pulled from each terminal digit section as new records are added. In this way the volume of records in each primary section is controlled, and large gaps in the file requiring backshifting of records are prevented. This volume control also simplifies file area planning.

Misfiles are substantially reduced with the use of terminal digit filing. Since the clerk is concerned with only one pair of digits at a time, the transposition of numbers is less likely to occur. Even if the tertiary digits are increased to three, e.g., 245-68-90, recalling three digits is easier than recalling seven. The use of preprinted, color-keyed folders further reduces misfiles. The clerk is immediately alerted to a possible error if a folder with one colored band is filed into a group of folders with another colored band.

The training period for new personnel is usually a little longer for a terminal digit system than for a straight numeric system, but most file clerks learn it in a few hours time. More units of shelving may also be required initially, since expansion must be planned by equipping the total file area from the start.

Middle Digit

Middle digit filing is an alternative to terminal digit filing. In middle digit filing with a six-digit number the middle parts of digits are the primary digits; the digits on the left are the secondary digits; and the digits on the right are the tertiary digits.

56   -   78   -   96

secondary   primary   tertiary

Shown below are sample sequences from a middle digit file.

56-78-96	99-78-96
56-78-97	99-78-97
56-78-98	99-78-98
56-78-99	99-78-99
57-78-00	00-79-00
57-78-01	00-79-01

From the first 4 numbers listed in the samples, one can see that blocks of 100 charts (i.e., 56-78-00 through 56-78-99) would be filed in straight numerical order. Thus it is simple to pull up to 100 consecutively numbered charts for study purposes, and conversion from a straight numerical system to a middle digit system is simplified. Middle digit filing provides a more even distribution of records than straight numerical filing, although it does not equal the balance achieved by a terminal digit filing system.

There are disadvantages to middle digit filing. Training is more involved than for straight numeric or terminal digit filing. Gaps result in the file when large groups of records are pulled for inactive storage. Middle digit filing does not lend itself well to numbers with more than six digits.

CONVERTING TO TERMINAL OR MIDDLE DIGIT FILING

Many facilities start terminal digit filing at the beginning of a new year or when they move into a new file area. If past records are not to be converted into terminal digit, medical records can be brought forward to the terminal digit area as the patients are readmitted to the health care facility.

If the past files are to be converted, the problem is simplified if the department is also moving because the conversion can take place simultaneously with the move. However, if the conversion takes place in the same area, all records must be moved out before section guides are installed. When converting, all records must be sorted first according to the primary digits (terminal digit); next by the secondary digits; and lastly by the tertiary digits.

Conversion can be either a concerted effort for a number of people, or it can be spread over a period of time with regular personnel if properly planned in advance. If the latter method is used, the routine work must be kept flowing smoothly.

During a conversion two important tasks may also be accomplished.

Misfiled records should be found, and all records not in the file should be accounted for. (If unable to locate the record, an empty folder should be placed in the file with the notation that the medical record was missing as of the date of the move.

PHYSICAL FACILITIES IN THE FILE AREA

The health information department must include sufficient space and equipment to store patients' medical records so they are easily accessible when requested. Adequate filing equipment, lighting, temperature control, supplies, and attention to safety in the file room all contribute to the productivity of filing clerks.

RECORD STORAGE EQUIPMENT

Open-shelf file units and five-drawer file cabinets are the most commonly used storage units for medical records. Open-shelf units are recommended over cabinets because they are less expensive than file cabinets, personnel can file or pull records faster because there is no opening or closing of drawers, and open shelves accommodate more records in a given floor area with less aisle space. Thirty-six inches is recommended for aisles between units, although thirty inches is adequate when there is a critical shortage of floor space. When file cabinets are arranged in a single row, a three-foot aisle between rows is adequate. When the cabinets face each other, five-foot aisles are required to allow room for opening two face-to-face drawers.

File cabinets provide a somewhat neater filing area, and protect records from dust and dirt. However, good housekeeping in an open-shelf filing area will alleviate the need to protect records from dust and dirt.

When purchasing storage units, one must determine the number of linear filing inches provided by the units and the number of filing inches currently being used to store medical records. Then the projected linear filing inches required for the next five or ten years should be added. Dividing this sum by the number of linear filing inches available in a storage unit determines the total number of units needed.

Example: A health information department currently using 1,435 linear filing inches to store its medical records wants to buy new open-shelf filing units. Each of the shelves in a new five-shelf unit measures 33 linear filing inches. With five shelves per filing unit, the total filing inches in one shelving unit would be 165 linear filing inches:

33 inches per x 5 shelves in = 165 filing inches in
  shelf   each unit each shelving unit

At present, 1,435 filing inches are required to store the medical records. It is estimated that an additional 300 filing inches should be added to allow for five-year expansion capabilities. Total filing inches required are 1,735. To determine the total number of file shelving units to purchase, divide the required filing inches by the number of linear filing inches in each shelving unit:

1,735 filing inches ÷ 165 inches per   =   10.5 shelving
                 shelving unit   units

In order to provide for all of the expansion file space, a total of 11 shelving units are needed.

Shelving may be purchased with more than five shelves per unit, some are as high as eight shelves. Consideration should be given to the fact that the higher the shelving, the more need there will be to provide step stools.

Pairs of units placed back to back in long rows are the most compact arrangement for storage units in the file area. Movable file units on tracks are also available and should be considered if storage space is a problem. In addition to saving space over conventional file shelving units, movable files increase operating efficiency; since the file area itself is more compact and personnel do not have to walk as far. Limited access to movable file area may be a major disadvantage for facilities with highly active files. As only one aisle is provided for several units of shelving, it is often impossible for two individuals to work in adjoining sections of the file. Health information departments with one or two persons responsible for filing may find movable files very beneficial to their efficient operation (Figure 3).

Automated filing systems have been developed which bring requested records to clerical personnel at the touch of a few buttons. The amount of clerical time and energy expended is reduced with automation, but the cost of such systems is very high and access may be inadequate for highly active files.

GUIDING THE FILES

Guides should be placed throughout the files to expedite the filing and finding of records. The number of guides needed depends upon the thickness of the majority of the medical records in the file. For records of medium thickness, a guide for every fifty records is adequate. For very thick records, more guides are needed. Active files generally require closer guiding than inactive files.

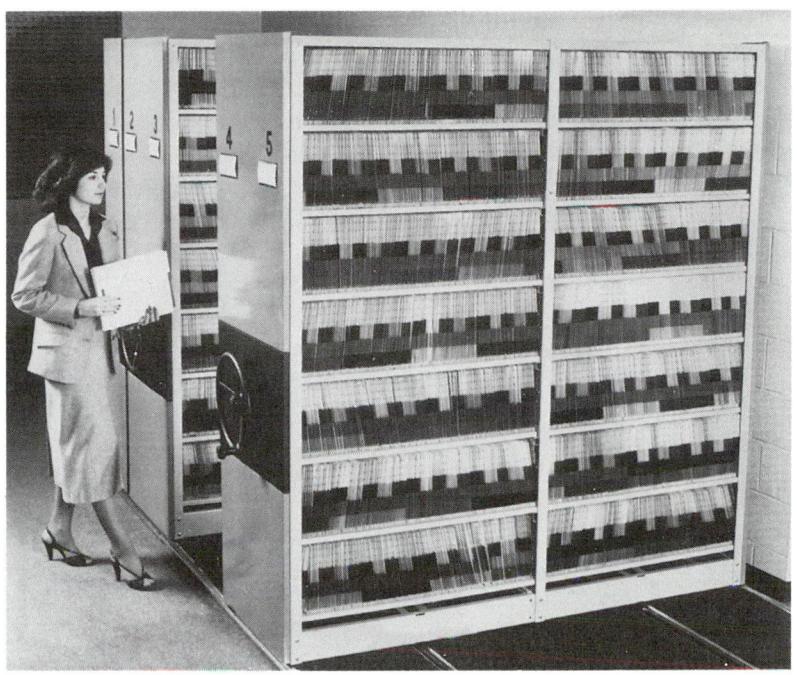

FIGURE 3. MOVABLE, OPEN-SHELF FILES

When purchasing guides, durability and visibility should be the primary concern. The tab or projection on the guide should project far enough beyond the records to ensure complete exposure of the numbers on the guide.

Usually two pairs of numbers appear on each guide in terminal and middle digit files. For example, guides for the primary digit 84 might be as follows:

$$\frac{00}{84} \qquad \frac{01}{84} \qquad \frac{02}{84} \qquad \frac{03}{84}$$

Note that the top number on the guide is the secondary number, and the bottom number is the primary number. In a terminal digit file, the first record to appear behind guide 00 would be 00-00-84, followed by the record 01-00-84.

To determine the total number of guides needed, the following formula may be used:

$$\frac{\text{TOTAL NUMBER OF RECORDS}}{\text{NUMBER OF RECORDS BETWEEN GUIDES}} = \frac{\text{TOTAL NUMBER}}{\text{OF GUIDES}}$$

If the total number of records is not known, an estimate may be made by multiplying the filing inches by the average number of records per inch. Records on several shelves should be counted to determine the average number of records per inch.

Once the total number of terminal digit guides has been calculated, the number pattern on the guides can be determined. There are 100 primary sections in the file area from 00

TOTAL NUMBER OF GUIDES NEEDED		PRIMARY SECTIONS		GUIDES IN EACH PRIMARY SECTION	PATTERN ON GUIDES
10,000	÷	100	=	10	00 00 01 00 (every 100 numbers) 02 00 etc.
5,000	÷	100	=	50	00 00 02 00 (every 200 numbers) 04 00 etc.
2,000	÷	100	=	20	00 00 05 00 (every 500 numbers) 10 00 etc.
1,000	÷	100	=	10	00 00 10 00 (every 1,000 numbers) 20 00 etc.
500	÷	100	=	5	00 00 20 00 (every 2,000 numbers) 40 00 etc.
400	÷	100	=	4	00 00 25 00 (every 2,500 numbers) 50 00 etc.
TOTAL NUMBER OF GUIDES NEEDED		PRIMARY SECTIONS		GUIDES IN EACH PRIMARY SECTION	PATTERN ON GUIDES

FIGURE 4. TERMINAL DIGIT GUIDE PATTERN

to 99. If the total number of guides necessary for the filing area is 100, one guide per primary section would be sufficient. The pattern on the guide would read 00-00, 00-01, 00-02, etc. Two hundred total guides would result in 2 guides per primary section, with one at the beginning and one in the middle of each section.

00-00	00-01	00-02
50-00	50-01	50-02

Thus, to determine the pattern on terminal digit guides, divide the total number of guides by the primary sections. The answer depicts the number of guides within each primary section, and these guides should be distributed evenly among the secondary numbers in that section.

A table for determining pattern of terminal digit guides is provided in Figure 4.

In a straight numerical filing system, guides must be continually changed. This is also true for middle digit filing. Because new numbers are issued in chronological order, new guides must be placed in the file to reflect the numerical increase of the two left-hand digits of the number. Similarly, as old records are permanently removed from the file, guides in affected sections of the file require change. Terminal digit guides, on the other hand, are more permanent, because their primary and secondary digits keep recurring as new numbers are assigned to patients

PROTECTIVE COVERS FOR RECORDS

In order to protect the pages from tearing during repeated handling, medical records should have protective covers such as chart covers, file folders, or large envelopes. For an additional small charge, chart covers can be equipped with fasteners

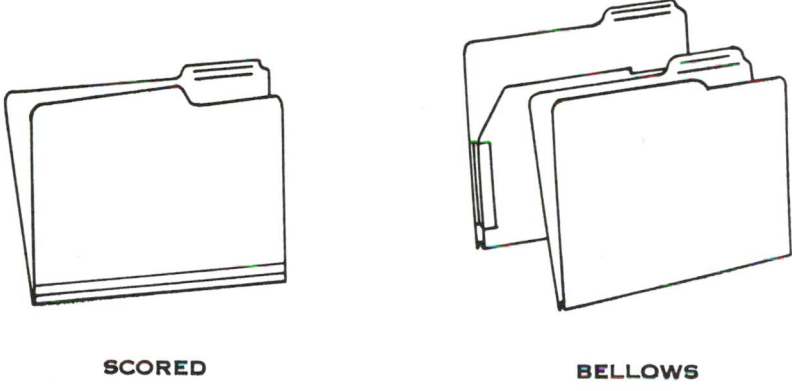

SCORED   **BELLOWS**

FIGURE 5. FILE FOLDERS

to hold the pages in place. These fasteners can be located at the top of the cover or on the left side as with books. The fold of a file folder should be scored or bellowed to allow for expansion (see Figure 5).

Chart covers may be purchased with preprinted numbers which provide a neat and legible appearance. If bar coding is used for record tracking, bar codes may also be preprinted. Alternatively, bar code labels may be affixed as the records are used, although this introduces a source for potential error. The patient's name should also be placed on the cover. A sequential list of years printed horizontally on the front right-hand side allows for checking the year of the most recent occasion of service and makes purging inactive records an easy process, as long as activity dates are consistently updated.

SAFETY

Safety factors are an important consideration in the filing area, and safety rules should be conspicuously posted. The prevention of falls is of prime importance, particularly when clerks are working with the upper shelves in open-shelf units. Skid-proof ladders are a wise investment. Work areas with table space should be interspersed throughout the files. There may be either pullout shelves in the record-storage unit or carts of some type to assist in processing records within the filing area. Adequate lighting reduces eyestrain. Proper conditioning of the air with regard to temperature, humidity, and dust control is essential for fire prevention and employee productivity.

Fire and other disaster prevention and control procedures are also essential. Records should not be stored on the floor, as there is potential for water damage from flooding or even routine floor washing. Sprinkler systems must be evaluated, and appropriate fire extinguishers placed conspicuously. All employees should be trained in what to do in the event of fire or other disaster.

ORGANIZATIONAL PATTERNS OF FILES

Storage and retention of medical records in a health care facility should facilitate the retrieval of requested records. There are two basic methods of filing records - centralized and decentralized.

CENTRALIZATION

Centralized filing means that all information about a patient is funneled into a single file held in a central location. In hospital applications, a centralized file usually means that the patient's inpatient, outpatient, and emergency records are filed in a single file in a central location.

The use of multiple-part forms for documentation of clinic and emergency records may make it possible to maintain centralized records while providing a mechanism for quick reference for telephone calls and unscheduled follow-up visits. Another alternative for areas rendering continuous care for a specified period, such as radiation or physical therapy, is to route their complete documentation to the unit record when treatment is concluded.

DECENTRALIZATION

Decentralized files result when certain parts of a record are filed in another location away from the central file area. In hospitals this may mean that the emergency record of a patient is filed in the emergency service, or outpatient records are filed in the outpatient area. This leaves only the inpatient records in a central file. Even when a "unit" is made of several inpatient admissions for a patient, the files are considered decentralized if outpatient or emergency room records are filed separately.

ADVANTAGES/DISADVANTAGES OF EACH

Centralization has many advantages:

- There is less duplication of effort with regard to creation, maintenance, and storage of records.
- There is less overall expenditure on space and equipment.
- A composite record containing all available information is of greater help to the health care team than one in which parts are scattered in several places.
- Procedures and policies for record activity are standardized.
- Personnel may become more proficient in various file room functions and procedures.
- Record control and security are easier to maintain.
- Supervision of file room personnel is more consistent.

In spite of obvious advantages, circumstances may make it expedient to decentralize records, either temporarily or permanently. This may occur when outpatients are being seen frequently so it is more efficient to store the record in the outpatient area. Another situation in which decentralization might be justified is when a health care facility operates from several sites, and a decentralized record system requires less transportation time and effort.

Other terms used for decentralization are "controlled/decentralized" (records are housed separately but controlled through uniform policies, procedures, methods, and forms) and "satellite" (records remain in a satellite location during active treatment, then are returned to the central file area).

Whatever the reasons for decentralizing records or the terminology used to describe it, one should be sure that the methodology chosen is best for the facility.

RECORD CONTROL

Regardless of whether files are centralized or decentralized, there must be centralization of authority over them. One person, logically the director of the health information department, should be authorized to establish and maintain control over all filing procedures and record usage.

REQUISITIONS

Routine requests for records, as from outpatient areas or for study purposes, should be delivered to the health information department by a specified time of day established by hospital policy. A common practice is to require that all routine requisitions for records be received in the department the afternoon before the day on which the records are needed. The exact time set for the deadline (noon or 4:00 P.M., for example) is dependent on the volume of requests received daily and the number of filing room personnel available to pull requisitioned records.

Patients care areas requesting records for scheduled appointments should bear the responsibility for filling out requisition slips which are readable and which have patients' names and numbers filled in correctly. Non-routine requests for records such as those from the emergency department must be processed as quickly as possible by health information personnel. Phone requests for records needed immediately are acceptable; file clerks can make out the necessary requisitions for these "STAT" requests. A facility policy should delineate how these records will be transported to their destination.

A requisition slip is usually a three-part form (see Figure 6). The minimum amount of information which must be included on the slip is the patient's name and medical record number, the name of the requisitioning patient care area or person, and the date on which the record is needed. In a large outpatient area of a hospital, or in a large ambulatory care facility, time of patient appointment may also be needed.

One copy of the requisition is fastened to the medical record when it is pulled from the file. This copy serves to route the record. Another copy becomes the sign-out which is placed in an outguide and filed to replace the pulled record. The outguide

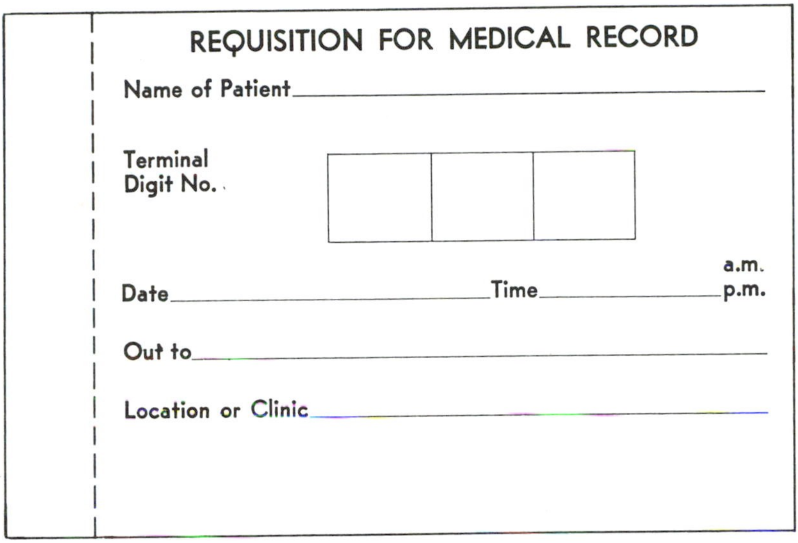
REQUISITION FOR MEDICAL RECORD

Name of Patient__________

Terminal Digit No.

Date__________ Time__________ a.m. p.m.

Out to__________

Location or Clinic__________

FIGURE 6. REQUISITION FORM

and sign-out are removed from the file when the record is returned. Still another copy of the requisition may be retained in the health information department as a reference to those records which have been sent to other areas of the facility and not yet returned.

A small card file box may be used to house the locator file which contains copies of requisition slips for all patient records removed from the department. The locator file is arranged in numerical order by medical record number. When the patient's record is returned to the health information department, this copy of the requisition slip is removed from the locator file and destroyed. If a medical record is not returned within the established time, the locator file provides a ready reference for reminding the requestor of the need for the record to be returned promptly to the health information department. In institutions in which scheduling of appointments is done via computer, the routing and/or sign-out slips(s) may be computer-generated and the locator file maintained in a computerized record tracking system.

OUTGUIDES

Outguides provide an important means of control over record usage. They are used to replace a record that has been removed from the files. The guide remains in the files until the borrowed record is returned and refiled. Folders or sign-out cards with

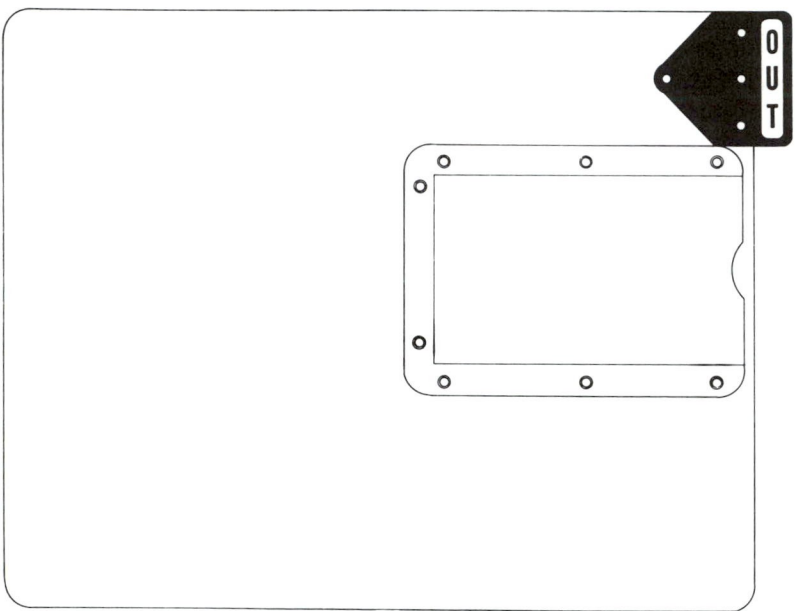

FIGURE 7. OUTGUIDES

pockets for storing requisition slips are popular for this purpose. The use of colored outguides is helpful to the clerk in spotting the correct location for refiling a record. Outguides with large plastic pockets may be used to hold loose or late reports until the record is returned to the files. Since outguides are used over and over again, sturdy construction is essential (see Figure 7).

CHARGE-OUT SYSTEM

The cardinal rule in the file area is that no record can be removed from file without being replaced by an outguide. This rule applies not only to extra-departmental personnel but also to employees of the health information department.

An individual receiving a record should assume responsibility for returning it in good condition and at the designated time. Certain rules should be established with regard to the length of time a record may be kept out of file. It is wise to require that medical records be returned at the close of each day; so if emergencies occur, records are available when needed.

An increasing problem in charge-out and return of records is the number of records required for various study purposes (claims audits, quality management, physician research, and so forth).

While physicians or other facility personnel may sign out records from the department to take to a work area during the day, all records must be returned to the department by closing time. If the same records will be needed again within several days, many health information departments set up separate temporary files within the health information department for these studies.

Persons who are not employees or members of the staff must review records in the health information department. Original records should never be removed from the facility except under subpoena or valid court order.

Transfer of records from the original requestor to another requires the use of a transfer card or slip. Use of transfers eliminates the need for such records to be sent back to the health information department before being forwarded to the second requesting party. Transfer notices are sent to the file area where they are placed in the outguide (see Figure 8).

AUTOMATED RECORD TRACKING SYSTEM

A computerized chart location system is an ideal method of tracking medical records. Commonly the patient name, medical record number, reason code, and user code are entered via a terminal to sign out a record to a user. The computer automatically records the date and time on each transaction. If the tracking system utilizes the same database as the master patient index, the computer may automatically provide the patient's name when the number is entered, so only verification of the accuracy of the name is required. Bar codes representing the patient's number may also be used on each medical record to speed up the process of checking medical records in and out. Bar codes may be pre-printed on record covers or a label may be applied. A bar code reader consisting of a small computer terminal with a wand is used to read the bar codes. The remaining information required to complete each transaction is entered via a keyboard.

COMMUNITY GENERAL HOSPITAL

TRANSFER OF MEDICAL RECORDS

Date_____

From_____

To_____

For: Clinic Appt._____Corres._____Room No._____

To Be Used By Dr._____

Please Send This Card to Medical Record Dept. Immediately

FIGURE 8. TRANSFER FORM

The installation of a computerized tracking system is highly recommended if the department's file activity justifies the expense. Such systems may be developed on inexpensive personal computers in smaller facilities or on mainframe computers in larger facilities. At a minimum, such a system should have the ability to inquire of chart location by medical record number, check records in and out by location and individual requestor, and display the status of any record. Inputs and outputs of automated record tracking systems are illustrated in Chapter 14.

LOCATING MISFILES

Regardless of the number of record control systems used in the health information department file area, occasionally a medical record will be placed in the wrong location or will not be signed out correctly. Various techniques are available to assist a person in locating a record that has been misfiled. Among these techniques are:

1. Look for transpositions within each set of two digits of the number. For example, the number 46-37-82 may be filed as 46-37-28 or 46-73-82.

2. Look for misfiles of "3" under "5" or "8" and vice versa as these numbers may look similar, and of "7" or "8" under "9", especially as covers become worn.

3. Check for a certain number in the hundred group just preceding or following the number, as 485 under 385 or 585, or under other similar combinations.

4. Check for transpositions of first and last numbers.

5. Check the record just before and just after the one needed. It sometimes happens that a record is put into another cover rather than between two covers.

6. Check immediately above and below where the record should be filed, as a distraction during filing may have resulted in misplacement.

COLOR CODING OF RECORD FOLDERS

Color coding refers to the use of color on folders to aid in the prevention of misfiles and in the location of misfiled records. Color bars in various positions around the edges of folders create distinct patterns of color in various sections of the file. A break in the color pattern in a file section signals a misfiled record. Color coding is most effective when used in conjunction with terminal digit and middle digit filing, although workable color-coding systems may be used for straight numerical filing.

One approach to color coding in a terminal digit or middle digit file utilizes ten different colors to signify the first primary digits 0 through 9. Two color bars or blocks appearing in the same position can be used to signify each of the two primary digits. In this case the top color bar represents the left-hand digit of the primary set, and the bottom color bar represents the right-hand digit of the primary set. If brown is the color assigned to the digit 8 and green is the color assigned to the digit 4, a chart numbered 16 94 84 in a terminal digit file is color coded with a brown band on top, with a green band directly beneath it. Additional color bars may be added to indicate secondary digits, and there are many combinations which may be used.

The entire folder may also be colored and signify the right hand primary digit or the left hand secondary digit to expedite visual location in large departments.

In setting up a color-coding system, it is generally advisable to limit color coding to two or three digits. This ensures a simple, easy-to-learn system. Folders already color coded may be purchased from commercial firms, or employees of the health information department may apply colored tape to the folders.

Figure 9 is a table which shows colors associated with two-digit primary numbers and one-digit primary numbers which are available through some vendors.

TWO-DIGIT PRIMARY NUMBERS	ONE-DIGIT NUMBERS	COLORED BANDS
00-09	0	PURPLE
10-19	1	YELLOW
20-29	2	DARK GREEN
30-39	3	ORANGE
40-49	4	LIGHT BLUE
50-59	5	BROWN
60-69	6	CERISE
70-79	7	LIGHT GREEN
80-89	8	RED
90-99	9	DARK BLUE

FIGURE 9. COLOR CODES FOR PRIMARY NUMBERS

OTHER FILING RULES AND PROCEDURES

Some basic rules to aid in efficient handling of medical records include:

1. When records are returned to the health information department, they should be sorted before being filed. This

facilitates the finding of needed but unfiled records, and makes refiling easier.

2. Except for facility personnel who have been instructed to use the file area during unattended hours, only health information department personnel should be authorized to handle records. During unattended hours, facility personnel returning records should leave them at a designated place in the file area or health information department.

3. Records with torn covers and those with loose papers should be repaired promptly to prevent further damage or loss of valuable information.

4. An audit of the files should be made periodically to locate misfiled records and check requisitions which indicate records have not been returned.

5. Medical records involving legal actions should not be stored in the general files; these can be filed in a locked file cabinet in the health information director's office. Outguides should be placed in the permanent file to indicate that these records are in a "special" file.

6. Filing-area personnel should be responsible for keeping the shelves neat and orderly. Disorderly files increase the likelihood of misfiles.

7. Medical records being processed or used by employees within the department should remain on desk tops or in specified files so they can be available at any time.

8. Written procedures for filing-area personnel are of assistance in their training and in maintaining control over the files.

9. Records which are voluminous should be separated into two or more volumes, but filed together in one location.

10. Laboratory slips, x-rays, and other "loose" or "late" reports received in the department should be date-stamped and sorted when received. Every effort should be made to incorporate them into the records as soon as possible. Care should be taken to be sure such reports are in the correct section of the record.

11. The person supervising the file area should keep a report of activities in the area. Items included in the report might include: number of requisitioned charts pulled each day, number of emergency calls, and number of records

which could not be found. Counts such as these provide useful information for planning work and for control over the files.

TRANSPORTATION OF RECORDS

There are several ways to transport records. In most facilities, the majority of records are hand-carried from one place to another. Health information departments should establish specific delivery and pickup schedules. Frequency of delivery and pickup is dependent upon the amount of record activity. Health information personnel cannot deliver individual records on short notice to requesting departments as a matter of routine unless department staffing includes "runners," or persons assigned to deliver records. Unless otherwise provided, departments requesting a record for emergency use should dispatch one of their own employees to pick it up.

Some facilities are equipped with pneumatic tube systems which rapidly transport single records to various departments. Strict rules regarding the use and maintenance of a tube system are essential. One of the drawbacks to such systems is the fact that tubes are often too small to transport a thick record.

Dumbwaiters, record elevators, and horizontal conveyors are often used to transport records. A patient registration area located directly above a health information department can make good use of a dumbwaiter or elevator.

Facsimile machines (FAX machines) are computer devices which transmit likenesses of documents over telephone wires. These may be used to transmit copies of records, often from one building to another. For example, a hospital may have several outpatient facilities throughout a city. Discharge summaries and other pertinent documents can be faxed to an outpatient center for the price of a telephone call and the FAX paper.

MEDICAL RECORD RETENTION POLICIES

In most facilities storage space is at a premium. Space costs money to acquire and maintain. Space that is not used for revenue-generating purposes is kept to a minimum.

The health information professional must develop a formal plan or record retention schedule for the automatic transfer of eligible records to inactive storage and later destruction of the medical record itself.

The definition of inactivity with reference to medical records in a given health care faculty depends on (1) the amount of filing space available in the health information department and (2) the yearly expansion rate of current files (number of filing inches needed for each year's records). In establishing a plan for the disposition of inactive records, one must consider (1) volume of research; (2) readmission rate for inpatients and outpatients; (3) statutes of limitation in the state in which the health care faculty is located; and (4) cost involved in microfilming, inactive storage, and destruction of records.

INACTIVE MEDICAL RECORDS

Practically speaking, the chief criterion for determining record inactivity is the amount of space available in the department for the efficient storage of newer medical records. If there is no more space for active record storage, an effort should be made to systematically retire old records to inactive status at the same rate as new records are being added.

Inactive records can be (1) stored in another area of the facility, (2) commercially stored, (3) destroyed in compliance with record retention statues, or (4) microfilmed, or (5) stored on disk.

Files for inactive records may be established in areas of the facility physically separate from the health information department. As old records are removed from the active files, they should be replaced by transfer slips to the inactive files, or their location may be noted in the computerized tracking system. This will eliminate unnecessary searching.

Some facilities utilize commercial storage companies to house inactive records. These companies make deliveries to the facility upon request. When this method is employed, it is advisable to have a contract drawn up stipulating the arrangements made for storage and retrieval, especially the requirements for confidentiality of the records.

DESTRUCTION OF MEDICAL RECORDS

Although some hospitals destroy inactive medical records by shredding or burning, most health care facilities microfilm medical records because they lack the storage space required to

Patient health information must be available to meet the needs of continued patient care, legal requirements, research, education, and other legitimate uses.

Each health provider should develop a retention schedule for patient health information that meets the needs of its patients, physicians, researchers, and other legitimate users and complies with legal, regulatory, and accreditation requirements. Providers should develop guidelines that specify what information should be kept, the time period for which it should be kept, and the storage medium (paper, microfilm, optical disk, magnetic tape, or other). In the absence of specific state requirements for record retention, providers should keep health information for at least the period specified by the state's statutes of limitations. A longer retention period is prudent, since the statute may not begin to run until the potential plaintiff learns of the causal relation between an injury and the care received. If the patient was a minor, the provider should retain health information until the patient reaches the age of majority (as defined by state law) plus the period of the statute of limitations.

Unless longer periods of time are required by state or federal law, the American Health Information Management Association recommends that patient health information be retained for the following minimum time periods:

Paitent health records (adults)	10 years after the most recent encounter
Patient health records (minors)	Age of majority plus statute of limitation
Diagnostic images (such as x-ray film)	5 years
Disease index	10 years
Fetal heart monitor records	10 years after infant reached age of majority
Master patient index	Permanently
Operative index	10 years
Registers of births	Permanently
Register of deaths	Permanently
Register of emergency department patients	Permanently
Register of surgical procedures	Permanently

As the health care industry moves from paper to computer-based patient records, retention policies must be re-examined. Development of longitudinal patient records will require the storage of core clinical information during the patient's lifetime.

Source: American Health Information Management Association, 1994

FIGURE 10. PATIENT HEALTH INFORMATION

maintain medical records for recommended retention periods. In 1994, the American Health Information Management Association published a position statement on the retention of health information. It is shown in Figure 10.

If the adoption of a record retention policy as suggested by this statement reduces the previous period of retention by a health care institution, it is recommended that any new policy be developed with the full knowledge and participation of the medical staff, legal counsel for the institution, and any past or present liability insurance carrier affording coverage during any time in which the affected records were made.

MISCELLANEOUS RECORD RETENTION

The needs of the individual hospital, the statute of limitations for the specific state, and possible future use of each type of record should be carefully considered before reaching a decision regarding retention periods for the individual health care facility.

Nurses' Bedside Records

As nurses' notes are primarily a means of communication between the physicians and nurses, they have served their most important function during the episode of care. Therefore, to reduce the bulk and make medical records less cumbersome to handle, some hospitals remove the nurses' notes from records of adult patients when health information personnel assemble and check the medical record after discharge of the patient. The nurses' notes are then filed in chronological order in some place less accessible than the current files until the statute of limitations has expired, and they are destroyed. By filing these records in chronological order, they can be easily found if needed; and it is a simple matter to destroy the oldest each year. Since the statute of limitations does not expire until after a minor has reached majority, it may be easier to retain them in the medical record and handle them in the same manner as the rest of the record. The practice of separating nurses' notes is not common due to the number of claims and quality assurance reviews conducted on medical records.

Emergency Department Records

Emergency department records need only be preserved for the duration of the statute of limitations for negligence or malpractice suits in the individual state unless needed for proof of hospital services or when a legal   action is pending. The medical information which they contain is often of an episodic nature so they are of little value except for the protection of the hospital as a record of what was done. However, if the patient was in a serious condition, the emergency department record should become part of the patient's medical record after admission to the hospital and thus be kept as long as the medical record.

Registers: Patient and Delivery Room

Patient and delivery room registers should be kept permanently, because they list all patients admitted to or born in the hospital in chronological order. Either or both of these registers may be required by state or local law. Even if they are not, they serve as a double check against the master patient index and will be invaluable if an index card is lost or misfiled. If space is at a premium or the paper on which these registers are written is deteriorating, they may be microfilmed.

Indexes

The period disease and operation indexes need to be retained is governed by the length of time covered by specific studies by the medical staff in each facility. If studies are frequently made covering a 25-year period, these indexes should be kept that long. Otherwise, these indexes would have served their maximum period of usefulness in 10 years.

The physicians' index has generally served its purpose within a maximum period of 5 to 10 years. A chief use of the index is in supplying information when physicians are applying to specialty boards, but this information is usually requested within a five-year period. If there is a possibility that the governing board of the hospital might want to know the amount of work individual physicians bring to the hospital, an annual summary could be compiled and preserved rather than keeping the index after its period of general usefulness has passed.

MISCELLANEOUS

Daily Analyses of Hospital Services should not be needed after a two-year period and monthly analyses after a five-year period. Annual reports compiled from these records should be kept permanently.

Birth and Death Certificates should be preserved permanently. If filed in the medical record at discharge of the patient, they will automatically be preserved as long as needed.

Narcotic records normally do not come under the supervision of the health information department, unless a facility does not have a registered pharmacist. Narcotic "records shall be kept, subject to inspection, for a period of two years from the date of dispensing or distributing of such drugs as opium, isonipecaine, coca leaves, opiate, and compound, salt, derivative, or preparation thereof." (U.S. Treasury Department, Bureau of Narcotics, Regulations No. 5 Section 2550; Section 2554. (c.) (1), (2), (4), (d); and Section 2556.)

MICROFILMING

Microfilm or microrecords are the result of a photographic process which reduces an original document to a very small size, resulting in high density information recording and thus considerable space saving. Because microfilm is self-reproducible, microfilming also reduces paper handling as a microfilm copy can be easily made while the original master remains in the file.

Microphotographic camera lenses are made which can reduce the size of the image by various amounts stated in terms of a reduction ratio. If the reduction ratio is 24 to 1, stated as 24X, the original document is reduced to an image 1/24 its original size. Reduction ratios range from 5X to more than 2,400X. Medical records are commonly microfilmed at a reduction ratio of 24X which results in a storage savings of 95 percent.

The magnification ratio specifies how much the microrecord will be enlarged. Ideally, the magnification ratio should match the reduction ratio so that the enlarged microrecord will be the original size of the document filmed. The film used in the microfilm process is available in four sizes: 16 mm, 35 mm, 70 mm, and 105 mm; 16 mm film is used for recording documents up to 14 inches in width.

In 1951 Public Law 129 was amended by Congress which allowed for the admission and acceptance of microfilmed records as primary evidence. This law was re-affirmed in Section 1732(b) in 1958. Thus the use of microfilm as primary evidence is now legal throughout the U.S. regardless of whether a state has a law to that effect or not. The application of microfilming to the health care industry for patient, departmental, and corporate storage of records has become a common practice.

FACTORS TO CONSIDER IN DECIDING TO MICROFILM

Factors to consider in deciding to microfilm are the cost, quality of original documents, and readability. Microfilming can be expensive and time consuming because of the equipment needed for the process. Equipment needed for in-house micro-filming includes cameras to photograph the records, jacket inserters which provide enlarged viewing of film images for inspection and selection, microfilm lay-up equipment which prepares microfiche masters, and film duplication equipment which replicates the microform. In any system there are costs for preparing records for microfilm and management costs for inspecting and indexing microrecords. To use microrecords, readers to enlarge the microrecord for reading, reader-printers for printing hard copies and storage equipment are required at a minimum. Film and filing supplies and storage equipment are also required.

Original documents that have deteriorated will result in microfilm of poor quality. Carbon copies and deep shades of colored paper do not photograph well. Colors on original paper can usually be photographed but in black and white only.

From the user's standpoint, viewing microrecords on readers can be difficult. In any event, readers should be widely located throughout the facility. But even with wide availability of readers, the user must still go to a fixed location to view the microfilmed record.

MICROFILMING PROCESS

Preparation of Records

The first step in microfilming is the preparation of the re-cords. Each facility must decide whether the entire medical record is to be filmed, or whether some pages are to be excluded. A distinction must also be made between the medical record per se, which pertains to the care and treatment of the patient, and administrative records.

Often forms kept for the protection of the hospital at the time of patient hospitalization, such as clothing lists, may be discarded. Blank sheets should be eliminated. Anything not vital to the patient's continuing care or not needed for study or legal reasons may be removed. In general, care should be exercised in preparing records. The cost of filming is low enough that documents of any potential future value should be retained. In any event, the procedures for stripping records must be clear; when in doubt, clerical personnel should be instructed to consult the health information director. For a final decision, the hospital's legal counsel should be consulted.

Other steps in preparing a record for microfilming include:

1. Pulling all staples or removing other types of fasteners.
2. Checking all sheets in the medical records to see that they are arranged in a standard sequence.
3. Indicating two-sided records that must be copied on both sides.
4. Removing all blank sheets and miscellaneous records not being preserved by the hospital.
5. Checking all names and medical record numbers.
6. Making a target sheet containing them medical record number. This separates one record from another.
7. Indexing each admission; separating and indexing outpatient and emergency records if necessary.

Filming the Record

The actual filming of records is a relatively simple process after preparation is completed. While personnel can be trained to operate a camera, processor, and unitizing equipment, the speed and quality with which the work is done depends upon the operator's dexterity and attitude. If space, personnel, or costs prohibit filming in-house, medical records may be sent to a microfilm service company. The entire job can be done on a contract basis or the actual filming may take place in the facility with the film being processed, inspected, and unitized under service contract.

If any part of the filming process is to be done by a microfilm service company, a formal contract should be made between the health care facility and the service company. Items to be included in the contract are: cost (usually based on a rate per 1,000 exposures); type of index system to be used on the microfilm; photography by trained technicians; processing and inspection of microfilm; retake of documents if needed; confidentiality of information; access to records being filmed, if required; transportation of records to be microfilmed and delivery of completed microfilm; and provision for destruction of original records. Original records should not be destroyed until the health information director or designee has spot-checked each batch of returned microfilmed records.

There are several types of cameras available if filming is to be performed by the facility. A rotary camera is the least expensive. With a rotary camera, documents move through the camera on a roller-transport system, which can make images at speeds exceeding 500 documents per minute. Approximately 2,500 images can be microfilmed on a single 100-foot roll of 16 mm film. A rotary camera can be used for filming either one side of a document or the front and back of a document at the same time. A planetary camera is used to film x-rays and other oversized documents which require high resolution or density, using 35 mm film. The rotoline camera is used for continuous forms such as EEGs, computer printouts, or monitoring strips. A step and repeat camera is used to produce microfiche only. One page of the record after another is exposed directly onto film which is 4 inches wide. The film is then cut into 6-inch lengths which result in the standard 4 x 6-inch microfiche.

Processing

Once medical record documents are photographed, the film is processed and may be left in its original roll form or converted into a unitized microform.

There are a wide variety of microforms available: roll film, microfilm jackets, microfiche, ultrafiche, aperture cards, and computer output microfilm (COM). When selecting a microform, a major consideration should be in selecting the microform which matches the needs of the user. Other criteria include: type of information to be stored, overall cost, accessibility, capability and cost of making duplicates, and frequency of updating the record.

Roll film is the least expensive microform to prepare and results in the greatest storage density. A 100-foot roll of 16 mm film containing up to 2,500 letter-size images is stored in a box measuring 4 x 4 x 1 inches. Roll film can be updated by splicing new images onto the roll of film. This procedure is not often used for medical records, however, as it destroys the security of the roll film, and sometimes its legal acceptability. As a permanent record, roll film is excellent; since documents committed to roll film are "locked in" and cannot be misfiled.

In high reference files, roll film can be packaged in either cartridges or cassettes that facilitate film loading onto microfilm readers.

Retrieval of information from roll films is highly dependent on file organization and film indexing. The contents of a roll must be noted on the storage carton, cassette, or cartridge. On the roll film itself, the target sheets containing the medical rercord number in large characters mark the beginning of each record. Other methods of indexing roll film are image count, bar or code line, and photo-optical binary code. In the image count method, marks (blips) below each image are counted electronically and used by the machine to control image retrieval in a linear sequence. In the bar or code line method, bars or lines between the frames have positional value as related to a scale along the edge of the reader or reader-printer screen. And, in the photo-optical binary code method, document numbers or index terms are recorded in optical binary code adjacent to each document. This method must be used with an electronic logic system for retrieval.

Since roll film cannot be easily updated, it is not recommended for use with either the serial-unit or unit methods of numbering. The integrity of the unit record cannot be maintained with roll microfilm. The best application of roll microfilm is in situations where serial numbering is used.

Unitized microforms are more costly than roll film, but the additional cost is often fully justified in terms of greater file flexibility, more rapid record retrieval, and the ability to provide a copy of the unitized microform rapidly and inexpensively.

There are several types of unitized microforms. Microfilm jackets are composed of two panels of very thin transparent material, joined horizontally by lines of adhesive which form channels. Microfilmed roll film may be slid into the channels. Jackets are advantageous in that they may be updated by inserting new images into the channels. A microfilm jacket that is 4 x 6 inches in size can hold 60 images - 5 rows of images, 12 images per row.

Microfiche is a transparent rectangle of film containing micro-images. Unlike microfilm jackets where images cut from roll film are inserted into channels, the images are photographed directly onto the film. The standard size of microfiche is 4 x 6 inches, which holds 98 images, filmed at a reduction ratio of 24X.

Ultrafiche is a variation of microfiche in which a much greater reduction ratio (90X to 2,400X) is used so thousands of images may be stored on a standard 4 x 6-inch card.

For any of the unitized microforms, an identifying header which is usually the medical record number, is lettered across the top margin of the microform. Color-coding may also be added across the entire top margin to aid in filing and retrieval.

Yet another microform, computer output microfilm (COM), was developed in response to the large quantities of paper that computers generate. COM takes information stored in a computer on magnetic tape, translates it into readable form, and displays it on a computer display screen. A microfilm camera, called a recorder, photographs the displayed information, reducing it to microrecord size. A processor develops the film.

Retrieving Information from Microfilm

Once medical records have been microfilmed, they must be placed on a projector, called a reader, for viewing. There are several types of readers available. The type selected will depend upon the needs of the user, the type of microform, and cost.

A portable reader weighs less than 50 pounds. Many are battery powered, and some may only be used with microfiche. Because of their low price, many facilities use them to supplement existing microfilm equipment.

Stationary readers may be desktop or free-standing. They provide a wide viewing screen and a wider choice of option features than portable readers. Some accept a number of different microforms.

A reader-printer may be used for both viewing and producing a hard copy of a microform. Reader-printers are available for both low-volume and high-volume reproduction units to reproduce documents ranging in size from 8-1/2 x 11 inches to 20 x 30 inches.

Computer assisted retrieval (CAR) is a method of locating and retrieving documents through the use of computer indexes. Computer assisted retrieval is applicable to records stored in hard copy, magnetic tape, or microfilm. The software indexing system for CAR pinpoints the location of any record in the file by file code. Computerized microfilm indexes are usually very detailed and comprehensive. On a microfilm file, a separate index for each document may be maintained; or groups of documents may be batched as one. CAR may be justified in microfilm systems where there is a high reference and retrieval rate.

DISK STORAGE

Recently, health information departments have been investigating the merits of magnetic disk (or tape) storage and optical disk storage. While these storage technologies are not new, their application to large volumes of archival data retention is new.

Magnetic storage allows computer-entered data to be saved on magnetic disk or tape. The magnetic medium affords speed of data access and erasability. Magnetic disk storage media generally hold more data and allow faster access than magnetic tape. While the erasability of data on a magnetic medium makes it practical for updating data, the average life of a magnetic medium is only a few years. Furthermore, the storage capacity of each disk or tape is rather limited, requiring human action to obtain a disk or tape from a storage "library" and place it "online" to be read by a computer. Until recently, entry of data into a computer to be saved on a magnetic storage medium has also been time consuming - requiring considerable keyboarding (typing on a computer keyboard) unless data were already input as data originated.

Optical disk storage utilizes a laser to etch data onto a prepared surface of glass or other permanent material. Optical disks have over eight times the storage capacity of magnetic disks, with the same or greater speed of access. The non-erasable quality (referred to as Write Once, Read Many - or WORM storage) makes it preferable for data retention purposes. Updating is accomplished by storing new data in a new location on the disk rather than storing the new data over old data as in magnetic media. (Erasable optical disks are also available and they combine the updating quality of magnetic media with the durability of the present WORM media.)

Inputting data onto an optical disk may be performed in the same manner as for magnetic media (i.e., entering data via a computer keyboard and having the data passed to the storage medium electronically), or data may be scanned. Scanning is a process in which the physical document is reduced to digital elements (called "bits" in computer terminology) by passing the document through a computerized document scanner.

In addition to scanners, optical disk technology may be accompanied by a "juke box" which serves to move, without human intervention, optical disks online (i.e., into position to be accessed by the computer).

Optical disk technology is currently high priced with costs from $150,000 to more than $1 million. As with most other computer technology, prices will drop. Savings in space, microfilming costs, personnel time, and copying costs should accrue from optical disk storage for medical data retention.

Microfilm was the first alternative medium to paper to be accepted by the courts for storing business records. Because its copying technology is photographically based, microfilm is difficult to alter. This fact combined with the presumption of reliability accorded records made in the regular course of business has led to the widespread acceptance of microfilm by legislatures and courts as a medium that is accurate, reliable, and trustworthy.

Despite the fact that data stored on magnetic media can be easily altered, the courts generally have admitted computerized records kept in the regular course of business on magnetic media. However, the foundational requirements have varied significantly depending on the jurisdiction in which the trial is held.

Given that both magnetic and optical storage are digital and electronic-based and magnetic storage has a history of being legally admissible, it is logical that there is legal foundation for admitting optically stored records in court. Commercial application of optical storage did not begin until the mid-1980s, thus relevant case law will be minimal for some period of time.

SUMMARY

While the methods of numbering medical records and the systems of filing all have the same objective, that is, a continuous record of the patient available at all times, the centralized unit or serial-unit system automatically attains this objective because all records of a patient are filed together in one folder and in one department. If a centralized unit system is coupled with terminal digit filing in health care facilities where the activity of the records is very great, efficient and improved service for the patient, physicians, and other personnel should be the result.

Because the space required for the filing of medical records grows rapidly, the health information practitioner must face the problem of retention of records realistically. It is economically impractical to continue to use valuable space for records that are seldom used or needed. Therefore, periodic surveys should be made by the department head to review the types and frequency of requests made for medical records. Results of these surveys can assist in making decisions regarding storage space, retention schedules, and miniaturizing (storing on microfilm, magnetic media, or optical disk).

STUDY QUESTIONS

1. Describe the serial and unit numbering systems, and list their advantages and disadvantages.
2. Place the following six medical record numbers in sequence according to each filing system: 312497, 312498, 312398, 312399, 322301, 322302:
   a. straight numeric
   b. terminal digit
   c. middle digit
3. List reasons why open-shelf filing units are preferable to file cabinets for medical record storage in the file area.
4. Depict the pattern which will appear on the terminal digit file guides in a file area requiring 2,500 total guides.
5. Define centralized and decentralized filing, and summarize the advantages of centralization for medical records.
6. Describe the functions of a three-part requisition slip.

7. Describe an automated chart location system.

8. List techniques which may be used in locating misfiled records.

9. List the items one must consider when developing a plan for the destruction of inactive medical records.

10. List reasons for microfilming medical records.

11. Discuss the legality of alternate forms of medical records.

12. List factors to consider in microfilming medical records.

13. List the steps in preparing records for filming.

14. Describe the different types of microforms available and the advantages and disadvantages of each.

15. Distinguish between magnetic media and optical disk storage.

REFERENCES

Accreditation Manual for Hospitals, Oakbrook Terrace, Illinois: The Joint Commission on Accreditation of Healthcare Organizations, 1994:38.

Avedon, Don M., "Selecting a Service Bureau," *Journal of Micrographics,* (September-October, 1976).

Bloomrosen, Meryl, "Successful Computer Applications in a Medical Record Department," *JAMRA*, Vol, 53, No. 3, (June, 1982): 34-44.

Broberg, Barbara A., "Records Evaluation for Conversion to Microfilm," Journal of Micrographics, (September-October, 1979).

Campbell, Robert J., "Automated Microfilm Retrieval: A Refresher Course," *Modern Office Procedures*, (October, 1980).

Capozzoli, Elisabeth, RRA, MBA, "An Automated Approach to Medical Record Teaching," *Topics in Health Record Management*, Vol. 2, No. 2, (December, 1981).

"Computers and the Medical Record Department," *Topics in Health Record Management*, Vol. 2, No. 2, (December, 1981).

Counterpoint, "Social Security Number Not National Identifier," *JAMRA,* Vol. 55, No. 4, (April, 1984): 11.

Edland, Linda B., "CAR: The Vehicle for Records Delivery," *Office Administration and Automation*, (September, 1983).

Flanagan, James B., "Look at cost and performance when selecting an optical disk system,"Medical Records Briefing, Vol. 4, No. 7, (June 1989).

Flanagan, James B., "Optical disks: The medical records manager's newest tool has a language all its own," *Medical Records Briefing,* (May 1989).

Flanagan, James B., "Organizational and procedural impact of an optical disk system," *Medical Records Briefing,* Vol. 4, No. 7, (July 1989).

Guide to Microreproduction Equipment, (National Microfilm Association).

Handbook of Hospital Microfilming, (Winston-Salem, NC: Decodex, Inc., 1979).

Johnson, Mina M., and Norman F. Kallaus, *Records Management*, Chapter 12, (Cincinnati, OH: Southwestern Publishing Company, 1982).

Legality of Microfilm, (Chicago, IL: Cohasset Associates, 1980).

Medicare Conditions of Participation, Health Care Financing Administation, 1989.

Mishelevich, David J., MD, PhD, et al., "Medical Record Control and the Computer," *Topics in Health Record Management*, Vol. 2, No. 2, (December, 1981).

Nofel, Peter J., and Christine Fehlner, "Big Business Likes Its Record Small," *Modern Office Technology,* (April, 1984).

Presby, Leonard, "Eight-Step Study Shows Pros, Cons of Microfilming Medical Records," *Hospitals,* (August 16, 1977).

Rogers, Tillie, "Problems with a Family Numbering System," *Medical Record News*, (February, 1975).

Statement Against Use of Social Security Numbers for Hospital Medical records, (American Hospital Association, 1974).

Statement on the Preservation of Patient Medical Records in Health Care Institutions, (American Medical Record Association and American Hospital Association, 1974) (Under Revision).

Terry, George R., and John J. Stallard, *"Office Management and Control,"* 8th Ed., (Homewood, IL: Richard D. Irwin, Inc., 1980).

Tomes, Jonathan P., *Healthcare Records Manual,* Boston, (Massachusetts: Warren Gorham Lamont, 1993).

"The Wonderful World of Color - Makes Records Management Easier," (Information and Records Management, October 1976).

Waters, Kathleen A., and Gretchen Frederick Murphy, *"Medical Records in Health Information,"* (Aspen Systems, 1979).

chapter 9

NOMENCLATURES AND CLASSIFICATION SYSTEMS

Information contained in medical records is of limited value if it is not categorized and processed in some meaningful way. Health care institutions need to be able to study patterns of illness and injuries treated for clinical, financial, and administrative purposes. Comparing health care data between individual facilities within a defined area or country, or even among countries is vital to the growth of medical information around the world. The information would be meaningless, however, without the use of standardized systems for the identification and classification of disease processes. Over the years, a number of standard systems have been developed for classifying and recording disease information for comparison purposes.

NOMENCLATURES AND CLASSIFICATION

Two terms are often associated with health care data - nomenclature and classification. Although often used interchangeably, the terms have different meanings when used for the comparison of disease data and should not be confused or misapplied.

An accurate study of the diseases treated in an institution cannot be made unless a nomenclature of diseases has been carefully followed. The word "nomenclature" comes from the Latin nomen, meaning name, and clature, a calling. The term thus signifies, literally, a calling of names. It is defined as a system of names used in any science or art. Thus a medical nomenclature is a recognized system of preferred terminology for naming disease processes. In the past, variations in disease terminology have made comparative studies difficult. One disease may have been denoted by several terms; likewise, one term may have been applied to two or more different disease.For instance, Parry's disease, Grave's disease, Flajani's disease, and Basedow's disease are all toxic diffuse goiter. Recklinghausen's disease may be multiple neurofibroma or osteitis fibrosa cystica.

A classification system, on the other hand, emphasizes grouping of related entities to produce necessary statistical information. A medical classification system provides a method of arranging related disease entities in groups for the reporting of statistical data. Unlike nomenclatures, classification systems usually contain all terms - not just terms deemed proper by a nomenclature - to facilitate categorization. A medical classification system standardizes the medical conditions or procedures which are to be grouped together while a medical nomenclature standardizes terminology. An effective classification system follows three basic rules:

1. The set of categories should be derived from a single classification principle, such as anatomic sites, etiology, or medical specialty.
2. The set of categories should be exhaustive, permitting every possible diagnostic or operative term to be placed within a category of the classification system. In other words, there is a place for everything.
3. The categories within the classification system should be mutually exclusive, so it is not possible to place a given diagnostic or treatment term within more than one category of the system. Thus, everything has a place in the system.

If used properly, nomenclature and classification systems should complement each other in the recording of medical information.

NOMENCLATURES

The number of persons working in the health care field is mushrooming. This fact, coupled with an increase in the number and kinds of health care specialists, makes it vital that there is clear communication about the patient's condition. Use of standardized terminology to describe clinical progress and treatment procedures is important for ensuring that all persons involved directly or indirectly in patient care have a common understanding of the patient's disease.

Numerous attempts have been made over the years to accurately describe and identify all the disease entities known to man. One of the earliest successful efforts was initiated in 1889 when an international commission on nomenclature was appointed by the Anatomical Society. In 1895, the report of the commission was accepted at a meeting in Basle, Switzerland. This report is now known as the Basle Nomina Anatomica (BNA). It was necessary because at that time 50,000 anatomical terms were found in the literature for about 4,500 structures. Revisions of this work have continued to appear, and the majority of the nomenclatures of disease have based the terminology of their anatomical classification on this report.

EARLY NOMENCLATURES IN THE UNITED STATES

Although several early nomenclatures were published in the United States, the *Standard Nomenclature of Diseases and Operations* was the first medical nomenclature to be accepted universally.

The *Standard Classified Nomenclature of Disease,* the forerunner of the *Standard Nomenclature of Diseases and Operations,* originated in 1928 when the New York Academy of Medicine called a conference to formulate a nomenclature that would be acceptable as a standard throughout this country. Diseases were to be arranged in a logical and orderly manner, with no overlapping, so statistics from various hospitals would be comparable. At this meeting the National Conference on Nomenclature of Disease was formed. By fall of 1930 the basic plan providing for a dual classification was adopted. Each disease was classified according to both anatomical location and the etiology, or cause. Code numbers, comparable to the classification number on books in a library, were also adopted. The first official edition was published in 1933 and the second edition in 1935. In 1937, the copyright and editing responsibilities were transferred to the American Medical Association (AMA). In 1942 the third edition of the *Standard Nomenclature of Diseases* and the first edition of the *Standard Nomenclature of Operations* were published in one volume, entitled *Standard Nomenclature of Diseases and Standard Nomenclature of Operations*. After the AMA had indicated its willingness to be responsible for continuing the revision of the *Standard Nomenclature*, publication of other systems was halted to attain uniformity. The last (fifth) edition of *Standard Nomenclature of Diseases and Operations* was published in 1961.

Several early nomenclatures are described on the following pages.

Standard Nomenclature of Diseases and Operations (SNDO)

The *Standard Nomenclature of Diseases and Operations* was designed to be used as a medical nomenclature and to provide an authoritative list of acceptable terms for describing a patient's illness and treatment. Its code numbers facilitated the retrieval of data for research and statistical purposes for more than thirty years in North America. Though its last revision was in 1961 and new terms and conditions are not included, the terminology is considered to be acceptable and almost classic.

Several reasons are given for the AMA's not continuing to republish the SNDO, including the cost of the updating process and the fact that its meticulous attention to detail and stringent coding rules made it difficult to use worldwide. A brief discussion of SNDO follows because there are several decades of medical data indexed by the system which health information practitioners may need to access.

SNDO is a dual system of classification. Each disease entity is described in two ways: first, according to the disease site, or topography (organ or portion of the body concerned); and second, according to the cause of the disease or etiology. Similarly, operative procedures are classified according to the topography and operative technique or procedure performed on that site. The following sample entries serve to demonstrate this point:

61 - 942   Arteriosclerosis of aorta
site etiology   *etiology   site*

461 - 16   Biopsy of aorta
site procedure   *procedure   site*

Every disease and operative code number consists of two parts separated by a hyphen. In both the disease and the operative codes, the portion to the left of the hyphen represents the topography. The etiology is shown in the digits to the right of the hyphen in a disease code, while the procedure is shown in the digits to the right of the hyphen in an operative code. Every disease code must contain a minimum of six digits, to a maximum of ten digits.

To retrieve records from a SNDO index, the health information practitioner should be familiar with the following characteristics of SNDO: decimal digits are used to add further detail to the topography or etiology portion of a code; the meanings of the decimal digits differ from category to category; open end codes and master codes require completion by referring to the classification listings in the front of SNDO; and neoplastic disease codes contain behavior letters to show pathologic behavior.

Example:

640-8091.OH - Adenocarcinoma of stomach with metastasis, differentiation not determined.

640 - Stomach

8091 - Adenocarcinoma

.O - With metastasis

H - Differentiation not determined

Current Medical Information and Terminology (CMIT)

Current Medical Information and Terminology is a system developed to name and describe diseases for reference in clinical recording and reporting. Each disease is described according to: additional terms, synonyms, and eponyms; etiology; symptoms; signs; complications; laboratory data; x-rays; and pathology. Each entry is assigned a six-digit code applicable to computerized indexing. The fifth edition of CMIT was published in 1981 and the American Medical Association, its publisher, has no plans to continue the project.

Standard Nomenclature of Athletic Injuries

In 1964 the American Medical Association began the development of a standard nomenclature relating to degree and type of injury in sports, so meaningful records and statistics concerning sports injuries and their cause and prevention could be maintained. For each term, descriptive information is provided to assist sports medicine practitioners to differentiate one clinical entity from another. A revised nomenclature was published in 1976, but there are no further plans for revision.

Systematized Nomenclature of Pathology (SNOP)

The *Systematized Nomenclature of Pathology* was published in 1965 by the American College of Pathologists. It provides a system for classifying pathological specimens. The Joint Commission on Accreditation of Healthcare Organizations previously encouraged hospitals to use a recognized disease nomenclature to describe surgical specimen and autopsies. Thus, SNOP was used for a number of years. (Now, however, the JCAHO encourages hospitals to have standardized codes, classifications, and terminology throughout the organization). The SNOP coding system is the first system to code diseases on a multifield basis. The principle used by SNOP is that a disease may be defined in terms of topography - part of body affected by disease; morphology - structural change in tissue; etiology - the cause of the disease or injury; and function - physiological or chemical disorders and alterations resulting from a disease or injury.

Example: Orchitis due to mumps

> T-7800   Testis NOS
>
> M-4800   Inflammation NOS
>
> E-3250   Mumps virus
>
> F-0414   Mumps

Although the primary aim of this nomenclature was to help pathologists organize and utilize their material, SNOP has also been used for the coding and indexing of medical records by some health information departments.

NOMENCLATURES IN USE TODAY

The following sections describe nomenclatures still in use by various healthcare providers.

Systematized Nomenclature of Medicine (SNOMED)

In 1977 the College of American Pathologists published the *Systematized Nomenclature of Medicine* which represented a major expansion of SNOP. This was revised in 1982 and a third edition is scheduled for late 1989 or early 1990. SNOMED is the most recent and most comprehensive nomenclature in the health field.

SNOMED has seven axes. Axis 1 is a hierarchical anatomic nomenclature called "Topography." Axis 2 represents abnormal anatomy called "Morphology." Axis 3 lists all causes and causal agents of disease, dysfunctions, and morphological alterations that occur in the human body and is called "Etiology." Axis 4 contains the normal and abnormal functions, functional states and physiological units of the body and the major organ systems and is called "Function."

Because combinations of the first four axes are necessary to obtain a disease, the fifth axis, called "Disease," is an organized list of classes of diseases, complex disease entities, and syndromes. SNOMED can actually express all the necessary diagnostic detail to manage the patient's signs, symptoms, problems, and disease components as well as place the final diagnosis in the disease classification axis for statistical reporting. Figure 1 provides an example of SNOMED as a nomenclature and as a classification system.

Nomenclature				Classification
Topography +	Morphology +	Etiology +	Function =	Disease
Crystalline lens +	Cataract, Mature +	Acquired +	Low vision =	Disease of lens
T-XX700	M-51120	E-0024	F-X0050 =	D-X080

FIGURE 1. INTEGRATION OF CODABLE FINDINGS
INTO A CLASSIFICATION OF DISEASE

The sixth axis, called "Procedures," is used to describe the actions of the health care team. It contains a list of administrative, diagnostic, therapeutic, and preventative procedures. Axis 7, called "Occupation," has been added to permit its comparison and correlation with medical databank information.

The structure of SNOMED allows practically all health care information recorded on patients' records to be stored for data retrieval. Because SNOMED was designed for computer storage and automatic encoding of medical text, it has not been widely used. Some anatomic pathology laboratories are utilizing automatic encoding programs to assign SNOMED codes.

Standard Nomenclature of Veterinary Diseases and Operations (SNVDO)

A standard nomenclature in veterinary medicine was developed in 1964 out of the National Cancer Institute's attempt to acquire retrospective data on animal neoplasia. A second abridged edition of SNVDO was published in 1975 by the Public Health Service. It is used in most veterinary medical schools to assign acceptable terminology and a unique descriptive code number to conditions common to domestic animal species in the United States and Canada. SNVDO classifies diseases according to the portion of the body affected (topography) and to cause of the disorder (etiology). A diagnostic code contains three parts:

Characters 1-4 represent the part of the body affected

Characters 5-8 represent cause of the disease process

Character 9 represents a particular pathologic state if it exists and is usually considered part of the etiology.

Example: Adenocarcinoma of biliary passages, differentiated, 6820-8091F

6820- topography - biliary tract

8091- etiology - adenocarcinoma

F - malignant neoplasm differentiated

An operative code number contains three characters to denote the location of the site of the surgical procedure, the last character being dropped from the topography code. Two digits are used after a hyphen to represent the procedure. For example, open reduction of femur would be assigned code: 235-54 with 235 representing the femur site and 54 open reduction, generally or unspecified including fixation. The structure of SNVDO and many of its codes are based on the *Standard Nomenclature of Diseases and Operations*.

Systematized Nomenclature in Veterinary Medicine (SNOVET)

In 1984 a fascicle of SNOMED for veterinary medicine was created by the College of American Pathologists with input from the American Veterinary Medical Association (AVMA). The purpose of SNOVET was to provide a nomenclature that would interface with SNOMED for purposes of comparative studies and scientific research. Because the 1984 edition of SNOVET is not comprehensive enough to be used without SNVDO, the AVMA has worked out a copyright agreement to develop its own comprehensive version of SNOVET following the completion of the third edition of SNOMED.

Specialty Nomenclatures

Some specialty groups have developed nomenclatures to improve communications, storage, and retrieval of specialty information. These nomenclatures describe the diseases and disorders associated with the specialty and provide useful information to assist coders in correctly classifying various diagnoses.

In 1973 the New York Heart Association published the seventh edition of the *Nomenclature and Criteria for Diagnoses of Diseases of the Heart and Great Vessels*. This nomenclature describes diseases of the heart and great vessels and lists criteria required for the diagnosis.

The Council for International Organization of Medical Science and the World Health Organization issued the first edition of *Diseases of the Lower Respiratory Tract* (bronchi, lungs, and pleura) and the *International Nomenclature of Diseases* (IND) in 1979. This nomenclature identifies recommended terms and describes each disease or syndrome for which a name is recommended. It serves as a complement to *International Classification of Diseases* (ICD); and the names recommended in the IND will be used, as appropriate, in the tenth revision of the ICD. See the description of ICD later in this chapter.

Current Procedural Terminology (CPT)

Current Procedural Terminology, Fourth Edition (CPT-4) is a comprehensive listing of medical terms and codes for the uniform designation of diagnostic and therapeutic procedures. Its purpose is to provide standard terminology and coding for consistency and comparability in reporting for third-party reimbursement. The federal government has incorporated CPT-4 in its *HCFA Common Procedure Coding System* (HCPCS) used for reporting reimbursable physician services rendered to patients. See the description of HCPCS later in this chapter.

The federal government has also incorporated CPT-4 into its reimbursement system for physicians' office services. The system is described in chapter 12.

The American Medical Association (AMA) has been publishing CPT-4 since 1966, and the association revises it annually to keep it current with changes in medical practice. Health information professionals, physicians' office managers, or anyone else interested in the system can make suggestions for updates. An advisory panel of physicians reviews suggestions and decides on revisions and new codes. Often the changes are numerous; sometimes hundreds of codes are changed or added. It is critical that any user of CPT-4 obtain updated code books or at least incorporate each year's revisions into existing books.

New terms in any edition are denoted with a O symbol, revised terms with a ^ symbol, and deleted terms are listed in parentheses in the main section of the book. An appendix also provides a listing of all changes in the edition for use in updating computerized listings of the terms and their codes.

The main body of CPT-4 consists of six sections: evaluation and management services (E/M), anesthesiology, surgery, radiology, pathology/laboratory, and medicine. Any procedure or service in any section of the book, however, may be used to designate the services rendered by any qualified physician.

Most physicians report a significant portion of their services using codes from the E/M section, which is divided into general categories such as office visits, consultations, nursing facility services, emergency department services, and hospital inpatient services. The E/M codes take into consideration whether the patient is new or established, the extent of history and physical take, and the level of medical decision-making required.

Each of the six sections starts with specific guidelines. For example, the guidelines for the E/M section define terms such as new and established patient and advises users on identifying the correct code. The guidelines also list codes to use for reporting services of procedures not defined elsewhere in the manual, often new procedures. When an unlisted procedure code is used for billing, a special report describing the medical appropriateness of the service or procedure may be required.

Each section's guidelines describe the use of "modifiers" that alter the code for a procedure or service in some way. Modifiers may show any of the following:

- the service or procedure was performed by more than one physician and/or in more than one location, - the service or procedure was performed more than once,
- the service or procedure has both a professional and a technical component - only part of the service was performed,
- a bilateral or adjunctive service was performed,
- the service or procedure was performed more than once, or
- unusual events occurred.

Although the format of CPT-4 is designed to provide stand-alone descriptions of procedures, to conserve space many procedure descriptions are not printed in their entirety. When this occurs, the incomplete description is indented under the main entry; a main entry is always followed by a semicolon.

> *Example*: 31505 Laryngoscopy, indirect (separate procedure); diagnostic
>
> 31510 with biopsy

The common portion of the description for code 31505 (the part before the semicolon) is part of both codes 31505 and 31510. The full description for code 31510 reads: "laryngoscopy, indirect (separate procedure); with biopsy."

The CPT index is arranged alphabetically and contains four kinds of entries: procedure or service, organ or other anatomic site, condition, and synonyms, eponyms, and abbreviations. Each entry is considered a main term and may be followed by subterms indented below the main term. To look up a code, the user first finds the main term in the alphabetical index, then reviews any subterms that follow.

The index refers the user either to a single code, a choice of two codes, or a range of codes. Even if the index refers the user to a single code, all codes should be checked in the main body of the book to determine whether the code most completely describes the procedure. Once the user has selected the most accurate code, it is important to consider whether a modifier is needed.

NOMENCLATURE USAGE

Regardless of the nomenclature used, disease and operative terms must be expressed with sufficient clarity and specificity for the data to be correctly identified and coded.

Every diagnosis must contain a specific site and etiology; and every operation a site and a procedure, insofar as possible. If the physician is unable to specify site or etiology because of inconclusive results from x-rays, laboratory tests, or other examinations, the statement should be made that a particular disease is suspected or that the diagnosis is incomplete. If the physician can state only symptoms and no disease, the diagnosis should be stated as deferred or unknown. The following examples illustrate some of these points.

INCORRECT TERMINOLOGY	CORRECT TERMINOLOGY
1. Embolism of artery *(no topography)*	Embolism of pulmonary artery
2. Emphysema *(no etiology)*	Emphysema due to infection
3. Arthrotomy *(no topography)*	Arthrotomy of knee joint
4. Headache *(symptom)*	Undiagnosed disease manifested by headache
5. Plastic operation of the arm with full-thickness skin graft *(incomplete operation)*	Plastic operation of arm with full-thickness skin graft Excision of skin of leg for graft, donor site
6. Infarction of myocardium from arteriosclerotic coronary thrombosis Polydipsia	Infarction of inferior myocardium from arteriosclerotic coronary thrombosis Diabetes mellitus, Polydipsia

(The symptom, polydipsia, cannot be explained by the infarction; therefore, another disease must be present.)

7. Hives	Urticaria

(Hives is a lay term. Urticaria is the correct term for this condition.)

8. Pott's disease	Tuberculosis of the vertebra

(An eponym is a name of a disease, organ, operation, etc., in which the name of a person is included. Certain eponyms are so commonly used that they are acceptable as a diagnoses, e.g., Laennec's cirrhosis. In most cases, eponyms are not an accurate substitute for a diagnosis stating site and etiology.)

The above examples point out some of the common errors in diagnostic and operative terminology. In may instances, the physician unknowingly makes these errors and will be willing to provide more specificity. The health information practitioner may assist physicians in documenting their patients' diagnoses. Only the physician who actually treats the patient is in a position to make the diagnosis.

STATISTICAL CLASSIFICATIONS

Classification systems are used to organize health care data for easy and meaningful retrieval. Frequently, the health information practitioner is responsible for selecting an appropriate classification system for classifying, storing, and retrieving patient health information from patient/client medical records.

HISTORY OF CLASSIFICATION SYSTEMS

Attempts to group data on disease processes in a relevant manner date back many years. The early Greeks, following the pathology of Hippocrates, classified diseases into the four humors - blood, which being from the heart, represents heat; black bile, which being from the spleen and stomach, represents wetness; yellow bile, which secreted by the liver, represents dryness; and phlegm, which from the brain and diffused through the whole body, represents cold.

In the seventeenth century, Captain John Graunt, of London, began directing the attention of the world to morbidity and mortality statistics in his *London Bills of Mortality*. This was the first real attempt to study disease from a statistical point of view.

As early as 1837, William Farr, Registrar General of England and Wales, worked to achieve better classification and international uniformity in the use of statistics. The general arrangement and the principle of classifying diseases by anatomical site proposed by Farr have survived as the basis of the *International List of Causes of Death*. Thus the foundation was laid for our present-day vital statistics.

INTERNATIONAL CLASSIFICATION OF DISEASES (ICD)

Dr. Jacques Bertillon developed the *Bertillon Classification of Causes of Death* in 1893. In 1898 the American Public Health Association recommended that the *Bertillon Classification* be adopted by registrars in Canada, Mexico, and the United States; and that the classification be revised every ten years.

Revisions, entitled the *International Classification of Causes of Death,* were completed in 1900, 1920, 1929 and 1938. In 1948, under the auspices of the World Health Organization, the sixth revision was published and included, for the first time, lists for the tabulation of morbidity as well as mortality. Hospitals began experiments using this system for classifying diseases.

In 1956 the American Hospital Association and the American Medical Record Association, supported by a research grant from the Public Health Service, undertook a pilot study using a modified version of the *International Statistical Classification of Diseases, Injuries and Causes of Death with the Standard Nomenclature of Diseases and Operations* being used as a control. The findings of the study revealed that the modified version was suitable for hospital indexing purposes. Coding and posting took less time; and in answering requests for certain disease entities, more pertinent records were found by using the listing, although more nonpertinent records were also found.

As a result of this study, a committee consolidated the findings for use as a hospital indexing tool. The completion of this task in 1959 resulted in U.S. Public Health Service Publication 719, the *International Classification of Diseases, Adapted for Indexing Hospital Records by Diseases and Operations* (ICDA). In 1962, modifications were made to provide greater detail; and some changes were made at the three-digit category level. A classification of surgical operations was also introduced.

U.S. Adaptation of ICD (ICDA-8)

Although the World Health Organization took into consideration the increased specificity required for indexing hospital records in preparing the eighth revision of ICD, it was recognized that the basic classification might provide inadequate detail for diagnostic indexing in some countries. In the United States, an advisory group to the Public Health Service recommended the preparation of an adaptation that gave greater detail and specificity. The *Eighth Revision, International Classification of Diseases, Adapted for Use in the United States,* published in 1968, served as the basis for coding diagnostic data for official morbidity and mortality statistics in the United States and also proved to be suitable for indexing hospital records by diagnoses and operations.

The evolution of an international listing of causes of death into a comprehensive classification of both morbidity and mortality has resulted in improved international cooperation in the field of vital and health statistics. This, coupled with better medical education has caused an exchange of information that has greatly contributed to the betterment of health standards all over the world.

Hospital Adaptation of ICD (H-ICDA)

A variation of the ICDA-8 classification system was published in 1968 by the Commission on Professional and Hospital Activities (CPHA) for use with its Professional Activities Study (PAS) data recording system. The *Hospital Adaptation of ICDA* followed the basic format of ICDA-8 with certain modifications. Those hospitals using the PAS data system were required to use the H-ICDA for coding and indexing patient information. In 1973 a second edition of the H-ICDA was published for use by PAS-participating hospitals. This edition was used until 1979 when it was replaced by the *International Classification of Diseases, Ninth Revision, Clinical Modification.*

Ninth Revision of ICD (ICD-9)

Although participating countries had been working individually to update ICD, representatives came together in 1975 in Geneva, Switzerland, to make the final decision for a ninth revision. The resulting publication, *International Classification of Diseases, Ninth Revision,* became effective as the World Health Organization's statistical classification in 1979. The current ICD is primarily a universal classification system for grouping illnesses. Its secondary purpose is for use in hospital disease indexing. The ICD-9 includes a tabular list of diseases, alphabetic index, and a new procedure classification. Coding was expanded into greater detail by the addition of a fifth digit in specified disease categories. Dual classification numbers were introduced which combined two descriptions of disease entities into a single code number.

CLINICAL MODIFICATION OF ICD (ICD-9-CM)

In 1977 the National Center for Health Statistics began the development of a modification of the ICD-9 for use in the United States. The *International Classification of Diseases, Ninth Re-*

vision, Clinical Modification resulted. The term "clinical" emphasized its intent to be a classification of morbidity data. It was to be used for reporting, compiling, and comparing health care data to assist in evaluating the appropriateness and timeliness of medical care, planning health care delivery systems, determining patterns of patient care among health care providers, analyzing payments for health service, and conducting epidemiological and clinical research.

The ICD-9-CM is published in three volumes. Volume 1 *Tabular List* contains a numerical list of the disease code numbers in tabular form. An alphabetic index to the disease entries in Volume 1 is provided in Volume 2 *Alphabetic Index*. A third volume contains the classification system for surgical, diagnostic, and therapeutic procedures. This volume is not part of the international version (ICD-9). Volume 3 *Procedures* contains both a tabular list and an alphabetic index for classification of procedures. The first two volumes of ICD-9-CM codes may be collapsed back to their ICD-9 counterpart. The ICD-9-CM procedure classification draws heavily on the fascicles of ICD-9, but compatibility with the ICD-9 *Classification of Procedures in Medicine* was not maintained when a different classification axis was deemed clinically more useful.

Structure of Code Numbers

The Volume 1 *Tabular List* of ICD-9-CM is divided into 17 chapters. Within each chapter, the disease classification is made up of three-digit categories which may represent a single disease entity or a group of closely related conditions. For example, 001 represents codes for cholera, while 002 represents typhoid and paratyphoid fevers.

Most three-digit categories have been divided into four-digit subcategories by adding one decimal digit. The addition of a fourth digit of 0 to the code 001, for example, shows cholera due to vibrio cholerae (code 001.0).

Some subcategories have been further subdivided into five-digit subclassifications by adding a second decimal digit. As shown in Figure 2, fifth digits for code 451.8 show specific sites of phlebitis and thrombophlebitis. Fourth and fifth digits provide specificity or more information regarding etiology, site, manifestations, or complications. Therefore, the code with the greatest number of digits should always be used.

Residual subcategory codes with titles of "other" and "unspecified" have been included to classify those conditions not accorded a separate title in the subcategories. These are usually numbered .8 for "other" and .9 for "unspecified." The most specific code possible should be used.

In addition to its 17 chapters, the Volume 1 *Tabular List* also contains the following two supplementary classifications:

- The *Classifications of Factors Influencing Health Status and Contact with Health Service*. These codes are used for circumstances other than a disease or injury classifiable in the main part of the tabular list. Such circumstances can arise in these three ways:

1. when a person who is currently not sick uses health services for some purpose, such as acting as an organ donor, receiving prophylactic vaccination, or healthy live-born infants;

2. when a person with a known disease or injury encounters the health care system for a specific treatment of that disease or injury, such as dialysis for renal disease or chemotherapy for malignancy; and

3. when some circumstance or problem influences a patient's current illness or injury but is not in itself a current illness or injury, such as a personal history of carcinoma.

Codes in this supplementary classification are termed "V codes", because they contain a "V" as the first character, followed by two numbers and a decimal digit. For example, V70.0 describes a person for whom a routine general medical examination was performed at a health care facility; V46.1 describes a patient who is dependent on a respirator.

- The Classification of External Causes of Injury and Poisoning. These codes are used to classify environmental events, circumstances, and other conditions as the cause of injury and other adverse effects. They are used with codes from the main body of ICD-9-CM, indicating the nature of the condition.

Codes in this classification are termed "E codes", because they begin with an "E" followed by three digits and a decimal digit. For example, code E923.0 describes an accident caused by fireworks; E930.0 is the adverse effect of penicillin in therapeutic use.

451 Phlebitis and thrombophlebitis
Includes: endophlebitis
inflammation,vein
periphlebitis
suppurative phlebitis

Use additional E code, if desired, to identify drug, if
drug-induced

Excludes: *postoperative NOS (997.2)*
that complicating:
abortion (634-638 with .7, 639.8)
ectopic or molar pregnancy (639.8)
pregnancy, childbirth, or the
puerperium (671.0-671.9)
that due to or following:
implant or catheter device 996.91-996.62)
infusion, perfusion or transfusion (999.2)

451.0 Of superficial vessels of lower extremities

Saphenous vein (greater) (lesser)

451.1 Of deep vessels of lower extremities

451.11 Femoral vein (deep) (superficial)

451.19 Other

Popliteal vein   Tibial vein

451.2 Of lower extremities, unspecified

451.8 Of other sites

Excludes: *intracranial venous sinus (325)*
nonpyogenic (vein) (437.6)
portal (vein) (572.1)

451.81 Iliac vein

451.82 Of superficial veins of upper extremities

Antecutbital vein
Basilic vein
Cephalic vein

451.83 Of deep veins of upper extremities

Brachial vein
Radial Vein
Ulnar vein

451.84 Of upper extremities, unspecified

451.89 Other
Axillary vein
Jugular vein
Subclavian vein
Thrombophlebitis of breast
(Mondo's disease)

451.9 Of unspecified site

FIGURE 2. STRUCTURE OF ICD-9-CM DISEASE CODES

Reporting E codes is not a requirement for Medicare reimbursement. The UB-92 has space for one E code, and the individual payers may ask hospitals to report E codes when appropriate. Some states also require the reporting of E codes and develop their own guidelines for doing so.

The ICD-9-CM procedure classification uses codes that are based on two digits with a decimal digit, plus a second decimal digit which is added where necessary to provide further speci-

---

13.7   Insertion of prosthetic lens [pseudophakos]

   13.70   Insertion of pseudophakos, not otherwise specified

   13.71   Insertion of intraocular lens prosthesis at time of cataract extraction, one-stage

   Code also synchronous extraction of cataract (13.11-13.69)

   13.72   Secondary insertion of intraocular lens prosthesis

---

FIGURE 3. STRUCTURE OF ICD-9-CM PROCEDURE CODES

ficity of site or procedure. As with the fourth and fifth digits in the disease classification, when a fourth digit breakdown is provided it must be used.

Coding Conventions

The ICD-9-CM includes a number of coding conventions which must be followed for accurate coding. These conventions include the use of instructional abbreviations, symbols, and notations in both the Tabular Lists and Alphabetic Indexes. These are explained in the Introduction to the classification itself and must be followed strictly for accurate coding.

Coding Guidelines

Many third party payers utilize ICD-9-CM codes for reimbursement purposes. The definitions in the UHDDS (see Chapter 14, Health Care Statistics) should be followed to sequence codes for reporting inpatient information to third party payers. The entire medical record should be reviewed to identify the principal diagnosis. This may differ from the admitting diagnosis/problem because after study the condition necessitating admission may be more specifically delineated. The first listed diagnosis entered by the physician at the time of discharge is not necessarily the principal diagnosis, but may be the primary diagnosis. The primary diagnosis has been used in vital statistics records to refer to the underlying condition or cause of death or morbidity. There is no universal agreement as to the definition, for "primary" is also used interchangeably with "most significant" to identify the diagnosis that utilized the most resources.

When using ICD-9-CM for reporting ambulatory care encounters for reimbursement, coding guidelines are different in some respects. ICD-9-CM is used only for reporting conditions; CPT-4 is used for reporting procedures. When listing ICD-9-CM codes on claim forms, the code for the diagnosis, condition, problem, complaint, or other reason for the encounter shown to be chiefly responsible for the outpatient services provided during the encounter should be listed first. Additional codes that describe co-existing conditions are then listed.

In addition to the definitions of the UHDDS, official guidelines for ICD-9-CM coding are developed by four cooperating parties. The cooperating parties are the American Hospital Association, American Health Information Association, Health Care Financing Administration, and National Center for Health Statistics. For guidelines to be official they must be unanimously approved by these cooperating parties.

Individual health care facilities should develop coding policies which specify the procedures which are to be assigned codes at that facility. Some health care facilities will not assign codes to many of the diagnostic and nonsurgical procedures because data on chest x-rays, audiometry testing, and so forth are available elsewhere, not required for reporting purposes, or not needed by the facility.

OTHER CLASSIFICATIONS

As the delivery of health care in the United States becomes more specialized, a need emerges for specialized patient information to follow up and evaluate the effectiveness of treatment measures. The health information practitioner must be aware of the various specialized classification systems available for the collection of statistical information. Only through the use of an appropriate coding and indexing system will the resulting collection of data be meaningful to the health care facility. Several of the more common coding systems are discussed below.

ICD-ONCOLOGY

One area requiring specific detailed information on the effectiveness and outcome of treatment is oncology - the study of tumors or neoplasms. For adequate statistical information and follow-up of patients, a detailed classification had to be devised to record the numbers and types of tumors in the United States.

In 1968 the *Manual of Tumor Nomenclature and Coding* was published by the American Cancer Society. Commonly referred to as MOTNAC, it combined segments of the *Systematized Nomenclature of Pathology* (SNOP) and the ICDA-8 into one detailed classification system for specialists in oncology.

In the same year, the World Health Organization requested the International Agency for Research on Cancer to begin work on the "Neoplasm" chapter for the ninth revision of the *International Classification of Diseases* (ICD-9). The recommendation was made to the World Health Organization to publish a supplemental neoplasm classification with ICD-9-CM based on MOTNAC for use by the field of oncology. The recommendation was endorsed by the World Health Organization and resulted in publication of the *International Classification of Diseases for Oncology* (ICD-O) in 1976. A field trial for the next edition is underway at the time of this writing. The purpose of the ICD-O is to provide a classification system for the field of oncology which contains sufficient detail to code the extensive topography, histology (morphology), and behavior of neoplasms.

The ICD-O is divided into three sections. The site or location in the body which contains the tumor is assigned a four-digit code number (from 140.0 to 199.9). The "Morphology-Numerical List" contains code numbers which are used to specify the type of tumor found and its behavior. The morphology terms have five-digit code numbers which run from 8000/0 to 9990/6; the first four digits indicate the specific histologic terms, and the fifth digit after the slash is a behavior code. An optional sixth digit may be added to the morphology code number which indicates differentiation of the tumor mass. Anatomical sites and morphological terms are listed in the ICD-O "Alphabetic

Index" for ease in selecting the appropriate code numbers to identify the neoplasms. The code numbers for topography, morphology, and behavior also appear in ICD-9-CM.

INTERNATIONAL CLASSIFICATION OF IMPAIRMENTS, DISABILITIES, AND HANDICAPS

This manual is published by the World Health Organization to measure the consequences of disease. It contains three classifications, each relating to a different plane of experience consequent upon disease:

> Impairments (I code) concerned with abnormalities of body structure and appearance and with organ or system function, resulting from any cause: in principle, impairments represent disturbances at the organ level.

> Disabilities (D code) reflecting the consequences of impairment in terms of functional performance and activity by the individual; disabilities thus represent disturbances at the level of the person.

> Handicaps (H code) concerned with the disadvantages experienced by the individual as a result of impairments and disabilities; handicaps thus reflect interaction with and adaptation to the individual's surroundings:

DIAGNOSTIC AND STATISTICAL MANUAL OF MENTAL DISORDERS (DSM-IV)

Those facilities specializing in the treatment of substance abuse and mental disorders can record detailed psychiatric data by using the *Diagnostic and Statistical Manual of Mental Disorders*. First published in 1952 by the American Psychiatric Association, the classification was an expansion of the mental disorders section of the ICD, and revisions are planned to coincide with the revisions of ICD. The publication of DSM-III coincided with that of ICD-9; the publication of DSM-IV was planned to coincide with ICD-10.

In 1983, however, the American Psychiatric Association was asked to contribute to the development of the mental disorders chapter of ICD-10 and found that the burgeoning literature in the field necessitated revisions before the anticipated publication of ICD-10 and DSM-IV in 1993. *The Diagnostic and Statis-*

tical Manual of Mental Disorders (Third Edition-Revised) (DSM-III-R) was published in 1987. While nearly all of the DSM-III codes were ICD-9-CM codes, a small number were non-ICD-9-CM codes, and caused some problems for record-keeping systems with responsibility for reporting to federal agencies. In order to remedy this for DSM-IV, the Mental Health Section of the American Health Information worked with the American Psychiatric Association (APA) to ensure all DSM codes are ICD-9-CM codes. However, there are still some differences in the fifth digits. Some fifth digits available in ICD-9-CM are not available in DSM-IV. Through extensive review of current literature, the APA has determined certain ICD-9-CM fifth digit codes (developed over 15 years ago) are not longer clinically meaningful.

The fifth digits for alcohol dependence are an example. The DSM-IV has recognized it is clinically more useful to note information regarding the period of remission - whether the remission has lasted less than a year (early) or more than a year (sustained) - than specifying the patterns of use (continuous or episodic) as in the ICD-9-CM. Therefore the DSM-IV code for alcohol dependence is 303.90.

Since ICD-9-CM coding is required by most third-party payers, it is important for each facility to evaluate its needs in establishing a coding policy. Frequently, mental health facilities will require that the diagnoses be recorded in the terminology of DSM-IV but will code all diagnoses according to ICD-9-CM. There is a DSM-IV to ICD-9-CM crosswalk available for the facilities who use dual coding procedures.

DSM-IV is a statistical classification and glossary of mental disorders, as well as a basis for research, education, and administrative information. The primary purpose of DSM-IV is to provide clear descriptions of diagnostic categories in order for clinicians to diagnose, communicate about, study, and treat various mental disorders. DSM-IV is not based solely on the etiology of mental disorders as this is not always known. Rather DSM-IV utilizes primarily both a descriptive and etiologic approach to the classification of mental disorders. All disorders without known etiology or pathological process are grouped together on the basis of shared clinical manifestations.

DSM-IV provides specific diagnostic criteria as guides for making each diagnosis to enhance diagnostic reliability (Figure

4). DSM-IV recommends the use of a multiaxial system for evaluation to ensure that information of value in planning treatment and predicting outcome is recorded in each of five axes. The first three axes are available to code both psychosocial context and level of functioning.

The five axes are:

Axis I: Clinical Syndromes
           Other Conditions That May
           be a Focus Clinical Attention

Axis II: Personality Disorder
           Mental Retardation

Axis III: General Medical Conditions

Axis IV: Psychosocial and Environmental Problems

Axis V: Global Assessment of Functioning (GAF)

FIGURE 4. DSM-IV MULTIAXIAL SYSTEM

CLASSIFICATION IN MENTAL RETARDATION

Since 1921 when its first manual on classification and terminology was published, the American Association of Mental Deficiency (AAMD) has been concerned about differences found within the population of retarded individuals. In 1983 the eighth edition of Diagnostic and Statistical Manual of Mental Disorders was published to reflect current thinking in the field and to make it consistent with ICD-9 and DSM-III, particularly with reference to medical classification.

The AAMD system provides for making a diagnosis of mental retardation by level (same as ICD-9-CM codes), a diagnosis by etiology such as lead poisoning or Down's syndrome, and a diagnosis of concurrent problems of the individual who is diagnosed as retarded such as blindness. ICD-9-CM codes may be used for all of these diagnoses, or AAMD codes may be used for etiology because parts of the AAMD medical classification system have greater specificity with reference to etiology than are found in either ICD-9-CM or DSM-III. The AAMD classification system also contains a glossary to provide some homogeneity to the professional language in the field of mental retardation. The classification is designed to facilitate communication for diagnostic, treatment, and research purposes, and to facilitate prevention efforts through identification of the causes of mental retardation.

ROENTGEN CLASSIFICATION

Other departments within the hospital may find it necessary to retain statistical information for purposes of follow-up and evaluation of patient care. Routine collection in the diagnostic radiology department, or through the hospital's quality assurance department/service, of information about important aspects of diagnostic radiology or therapy services was in the past required by the Joint Commission on Accreditation of Healthcare Organizations. Therefore, radiology departments maintain an index for data collection purposes. The American College of Radiology developed the *Index for Roentgen Diagnosis,* which serves as a classification system for diagnostic radiology departments. Its third edition was published in 1986.

Two sections comprise the *Index for Roentgen Diagnosis* - the listing of diagnostic code numbers and an alphabetic index. The code number describes both the anatomical site of the x-ray and the pathological process or disease. The anatomy code ranges from two to four digits before a decimal point, while the two to five decimal digits after the decimal point refer to the disease process.

Example: 844.316 - Benign prostatic hypertrophy:

8	- Genitourinary system
84	- Male urethra, genitalia
884	- Prostate
.3	- Neoplasm, neoplastic-like condition
.31	- Benign neoplasm, cyst
.316	- Prostatic hyperplasia

A minimum of two anatomy and two pathology digits should be used. The extent of detail to be incorporated into an individual facility's index is left to the discretion of each health care institution.

HCFA COMMON PROCEDURE CODING SYSTEM (HCPCS)

The Health Care Financing Administration (HCFA)'s Common Procedure Coding System (HCPCS) was designed to promote uniform reporting and statistical data collection of medical procedures, supplies, products, and services. The procedure codes, along with ICD-9-CM codes for diagnoses, are used to obtain reimbursement under Part B (physician services) of Medicare.

The codes are divided into three levels (or groups) as described here:

- Level I: Codes copyrighted by the American Medical Association's *Current Procedural Terminology* (CPT-4). These are five position numeric codes primarily representing physician services.
- Level II: Codes approved and maintained jointly by the AlphaNumeric Editorial Panel, consisting of HCFA, the Health Insurance Association of America, and the Blue Cross and Blue Shield Association. There are five-position alpha numeric codes representing items and nonphysician services that are not represented in the Level I codes, such as traction equipment.
- Level III: Codes developed by individual Medicare carriers to use at the local (carrier) level. Level III codes are five-position alpha numeric codes that represent physician and nonphysician services that are not represented in the Level I or II codes. These codes, similar to CPT's unlisted procedure codes, serve as the basis for updates to Level II.

HCPCS also contains modifiers, which are two-position codes used to indicate that a service or procedure which has been performed has been altered by some specific circumstance but has not changed its definition or code.

AMBULATORY CARE CLASSIFICATIONS

Ambulatory care is another aspect of the health care delivery system which presents its own unique problems and needs for data retrieval. The coding system associated with the CPT-4 nomenclature, previously described, is used for reporting ambulatory care claims data, but other systems have also been designed to meet special ambulatory care needs.

International Classification of Health Problems in Primary Care (ICHPPC)

The *International Classification of Health Problems in Primary Care* was developed in 1975 by the Classification Committee of the World Organization of National Colleges, Academies, and Academic Associations of General Practitioners/Family Physicians (WONCA), and published by the American Hospital Association. ICHPPC was designed to meet the particular needs of the ambulatory care community and closely paralleled the ICD-8 classification system.

In 1979 the second edition of the *International Classification of Health Problems in Primary Care* (ICHPPC-2), published by the Oxford University Press, became available, following publication of the ICD-9 and closely paralleling it. Both a "Tabular Classification of Health Problems" and an "Alphabetical Index" are included in ICHPPC-2. The tabular classification lists the four-digit code numbers used in ICHPPC-2, and also provides a cross reference to corresponding code numbers in ICD-9. If a fourth digit is not necessary to fully describe the diagnosis, a three digit code number and slash mark are assigned instead. For example, osteoporosis is assigned code number 7330, while transient cerebral ischemia is assigned 435/.

In 1983 ICHPPC-2-Defined was issued. The major new feature was that an attempt was made to define by selection criteria the majority of terms used in the classification. For each defined rubric, one or more criteria are identified which must be fulfilled to code a problem under that diagnostic tile. For example, the ICHPPC code 4273 Atrial fibrillation or flutter. Inclusion in this rubric requires one of the following (1) demonstration of characteristic findings by electrocardiogram, or (2) totally irregular heart rate with a pulse deficit.

Reason for Visit Classification (RVS)

Another ambulatory care classification system is the *Reason for Visit Classification System,* developed in 1977 by the American Medical Record Association. RVS is based on a survey of patients of ambulatory care facilities conducted by the National Center for Health Statistics, entitled *National Ambulatory Medical Care Survey: Symptom Classification.* The classification is designed to collect statistical information on the symptoms, complaints, and problems which motivated the patient to seek medical care.

The *Reason for Visit Classification System* consists of two major sections: the "Tabular List of Inclusive Terms" and the "Alphabetic Index of Terms." The tabular list is divided into seven modules: (1) Symptoms; (2) Diseases; (3) Diagnostic, screening and preventive; (4) Treatment; (5) Injuries and adverse effects; (6) Test results; and (7) Administrative.

Descriptions of signs and symptoms are included as they might be told to the physician in the patient's own words. For example, entries such as "runny nose," "sniffles," and "postnasal drip" are included under S400.0 Nasal congestion.

Code numbers contain three digits before the decimal point, with one decimal digit for greater detail. Fourth-digit decimal categories may be expanded at the facility's discretion to allow for greater detail and flexibility.

Reason for Encounter Classification (RFEC)

The World Health Organization developed the *Reason for Encounter Classification* (RFEC) to classify the reasons patients seek care at the primary level. It incorporates an expanded version of the existing *Reason for Visit Classification* and the rubrics in the diagnoses and diseases component are the same as those in the *International Classification of Health Problems in Primary Care.*

The RFEC is designed along two axes: chapter and component. Thirteen chapters have titles related to body systems, and the other three are "General," "Psychological," and "Social." Each chapter is subdivided into seven components each of which is represented by two digits in the RFEC code. The seven components are (1) Symptoms and complaints; (2) Diagnosis and screening prevention; (3) Treatment, procedures, and medication; (4) Test results; (5) Administrative; (6) Other; and (7) Diagnoses, diseases.

The 3-character biaxial classification system has five process components, numbers 2 to 6 which have two-digit codes that are identical in all chapters. For example, the code D50 indicates the reason for the encounter is Medications, for the digestive system; A50 is Medications, general; and K50 is Medications, circulatory. RFEC has a strong nondisease orientation and is an easy classification to use.

The pilot study revealed that the RFEC can be used not only to clarify the patient's subjective statement of his or her reason for the encounter but also to interpret that reason or problem at the highest diagnostic level possible for primary care providers.

NURSING DIAGNOSES

Nurses have traditionally used medical diseases as the basis of nursing treatment. However, in the early 1970's, nurses began to identify a need for a classification of nursing diagnoses. In 1976 the American Nurses Association stated that "nursing diagnosis describes actual or potential health problems which nurses are capable of treating and licensed to treat." The physician may diagnose Parkinson's disease while the nurse diagnoses the problems that are consequences of the disease - difficulty ambulating, dependence in feeding, and poor oral secretion control.

One classification system published in 1983 as part of the book *Nursing Diagnosis—Application to Clinical Practice,* is the "Manual of Nursing Diagnoses." In this system, each of 43 diagnostic categories are described with the following: definition, etiological and contributing factors, defining characteristics, focus assessment criteria, nursing goals, and principles and rationale for nursing care. Each diagnostic group is then further explained by one or more specific nursing diagnoses that are further explained with assessment data, outcome criteria, and interventions. For example, alterations in comfort is a diagnostic category. Within this category, acute pain, chronic pain, and pain in children are specific nursing diagnoses.

No universally accepted classification of nursing diagnoses is currently available.

CASE-MIX CLASSIFICATIONS

The purpose of a statistical compilation of disease and procedural data is primarily to furnish quantitative data on the incidence of certain disease/procedures (morbidity) and the causes of death (mortality). Health care facilities and third party payers in the United States, however, have other data needs; so for the last twenty years researchers have been trying to develop a useful classification system to measure the case mix (categories of patients and type) treated by a health care institution. To date, numerous approaches have been developed including related groupings of diseases and severity of illness systems.

Diagnosis-Related Groups (DRGs)

Diagnosis-Related Groups (DRGs) represent an inpatient classification scheme to categorize patients who are medically related with respect to diagnoses and treatment, and who are statistically similar in their lengths of stay. DRGs are statistically consistent - patients in a DRG tend to consume similar amounts of hospital resources as measured by length of stay and cost. They are also medically meaningful - physician input was used to ensure that patients in a DRG have similar clinical conditions or treatment. Twenty-five major diagnostic categories (MDCs) cluster patients such as:

MDC 11 Diseases and disorders of the kidney
and urinary tract

MDC 12 Diseases and disorders of the
male reproductive system

MDC 13 Diseases and disorders of the female
reproductive system

MDC 14 Pregnancy, childbirth, and puerperium

Decision trees are utilized to display the divisions in the Major Diagnostic Categories and the specific DRGs, of which there are nearly 500. Patients in most MDCs are divided into two groups depending upon the presence or absence of qualifying surgery. Each procedure in ICD-9-CM was classified by physician panels as "OR" (operating room) or "non-OR" (non-operating room). After MDCs are divided into medical and surgical categories, medical patients are further divided based on the specific principal diagnosis, while surgical patients are further divided based on the specific surgical procedure performed. The medical classes in each MDC usually include a class for neoplasms and classes for symptoms and specific conditions relating to the organ or system involved. Since patients can be assigned to only one DRG per episode of care, assignments are based on the Uniform Hospital Discharge Data Set definition of principal diagnosis.

Patients with multiple procedures are assigned to the surgical DRG highest in the hierarchy within the MDC. Thus a patient having a breast biopsy and a radical mastectomy is assigned to the mastectomy DRG. Other partitions depend on the procedure, age of patient in some instances, and/or qualifying complications/comorbidities (CC). A complication is a secondary condition that arises during hospitalization and is thought

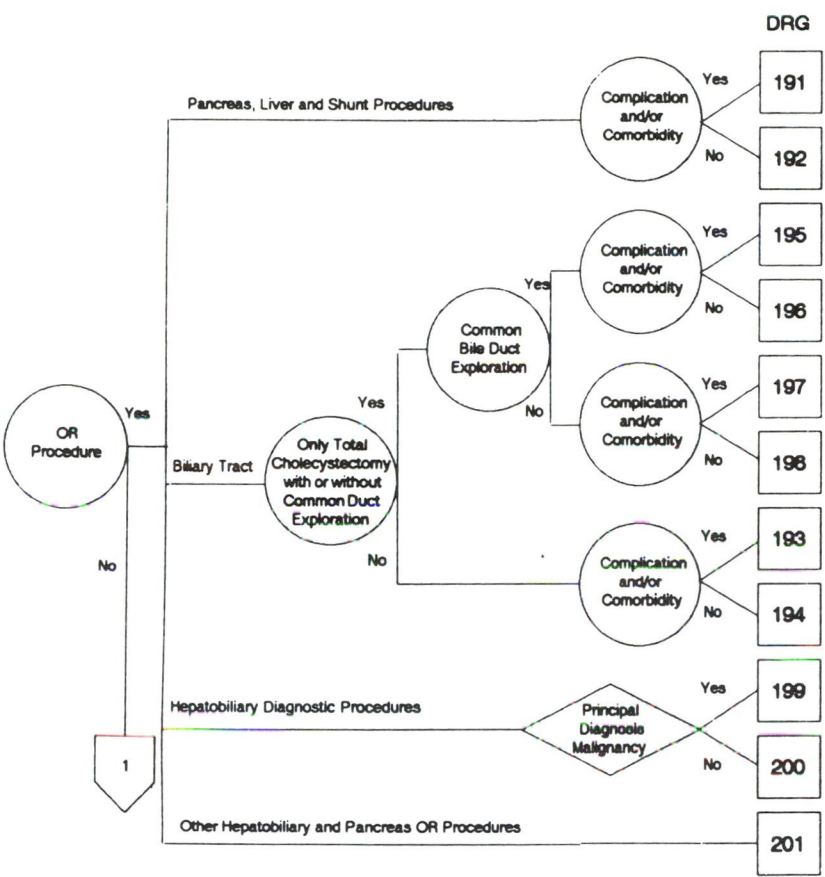

FIGURE 5. EXAMPLE OF DRG DECISION TREE

to increase the length of stay by at least one day for approximately 75 percent of the patients. A comorbid condition is a condition that existed on admission and is thought to increase the length of stay at least one day for approximately 75 percent of the patients.

The DRG system facilitates analytical use of the hospital's medical record data. Many third-party payers, including the Medicare program, use DRGs to reimburse hospitals. Rates are set prospectively by DRG thus allowing the government or the insurer to fix prices in advance.

DRG assignment is usually performed by a computer with grouper software, but may be performed manually utilizing the decision trees and listings of OR procedures, complications, and comorbidities.

Example: A patient is admitted with adult onset diabetes and acute abdominal colic. Workup reveals gallstones, and a cholecystectomy and common duct exploration are performed for acute cholecystitis and cholelithiasis. The patient's diabetes is out of control for most of hospital stay. Because the affected body system is the hepatobiliary system and pancreas, and because the patient had an OR procedure, the decision tree in the surgical partition of MDC 07 is used. On this decision tree, the patient is tracked through total cholecystectomy and common bile duct exploration and no complication/comorbidity (adult onset uncontrolled diabetes is not defined as a comorbid condition or complication) so DRG 196 is assigned (Figure 5).

Ambulatory Patient Groups (APGs)

Ambulatory Patient Groups (APGs) describe an ambulatory patient case mix classification system currently under development and study. Development of APGs began as early as the late 1970s with the initial version released in 1980. As constructed in the original project, APGs provided the ability to compare productivity and performance in the ambulatory setting for the first time. In preparation for an ambulatory care prospective payment system, the Health Care Financing Administration Office of Research and Demonstration has supported a grant for further development of APGs. The objectives of this grant were to include the use of ICD-9-CM and CPT-4 codes as the rubrics of the classification system, to develop a classification that could be used to examine resource consumption beyond physician time, and to link APGs to inpatient DRGs.

Under APGs, the visit is the basis of the payment. The APG system uses three techniques for grouping different services provided during the same visit into a single payment unit:

- Significant procedure that is normally scheduled, is the reason for the visit, and dominates the time and resources expended during the visit.

- Ancillary tests that are ordered by the primary physician to assist in diagnosis and treatment and ancillary procedures that do increase the time and resources expended, but do not dominate the time and resources.

- Multiple significant procedure and ancillary discounting is applied when multiple unrelated significant procedures are performed or when the same ancillary service is performed multiple times.

The system includes groups for both medical and surgical/procedural services. The CPT code determines the significant procedure APG assigned, and the ICD-9-CM code determines the medical visit APG. For example, a patient treated in the ambulatory clinic with a diagnosis of hernia would be assigned to a medical visit APG if he has the condition assessed, diagnosed, or has medication given. If the patient has the hernia treated surgically, the APG would be one for significant procedures.

Although the use of APGs is currently limited, health information practitioners should be aware that APGs may be adopted in the future to provide a prospective payment system for ambulatory care. Coding of ambulatory care records should, therefore, be subject to the same quality controls as are applied to inpatient records.

Pediatric Modified Diagnostic Related Groups (PM-DRGs)

Pediatric Modified Diagnostic Related Groups (PM-DRGs) were developed during 1984-87 as part of a research project entitled "Children's Hospitals Case Mix Classification Project." Research determined original DRG system does not articulate well the more complex and costly children's conditions often treated at specialty hospitals. Thus DRGs, when used as the basis for payment, create a risk to providing adequate resources for those children needing special health care treatment, and for the facilities providing that care. PM-DRGs represents a refinement of the present DRGs, not a departure from them.

Resource Utilization Groups (RUGs)

The patient classification system called Resource Utilization Groups is a case-mix system for long term care. The latest edition, RUGs III, uses forty-four categories for patients which are based on the amount of assistance required in activities of daily living and clinical characteristics. Patients are first placed into one of the following seven clinical categories: special rehabilitation, special care, extensive services, clinically complex conditions, impaired cognition, behavior problems, and reduced physical functioning. These seven categories are then subdivided into activities of daily living variables. To arrive at the appropriate classification, a resident assessment instrument, called the Minimum Data Base +, is used.

Severity of Illness

The patient's stage of disease severity is not directly reflected in DRG assignment. Patients with multiple complications or comorbid conditions are assigned to the same DRG as those with one complication or comorbid condition. Many health care professionals believe severity of illness must be considered to achieve equitable prospective payment and that tertiary hospitals treating proportionately more patients at the higher levels of severity may be exposed to great financial risk under a prospective payment system not adjusted for severity. The government has recognized these inequities and plans to adjust its Medicare DRGs for severity for fiscal year 1995 or 1996.

Measuring severity of illness, however, is not easy, as there are many factors to consider. Much research is being conducted in order to develop a system that can truly describe sicker patients and how to reimburse for them. Most of the severity measurement systems take the form of computer programs sold by software vendors. The available systems vary on a number of dimensions, including:

- The conceptual basis for the disease and severity classifications.
- The number and type of clinical indicators and other variables used to group patients into categories, and the objectivity of those variables.

- Point in time when patient severity is rated - at admission or after discharge.
- Use of patient records abstraction versus discharge codes, and the associated personnel costs of each method.
- Disease specific vs. non-disease specific severity criteria and groupings.
- Number of severity categories, and use of one overall patient rating vs. ratings for each comorbidity.
- Availability of national normative data for comparative purposes.

There are six most prominent and widely studied severity of illness systems.

Acuity Index Method (AIM) defines subgroups within each DRG that are homogeneous in terms of resource use. Each DRG is divided into five levels of severity with different predicted lengths of stay. Based on abstracting medical records of discharged patients, the patients are assigned to a level based on the relationship between the primary diagnosis and various other factors, including secondary diagnosis, surgical procedures, age, and sex. It is designed for use on a health care facility's mainframe computer.

Acute Physiology and Chronic Health Evaluation (APACHE) is available in two forms. APACHE II is for use in analyzing intensive care unit (ICU) patients only. APACHE IIB is more recently developed for use with all hospital patients. The purpose of the original software was to measure acuity levels in ICU patients to evaluate the efficacy of their care. The basis for the system is clinical findings from the medical record recorded within 24 hours of hospitalization. A severity score is obtained by combining 12 physiologic variables, such as temperature, blood pressure, pulse rate, and blood tests with adjustments for age, existence of prior severe organ system deficiency, and elective surgical or non-elective status. These variables create a score of 0-71 which is independent of the patient's diagnosis. APACHE II permits hospitals to evaluate the appropriateness of their ICU utilization, to compare their mortality rates, and to test the effectiveness of different therapies. Researchers have studied the validity of APACHE II extensively, and, of all the severity of illness systems, it has the widest acceptance for its limited purpose. APACHE IIB was designed to broaden the scope of the system.

Computerized Severity Index (CSI) produces a severity measure for use with DRGs to explain differences in resource use among patients. It uses objective clinical findings in the patient record, including lab values, signs and symptoms, vital signs, plus diagnosis, sex, age, and some information on performed procedures, to assign hospital inpatients to one of 700 disease conditions, each with four levels of severity. The software assigns an individual severity score for the primary diagnosis and for each complicating condition and comorbidity, and also assigns an overall severity level measuring the interactive effects of the conditions. CSI compiles the overall score by using a weighting system based on physician input and empirical analysis. CSI's 1-4 severity score is added as a sixth digit to the 700 disease criteria sets collapsed from the 10,000 item ICD-9-CM system. These disease criteria sets are described in a companion volume to the ICD-9-CM manuals. Health information personnel can enter the clinical findings on patients into the computer and determine the CSI score at any point in the hospitalization. They can obtain a score representing the maximum overall severity rating throughout the hospital episode and a score during the last 24-48 hours for each disease condition.

Disease Staging is a system which refines diagnostic classifications by producing clusters of similar patients useful for comparative studies and quality assessment. In Disease Staging diseases are divided into four major stages based on the progression that occurs in the absence of treatment. Patients are assigned a disease stage for each of up to 12 diagnoses. An additional program, called Q-Scale, assigns an overall severity score to each patient.

MedisGroups II measures the potential for organ failure and the probability of response to treatment in order to evaluate the quality of care. MedisGroups uses objective clinical findings gathered from patients' first 48 hours of hospitalization to categorize them into five severity groups from 0-4. Health information personnel trained by the developers of the system identify key clinical findings from a possible set of about 200 tests, procedures, and vital signs in patient records, and key them into the computer. The software assigns a severity score from 1-3 to each finding, based on a proprietary scheme for weighing the findings for relative importance. The Medis-

Groups classifies the patients into severity groups 0-4, based on potential for organ failure and probability of responding to treatment. Hospitals repeat the rating process later in the hospitalization to track patients' response to treatment and to check quality of care and utilization efficiency. The MedisGroup rating is not disease specific and therefore the rating must be combined with another patient grouping system, such as DRGs or diagnostic discharge codes, to compare treatment patterns between similar classes of patients. MedisGroups offers its users access to its database of severity adjusted patient records, which enables users to compare their utilization, costs, clinical outcomes, and other variables with other users.

Patient Management Categories (PMC) is an alternative to DRGs that divides patients into clinically specific types that require distinct and consistent diagnosis and treatment. Each of over 800 patient management categories is associated with a specific list of ICD-9-CM codes for diagnoses and procedures. The PMCs are divided into groups, or modules, based on clinically defined disease categories. A patient is assigned to one or more PMCs in different modules, based on clinically defined disease categories. A patient is assigned to one or more PMCs in different modules based on the codes appearing on the discharge abstract. If the patient can be assigned to more than one PMC within a module, the patient is assigned to the one that is most severe or difficult to manage. PMC users also can get Relative Cost Weights software, which provides costed-out dollar estimates for serving each patient category enabling users to evaluate their efficiency against physician-developed norms of necessary care. Patients receive one overall cost weight that considers the interaction of their conditions and their discharge mortality status. PMC also offers its users access to its database of patient records to compare their costs and clinical outcomes by patient category with national norms.

In 1988, HCFA issued a software program to help hospitals adjust their mortality data to account for severity of illness. The software, called **Medicare Mortality Predictor System (MMPS),** is based on a version of the APACHE severity measurement system. The program uses a database of 6,000 patients in four disease categories with high mortality: congestive heart failure, acute myocardial infarction, pneumonia, and stroke. The program contains information for patients in the database on severity of illness and on their in-hospital and 30-day mortality. By entering the same clinical information about their patients in these categories, hospitals can use the software to compare them with the severity-adjusted national database and see whether their severity-adjusted mortality rates are higher or lower than the national sample.

CHOOSING A CLASSIFICATION SYSTEM

The classification system or systems chosen by a particular health care facility must be capable of supplying the information specified by federal and state regulations and accreditation requirements, as well as information desired by the facility's administration and medical staff. The type and amount of information to be collected will help determine the system or combination of systems to be used for the storage and retrieval of data. For example, an acute care facility might use the ICD-9-CM classification system to collect data on inpatients, ICD-O in the tumor registry, the *Index for Roentgen Diagnosis* in the Radiology Department, SNOMED in Pathology, CPT-4 for outpatient procedures, and DSM-III-R in the mental health area.

The original regulations for the prospective payment system specified:

> "that all hospitals subject to the prospective payment system will be paid for inpatient services provided, a specific amount for each discharge based on the case's classification into one of 467 diagnosis-related groups. Every hospital discharge case will fit into a DRG category and no case will apply to more than one category. The assignment is based on the principal diagnosis, secondary diagnosis (if any), procedures performed, and age, sex and discharge status of the patient. The DRGs provide coverage of the complete range of diagnoses represented in the *International Classification of Diseases 9th Revision, Clinical Modification (ICD-9-CM)* without overlay."

Acute care hospitals participating in the Medicare program, therefore, must supply ICD-9-CM codes to obtain reimbursement for inpatient services. They also must monitor changes in the DRG system as announced by HCFA each year in the Federal Register and update their systems accordingly.

Health information practitioners need to continually review health care literature to identify the changes being made in existing health care classification systems and to monitor the development of new systems. As alternate forms of health care delivery become more common, health information practitioners will be required to assess the data needs of these facilities to identify classification systems appropriate for their data needs. Cost of data collection, storage, and retrieval must also be a major factor in choosing one or more classification systems.

ENCODING SYSTEMS

An encoder is defined in *Webster's Unabridged Dictionary* as a "cipher machine." Today's use of the word has expanded its usage to mean the conversion of data from one type to another type. An example of this may be found in the simple act of coding a disease or condition. Computer-assisted encoders are software for use either on a facility's mainframe computer system or on a microcomputer. A logic driven encoder prompts the coder through a series of choices displayed on the screen until a code is assigned for each diagnosis and procedure (Figure 8). Book-driven encoders display the correct pages of the ICD-9-CM Alphabetic Index and Tabular Lists so the coder does not spend time thumbing through the code books but still is able to check all inclusion and exclusion notes to ensure assignment of the correct code.

Consistency among coders is one of the major advantages computerized coding systems offer. Encoders also promote accuracy, for the coder must go through each step of the ICD-9-CM decision process. There is no way to short-circuit the procedure by omitting a step.

Experienced coders may assign common codes more quickly working from memory and familiar code books than by working with an encoder. However, when working from memory, a coder may consistently assign an incorrect code number. Computer assisted encoders, however, only assign codes to diagnoses input by the coder. The coder must analyze the discharge information in the medical record to ensure that the physician has identified the appropriate principal diagnosis according to

Sex: M

Age: 74

Disposition — Choose one:

[NL]   Home — Self-Care/Home Health Service or still in hospital
2   Left against medical advice
3   Transferred to acute care facility
4   Expired
5   SNF, ICF, or other facility

Choice: NL

Principal Diagnosis
Enter Key Word: Cor

1 Cor

Which Line?

Principal Diagnosis

Cor

Cor

1. Cor Biloculare
2. Cor Bovinum or Bovis (coded as cardiac hypertrophy)
3. Cor Pulmonale
4. Cor Pulmonale with Pulmonary Hypertension
5. Cor Triatriatum or Triatrium
6. Cor Triloculare
Which Line?

Principal Diagnosis

Cor
Cor Pulmonale

Cor Pulmonale

1. Acute
2. Chronic
3. With Pulmonary Embolus
4. Unspecified

Which Line?

Principal Diagnosis

Cor
Cor Pulmonale
Acute

ICD-9-CM   Review Code
  415.0   Acute cor pulmonale

Press any key to continue

FIGURE 6. LOGIC-DRIVEN ENCODER

UHDDS definitions. Additionally, the documentation in the record must indicate that the diagnosis selected is that condition which, after study, occasioned the admission of the patient to the hospital for care.

Encoders can accurately assign a code to the diagnosis selected and even query the coder to ensure that the coder does not want to select a different diagnosis as the principal one (Figure 9). However, the coder makes the final decision on the identification of the principal diagnosis and other diagnoses to be reported. The encoder cannot tell which diagnoses listed by the physician affect the current stay. Yet, only those diagnoses

DRG

336   Transurethral Prostatectomy (70+/cc)
      HCFA wt. 0.9974 Mean LOS 8.4 Outlier LOS (22 days)

Diagnoses

1. * 185   Malignant neoplasm of prostate
2. * 25030 Diabetes mellitus with coma, non-insulin
            dependent or unspecified (Type II)

Select alternate principal Dx or NL to continue

Procedures

602 Transurethral prostatectomy

DRG

468 *** O.R. Procedure Unrelated to Diagnosis MDC ***

      HCFA wt. 2.0818 Mean LOS 11.2 Outlier LOS 33 days

      *Note this may not be an error in coding, but
      you should carefully examine your selection of
      principal diagnosis and make sure you have
      included all surgeries.

Diagnoses:

1. * 25030 Diabetes mellitus with coma, non-insulin
           dependent or unspecified (Type II)
2.   185   Malignant neoplasm of prostate

Select alternate principal Dx or NL to continue
Procedures
* 602 Transurethral prostatectomy

FIGURE 7. ASSIGNING DIAGNOSIS CODE WITH ENCODER

which affect the patient stay are to be reported according to the UHDDS definitions. Diagnoses that relate to an earlier episode of care which have no bearing on the current hospital stay are to be excluded.

Some vendors have developed encoders which encourage selection of the diagnosis with the highest reimbursement as the principal diagnosis. This practice constitutes Medicare fraud when the medical record documentation indicates a less costly diagnosis as the principal diagnosis.

For accurate coding, either manually or with an encoder, the critical skill is searching the medical record to identify the diagnosis which fits the UHDDS definition of principal diagnosis, and all other diagnoses and procedures which affect the hospital stay.

Computer support of the coding function is expensive; for in addition to hardware and software costs, an annual license fee may be assessed. After assessing the volume of coding to be completed and the proficiency and depth of a hospital's coding staff, each health information practitioner must decide whether computer-assisted encoders will improve the accuracy of coding performed and can be cost justified.

SUMMARY

Many disease and operation nomenclatures and classification systems have been used in the United States throughout the years. As our health care delivery system has become more specialized, specialty classification systems have been developed for use in recording valuable medical statistical information. Although federal and state requirements may somewhat mandate the choice of a classification system, special information needs of a health care facility often require the health information practitioner to utilize additional classification systems. The health information practitioner must constantly stay abreast of changes and innovations in published classification systems and nomenclatures. No single classification will satisfy everyone's needs. A careful appraisal of the needs of the facility and an up-to-date knowledge of available classification systems will result in selection of an appropriate classification system by the health care institution.

STUDY QUESTIONS

1. Define nomenclature and classification systems, and explain how each may be used to complement the other in recording medical information.

2. State the purpose, and describe the structure of the code numbers used in each of the following nomenclatures and classification systems:

    a. SNOMED   e. ICD-O

    b. SNVDO/SNOVET   f. DSM-IV

    c. CPT   g. HCPCS

    d. ICD-9-CM

3. State the purposes of case-mix classifications, and describe the structure of:

    a. DRGs

    b. APGs

    c. RUGs

    d. Severity of Illness Systems

4. List some considerations which should be made when selecting an appropriate classification system for use in a health care facility.

5. Identify the strengths and weaknesses of computer assisted encoders.

REFERENCES

American College of Radiology, *Index for Roentgen Diagnoses,* 3rd Ed., (Chicago: American College of Radiology, 1975).

American Medical Association, *Current Procedural Terminology,* 4th Ed., (Chicago: January 1994).

American Medical Association, *Standard Nomenclature of Athletic Injuries,* (Chicago: 1976).

American Psychiatric Association, *Diagnostic and Statistical Manual of Mental Disorders,* 4th Ed., (Washington, D.C.: 1994).

A Reason for Visit Classification for Ambulatory Care, Series 2, No. 78, (Hyattsville, MD: U.S. Department of Health, Education, and Welfare, February 1983).

Barnes, Cathleen A., "Disease Staging: A Clinically Oriented Dimension of Case Mix," *Journal of the American Medical Record Association,* (January 1985): 22-27.

Campbell, Claire, *Nursing Diagnosis and Intervention in Nursing Practice,* (New York City: John Wiley and Sons, 1978).

Carpenito, Lynda Juall, Nursing Diagnosis - *Application to Clinical Practice,* (Philadelphia: J.B. Lippincott, 1983).

College of American Pathologists, *Systematized Nomenclature of Medicine,* (Skokie, IL: 1979).

College of American Pathologists, *Systematized Nomenclature of Pathology,* (Chicago: 1965).

Cote, Roger A. and Stanley Robbory, "Progress in Medical Information Management: Systematized Nomenclature of Medicine (SNOMED)," *Journal of the American Medical Association,* (February 22/29, 1980).

Council for International Organizations of Medical Sciences and the World Health Organization, *International Nomenclature of Diseases - Diseases of the Lower Respiratory Tract,* (Geneva, Switzerland, 1979).

Federal Register, Vol. 53, No. 190, (Friday, September 30, 1988/Rules & Regulations): 38590.

Finkel, Asher, *Current Medical Information and Terminology,* 5th Ed., (Chicago: American Medical Association, 1981).

Finnegan, Rita, *Coding for Prospective Payment,* (Chicago: American Medical Record Association, 1992).

Fries, Brant E. and Leo M., Jr., "Resource Utilization Groups: A Patient Classification System for Long-Term Care," *Medical Care,* Vol. 23, (February 1985): 110-122.

Gardner, Elizabeth, "Measuring Degrees of Illness," *Modern Healthcare,* (December 16, 1988): 22-30.

Gebbie, Kristine M. and Mary Ann, *Classification of Nursing Diagnoses,* (St. Louis, MO: The C.V. Mosby Company, 1975).

Gonnella, Joseph S., Mark C. Hornbrook and Daniel Z. Louis, "Staging of Disease: 4A Case-Mix Measurement," *Journal of the American Medical Association,* (February 1984).

Grossman, Herbert J., *Classification in Mental Retardation,* (Washington, D.C.: American Association on Mental Deficiency, 1983).

Health Care Financing Administration Common Procedure Coding System, Health Care Financing Administration, (Washington, D.C.: U.S. Dept. of Health and Human Services, 1980).

Horn, Susan Dadakis, "Measuring Severity of Illness: Comparisons Across Institutions," *American Journal of Public Health,* (January 1983): 25-31.

International Classification of Diseases for Oncology, World Health Organization, (Geneva, Switzerland: 1976).

Joint Commission on Accreditation of Healthcare Organizations Accreditation Manual for Hospitals, (Chicago: Joint Commission, 1994).

Lamberts, Henk, Sue Meads and Maurice Wood, "Classification of Reasons Why Persons Seeking Primary Care: Pilot Study of a New System," *Public Health Reports,* (November-December 1984).

Manual of the World Health Organization International Statistical Classification of Disease, Injuries, and Causes of Death, (Geneva, Switzerland: World Health Organization, 1977).

Meyer, Harris, "System Developers Vie for Review Market," *American Medical News,* (June 19, 1987): 25-26.

Nomenclature and Criteria for Diagnosis of Diseases of the Heart and Great Vessels, 7th Ed., (New York Heart Association, 1973).

Shlala, Tom, "AVGs: Impact on the Medical Record Department of Acute Care Facilities," *Journal of American Medical Association,* (January 1988): 25-29.

Simmons, DeLanne A., A Classification Scheme for Client Problems in Community Health Nursing, Publication No. HRA 60-16, (Washington, D.C.: Department of Health and Human Services, 1980).

Standard Nomenclature of Veterinary Diseases and Operations, 2nd Ed., (U.S. National Institutes of Health, U.S. Department of Health, Education, and Welfare, 1975).

Thompson, James, Delray Green and Harry L. Savitt, "Preliminary Report on Crosswalk from DSM-III to ICD-9-CM," *American Journal of Psychiatry,* (February 1983).

"Training session: Understanding CPT fundamentals," Briefings on Practice Management, November 1993.

"This year brings few DRG changes...but watch for next year's refinements," Medical Records Briefing, October 1993.

World Health Organization, *International Classification of Impairments, Disabilities, and Handicaps* (Geneva, Switzerland: WHO, 1980).

World Organization of National Colleges, Academies, and Academic Associations of General Practitioners/Family Physicians, *International Classification of Health Problems in Primary Care,* 3rd Ed., (New York City: Oxford University Press, 1983).

chapter 10

INDEXES AND REGISTERS

The maintenance and retrieval of health information are an important function in any health care facility. Two tools employed to facilitate the maintenance and retrieval of health information are the index and register. According to the American Heritage Dictionary an index is "Anything that serves to guide, point out, or otherwise facilitate reference." A register is "A formal or official recording of items, names, or actions."

Hospitals usually maintain an admission register, death register, birth register, operating room register, emergency room register, number index, master patient index, physicians' index, and disease and operative indexes. Some hospitals also maintain cancer or other diagnostic or procedural registries.

Until the early 1970s, most indexes and registers in health care facilities were compiled by manual methods. Certain kinds of information about the patient and/or patient care were extracted from the medical record and hand-posted on ledger sheets or cards.

Today, indexes and registers are computerized in almost all facilities, although historical information is retained in manual form. Computerization of this information has improved the process of planning for future needs, compilation of data, and study of diseases and their outcomes. These systems allow for manipulation of data in ways that would have been burdensome or virtually impossible in a manual system. This availability of information through computerization has brought health information departments into the information age and changed the role of health information practitioners to health information management professionals. As with any system, a key component of this role is understanding how the data is collected, its shortcomings, and its appropriate use.

Indexes and registers contain much valuable information. The most familiar and traditional use of indexes and registers is to direct the location of health information for use by physicians in patient care management and research. Administration of the facility, however, has become a prominent user as more information for management and financial decisions are needed. Health care facilities are also being required to provide patient care information with great frequency by agencies that fund such care. Third-party payers want to be assured that the episodes of patient care they are paying for was necessary and appropriate. Peer review organizations, accrediting agencies, and licensing bodies request health information to review the quality of the care delivered.

These increasing demands for health information require the health care facility to maintain an effective and efficient information system using appropriate indexes and registers. The use of computers with their ability to accept, store, and produce data with efficiency and ease is a must.

MASTER PATIENT INDEX

The master patient index (MPI) identifies all patients who have ever been admitted or treated by the health care facility. The master patient index is the key to locating patient records and is one of the most important tools in the health care facility. Traditionally, the master patient index was maintained by preparing an index card for each patient admitted or treated at a health care facility. The index cards were arranged alphabetically in a vertical file or filed phonetically by last name. The patient index card may have been prepared in the patient registration area at the time of admission or later by health information personnel. The index was maintained in the health information department.

Computerization of the master patient index is now current practice. Computerization allows the registration areas at the time of patient registration to obtain the medical record number of any patient previously registered or enter the required information to register a new patient. An identification number may be automatically assigned to the new patient. Although patient registration areas may access the master patient index and assign numbers, control of the data generally is the responsibility of the health information management department which is responsible for maintaining the accuracy of the MPI.

The American Hospital Association recommends that hospitals retain certain basic information after the medical record has outlived the statute of limitations for that state or the time period established by the hospital for the destruction of records. Therefore, the patient index remains as a permanent record of all patients who have ever been admitted to the hospital.

CONTENT OF THE PATIENT INDEX

The master patient index contains only information of an identifying nature necessary for prompt location of a particular medical record (Figure 1). This information should as a minimum include: full name, address, identifying number, social

```
X Y Z HOSPITAL                              MPI INQUIRY SCREEN - 1 MAR 1989
ENTER FULL NAME OR FIRST 3 CHARACTERS LAST NAME:————————————

SEQ  #          HOSPITAL  #              ————NAME————-
BIRTHDATE
   1            348729            Smith, Arthur E.         12-16-74
   2            284195            Smith, Caroline          08-04-38
   3            318366            Smith, Claude R.         02-18-50
   4            338750            Smith, Dorothy Marie     10-05-45
```

```
X Y Z HOSPITAL                               MPI PT ID SCREEN - 1 MAR 1989
NAME: Smith, Claude R.                               HOSPITAL #: 318366
ADDRESS: 204 East 5th St.
CITY, STATE, ZIP: Town, IL 60610
SEX: M          BIRTHDATE: 02-18-50          MOTHER'S MAIDEN NAME: Jones
ENTER U TO UPDATE, V TO VALIDATE, OR RETURN FOR NEXT INQUIRY:
```

FIGURE 1. MASTER PATIENT INDEX COMPUTERIZED ENTRY SCREEN

security number, and birth date (month, date, and year; in cases where patients have the same name, the date of birth provides additional information for identifying and obtaining the correct health record). Other identifying information may include sex, mother's maiden name (to further assist in identifying people with common names), and race/ethnicity. Sometimes the master patient index includes other information such as admission and discharge dates, result (discharged or died), and attending physician's name, although such information is generally found in the patient's record and does not need to be duplicated in the MPI.

Identifying information may be given out only in accordance with health care facility policy in response to legitimate requests. It is inadvisable to record service or diagnostic/procedural information in the master patient index. Guidelines for developing release of information policies are included in Chapter 15 — Legal Aspects of Medical Records.

ARRANGEMENT OF THE MASTER PATIENT INDEX

Prior to computerization, facilities often used index cards or even bound volumes for the MPI. When bound volumes were used, the book was divided into alphabetic sections. Names were listed under the first letter of the surname in chronological order by date of admission. When index cards were used, facilities placed patient data in a vertical file, with a separate card for each patient. Some facilities file cards by year of admission, a practice that was impractical because patients often forgot the dates of their last admissions or whether they had been patients at all.

Over the last three decades, facilities have changed their MPIs from manual ones to computerized systems. The level of sophistication and the depth of data in today's MPIs vary. The computerized MPI allows staff to access data in a variety of ways — alphabetically, by medical record number, by billing number, phonetically, by birth date, and by social security number. A computerized master patient index also solves space and retrieval problems, assists in maintaining accuracy, and can provide other departments with immediate access to the MPI.

If the patient does not provide complete identifying information or a previous entry contained an error, duplication of patient registration may occur in a computerized system just as in a manual system. Therefore, it is important to monitor for patients with more than one medical record number.

Regardless of the type of MPI the facility maintains, it is important for the health information management professional to know basic guidelines for alphabetizing and phonetically arranging and accessing data. The following pages give guidelines for both types of filing and accessing data.

Guidelines for alphabetical data

The following guidelines are suggested for both computerized and manual master patient indexes.

1. Place surname first, then given name followed by middle or maiden name or initial, and file in strict alphabetical sequence.

2. Arrange names in alphabetical order like words in a dictionary, following letter by letter to the end of the name and then by given name and initials. The telephone directory serves as a ready reference when in doubt.

3. If there is more than one person with the same surname and given name, the data should be arranged alphabetically by middle initial. If no middle initial is given, the names are arranged according to birth date, filing the oldest card first.

4. Names with prefixes of D', de, De, Des, Di, Du, La, Mc, Mac, Van, Von, etc., are filed alphabetically as D'Armand (D-A-r-m-a-n-d), De Tarnowski (D-e-T-a-r-n-o-w-s-k-i), etc.

5. Names beginning with St., as St. Peter, are filed as S-a-i-n-t.

6. Compound or hyphenated names are filed as one word; thus Craig-Stuart would be filed under C-r-a-i-g-S-t-u-a-r-t, following the name through, letter by letter.

7. Names with religious titles such as Reverend, Mother, Father, Brother, and Sister are filed under the surnames, the titles being disregarded, and then given name. Sister Mary Douglas is filed as Douglas, Mary. Religious titles should not be filed in groups such as all Sisters together, for this method is not efficient.

8. If an initial is given instead of a patient's first or middle names, the rule is "file nothing before something." Thus, M. Brown would precede M. Kay Brown and Mary Kay Brown.

9. Because of difficulty in distinguishing between two names with the same sound, it is permissible to combine Mac

and Mc without distinction as to spelling, filing Mc as if spelled Mac. Whichever filing method is adopted, it must be adhered to throughout the file to maintain uniformity.

10. It is customary for people of Spanish descent to combine the name of the mother with the name of the father. For instance, with the name Soto Ramariz, Soto is the surname of the father, and Ramariz the maiden name of the mother. They are filed in alphabetical sequence of first the father's name and then the mother's maiden name. Thus, the name of Maria Dolores Soto Ramariz would be filed in the S section of the file in the following order: S-o-t-o-R-a-m-a-r-i-z, Maria Dolores.

11. If a patient's name has changed since a previous admission, a cross-reference should be made to the former name. For instance, if O'Brien, Mary Catherine is admitted, a cross-reference should be made to her previous admission as McCarty, Mary Catherine. All information recorded on the original card is entered on the new card and the original card is cross-referenced to the new card.

12. When looking for a given person's name card, one must keep in mind that there may be many spellings of the same name; search must be made under every possible spelling of the name before stating there is no card for that name. For instance, there are approximately 35 ways of spelling the name Baer, 10 or more ways of spelling Burke, etc. Again, the telephone directory is an excellent reference for alternate spellings of common names.

13. Card files should be audited regularly for misfiles, and additional training of master patient index clerks provided as necessary.

14. When a computerized MPI allows many different points of patient registration, it is imperative that the above guidelines be adopted for use when entering the patient's name so that all like entries will be entered consistently.

Phonetic Filing

Facilities located in communities having large populations with foreign names may use the phonetic system for filing patient index cards. This phonetic capability for searching the MPI is often available in computerized systems. When this method is used, the patient's index card is filed behind the appropriate guide for the initial letter of the surname, but according to sound rather than according to spelling. Thus, all surnames that sound alike but are spelled differently are filed together.

The English alphabet, with the exception of the vowels a, e, i, o, u and the letters w, h, and y, which are not coded, is reduced to six key letters with a corresponding three-digit numeric code as follows:

Key Letters	Code Number	Equivalent
b	1	p, f, v
c	2	s, k, g, j, q, x, z
d	3	t
l	4	none
m	5	n
r	6	none

Instead of indexing each name by its exact spelling, as in a straight alphabetical file, name variations are brought together by the code number which represents the key letters. The first letter of the surname is not coded but serves as a prefix to the three-digit code number, and coding is limited to succeeding key letters or their equivalents. For instance, to code the surname Martin:

> M - prefix, not coded
>
> a - vowel, not coded
>
> r - 6 (key letter)
>
> t - 3 (an equivalent)
>
> i - vowel, not coded
>
> n - 5 (an equivalent)

The name Martin is, therefore, coded 635. All variations in the spelling of the name Martin are coded 635 and will be filed together: Mardan, Marden, Mardyn, Martan, Marten, Martin, Martyn, Merten, Merton, Morden, Morten, Mortin, Morton, Murten. Thus it can be seen that names of like or similar sound will generally code the same, be grouped together in a file, and be found more quickly than if it is necessary to hunt through a completely alphabetized patient's index file.

In a manual file section like the illustration in Figure 2 all names beginning with the letter S are grouped together according to their codes behind the main guide S.

Equivalent letters at the beginning of a name are treated as one letter. For example, s, c, and h are treated as one letter in Schmidt. The letters shown on the left-hand side of the file and on the left-hand side of the following listing represent the key letters of the surname to be coded, while the number alongside represents the resulting codes for those key letters.

The second-position and third-position guides are auxiliary guides for the given names and are used when there is a large group of cards with the same given name initial letters. As an example, the following names may be found in this file behind the specific guides:

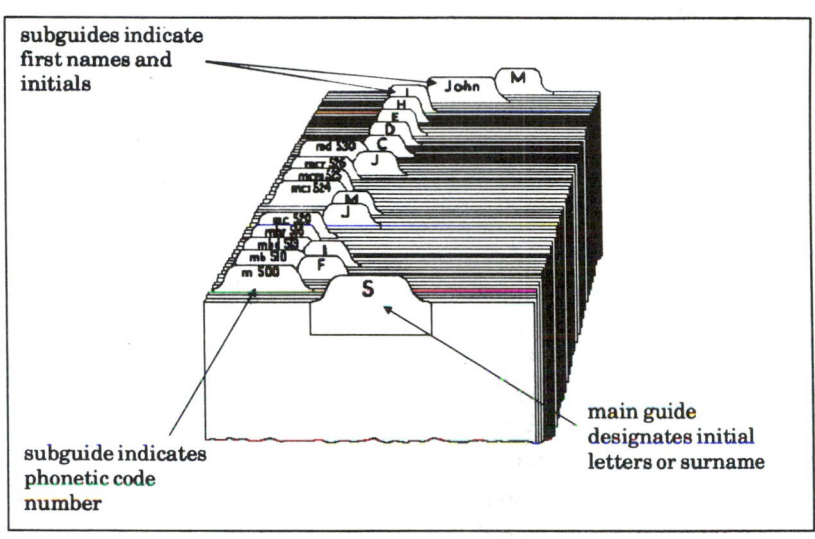

Courtesy Kardex Systems, Inc.

FIGURE 2. PHONETIC ARRANGEMENT OF PATIENT INDEX

mcr 562	Singer, Anna Marie
	Sanger, Fred C.
	Singer, Ralph R.
	Senger, William T.
md 530	Smith, Arthur E.
	Sinda, Andrew T.
	Shenit, Barbara Jean
C	
	Schmidt, Charles M.
	Smith, Claude R.

Duplication is avoided as names spelled incorrectly, as well as those with typographical errors, will be filed together if they sound alike.

The sponsors of this system state there are only five rules that must be observed in maintaining a phonetic file:

1. When two or more key letters or their equivalents occur together, treat them as one letter.

2. If a name contains less than three key letters, add zeros to arrive at the code number. The name "Jackson" is completely coded with the number 25, so a zero (also called a cipher) is added to assign the name of a 3-digit code, J-250.

3. If two of the same key letters, or a key letter and its equivalent, are separated by h or w, code one key letter.

4. When a repeated key letter or its equivalent is separated by a, e, i, o, u, or y, the key letters or their equivalents are considered separately.

5. After coding of the surname, arrangement between the key letter guides should be alphabetical according to given name.

With a phonetic file the user does not have to think of the various other ways the particular name being searched might be spelled. The sponsors of this system claim that this method detects duplication in the files and discloses 90 percent of all transposition of letters. This system has one great disadvantage in that rules for phonetic filing must be learned, and when persons who know how to file and retrieve are not present, access to the file is limited.

Many computer systems incorporate a phonetic filing option so that when a patient's name is typed into the computer system, a display of all possible names and identifying information (converted to alphabetical order) may be provided.

THE NUMBER INDEX

The number index is important as the patient identification number control. It is the origin of the numbering system whether it be serial, unit, or serial-unit. It is a chronological list of the patient identification numbers issued to patients and the name of the patient assigned each number. It must be remembered that a number index is a numerical listing of numbers. Therefore, if unit numbers are used, all admissions of any one patient will not be shown; while an admission register, being a chronological listing of admissions, provides a record of all admissions.

In the past, the number index may have been a loose-leaf book, vertical or visible file, or a computer listing. If the facility kept a loose-leaf book, the sheets should have been bound at the end of the year to prevent loss.

Now, computers store the number index and automatically assign a medical record number when a patient is being registered for admission. Automated assignment of identification numbers reduces the chance of skipping numbers or assigning the same number to two patients.

Because the number index is the source of facility numbers and, therefore, used as a reference when there is doubt about the accuracy of a number, the number index should be monitored to assure its accuracy and completeness.

DISEASE AND PROCEDURE INDEXES

A disease index lists diseases and conditions according to the classification (coding) system used by the facility. A listing of surgical and procedural code numbers comprises the operation index.

CONTENT OF THE DISEASE AND PROCEDURE INDEXES

Today's requests for patient information are often detailed, and provision should be made in the disease and operation indexes to respond to these requests as quickly as possible. In general, the indexes should provide sufficient detail to complete required medical and statistical reports and requests. Licensing and accrediting agencies require data for their surveys, and provision for this should be made in the index. Data routinely entered under code for each disease affecting a patient or procedure performed on a patient includes:

1. Patient's sex.

2. Patient's age.

3. Patient's race/ethnicity.

4. Name of attending physician and surgeon.

5. Service on which the patient was hospitalized.

6. End results of hospitalization — this category specifies whether the patient died or was discharged. If the patient died, it may be of interest to record whether or not an autopsy was performed.

7. Date of admission and/or discharge, length of stay, and charges and costs. Length of stay data may be useful for evaluating utilization factors. The date of admission or discharge may assist in locating a particular record.

8. Associated diseases and procedures.

A disease and procedure index may be set up either for simple indexing or cross-indexing, depending on the facility's needs. Simple indexing means that entries for each disease and operation a patient has are made under their respective code numbers with no reference to other code numbers assigned to that patient. With cross-indexing, reference is made to the code numbers for all diseases and operations a patient had during hospitalization, for each separate entry posted in the index. If cross-indexing is done, space must be set aside for the recording of codes for associated diseases or operations.

Computerized disease and procedures indexing systems provide cross-indexing automatically. Automated systems also allow for data to be retrieved by diagnosis or procedure, with the flexibility of retrieving any data field entered for a patient. Some basic computer systems contain a limited number of items, displayed in predefined reports. Other automated systems include flexible or ad hoc reporting which allows the user to define parameters and data fields to be included and thereby create specially designed reports.

COST OF INDEXES

The disease and operation indexes are the most expensive indexes in the department to maintain. The person abstracting and entering data must not only be a capable individual but also extremely accurate in making the entries. The more data indexed from any one record, the greater the cost to the department in terms of personnel time.

Another expense is the retrieval of data from the index. A physician may request a list of all cases of cholecystitis in female patients. If the sex of patients has not been indexed, all of the records with a diagnosis of cholecystitis will have to be pulled. The pulling of many nonpertinent cases takes time and is, therefore, costly. If the index is in a computer system with flexible reporting capability, however, the health information manager can manipulate the data to provide any information that is in the system in a format most useful to the person making the request.

The health information professional must determine how often the index is being used and for what purposes. The amount and kinds of data needed to be indexed can be determined by studying the patterns of usage. A physician or a medical staff committee might use the disease and operation indexes to retrieve medical records for the following purposes:

1. To review previous cases of a given disease in order to provide insight into the management of a current patient's health problems.
2. To test theories and compare data on certain diseases and/or treatments in order to conduct research and prepare scientific papers.
3. To procure data on the utilization of facilities and to establish a facility's need for new equipment, beds, staff, etc., in various departments.
4. To evaluate the quality of care in the facility.
5. To conduct epidemiological and infection-control studies.
6. To accumulate risk management data, such as the incidence of medical and surgical complications.

In addition to physicians' uses of the indexes, numerous requests for patient care data are received from administrators and other authorized personnel, planning agencies, educational programs, fiscal intermediaries, and health care agencies and organizations. Examples of other uses of these indexes include:

1. Providing patient care data required for licensing and accreditation surveys.
2. Providing data on medical practice in the facility in order to qualify for accredited internship and residency programs.
3. Determining whether the treatment and procedures provided were necessary and appropriate for the diagnosis.
4. Providing educational material for students, grand rounds, and medical staff meetings.

Disease and operation indexes should be tailor-made to meet the needs of the institutions they serve. Consideration should be given to the need for the index, who will use it, and what information will be requested. Careful planning will result in an index that will serve the medical and facility staff well and promote the efficiency of the indexing operation itself.

AUTOMATED INDEXES

In today's facilities, disease, operation, and physician indexes are computerized. An in-house computer or a commercial discharge data service may be used. Some state hospital associations or third-party payers also process discharge data on a per discharge basis.

Use of computerized capabilities within the facility should be compared to the cost of using outside data services. In-house data processing allows the health information practitioner to design an abstracting and indexing system specific to the facility's individual needs.

DISCHARGE DATA ABSTRACTING

Abstracting is compiling the pertinent information from the medical record. A data entry source document called a case abstract or discharge data abstract may be used to collect the data. The items appear on the abstract form in somewhat the same order as in the medical record, so the transfer of data from the record to the abstract can be performed quickly and accurately (Figure 3).

To ensure timely data, it is ideal to abstract (or index) the medical record immediately after it has been assembled and coded and before it is filed in the incomplete file. However, a record may not be complete enough to code at that time or the physician may want to add or change a diagnosis. Therefore, abstracting after the physician has completed the record results in more complete and accurate data.

To ensure that every record is abstracted, the health information practitioner needs a control system. As records are abstracted, the staff may check off the discharge list to show which records have been processed. A computer system, however, makes it easy to print a list for control purposes.

A paper abstract is prepared for each discharged patient, batched, and sent to the in-house data processing department or to the service discharge date for compilation. Any errors detected by computer edits result in the abstract being sent

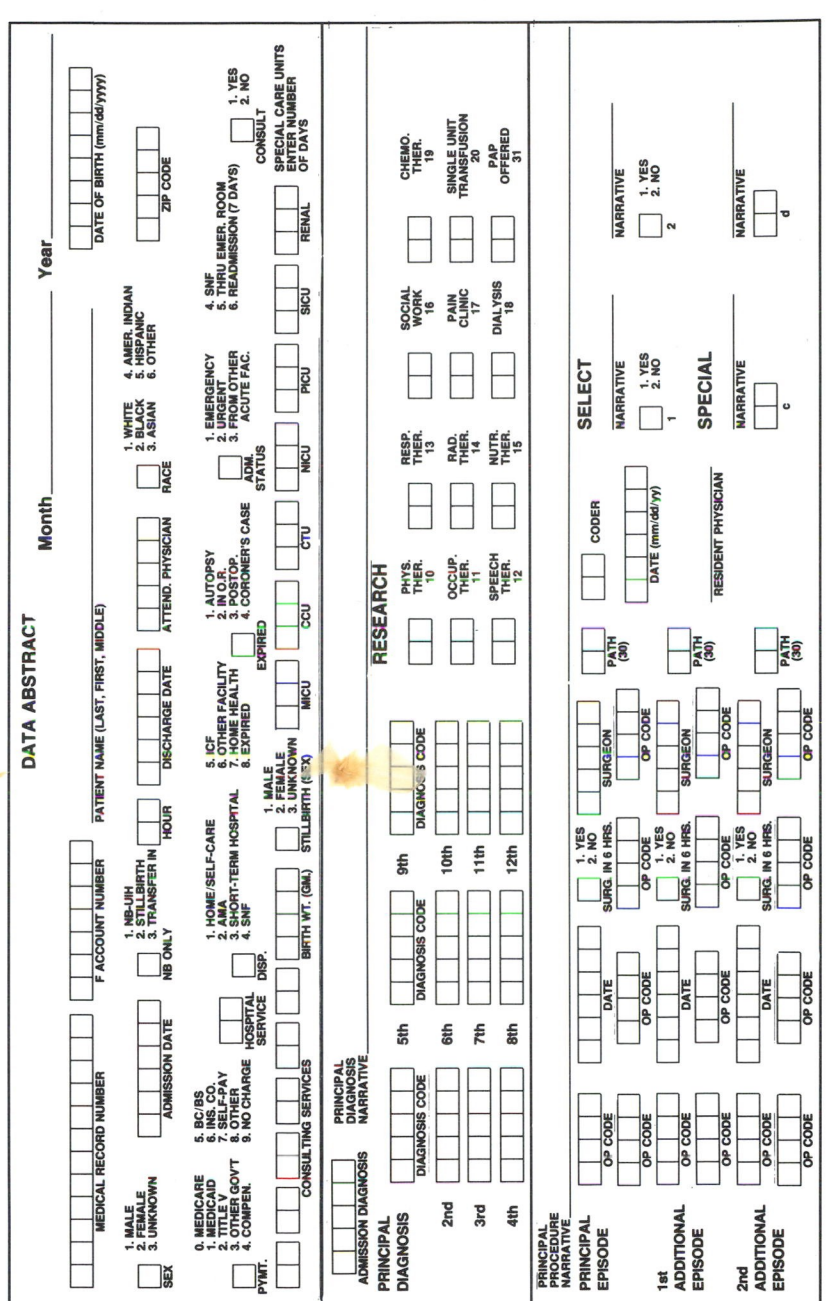

FIGURE 3. HOSPITAL-DESIGNED DISCHARGE DATA ABSTRACT

back to the health information department for review, correction, and resubmission. The corrected data are then compiled to produce the disease and operation indexes (Figure 4) and provide meaningful reports reflecting the treatment rendered in that facility.

REPORT PERIOD: 01/01/85 - 01/31/85 DATE PREPARED: 03/01/85
01 - 000001 MCAUTO TEST HOSPITAL 8 PAGE 1
SEQ: PROC CODE - MED REC NUMBER OPERATION INDEX - 215 600-CR1600

DIAG (1)	OTHER DIAGNOSES (2A)	(2B)	(2C)	ATTNDG SURGEON DPT/SRV (3)	OTHER PHYS (4)	INDEX PROC (5)	PROCEDURES (5A)	(5B)	(5C)	DISCH DATE (6)	HOSP DAYS LOS (7A)	SPEC UNIT (7B)	(7C)	DISCH STATUS (8)	OPTIONAL AREA (9)	MED. REC. NO. PATIENT NAME ABSTRACT NO. (10)	AGE SEX (11)	(12)	PAY A/B (13)	(14)	(15)	TYPE	UNITS
						SUBMUCOUS RESECTION OF NASAL SEPTUM AS PRINCIPAL PROCEDURE																	
470 P	7380	486	7380 A	B180 B180 QQ	0124R	215	215	2187		0105	4		1	1	1 01/02	648606 280019 $499	16 F	1 1	4	2 1	2 1		
						OTHER RHINOPLASTY AS ASSOCIATED PROCEDURE																	
470 P	7380	486	7380 A	B180 B180 QQ	0124R	2187	215	2187		0105	4		1	1	1 01/02	648606 280019 $499	16 F	1 1	4	2 1	2 1		
						TONSILLECTOMY WITH ADENOIDECTOMY AS PRINCIPAL PROCEDURE																	
47410P			47410A	A252 B179 QQ	B179C	283	283			0130	1			1	1 01/29	649960 280001 $175	6 F	1 1	6	2 2	2 1		
						LARYNGOSCOPY AND OTHER TRACHEOSCOPY AS ASSOCIATED PROCEDURE																	
490 P	7863	40290	7863 A	A250 A250 AA	B176C	3142	3324	3142	4223	0117	11		1	3	1 01/07	649223 280013 $1111	60 F	1 1	4	2 3	3 2		
						SEGMENTAL RESECTION OF LUNG AS PRINCIPAL PROCEDURE																	
1629 P	496	5239	25000 1629 A	B176 B178 BN7	B177C B178S B178C	323	323 3324 3426 9219	9605 3422 9399		0128	73	40	4	7A	1 11/16 1 11/20 1 11/21 N 12/18	647302 280007 $13459	74 M	2 2	1 4	2 1	2 1		
						ENDOSCOPIC BRONCHIAL BIOPSY AS PRINCIPAL PROCEDURE																	
490 P	7863	40290	7863 A	A250 A250 AA	B176C	3324	3324	3142	4223	0117	11		1	3	1 01/07	649223 280013 $1111	60 F	1 1	4	2 3	3 2		
						AS ASSOCIATED PROCEDURE																	

Reprinted with permission of the McDonnell-Douglas Health Information Systems Company

FIGURE 4. PRINT OUT FROM AUTOMATED OPERATION INDEX

On line data entry into a computer is also possible. In this situation a data entry clerk in the health information department abstracts data from the medical record and keys it directly into a computer in accordance with directions displayed on the computer's monitor. The directions are displayed in a similar form as on the paper abstracts. Because editing of data takes place immediately, time is saved in obtaining reports.

In an in-house system, a microcomputer may be used for all processing of the discharge data or, more commonly, data are entered into the facility's mainframe via a terminal. For commercial discharge services data may be collected on a disk that is sent to the commercial service at the end of the month, or data may be transmitted over telephone lines using a modem and data communications software.

Manual disease and procedure indexes are becoming rare in today's computerized health information departments.

Manual indexing requires posting disease and operation code numbers on each index card which are then filed in strict numerical order by codes. Another manual method is called group indexing. In that system, a range of code numbers is included on each disease and operation index card. Such a system keeps the index from becoming so large that it is unmanageable.

Small, non-automated indexes can be filed in equipment that allows the titles of all cards to be seen or in vertical indexes that have guides to indicate the range of numbers behind each.

RETRIEVAL FROM INDEXES

When a request is made for medical records with a certain diagnosis, care must be taken to ensure that all records with that diagnosis are secured. Pertinent records may often be found under more than one code number; therefore, health information personnel should discuss with the requester all code numbers which might provide relevant records, as well as other patient characteristics such as age groups, sex, service, etc.

PHYSICIANS' INDEX

TYPES

The physicians' index provides every medical staff member a record of patients treated. Entries in the physicians' index are usually the name and medical record number of the patient but may include other data such as the hospital service, length of stay, charges and costs. It may also identify those patients for whom a physician served as surgeon or consultant, the end results of hospitalization, and any other data which might be desirable. If an in-house computer or a discharge data service is used for indexing diseases and operations, producing a physicians' index is a simple process. Monthly or yearly listing of physicians and their patients' names can be maintained. (Figure 5).

Valuable use may be made of the patient data stored in the physicians' index, both by individual physicians and authorized medical staff committees. The following are examples.

1. The physician may survey trends in volume and changes in practice using data included in the index.

2. The credentials committee of the medical staff may use the physicians' index to identify physicians' activity profiles.

3. Data on physician use of the facilities can be compiled to identify appropriate members for medical staff appointments to such committees as operating room, perinatal, morbidity, etc.

4. Administration may use the index to identify needs for consultants in certain specialties and to note increases or decreases in individual physician's practices.

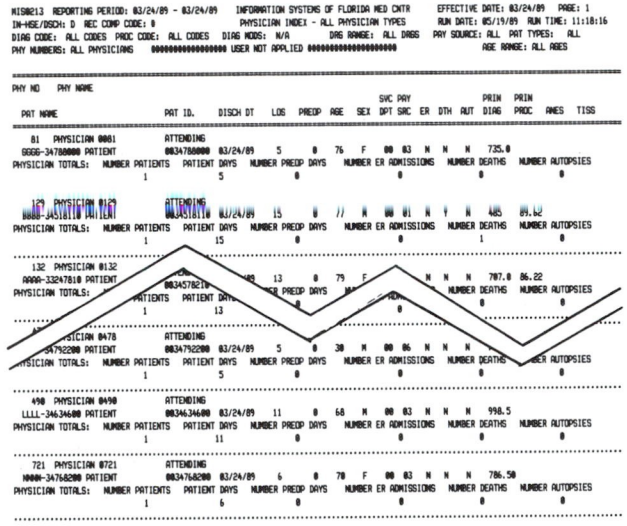

FIGURE 5. COMPUTER LISTING OF PHYSICIANS' CASES

A physicians' index is a confidential record. The information contained in it is available only to the governing board and chief executive officer, to committees of the medical staff directed to review the physicians' work, and to the physician who wishes to review personal work. The index may be subpoenaed by a court. It is sometimes used in malpractice cases or for income tax investigations.

Because of the confidential nature of this index, many facilities assign each physician a code number which appears on the card instead of the physician's name. In a computerized indexing system, a code number is essential to safeguard the confidential nature of the index. This code number should be different from code numbers assigned to the physician for other purposes, such as using the hospital's dictation system. Assigned code numbers should not be reused following resignation or death of a medical staff member. It is the responsibility of the health information professional to guard this index from unauthorized access.

Manual index cards are usually filed alphabetically by physicians' names in a visible or a vertical file or in numerical sequence according to the physician's code number. It is convenient to post to this index immediately after receipt of the discharged record.

Computerized indexes provide a variety of physician profiles. Printouts can be generated on demand or displayed on a terminal screen. Because of the confidential nature of this data, access to a computerized physicians' index is available only to those authorized to have such data by facility policy. A computer system is also beneficial as data may be abstracted once a patient has been discharged, and the computer used to manipulate that data to generate all necessary reports.

REGISTERS

Several registers which provide a chronological list of various data are maintained in a health care facility. These registers are developed and maintained in departments as a reference or control to basic information. Any department wishing to keep basic data to monitor their workload may maintain a register. Examples include radiology register, physical therapy register, implant register, trauma register, diabetes register, birth defect register, and emergency service register. A few of the more common registers are discussed here.

PATIENT ADMISSION AND DISCHARGE REGISTERS

Many states require that patient admission and discharge registers be kept within the facility. Automated systems generate these reports with ease. The admission register is arranged in chronological order by date and time of admission.

The discharge register may also be arranged in chronological order by date of discharge. Information recorded in a register should be kept to the useful minimum and be sufficient to meet legal requirements. It should include only items needed for quick reference. Items that might be included in admission and discharge registers are:

Admissions	Discharges
Medical record number	Medical record number
Admission type	(same as assigned at admission)
Admission	Patient's name
Patient's name	Date of discharge or death
Date of admission	Discharge status
Physician	Physician

An analysis of survey forms and questionnaires received routinely by the facility is helpful in determining essential data for inclusion in these registers.

These registers should be kept permanently as they are a chronological list of all admissions and discharges to and from the facility. In a manual indexing system, they serve as a back-up to the master patient index if a card is misfiled. At predetermined intervals the registers may be microfilmed. In many facilities copies of daily admission and discharge lists are retained and serve as the admission/discharge register. In most facilities, admission and discharge registers are computerized and accessed through a terminal or retained in the form of computer printouts.

OPERATING ROOM REGISTER

This register is kept in the operating room and should be preserved for ten years. Data included are the date of operation, patient's name and medical record number, and the names of surgeons and assistants. The register, which is frequently computerized, provides statistical data for case-load analysis and administrative reports. After ten years these registers are no longer needed, for any information regarding an individual may be found in the medical record.

REGISTER OF BIRTHS AND DEATHS

Some states do not provide a copy of the birth, fetal death, or death certificate for the medical record. Information from birth certificates may be copied into a register of births, and information from death certificates into a register of deaths. This practice provides readily accessible information without referring to a medical record. In many states the law requires these registers, and the health information director should investigate a specific state's requirements.

If the state requires fetal death certificates and a register of births is used, fetal deaths may be entered in red ink, in chronological order with the live births; or special pages may be set aside for fetal deaths in the back of the book. Whichever method is used, the procedure should be described in the front of the register, so everyone will know how fetal deaths are recorded.

EMERGENCY SERVICE

A register to monitor the patients who enter the emergency service must be maintained to provide data for administrative reports and to fulfill the standards of the Joint Commission on Accreditation of Healthcare Organizations.

The Joint Commission specifies that a control register shall be continuously maintained and shall include at least the following information for every individual seeking care: identification, such as name, age, and sex; date, time and means of arrival; nature of the complaint; disposition; and time of departure. The names of individuals dead on arrival are also entered in the register.

Information from the register may aid in planning emergency service staffing and can be used to select records for evaluating the appropriateness and quality of care rendered in the emergency service.

In a computerized system, emergency department records are abstracted and the information necessary for planning can be manipulated through flexible reporting. Detailed data can be abstracted to provide information for planning and studies of emergency care.

CANCER REGISTRY

A cancer registry is established for the collection and maintenance of comprehensive patient care data on all cancer patients. The two main objectives of a cancer registry are to provide lifetime follow-up of the cancer patient and to provide meaningful information to the physician for patient care evaluation and research.

Since 1913 the American College of Surgeons has recognized the need for improved care of cancer patients. In 1956, as part of its goal to provide cancer patients the best possible care available, the Commission on Cancer of the American College of Surgeons established requirements for the approval of a hospital cancer program. These include a functioning cancer registry, cancer committee, cancer conferences, and patient care evaluation studies.

TYPES

Basically there are three types of cancer registries: hospital-based, central registry, and special-purpose registry. A hospital-based registry operates exclusively for cancer patients treated at a particular health care facility. A central registry can either be population-based or the main registry for a group of hospital-based registries. The central registry collects data from its designated territory, thus accumulating enough information to study trends in cancer occurrence, treatments, and results. Special purpose registries collect data on one type of cancer such as leukemia, lung cancer, breast cancer, Hodgkin's disease, etc.

Regardless of the type of registry, the collection and analysis of data on all cancer patients to improve cancer management, now and in the future, remains the basic purpose of a cancer program.

FORMAT OF THE CANCER REGISTRY

Cancer registries collect data on all inpatients and outpatients seen at a facility regardless of where the patient was originally diagnosed. Case identification is a process to assure that all reportable cancer cases in the facility are accounted for. The health information department is the most likely department for case identification. The disease index is the source for case finding, as it is a complete list of patient discharges grouped according to diagnosis using the facility's classification system.

Another means to identify cancer cases is through the pathology, radiology, and outpatient departments, as these departments often perform tests and provide therapy to cancer patients. Procedures should be established for the registrar to routinely examine these departments' registers or to obtain copies of pertinent pathology reports.

A properly functioning cancer registry has four basic components to store and retrieve data in a timely manner.

Master Index File

The cancer registry master index file serves the same purpose as the hospital's master patient index. It is an alphabetical listing of all patients entered into the registry. The information usually includes the patient's name, sex, race, birth date, hospital number, accession number, diagnosis date(s), age at diagnosis, diagnosis (primary site and type), and date of death.

There are many computerized systems available for cancer registries. These systems provide for abstracting of cancer cases and in turn generate a master index file. If the file is manual, the data is recorded on a card for each patient.

Accession Register

The accession register is a loose leaf bound book, or computer printout containing a chronological list of all cancer cases. The cases are assigned a registry or accession number by year of accession. For example, the numbering system for cases accessed in 1990 would appear 90-001, 90-002, and so forth. Additional information includes: patient's name, hospital number, diagnosis - primary site, and date of diagnosis. The accession register is used to assess registry work load, monitor case identification, and audit the registry file for lost abstracts.

Case Files

Case files are the abstracts which have been prepared on "analytical cancer patients," which are those who were diagnosed and/or who received all or part of their first course of treatment at the reporting facility. Nonanalytical cases do not need to be abstracted; however, the cases should be accessioned and entered into the master patient index.

The data abstracted on analytical cancer patients must meet the minimum requirements set by the American College of Surgeons for cancer program approval. Information required includes: identifying information such as age, sex, race, place of residence; the medical history of the cancer to include primary site, date of initial diagnosis, histology, stage, etc.; procedures performed such as biopsies, x-rays and surgery, to include names, dates, and results; treatment used such as surgery, radiation, chemotherapy; and follow-up information as to subsequent treatment, and patient status.

In a manual cancer registry, it is best to file abstracts by primary site, alphabetically under year of accession. Because requests for information are usually for a specific site or cancer, this method of filing allows for timely retrieval of abstracts.

For patients with multiple primary sites, one abstract for each primary site diagnosed or treated at the facility is prepared and cross-referenced. The abstracts are updated with each readmission or annual exam.

Follow-up File

One of the major functions of the cancer registry is to assure that cancer patients receive regular and continued observation and management. Once a patient is abstracted, follow-up is continued for the lifetime of the patient. Each month the registrar refers to the follow-up file to determine which patients are to be checked that month. This file identifies cases due for follow-up and is sometimes called a "tickler" file. The file consists of two sets of guides with subdivisions for every month of the year. The first set of guides is used for filing the index cards of those patients due for follow-up in the current year. Once the patient has been successfully followed up, the card is filed behind the appropriate month for the following year. For example, after a patient is seen by the physician in August, 1993, the card will be filed behind the August, 1994 guide to remind the registrar that this patient is due for another follow-up examination at that time. This process continues for the lifetime of the patient.

A readmission constitutes a follow-up, so if a patient is due for follow-up in April, 1994, but is admitted to the facility in February, 1994, there is no need to generate a follow-up in April of the same year. Instead, the patient's card is filed behind the February guide for 1995.

Information contained on the follow-up card includes: patient name, address and phone number, medical record number and accession number, names and addresses of relatives or contacts, diagnosis, and follow-up dates. Patients having more than one primary site require only one card with each primary site and the date of diagnosis listed for cross-reference purposes.

The following sequence of events constitutes the follow-up procedure.

First, the health record is reviewed, because it will often provide information on any checkups. Next, the attending physician is sent a form letter requesting information on the health of the patient. The letter should be prepared so the physician only has to place a check next to the applicable statements. If the physician does not return the form, a second letter is routinely sent about a month later. If the physician has lost contact with the patient, the registrar generally obtains blanket consent from the cancer committee to contact the patient. Because of the sensitive nature of the disease, care must be taken in the method of approach to the patient. No reference to the patient's diagnosis should be made and the importance of a regular examination is to be stressed. Some registrars assist patients in making appointments with their attending physicians. In many cases, patient contact involves a great deal of time, determination, and detective work. If a patient cannot be contacted by telephone or letter, other alternatives may be to:

- send a certified letter requesting receipt, signed by addressee only;
- contact an employer; check the post office; and
- check the obituary columns in the newspaper.

A hospital cancer program must strive to maintain a successful follow-up rate of at least 90 percent to meet one of the ACS approval requirements, so the facility must persist in the search for missing cancer patients.

THE TUMOR REGISTRAR

The responsibility for maintaining the cancer registry is usually assigned to the tumor registrar. This may be an RRA or an ART, or it may be someone trained on the job with supplemental workshops from the American College of Surgeons. The National Cancer Registrars Association (NCRA) certifies tumor registrars (designated as CTR) who have successfully completed the certification examination offered by NCRA.

The registrar must have a complete knowledge of the disease process and understand the methods and procedures used to diagnose cancer. The registrar must be familiar with the organization and composition of the medical record and know where to find pertinent information regarding the cancer. An effective registrar must have the ability to interpret diagnostic reports and discern what is important to record on the abstract. The registrar also must possess statistical and analytical skills in order to provide meaningful reports.

IN-HOUSE COMPUTERIZED CANCER REGISTRY

With an on-line computer system, the four main components of a cancer registry can all be maintained on a computer. The same functions performed in a manual cancer registry apply to an automated one. There are differences, though, in the time required to perform these operations and the quality of the work produced.

After a case has been identified for entry into the cancer program, the patient's name is entered via the keyboard, and the computer quickly searches for that name. If the patient has previously been registered, the registrar will know that the patient's current status needs to be updated. If there are no data in the system for the patient, the patient is automatically assigned an accession number by the computer and added to the master index file as a new cancer patient.

The data are coded for topography and histology using the *International Classification of Diseases for Oncology* (ICD-O). Staging (the measurement of the extent to which a neoplasm has progressed) is coded using the staging guide for the Surveillance, Epidemiology, and End Results (SEER) programs of the National Cancer Institute. In addition to SEER staging, cases must also be staged by the TNM (Tumor, Node, and Metastasis) system of the American Joint Committee on Cancer.

Computerized abstracting assures consistency in case summarizing, because the registrar is forced to search the medical record to answer the queries posed by the computer.

During the entry process, data appears on the screen so the registrar may immediately check the accuracy of the data entered. In addition, the computer is programmed to accept only certain codes for each data item.

As close to discharge of the patient as possible, a case summary is printed in natural language (not coded) as specified by the American College of Surgeons. For the purpose of facilitating patient care management, copies are produced for insertion in the patient's medical record, and for the attending physician; a copy is also kept in the cancer registry.

The follow-up function of a manual cancer registry is normally a time-consuming process. In the automated process, the computer generates a monthly list of patients due for follow-up. Letters to be sent to physicians are automatically printed from the computer. The letters are designed for easy physician response and to facilitate input directly into the computer. Letters sent to patients or relatives may also be generated from the computer. Through the use of word processing these letters can be specially written to meet unique needs of individual patients.

REPORT GENERATION

A computerized cancer registry makes data readily available to enhance patient care management. The quality of data is very dependable and researchers enthusiastically request information.

The computer generates three kinds of basic reports: the case summaries, routine reports such as the accession register and master index file which are referred to daily, and nonroutine reports to respond to various requests for information. Routine reports can be printed overnight. Because every data item in computer storage can be accessed independently, reports can be generated by cancer site, histology, survival rate by cancer site, etc. Storage is arranged so every data item is a key variable and can be accessed as such. The ability to create ad hoc reports is a key element.

MULTIHOSPITAL CANCER REGISTRY

A multihospital cancer registry collects cancer patient data for several participating hospitals in a geographic area. The most immediate and gratifying advantage of this arrangement is the elimination of duplicate effort. Often patients initially diagnosed at one facility receive therapy and subsequent follow-up at another facility. In a multihospital on-line system, all data for one patient is stored under one number, accessible by all facilities that treat that patient. Any facility can add data to a patient file, thereby maintaining a current registry. Only the facility which first entered data on the patient is responsible for follow-up. To maintain confidentiality, the system does not allow a facility access to a patient's file unless the patient is listed as being treated by the inquiring facility.

In a multihospital cancer registry, the data collected by each participating facility are standardized. Therefore, comparison and epidemiological studies are easy to prepare.

DATA QUALITY

Controlling the quality of coding, indexing, and abstracting is the responsibility of the director of the health information department.

To ensure data quality in a medical information system, specific procedures and controls must be defined within each process in the medical record data flow. Errors may occur when medical record data are entered in the record (documentation), when data are retrieved from the record (abstracting), when data are manipulated (coding), when data are processed manually or electronically (indexing), and when medical record data are used (interpretation), These procedures and controls may be categorized as:

1. Specifying Standards - The basis for measuring conformance to characteristics of excellence; reliability, validity, timeliness, completeness, accessibility, confidentiality, and security.

2. Quality Control - Measures performance, comparing it with standards and acting on the difference.

3. Audit - Reviewing the quality of outputs from a data system and the adequacy of quality control procedures for these systems.

For example, procedures should be developed which regularly provide for the independent development of a medical record abstract followed by comparison and reconciliation with the original abstract to evaluate the reliability of data maintained in the health information department.

Reliability studies which ask the question, "Would the same abstractor make the same decisions or judgments twice?", and studies which ask the question, "Would two different informed abstractors make the same judgments when completing an abstract?", must be performed regularly. The results obtained from such studies must be compared to the department's established standards for coding/abstracting and corrective actions implemented as necessary.

In addition, audits should be performed to assess the accuracy and completeness of indexes and data systems.

SUMMARY

Indexes and registers are important sources of information commonly compiled by the health information department staff.

The amount and type of data to be stored for each patient stay depends on the needs of the individual facility and its licensure and accreditation requirements. Information requests must be monitored to determine what data needs to be maintained, as maintenance of indexes and registers can be costly in personnel time as well as in storage or computerization activities.

In most facilities, internal or external computer support is available to assist the staff of the health information department to maintain indexes and registers effectively and efficiently. The health information professional must keep informed about the services discharge data services can provide and also medical record applications which may be completed on personal computers in small facilities.

Because of the important role indexes and registers play in patient care management and research, facility planning, and reimbursement activities, data quality must be regularly assessed as part of the department's quality management program. Additionally, procedure manuals and employee performance must be assessed regularly to ensure that timely, accurate indexes and registers are maintained in a cost-effective manner.

STUDY QUESTIONS

1. List the reasons why the master patient index is considered the most important tool in the health care facility.
2. State the purpose of a number index, and disease and operation index.
3. Discuss the alternatives of using manual, external data service, or in-house computer systems for the abstracting and indexing function of the medical record service.

4. Describe the function of registers, and identify four types of registers which may be maintained.

5. Describe the purposes of a cancer registry, and explain how the data collected are utilized.

6. Discuss procedures and controls which may be used in a health information department to assure data quality, and explain how each control functions.

REFERENCES

American Joint Committee on Cancer, *Manual for Staging of Cancer,* 3rd Ed., (Philadelphia: J.B. Lippincott Co., 1988).

Bender, Alan p. and Geary W. Olsen, "A Survey of the American College of Surgeons Hospital Based Tumor Registries," *Journal of the American Medical Record Association,* (January, 1984): 20-23.

Clive, Rosemarie E. and James Brent, MD, "CanSur: Modern Data Management for Improved Cancer Patient Care," *American College of Surgeons,* Vol. 66, No. 9, (September, 1981).

Commission on Cancer - American College of Surgeons, *Cancer Program Manual,* (1986).

Commission on Cancer - American College of Surgeons, *Data Acquisition Manual,* (1988).

Finnegan, Rita, MA, RRA, *Data Quality and DRG's,* (American Medical Record Association, 1983).

Glass, Peggy J., RRA, "Computer Patient Index, a Tool for Linkage of Medical Information," *Medical Record News,* (April, 1975).

Hollinsworth, G., "A Medical Record Department Responds to Increased Institutional Needs for Patient-Related Data," *Topics in Health Record Management: Computers and the Medical Record Department,* Vol. 2, No. 2, (December, 1981).

Joint Commission on Accreditation of Healthcare Organizations, *Accreditation Manual for Hospitals,* (Chicago: Joint Commission, 1994).

Markham, Daniel, et al., "A Computerized Cancer Registry Data System at a Major Teaching Hospital," *The Eighth Annual Symposium on Computer Applications in Medical Care,* (November 4-7, 1984).

Murray, Charles, MD, FACP, and Jean Wallace, "The Development and Use of a Computerized Cancer Data System," *Topics in Health Record Management: Computers and the Medical Record Department,* Vol. 2, No. 2, (December, 1981).

O'Sullivan, Vincent J., "Computers and the Cancer Registry," *Journal of the American Medical Record Association,* (November, 1984): 33-37.

Parkin, D.M. et.al., "Cancer Registration Using A Microcomputer," *Medical Informatics 10,* (Oct.-Dec., 1985): 301-309.

Stachura, Cheryl Tabatabai, "Software Reference Guide: Master Patient Index," *Journal of the American Medical Record Association,* (September, 1986): 20 -24.

Stachura, Cheryl Tabatabai, "Software Reference Guide: Registries," *Journal of the American Medical Record Association,* (June, 1987): 47-49.

U.S. Department of Health, Education, and Welfare, *Self-Instructional Manual for Tumor Registrars,* (U.S. National Institutes of Health, 1975).

Waters, Kathleen A. and Gretchen Frederick Murphy, *Medical Records in Health Information,* (Aspen, 1979).

Williams, Sandra E. and Philip Latessa, "Improving the Quality of Discharge Data," *Topics in Health Record Management,* (June, 1982): 41- 48.

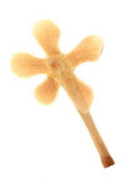

chapter **11**

HEALTH CARE STATISTICS

INTRODUCTION

Health information practitioners must realize how important the department's contribution is to those who use health care data. Medical records are the prime source of data used in compiling medical care statistics. Statistics about the professional work performed in the hospital or other health care facility are compiled and provided to users for a variety of reasons. These statistics, however, mean something only when the health information practitioner, the administration, and the medical staff have a mutual understanding about the definitions of terms used, how the data are collected, and how accurate the information is. Reports to agencies and organizations outside of the health care facility have meaning when everyone concerned understands the definitions and parameters of the data included.

Statistics are facts set down as figures. To serve their purposes, such figures must be relevant, and they must be reliable if anyone is to evaluate them accurately and use them for decision making. Preparing statistics involves the collection, analysis, interpretation, and presentation of facts as numbers. Because health information practitioners possess a broad range of knowledge about health care facilities, they are in the best position not only to collect and prepare the data, but to analyze and interpret the data. Health information practitioners need a broad knowledge of statistical methods and reasoning as well as an understanding of what computers can do with raw data. They must keep abreast of available technology for recording and retrieving data to supply more informative reports to the administration, medical staff, and outside agencies.

Statistics are only as accurate as the original documents from which they are obtained. The health information practitioner must decide whether or not the contents of medical records meet statistical needs. The practitioner must also be aware of other sources of data within the health care facility and be prepared to merge those data with data from the medical record. The kind and extent of data collected and the use made of the data vary from one health care institution to another. The administration and governing board use statistics to compare current operations with the past and as a guide in planning for the future. The medical staff uses statistics to appraise its own performance. Reports compiled for outside agencies and organizations on a local, state, and national level are used to list, accredit, license, and approve hospitals and other health care facilities and to disburse funds.

It is important to periodically review the data collected and the collection methods used. Why certain data are collected and reports compiled should be questioned. If health information practitioners do not routinely question their methods, the reasons for keeping data, and the way they present the data, they may be wasting valuable time preparing reports nobody reads. Keeping up with current reporting and data display needs will save unnecessary work and help modify collection techniques so information will be accurate and useful.

DATA SETS

To promote uniform collection and reporting of data, minimum data sets for various types of health care delivery have been developed. Health care statistics mean something only if they can be compared to statistics of previous years or for other facilities. When making a comparison, the reason for the observed difference must be explained. Meaningful comparisons can be made and differences explained only if the definitions of the items compared and counted are identical. The factors comprising a measure must be clearly stated before the data can be used to make meaningful decisions. Data compiled and compared in one health care facility cannot be compared to data compiled in another facility unless uniform definitions of the factors involved are used. The most widely used data set is the Uniform Hospital Discharge Data Set (UHDDS). There are also data sets for ambulatory and long term care patients which are discussed in Chapters 4 and 5, and many states also collect specific data from institutions.

Uniform Hospital Discharge Data Set

A Uniform Hospital Discharge Data Set (UHDDS) was promulgated by the Secretary of the U.S. Department of Health, Education, and Welfare in 1974 as a minimum common core of data on individual hospital discharges in the Medicare and Medicaid programs. In the past fifteen years, the UHDDS has achieved widespread use as a minimum, common core of data within the Department of Health and Human Services (DHHS) in programs which require data on individual hospital discharges on a continuing basis. The data set is also used within other federal agencies and has gained acceptance and use as a standard in the nonfederal public and private sectors, such as hospital discharge abstracting services.

The UHDDS was revised in 1984 and again in 1986 to improve the original version in the light of current needs and developments. The current data set consists of the following items:

Number 1	Personal Identification - The unique number assigned to each patient within a hospital that distinguishes the patient and his or her hospital record from all others in that institution.
Number 2	Date of Birth - Month, day, and year of birth.
Number 3	Sex - Male or female.
Number 4a	Race - White, Black, Asian or Pacific Islander, American Indian/Eskimo/Aleut, Other
Number 4b	Ethnicity - Spanish origin/Hispanic, Non-Spanish origin/Non-Hispanic.
Number 5	Residence - Zip Code, Code for foreign residence.
Number 6	Hospital Identification - A unique institutional number within a data collection system.

Number 7-8   Admission and Discharge Dates - Month, day, and year of both admission and discharge.

Number 9-10   Physician Identification-Each physician must have a unique identification number within the hospital. The attending physician and the operating physician (if applicable) are to be identified.

9. Attending Physician - The clinician who is primarily and largely responsible for the care of the patient from the beginning of the hospital episode.

10. Operating Physician - The clinician who performed the principal procedure.

Number 11   Diagnoses - All diagnoses that affect the current hospital stay.

a. Principal Diagnosis is designated and defined as: the condition established after study to be chiefly responsible for occasioning the admission of the patient to the hospital for care.

b. Other Diagnoses are designated and defined as: all conditions that coexist at the time of admission, that develop subsequently, or that affect the treatment received and/or the length of stay. Diagnoses that related to an earlier episode which have no bearing on the current hospital stay are to be excluded.

Number 12   Procedures and Date - All significant procedures are to reported.

a. A significant procedure is one that is:

(1) Surgical in nature, or
(2) Carries a procedural risk, or
(3) Carries an anesthetic risk, or
(4) Requires specialized training.

b. For significant procedures, the identity (by unique number within the hospital) of the person performing the procedure and the date must be reported.

c. When more than one procedure is reported, the principal procedure is to be designated. In determining which of several procedures is principal, the following criteria apply:

The principal procedure is one that was performed for definitive treatment rather than one performed for diagnostic or exploratory purposes, or was necessary to take care of a complication. If there appear to be two procedures that are principal, then the one most related to the principal diagnosis would be selected as the principal procedure.

Number 13   Disposition of Patient
Discharged to home (routine discharge).
Left against medical advice.
Discharged to another short term hospital.
Discharged to a long term care institution.
Died.
Other.

Number 14   Expected Payer for Most of This Bill - Single major source that the patient expects will pay for his or her bill.

Blue Cross.
Other insurance companies.
Medicare.
Medicaid.
Workers' Compensation.
Other government payers.
Self-pay.
No charge (free, charity, special research, or teaching).
Other.

DETERMINATION OF COLLECTION NEEDS

As has been noted, both the administration and medical staff of a health care facility use statistics, so their needs should be anticipated and discussed with them. The concern about health care costs has increased the demand for financial data as it relates to clinical data. Therefore, the health information practitioner needs to consult regularly with the members of administration who are responsible for financial affairs to make certain the merged financial-clinical data will be available for regular or special request use. The latter may include, for example, cost of disease entities or costs per physician, medical staff unit, or diagnosis related group.

Each year hundreds of outside agencies request information from hospitals on some periodic, formal basis. Data may be requested about the hospital's operations (utilization, personnel, and finances) or about patient care. Some of these agencies are: American Hospital Association, state hospital associations, state hospital licensure and planning agencies, Joint Commission on Accreditation of Healthcare Organizations, Blue Cross and Blue Shield, American Medical Association, health data consortiums, Peer Review Organizations, Internal Revenue Service, insurance companies in the accident and health field, Social Security Administration and their intermediaries, and local and state welfare departments. The health information practitioner should study the reports and instructions for completing the forms received from these agencies before setting up or revising a data collection system.

Most health care facilities must be state licensed. Licensure renewal requirements vary from state to state and by type of facility, but include the provision of data about facility services. Health information practitioners should be familiar with their own state requirements.

Accreditation from the Joint Commission on Accreditation of Healthcare Organizations is very important to hospitals and other health care facilities; without accreditation it is difficult to obtain federal funds for patient services, offer residency training programs, and conduct other types of endeavors. The Joint Commission is undertaking a major research and development project that is intended to improve its ability to evaluate health care organizations and stimulate greater attention to the quality of patient care.

The Joint Commission is developing clinical and organizational criteria or indicators that would mean an ongoing cycle of data transmission to the accrediting agency. The program, called the Indicator Monitoring System, is currently voluntary, but JCAHO plans to make it mandatory for accredited hospitals sometime in the future. When that happens, hospitals will report a great deal of clinical data to the JCAHO as part of the accreditation process.

The indicator monitoring system is not JCAHO's only involvement in hospital data. The organization's 1994 Accreditation Manual for Hospitals includes a chapter on information management. That chapter calls for data to be consistently defined across the hospital, to be available when needed, and to be standardized as much as possible. The 1994 standards also require hospitals to participate in one external database, such as the JCAHO's indicator monitoring system.

There are other state and national organizations which approve specific programs or accredit other health care facilities. For example, the Department of Health and Human Services conducts reviews to certify facilities under the Medicare Conditions of Participation, if the facility has not received Joint Commission accreditation. The American Osteopathic Association accredits osteopathic hospitals. The health information professional needs to determine the information needed for such accreditating or licensing agencies and make it available when it is requested.

The American Hospital Association conducts an annual survey of all hospitals for its *Guide to the Health Care Field*. The survey asks for data on organizational structure, facilities and services, beds and utilization by inpatient service, financial status, personnel, and medical staff. The health information department contributes much of the data for the survey, and should ensure that it is using appropriate definitions and supplying accurate data.

Many states have health care data collection agencies. Some of these are located in the state's department of health services and some are independent commissions. The purpose of the agencies is to monitor and compare health care services/charges to foster a competitive environment that contains health care costs. Most state-required data is being collected via the UB-92, which is the uniform bill adopted by the National Uniform Billing Committee. It is required for billing Medicare and many other third party payers. Although the data is collected via this billing office-generated form, the health information department supplies the clinical data that is placed on the form and must ensure its accuracy. The health information practitioner may also use data from reports generated by state agencies in comparative reports prepared for administration and the medical staff.

Hospitals having approved residencies are required to complete a form for the *Directory of Residency Training Programs* published by the Division of Medical Education, Department of Graduate Medical Education of the American Medical Association. The health information practitioner may be requested to furnish data to the directors of the residency programs within the hospital or complete the form for them, but the director of each approved program should verify the information submitted.

Questions the health information practitioner must ask to determine what data to collect include: (1) What reports are needed by administration and medical staff routinely? (2) What reports are required by outside agencies? (3) What ad hoc requests for data are made? Who makes these requests, what data are requested, and how are the data used? Can these data needs be anticipated and planned for in advance? (4) Are there data needs that are not met? Are there data that the health information practitioner can supply that would highlight opportunities or threats to the health care facility that may go unnoticed without such data? (5) Is the data being displayed in a format that is understandable and usable? When a questioning attitude about statistics is developed and maintained, needed information can be more readily supplied and unnecessary data collection can be avoided. A review of statistics and reports compiled should be conducted annually.

GLOSSARY OF HEALTH CARE TERMS

Because of the need for uniformity in definitions through the country, the *Glossary of Health Care Terms* was developed by the American Health Information Management Association after much research into statistical reporting and consultation with representatives from twenty-two health-related organizations. The terms in the *Glossary,* first published in 1969, were initially those common to short term hospitals and their patients. The most recent edition was published in 1994. It broadened the original glossary of hospital terms to a glossary of health care terms. Reference is now made to terms used in health care corporations, health maintenance organizations, and many other health-related programs and facilities.

The *Glossary of Health Care Terms* should be available to those preparing statistical reports. When a definition is given on a report form, that definition should be followed; when a term is not defined, the *Glossary* should be used to identify the appropriate definition for the term to ensure uniform reporting. When *Glossary* definitions are used, more of the statistics collected have meaning, are reliable, comparable, and serve a useful purpose.

GLOSSARY DEFINITIONS OF EVENTS

Traditionally, much more data has been collected on inpatients in hospitals than on other types of patients in other facilities. This is changing, however, as new forms of health care delivery emerge and as cost and quality of care in these environments are scrutinized. Standard definitions of terms that describe the types of health care events are important in order to distinguish among them. Definitions provided in the *Glossary of Health Care Terms* are:

Inpatient Hospitalization - "a period in a person's life during which he is an inpatient in a single hospital without interruption except by possible intervening leaves of absence."

Inpatient Admission - "the formal acceptance by a hospital of a patient who is to be provided with room, board, and continuous nursing service in an area of the hospital where patients generally stay at least overnight."

Inpatient Discharge - "the termination of a period of inpatient hospitalization through the formal release of the inpatient by the hospital." The term inpatient discharge includes the end of a hospitalization by order of the physician, against advice, or by death. Unless other specified, discharges include deaths.

Outpatient - "a patient who receives care without being admitted for inpatient or resident care."

Health information practitioners should familiarize themselves with definitions of other terms associated with inpatient hospitalization, hospital outpatients, and other patients which are provided in the *Glossary*.

DATA COLLECTION

After it has been determined what data are needed and how they are defined, much of this data must be abstracted in some organized form from medical records. Collecting data from hospital medical records is usually performed retrospectively upon discharge,- but may be begun concurrently during the inpatient stay. The necessary data items may be hand-posted on work sheets, entered on abstracts for batch input into a commercial or in-house data processing system, or entered directly into a computer database. Manual data collection procedures utilizing work sheets with columnar headings for services, results, and optional data with hand entries for each patient by case number have been replaced in all but a few small hospitals by discharge data abstracts or real time input of data into a computer. Regardless of methodology, a procedure should be developed for identifying the medical records from which data is to be collected and for accessing those records.

In a concurrent review system, personnel visit the nursing station to collect data from the records. Data may be collected within 24 hours of admission, two days after admission and every third day thereafter, or in some other pattern the hospital finds workable. An admission list and current census are required for identifying and locating patients' records. Upon discharge, very little additional data collection is necessary. In a retrospective review system all data collection is performed upon discharge of the patient. A procedure must be developed to receive all records of patients discharged from the hospital by the following morning. A list of patients discharged each day serves as a checklist for records received. The admitting department, patient accounts department, nursing service, or health information department may be responsible for preparing the admission lists, census reports, and discharge lists; or, more likely, computer printouts of admissions and discharges are-distributed daily from a data processing system.

INPATIENT DISCHARGE ANALYSIS

Whether data collection is initiated during concurrent chart analysis and completed at discharge or performed entirely upon discharge, the data collected is fairly standard across hospitals. The data collection process goes by several names.

Manual data collection is frequently performed using an "Analysis of Hospital Service" form, and thus the process of completing this form is called analysis of hospital service or daily discharge analysis. The primary purpose of the analysis of hospital service is to describe the professional activities of the existing organized medical staff units and/or specialty clinical educational (residencies) programs of the hospital. Every discharge is entered on a Daily Analysis of Hospital Service form and a cumulative tally kept of results, and number of patients per medical staff unit, their days of hospital care, infections, deaths, autopsies, and consultations.

Automated data collection has combined the cumulative analysis of medical staff unit activity with collection of patient demographics, payment source data, codes for the disease and operative index, physician index data, and other clinical data. Abstracting is the term used to describe collection of data on discharged patients for computer entry. A "case abstract" or "discharge data abstract" form may be used to record the data for each patient. Chapter 10, Indexes and Registers, describes the process of abstracting and the use of discharge data abstracts used by a commercial discharge data service.

MEDICAL SERVICES AND ORGANIZATIONAL UNITS

All forms of inpatient discharge analysis collect data on "service." From the *Glossary of Health Care Terms* it can be seen that the word "service" has been overused and has many meanings. Heretofore, "service" has had at least three meanings: It could be a "division or unit of medical staff responsibility," a "group of inpatient beds," or a "group of discharged patients with related diseases or treatments."

The *Glossary* suggests that the term "care unit" be used in place of service. A care unit is defined as "an organizational entity of a health care facility." Hospitals are organized both physically and functionally into units. The *Glossary* suggests that the term "inpatient care unit" be substituted and used to describe the various types of patient care facilities in which inpatient beds are located and related services performed. A *medical care unit* is defined as "an assemblage of inpatient beds (or newborn bassinets) and related facilities and assigned personnel in which medical services are provided to a defined and limited class of patients according to their particular medical care needs." A special care unit is defined as "a medical care unit in which there is appropriate equipment and a concentration of physicians, nurses, and others who have special skills and experience to provide optimal medical care for critically ill patients, or continuous care of patients in special diagnostic categories."

Inpatient care units do not always correspond to organized "medical staff units," defined as "one of the departments, divisions, or specialties into which the organized medical staff of a hospital is divided in order to fulfill medical staff responsibility." For example, a hospital may have obstetric, newborn, pediatric, intensive care, medical, and surgical care units. This same hospital may have organized medical staff units of medicine, surgery, otorhinolaryngology, obstetrics and gynecology, and pediatrics.

Classifying discharged patients with related diseases or treatments using a system other than a standard classification which has universal applicability (such as ICD-9-CM) is not recommended by the *Glossary*. Using a non-standard classification system does not promote consistency between/among hospitals.

Assigning Patients to Medical Staff Units

When data are kept according to existing organized medical staff units, a true analysis of hospital service is available. The number of medical staff units in a hospital will vary according to the size of the hospital, the number of physicians on the medical staff, the type of treatment rendered to patients, and the type of medical staff organization. The medical staff units (departments, divisions, or specialties) or specialty clinical education programs (residency training programs) into which the medical staff of a hospital are organized should be included in the bylaws, rules, and regulations of the medical staff. When designing a discharge abstracting system, "service" should refer only to those units into which the medical staff is formally organized. In a facility with a structured medical staff, physicians will only treat patients within the medical staff unit of their specialty, so accurate statistics can easily be gathered about the care given by the physicians in that unit.

There are some hospitals where the medical staff is formally organized, but physicians may be granted privileges to render care in more than one medical staff unit. Evaluation of physicians' activities within each unit is more difficult. For purposes of internal evaluation in these hospitals, discharged patients should be assigned to the most appropriate medical staff unit given the patients' principal diagnosis and operations. If a medical staff does not have a formally organized family practice unit, patients of family practitioners should be assigned to the medical or surgical unit based on whether they received only medical care or surgical care as well.

When a hospital's medical staff is not organized into units, data should be classified by the medical care provided according to the three basic units: medicine, surgery, and obstetrics. Also, for statistical purposes, a newborn unit is necessary. Infants newly born in the hospital should not be grouped in the three basic units. This is true even if the newborn infant receives care from an obstetrician rather than a pediatrician. Certain arbitrary decisions will be necessary to determine if a patient should be classified as receiving medical or surgical care.

It is recommended that the determining factor be whether or not a surgical operation was performed in the operating room. The one exception to the rule is obstetrical surgery, e.g., cesarean section. If the surgical operation is related to pregnancy or delivery, the patient should be counted as obstetrical, not surgical.

Transfers Between Care Units

In larger hospitals, care units (beds) will be restricted to the care of patients assigned to a specific medical staff unit or clinical education program. In either case, or both, the statistics for each medical staff unit or clinical education program must be preserved. The integrity of these statistics is achieved by having the medical record, census figures, and all reports indicate clearly whenever patients transfer from one medical care unit to another during their periods of hospitalization. This information can be included in the discharge analysis work sheets or computer printouts by adding two columns per medical staff unit. One column will show patients transferred off the unit; the other will indicate the days before transfer. By this means, credit is given for patient care to each medical staff unit rather than just the unit discharging the patient; and the number of days of care rendered the patient on each unit can be tabulated.

Division of Adults and Children

In some hospitals, divisions by adults and children under each medical staff unit may be required. Pediatric patients and child patients are, however, not synonymous. To avoid confusion, the term "pediatric patients" should be used for those children cared for by the organized medical staff unit of pediatrics. If patients are divided into adult and child categories, the upper age limit used should be specified. Hospitals in the United States have no standard dividing line between children and adults. Most often, patients 13 years of age and younger are considered children; but, almost as often, patients 14 years of age and younger are considered to be children. Whenever possible upon admission, the actual age of each patient should be recorded. If grouping of ages is necessary, the purpose for which the information will be used should determine the ranges of each group. The narrowest grouping of age should be used whenever possible.

Newborn and Obstetrical Patients

The following information concerning newborn and obstetrical patients will be helpful when tabulating patients who are cared for by physicians on these care units:

Hospital Inpatient Newborn (alive at birth) - This category includes only infants born in the hospital. Infants who are born elsewhere are not hospital newborn inpatients but are hospital inpatients other than newborn.

Obstetrics - Includes all patients having diseases and conditions of pregnancy, labor, and the puerperium, whether normal or pathological. Pregnancy commences with conception, and the puerperium ends six weeks after delivery. If desired, obstetrical patients may be subdivided into one of the following four categories:

> *Delivered in Hospital* - Includes mothers for whom the pregnancy has terminated in the hospital, regardless of whether the infant is liveborn or is a fetal death.

> *Admitted After Delivery* - Includes mothers for whom the pregnancy terminated before reaching the hospital, regardless of whether the infant is liveborn or a fetal death. Some

may classify these mothers as "Not Delivered." Patients in this category include women who have delivered outside the hospital and are brought in for the puerperium, those patients with retained placentas, postpartum hemorrhages, and other puerperal conditions immediately following delivery.

Aborted - Includes mothers for whom the pregnancy has terminated in less than the time specified by the health agency for a viable infant.

Not Delivered - Includes pregnant women admitted for a condition of pregnancy but not delivered of a liveborn or stillborn infant in the hospital. Patients so classified have conditions such as threatened abortions which have been prevented from terminating and false labors.

MONTHLY AND ANNUAL REPORTS

Inpatient discharge analysis results in the compilation of monthly and annual reports. Final tallies from the manual Daily Analysis of Hospital Service form may be transferred to an Analysis of Hospital Service form such as displayed in Figures 1 and 2.

Other sources of statistics for these reports may include monthly data from therapeutic and diagnostic departments (surgery, clinical and pathologic laboratories, x-ray, physical therapy, etc.) and the daily census to be explained later in this chapter. The monthly analysis report concerning professional care rendered to patients reflects only those medical staff units of the hospital included in the Daily Analysis of Hospital Service.

Monthly and annual reports generated by discharge data services provide the hospital with many and varied reports. An administrative summary is often produced. It may include patient demographics, hospital performance indicators (rates related to admissions, discharges, deaths, occupancy, length of stay), expected source of payment, and other pertinent data. See Figure 3 for an example. Additional reports may be generated on specific areas of interest, such as emergency admissions, medical record with incomplete diagnoses, medical staff utilization, tissue results, zip code summary, and so forth. Disease, operation, and physician indexes are also generated.

Hospitals which develop their own systems produce reports similar to those produced by commercial services. In designing their own systems, hospitals have a greater amount of flexibility in designing reports from the data collected. Because of this,

ANALYSIS OF HOSPITAL SERVICE Month of

CLASSIFICATION or SERVICE (List each patient once only)	Number of Patients	Hospital Days	CONSULTATIONS			Infections	DEATHS			AUTOPSIES	
			Total	Rendered	Recorded		Total	Post-oper.	Anesthetic	Total	Over 48 hrs.
Medicine											
Surgery											
Obstetrics											
Delivered in Hospital											
Admitted After Delivery											
Aborted											
Not Delivered											
Newborn											
Term, Born Alive											
Immature, Born Alive											
Gynecology											
Ophthalmology											
Otorhinolaryngology											
Urology											
Orthopedics											
Dermatology											
Pediatrics											
Neurology											
Neurosurgery											
Psychiatry											
Thoracic Surgery											
Total Discharges											

RECAPITULATION OF PATIENTS IN HOSPITAL		
Patients in hospital midnight last day previous month		
Patients admitted during month (exclude newborn)		
Newborn this month		
Total patients treated this month		
Patients discharged this month (exclude deaths)		
Deaths this month		
Total patients in hospital last day this month		

RESULTS (List each patient once only)	Number of Patients
Discharged Alive	
Deaths - under 48 hours	
over 48 hours	
Total Discharges and Deaths	
Late Fetal Deaths (stillbirths)	

DEATHS

(List additional deaths on a separate sheet)

FORM C-619 PHYSICIANS RECORD CO. BERWYN, ILLINOIS - PRINTED IN U.S.A. (OVER)

Form courtesy of Physicians' Record Company

FIGURE 1. MONTHLY ANALYSIS OF HOSPITAL SERVICE (front)

many hospitals produce relatively few reports on a regular basis. Instead, reports are generated in an ad hoc, or as needed, basis. In a hospital-designed system, data abstracted from medical records may be more readily merged with financial data to produce reports showing the impact of clinical practice on hospital costs.

COMPARATIVE REPORT OF PROFESSIONAL PERFORMANCE				
Month_____19_____	THIS MONTH	THIS MONTH LAST YEAR	THIS YEAR TO DATE	LAST YEAR TO DATE
TOTAL PATIENTS DISCHARGED (including deaths)				
Adults and Children.				
Newborn Infants.				
DAYS OF CARE TO PATIENTS DISCHARGED (including deaths)				
Adults and Children.				
Newborn Infants.				
AVERAGE LENGTH OF STAY (based on days of care to patients discharged, including deaths) .				
Adults and Children.				
Newborn Infants.				
TOTAL DEATHS.				
Deaths - under 48 hours.				
over 48 hours.				
Net Death Rate.				
Maternal Death Rate.				
Infant Death Rate.				
Postoperative Death Rate				
Late Fetal Deaths (stillbirths)				
TOTAL AUTOPSIES (on discharged patients, exclusive of stillbirths)				
Gross Autopsy Rate.				
Coroner's or Medical Examiner's Cases.				
Coroner's or Medical Examiner's Cases Autopsied at Hospital.				
Net Autopsy Rate.				
TOTAL PATIENTS ADMITTED.				
Adults and Children.				
Newborn Infants (born alive)				
DAILY CENSUS OF HOSPITAL PATIENTS.				
Maximum on Any One Day This Month (including newborn)				
Minimum on Any One Day This Month (including newborn)				
Total Patient Days Care to Patients in Hospital.				
Adults and Children.				
Newborn Infants.				
Average Daily Census.				
Adults and Children.				
Newborn Infants.				
Average Percentage of Occupancy.				
Adults and Children.				
Newborn Infants.				
OPERATIONS PERFORMED (total patients operated upon)				
Postoperative Infection Rate (on clean cases)				
Normal Tissue Removed.				
Total Cesarean Sections Performed				
Cesarean Section Rate.				
Total Primary Sterilizations.				
Total Therapeutic Abortions.				
				(C-619 BACK)

Form courtesy of Physicians' Record Company

FIGURE 2. COMPARATIVE REPORT OF PROFESSIONAL PERFORMANCE (back of Fig.1)

COMPUTATION OF PERCENTAGES

Reports generated from inpatient discharge analysis include information in the form of percentages, rates, and ratios.

Whether the health information practitioner calculates hospital percentages by hand or interprets computer output, it is important to understand how percentages are calculated in order to ensure their accuracy.

PAS Professional Activity Study

Executive Summary

1. CLASSIFICATION OF PATIENTS

A.

	PATIENTS	TOTAL DAYS	AVG. STAY
GRAND TOTAL	918	7738	8.4
TOTAL EX NEWBORN	777	7091	9.1
TOTAL EX NEWBORN OB	592	6304	10.6

B TOTAL ABSTRACTS (INCLUDES STILLBORN) 918

C STILLBORN — TOTAL. — AUTOPSIED

D RACE

	TOTAL	%
WHITE, NON-HISP.	905	99
BLACK, NON-HISP.	9	1
ASIAN/PACIFIC IS.	2	+
HISPANIC		
OTHER		
NO VALID ENTRY	2	+

E SEX

	TOTAL	%
MALE	340	37
FEMALE	578	63
NO VALID ENTRY		

F ADMISSION

	TOTAL	%
EMERGENCY	326	42
URGENT	77	10
THRU ER	294	34
FROM OTH. ACUTE FAC.		
FROM SNF		
READMIT	423	54

G DISPOSITION

	TOTAL	%
ALIVE	886	97
HOME/SELF CARE	848	96
AGAINST ADVICE	5	1
SHORT TERM HOSP.		
SNF	15	2
IOF	3	+
OTHER FACILITY	2	+
HOME HEALTH SVC.	13	2
EXPIRED	22	3
AUTOPSIED	9	28
CORONER'S CASE	1	3
EMERGENCY ADM.	29	91
EMER. DEPT. ADM.	28	88
WITHIN 2 DAYS	6	18

OPERATED — TOTAL 9 — RATE 2

IN OR — PREOP — NEONATAL — NO VALID ENTRY

H DEATH IN 48

2. EXPECTED SOURCE OF PAYMENT

PAYMENT TYPE	TOTAL PRINCIPAL	% PRINCIPAL	TOTAL SECONDARY
MEDICARE	153	17	3
MEDICAID	30	3	
TITLE V (M&CH)			
OTHER GOVT. PAY	10	1	1
WORKMEN'S COMP.	7		
BLUE CROSS	517	56	120
INSURANCE CO.	129	14	7
SELF PAY	8	1	
NO CHARGE	55	6	
OTHER	8	1	
NO VALID ENTRY	1	+	

3. HOSPITAL PERFORMANCE INDICATORS

A PERFORMANCE INDICES

	THIS REPORT PERIOD	LAST REPORT PERIOD	THIS PERIOD 1 YEAR AGO
RESOURCE NEED INDEX	1.05	1.25	1.00
LENGTH OF STAY INDEX	.95	1.15	.95
FATALITY INDEX			
PERINATAL MORTALITY INDEX			
NEONATAL MORTALITY INDEX			

B OPERATED PATIENTS

	PATIENTS
OPERATED	407
OPERATED WITHIN 6 HRS.	58
MORE THAN 1 EPISODE	156

C PATIENTS WITH CONSULTATIONS

NUMBER	300
PERCENT	37

D SPECIAL CARE UNITS

	PATIENTS	TOTAL DAYS
INTENSIVE	15	119
CARDIAC	12	41
SPECIAL	1	5

E PATIENTS W/O MIN. WORKUP

NUMBER	102
PERCENT	11

4. LENGTH OF STAY DATA

A STAYS UNDER 3 DAYS (EXCLUDES DEATHS)

NO. OF 1 OR 2 DAY STAYS — TOTAL NUMBER 36

NO. OF NOT OVER — NIGHT STAYS 7

STAYS OVER 30 DAYS (INCLUDES DEATHS) — TOTAL NUMBER 122

B DATA BY DATE OF THE WEEK (EXCLUDES NEWBORN, OB)

GEOMETRIC MEAN STAY BY DAY OF ADMISSION

	ALL. PTS.	MON.	TUES.	WED.	THU.	FRI.	SAT.	SUN.
	6.7	6.0	5.8	6.9	5.8	8.0	9.8	6.3

IS STAY SIGNIFICANTLY OFF FROM?

		MON.	TUES.	WED.	THU.	FRI.	SAT.	SUN.
% ADMITTED ON		12	12	14	17	12	13	20
% DISCHARGED ON		7	16	14	15	16	19	14
% OPERATED ON DAY OF OR DAY AFTER ADMISSION		80	89	77	78	89	26	78

‡ Figure exceeds space provided (For percents, + means between 0 and 0.5%.)
† For explanation, contact Medical Records of CPHA.

Copyright 1981 by COMMISSION ON PROFESSIONAL AND HOSPITAL ACTIVITIES, Ann Arbor, Michigan   Form No. 931 (7-86)   Printed in U.S.A.

ES

Reprinted with permission of the Commission on Professional and Hospital Activities

FIGURE 3. SAMPLE COMMERCIAL DISCHARGE DATA SERVICE REPORT

A percentage is computed on the basis of the whole divided into 100 parts. Because of this, a percentage based on too few items may be misleading. A percentage should not be calculated when the whole is less than 20. Some percentages, therefore, should be calculated annually rather than monthly. A percentage results when fractional parts are converted into units of 100. Any two-place decimal fraction (e.g., 0.54) is a part of 100, and it can be expressed as a percent (per 100) by moving the decimal point two places to the right and adding the percent sign (54%). Any percentage (e.g., 24%) may be expressed as a decimal fraction (0.24) by moving the decimal point two places to the left and dropping the percent sign.

A fraction such as 1/8 may be written as a percentage by dividing the numerator (1) by the denominator (8), multiplying the quotient (0.125) by 100 (12.5%) - which involves moving the decimal point two places to the right - and adding the percent sign.

To convert a one-place decimal fraction (0.2) to percent, a zero must be added when the decimal point is moved two places to the right and the percent sign is added (20%).

It is impossible to work all percentages out to whole numbers. Therefore, each hospital should establish its own policy as to the number of decimal places to be used in computing and reporting percentages. Regardless of the policy established, the division process should always be carried out to one more place in the quotient than is desired. The quotient is then rounded to the desired number of places by applying the following rule: drop the last figure if it is less than the number 5; add one unit to the preceding figure if the last figure is 5 or more

The term "ratio" is frequently used instead of percentage. A ratio expresses the quantitative relation of one thing to another, such as the relation of births to deaths or of deaths to discharges. A ratio may be written as a proportion (e.g., 2:5; read "two to five"), or as a fraction (e.g., 2/5). A ratio thus can be reduced to a decimal fraction and from a decimal fraction to a percentage. A ratio can be expressed as parts of 100 (percentage) and a percentage can be expressed as a ratio. A ratio of 2:5, or 2/5 is 40%. After a percentage has been determined, the result may be referred to as a rate.

There is one bit of common-sense reasoning that will help when computing a rate. A rate should be considered as the number of times something did happen compared to the number of times something could have happened. When expressing this ratio as a percentage, the number of times a thing happened is divided by the number of times it could have happened. In the formulas for computing various percentages which follow, the numerator is stated above a line which means "divided by." Beneath this line is the denominator.

Careful attention must be given percentages. Many mathematical errors occur because of misplaced decimal points. All calculations should be double-checked to be sure they make sense. For example, a death rate of 45% would seem unreasonable. Upon checking the decimal placement, one may find the rate should have been 4.5%, or even 0.45%.

Care must also be taken in comparing percentages. If a percentage of given totals is desired or if the ratio between the total of the numbers being compared is to be found, the percentage should be figured on the given totals. It is incorrect to add percentages.

Example:

Service	No. of Patients	No of Deaths	% Deaths
Medicine	42	2	5
Surgery	63	5	8
Obstetrics	25	0	0
Newborn	25	1	4
Total	$\overline{155}$	$\overline{8}$	$\overline{5}$

If the individual percentages of deaths in the above example had been added, the result would indicate the percentage of deaths was 17%. Actually, 8 deaths out of 155 cases is 5%.

COMMON HOSPITAL PERCENTAGES AND RATES

The percentages and rates commonly computed in hospitals are defined and exemplified below. In a hospital that performs inpatient discharge analysis manually, the health information practitioner may be responsible for calculating these percentages and rates. Where such percentages and rates are computer generated, the practitioner should review the figures to ensure their accuracy. Since the data abstracted from the medical records are the data used in these calculations, erroneous results may be due to erroneous entries. Ensuring quality data entry is critical to ensuring that the results are accurate. Common hospital percentages and rates may be calculated monthly, quarterly, or annually. The frequency of calculation requires judgment by the health information practitioner after consulting with the administration and medical staff, as well as careful review of external requests.

DEATH RATES (MORTALITY)

Death rates have always been important information for hospitals in evaluating the quality of their medical care and for public health agencies to plan for health services. Changes in the regulatory guidelines of the Freedom of Information Act in 1985, however, have increased the significance of death rate data. The guidelines of the Freedom of Information Act require Peer Review Organizations [PROs] (which contract with the Health Care Financing Administration [HCFA] of the federal government to oversee the quality of medical care provided Medicare patients) to make available to the public hospital-specific data concerning Medicare patients. PROs are thus providing the public with hospital-specific mortality rates from various DRGs, the number of patients who develop postoperative infections, the average length of hospital stays, and the cost and volume of various procedures. Release of such data is part of HCFA's strategy to enhance competition by providing physicians and consumers with more information to ensure that services provided Medicare recipients are not reduced without regard to the quality of care, and to provide data to the PROs to increase their oversight abilities.

When the first "HCFA Mortality Data" were released, much media attention was directed on them with confusion and misinterpretation. Since then, modifications have reduced such problems, yet the data still present a challenge to health care executives and health information practitioners in particular. The data currently being released each year include for each hospital the number of Medicare beneficiaries treated, the percentage of beneficiaries who die within 30 days of admission, and the expected percentages of deaths calculated on the basis of overall national experience with patients of similar age, sex, incidence of complicating diseases, and prior hospitalizations. Data are presented on deaths occurring for any cause and for major medical disciplines, distinguishing between high and low probability of death.

Hospitals should respond to the release of this data with a well-thought-out plan. First, the data, which is pre-released to hospitals, should be reviewed against the hospital's records. Corrections should be submitted before public release. Hospitals should also compare the data with the hospitals' own mortality data. Press releases and other forms of data dissemination should be developed to further explain the data. For example, hospital data should be analyzed to determine variables not considered by HCFA, such as terminal patients with "no code" and "do not resuscitate" requests, or other complications.

Health information practitioners must understand the basic death rates and be ready to calculate other data pertaining to mortality as may be necessitated by subsequent releases of data from HCFA.

Calculation of Death Rates

Various death rates may be computed: gross death rate, net death rate, anesthesia death rate, postoperative death rate, maternal death rate, neonatal death rate, etc. Deaths are included in discharges because, like discharges, deaths are terminations of inpatient hospitalizations. The hospital death rate is defined in the *Glossary of Health Care Terms* as "the proportion of inpatient hospitalizations that end in death, usually expressed as a percentage."

Patients who are dead on arrival (DOA) are not included in these rates. Patients who die in the emergency room where there has been no decision to provide them with room, board, or continuous nursing service in an area of the hospital where patients generally stay overnight are not included when figuring this rate. When a patient dies while receiving lifesaving services in any unit (e.g., operating room, recovery room) of the hospital other than the emergency unit, this patient is considered a hospital inpatient and, therefore, a hospital death. Fetal deaths are not included when figuring the death rate. Their number should be counted separately. If newborn inpatients are included in the numerator, all newborn inpatient discharges (including deaths) must be included in the denominator.

Death rates can be computed for deaths occurring both before and after 48 hours of admission and are sometimes requested in this manner by reporting agencies. However, as an indicator of hospital care, such distinction is not really useful. The health information practitioner needs to know what data agencies are requesting on their forms in order to decide which rates will be computed regularly.

Hospital Death Rate (Gross Death Rate) - This is the proportion of inpatient hospitalizations that end in death, usually expressed as a percentage. The percentage is computed as follows:

$$\frac{\text{Number of deaths of inpatients in a period x 100}}{\text{Number of discharges (including deaths) in the same period}}$$

Example: A hospital had a total of 21 deaths during May. These included inpatient deaths of all ages, those occurring under and over 48 hours, and coroner's or medical examiner's cases. A total of 650 patients were discharged (including deaths) during the month. To figure the hospital death rate according to the formula, 21 x 100 divided by 650 = 3.23%. Therefore, the gross percentage of deaths, or the hospital death rate, for May was 3.23%. Some hospitals would round this figure to the nearest tenth of one percent which would be 3.2%. Hospitals reporting percentages in whole numbers would report 3%.

From this basic death rate, many others may be calculated.

Postoperative Death Rate - This is often computed in hospitals as the ratio of deaths within ten days after surgery to the total number of operations performed during the period. Rather than compute this rate, some hospitals prefer to examine the relationship between deaths and surgical operations such as all deaths following cholecystectomies.

Death Rates Relating to Pregnancy - These provide the medical community with valuable information on reproductive health, as well as data on trends in the U.S. and around the world. Many of these rates are not calculated routinely by individual hospitals because such deaths occur infrequently. Rather, the raw data may be submitted to external agencies who calculate the rates nationwide, or by state, region, or locale. Hospitals may calculate these rates annually or only upon special request.

For definitions of reproductive health terms, the *Glossary of Health Care Terms* relies on the *Standard Terminology of Reproductive Health Statistics in the US and Guidelines for Perinatal Care*. The *Standard Terminology* was approved by the American College of Obstetricians and Gynecologists (ACOG) in 1985 and was developed to promote uniform collection and interpretation of reproductive health statistics. The *Guidelines for Perinatal Care* was published by ACOG in 1983.

AUTOPSY RATES

The autopsy rate is the ratio of autopsies to deaths. Some hospitals consider only autopsies performed on inpatient deaths when computing this rate. This excludes autopsies performed by a hospital pathologist or physician on the medical staff on bodies of persons who were inpatients, but were discharged and died elsewhere. An autopsy performed by a hospital pathologist or medical staff physician authorized to perform autopsies is valuable for education and research purposes.

In the *Glossary of Health Care Terms,* the following definition of hospital inpatient autopsy is given: "Postmortem examination performed in a hospital facility by a hospital pathologist or a physician of the medical staff to whom the responsibility has been delegated, on the body of a person who has at some time been a hospital patient." However, not all hospitals have facilities for autopsying patients, and instead contract with other hospitals, local funeral homes, or other places for postmortem examinations. The *Glossary* provides a second term with a slightly different definition for those hospitals: "Hospital autopsy: Postmortem examination performed by a hospital pathologist or a physician of the medical staff to whom the responsibility has been delegated, wherever performed, on the body of a person who has at some time been a hospital patient."

Gross Autopsy Rate - This is the ratio during any given period of time of all inpatient autopsies to all inpatient deaths. The formula for computing the percentage is:

Total inpatient autopsies for a given period x 100
Total inpatient deaths for the period

Net Autopsy Rate - This is the ratio during any given time period of all inpatient autopsies to all inpatient deaths minus unautopsied coroners' or medical examiners' cases. The formula for computing the net autopsy rate is:

Total inpatient autopsies for a given period x 100
Total inpatient deaths minus unautopsied coroners'
or medical examiners' case

Example: During August, 42 inpatient deaths occurred. Among these were four deaths that had to be reported to the medical examiner (coroner); two of these bodies were removed from the hospital, and no hospital autopsy was performed; hospital autopsies were performed on the other two cases. These were two of the 14 hospital autopsies performed following inpatient deaths during the month. The net hospital rate for the month was 35% computed as follows: 14 x 100 divided by 40 = 35%.

Hospital Autopsy Rate (Adjusted) - Another way of calculating the autopsy rate is the adjusted hospital autopsy rate. Because this rate compares total hospital patients whose bodies are available for hospital autopsy, it is a more accurate indication of the hospital's resources for physician education.

The formula for computing the percentage is as follows:

$$\frac{\text{Total hospital autopsies x 100}}{\text{Number of deaths of hospital patients whose bodies are available for hospital autopsy}}$$

The bodies of hospital patients included are: (1) Those of inpatients except the bodies of those removed by legal authorities such as coroners, medical examiners, anatomical boards, etc. If, however, the hospital pathologist or delegated medical staff physician acts as an agent for the coroner or medical examiner and performs an autopsy of any of these cases, the autopsy and death are included in computing the percentage. (2) Other hospital patients including ambulatory care patients, hospital home care patients, and former hospital patients who died elsewhere, but whose bodies have been made available for the performance of hospital autopsies by the hospital pathologist or delegated medical staff physician. The number of these autopsies and deaths will be included when computing the percentage.

Other than hospital inpatients who die, it is impossible to determine the number of former hospital patients who die in any given period. "Available for hospital autopsy" in the formula implies that at least the following conditions prevail: (1) the autopsy is performed by the hospital pathologist or delegated medical staff physician on the body of a patient who was treated by the hospital at some time, (2) the report of autopsy will be filed in the patient's medical record and in the hospital laboratory or pathology department, and (3) the tissue specimens will be filed in the hospital laboratory.

Example: During September 25 inpatient deaths occurred. Among these were 3 deaths that had to be reported to the coroner; 2 of these bodies were removed from the hospital so no hospital autopsy was performed; 1 hospital autopsy was performed on the other case. This was 1 of the 15 hospital autopsies performed following inpatient deaths during the month. In addition to the 15 autopsies performed on inpatient deaths, hospital autopsies were performed on the following cases:

1. A child known to have congenital heart disease who died in the emergency room four hours after being brought in, and the parents authorized performance of a hospital autopsy.

2. A former inpatient who died in an extended care facility two months following discharge from the hospital, and the body was brought to the hospital for autopsy.

3. A former hospital patient who was discharged three months previously with an undetermined progressive illness who died at home, and the body was brought back to the hospital for an autopsy.

4. A patient who had been receiving radiation therapy treatment for three years died of an apparent myocardial infarction on the x-ray therapy table, and a hospital autopsy was performed on his body.

5. A hospital home care patient died at home, and the body was brought to the hospital for an autopsy.

6. A patient who had eight inpatient hospitalizations during the past four years died in an ambulance on the way back to the hospital. A hospital autopsy was performed on the body.

Therefore, these 6 deaths are added to the 25 available inpatient deaths and the 6 additional hospital autopsies are counted. The adjusted hospital autopsy rate, which truly gives an accurate picture of the service rendered by the hospital pathologist for teaching and scientific purposes, is computed as follows: 21 x 100 divided by 29 = 72.41%. The hospital autopsy rate (adjusted) for the month of September is 72.41 or 72%.

Deaths and autopsies performed on newborn patients are included when figuring the autopsy percentage, unless it is requested that they be excluded and figured separately. Also, the health information practitioner may be requested to keep figures on autopsies performed on patients who expire 48 hours or over after admission, postoperative deaths, maternal deaths, anesthesia deaths, and coroner's or medical examiner's cases which were autopsied in the hospital.

When specific autopsy (or other) percentages are not required by an outside agency or organization each hospital should establish criteria suitable for achieving its highest standard of patient care.

MORBIDITY RATES (INFECTION)

Although morbidity rates calculated in hospitals have generally implied infection rates, other forms of morbidity (disease) may be singled out for special study.

Prevalence and Incidence Rates

Epidemiology was born in relation to the study of the great epidemics of the world such as those of cholera, plague, typhus, and so forth. Epidemics are unusually frequent occurrences of a disease. Methods developed to study epidemics are applicable to the study of all important diseases such as AIDS, heart disease, influenza and other major respiratory infections, cancer, diabetes, arthritis, and so forth. In studying the impact on society of chronic diseases, two aspects of disease occurrence are most often considered: prevalence and incidence. Prevalence is the ratio of known cases of a chronic disease at a given point in time to the population at that time. It describes the magnitude of the chronic disease problem and is a useful indicator of needs for medical and social care to cope with current cases. Incidence is the ratio of newly reported cases in a defined period, such as a year, to the population at midperiod. Incidence measures the rate at which new cases are occurring in the population and is an indicator of the need for preventive measures. It may be used to describe both acute and chronic diseases.

As the guidelines of the Freedom of Information Act of 1985 are utilized more by the Health Care Financing Administration (HCFA), release of morbidity data as measures of "quality of care" may occur in the future. Complication rates, comorbidity rates, accident rates, and other forms of morbidity may be calculated in an attempt to describe the quality of care provided by a hospital.

Infection or Morbidity Rate

Hospitals currently equate morbidity rate with infection rate. Hospital bylaws should require that there be a hospital-wide committee charged with the responsibility to investigate,

control, and prevent infections. The primary purpose of evaluating infections is to determine the cause so repetition may be avoided. Medical judgment is needed to establish the incidence of infections and the proper control measures to be taken. The health information practitioner may be asked to pull records of patients suspected of having had a hospital infection or call to the committee's attention specific cases according to criteria set forth by the committee. However, the health information practitioner should not make the determination as to whether or not a hospital infection occurred. Only a physician can make the determination that an obstetrical infection, for instance, was not chargeable to the hospital or to the obstetrical unit, because it was due to recurrence of a previous urinary tract infection; or that a suppurating wound on a surgical case was chargeable to the surgery unit.

The hospital committee charged with infection control should establish procedures for the surveillance and reporting of infections.

Hospital Infection Rate - If this rate is desired by the medical staff, health information personnel should compute and report it on a regular basis. An infection rate for the entire hospital may be desired, and/or infection rates for specific medical care units where infections were reported may be requested. Infection rates may be calculated for specific types of infections; for example, a urinary tract infection rate may be calculated. In computing any of these rates, remember a rate is the number of times a thing (in this case infection) happens (in the hospital as a whole or on a specific medical care unit) compared to the number of times it could have happened (discharges including deaths for the hospital as a whole or from a specific medical care unit).

Postoperative Infection Rate - This rate represents the ratio of all infections in clean surgical cases to the number of surgical operations. Not all hospitals use this rate on a regular basis; therefore, the health information practitioner must make a decision based on need in a particular hospital. The medical staff can give guidance to what constitutes clean surgical cases.

The *Glossary of Health Care Terms* gives a definition of a surgical procedure and of a surgical operation. A surgical procedure is defined as "any single separate systematic process upon or within the body which can be complete in itself, normally performed by a physician, dentist, or other licensed practitioner, either with or without instruments, to restore disunited or deficient parts, to remove diseased or injured tissues, to extract foreign matter, to assist in obstetrical delivery, or to aid in diagnosis." A surgical operation is defined as "one or more surgical procedures performed at one time for one patient via a common approach or for a common purpose."

A formula which may be used for computing the postoperative infection rate is:

$$\frac{\text{Number of infections in clean surgical cases for a period x 100}}{\text{Number of surgical operations for the period}}$$

Example: During the month of May, 626 operations were performed. The infection committee reported 1 postoperative infection in a clean surgical case for the month. According to the formula, this is 1 x 100 divided by 626 = 0.159%. Therefore, the postoperative infection rate for May was 0.16% or 0.2%

LENGTH OF STAY CALCULATIONS

Length of stay for one inpatient refers to the number of calendar days from admission to discharge. Length of stay data is extremely important for evaluating and managing the utilization of hospital resources.

Length of Stay (for one inpatient) - To compute a patient's length of stay, the date of admission is subtracted from the date of discharge when the patient is admitted and discharged in the same month, with appropriate adjustments when hospitalization extends over one or more month endings. For example, Joe Jones was admitted June 27 and discharged June 30. His length of stay is 3 days. If he was admitted and discharged the same day, his length of stay is one day because a partial day's stay is never reported as a fraction of a day. If he was admitted June 27 and discharged July 3, his length of stay is 6 days.

Total Length of Stay (for all inpatients) - or **discharge days**, is the sum of the days' stay of any group of inpatients discharged during a specific period of time. This total has also been termed "days of care rendered to patients discharged or died." Total discharge days are necessary to compute the average length of stay. The total inpatient service or census days (days' of care rendered to patients in the institution) are not to be used when computing this average.

Average Length of Stay (Average Stay) - This figure reflects the average hospitalization stay of inpatients discharged during the period under consideration. The average length of stay for newborn inpatients is reported separately.

The formula for computing the average length of stay is:

$$\frac{\text{Total length of stay (discharge days)}}{\text{Total discharges}}$$

Example: A hospital discharged 1,251 patients (including deaths; excluding newborns) during April. Their combined length of stay was 6,792 days. According to the formula, divide 6,792 by 1,251 which equals 5.4. The average length of stay of the patients discharged from this hospital during April, therefore, could be rounded off at 5 days.

INPATIENT CENSUS AND RATES COMPUTED FROM IT

TERMS AND DEFINITIONS

Whether or not the health information practitioner is responsible for compiling the census of the hospital the principles involved should be understood. The best starting point is to define the terms used. The terms below and their definitions are from the *Glossary of Health Care Terms*.

Census - the number of inpatients/residents present at any one time.

Daily Census - the number of inpatients/residents present at the census-taking time each day, plus any inpatients/residents who were both admitted and discharged after the census-taking time the previous day.

Inpatient/Resident Service Day - a unit of measure denoting the services received by one inpatient/resident in one 24-hour period.

Total Inpatient/Resident Service Days - the sum of all inpatient/resident service days for each of the days in the period under consideration.

Average Daily Inpatient/Resident Census (average daily census, average census, average daily number of inpatients) - average number of inpatients/residents present each day for a given period of time.

The census may be compiled by the admitting/registration department, nursing service, patient accounts or health information department; and it may be collected manually or by computer. When it is done manually, nursing service personnel usually compile the census for each floor or each inpatient care unit of the hospital at a specified census-taking time, usually midnight. It may be taken at any convenient time, but it must be taken at the same hour each day. A census report from each nursing unit is sent to the department responsible for combining them into a complete master census. If the census is done by computer, the necessary data (admissions, discharges, and transfers) are entered into the computer as they occur.

The newborn infant census is reported separately. The newborn nursery census is the number of newborn inpatients occupying hospital newborn bassinets. Hospital newborn bassinets include bassinets, incubators, and isolettes in a newborn nursery and/or a newborn intensive care unit.

CALCULATION OF INPATIENT CENSUS AND INPATIENT SERVICE DAY

Inpatient Census - This is the number of patients remaining in the hospital at the census-taking time for a specific day, plus the admissions for the next day, equal the patients remaining at the next census-taking time.

Inpatient Service Day - This measures the services received by one inpatient in one 24-hour period. The "24-hour period" is the time between the census-taking hours on two successive days. When the census-taking time is midnight, the 24-hour period will be 12:01 A.M. through 12:00 P.M., which is the same as the calendar day. One inpatient day must be counted for each inpatient admitted and discharged the same day - between two successive census-taking hours. If this is not done, credit for the medical services rendered to these patients will be lost. The days a patient does not occupy a bed due to leave of absence are excluded because the patient isn't present at the census taking hour. An absence of less than one day is not considered a leave of absence in compiling statistics. The unit of one inpatient service day should never be reported as a fraction of one day.

Computing the Census for Adults and Children

Example: The census-taking time is midnight.

	Number of patients in the hospital at midnight April 29	455
Plus	Number of patients admitted April 30	+ 21
		476
Minus	Patients discharged (including deaths) April 30	- 18
	Patients in hospital at 12 P.M(Midnight) April 30	458
	INPATIENT CENSUS	
Plus	Patients both admitted and discharged (including deaths) on April 30	+ 3
	INPATIENT SERVICE DAYS, April 30	461

These three patients do not show on the midnight census because they were added when they were admitted and subtracted when they were discharged, both of which occurred between census-taking times. Each, however, received one inpatient service day (one patient day's care). To account for the services rendered these patients, 3 inpatient service days must be added to 458, the midnight census of adults and children for April 30. The total inpatient service days for adult and child patients on April 30 is, therefore, 461.

In this example, the inpatient census was compiled for adults and children only. The newborn infant census must also be figured. If 80 newborn inpatients remained at midnight on April 29 and 9 newborn infants were admitted and 4 discharged on April 30, the midnight newborn census on April 30 is 85. No newborn inpatients were both admitted and discharged (including deaths) April 30. Therefore, the newborn inpatient service days and the inpatient census are both 85.

Computing Medical Care Unit Census and Service Days

If hospital administration or medical staff desires to study the inpatient census and/or inpatient service days on any specific medical care unit, e.g., intensive care unit, the census for that unit can be separated for purposes of the study or for any valid reason just as the newborns are separated from adults.

The census for a medical care unit shows transfers on and off the unit as subdivisions of patients admitted to and discharged from the unit. An intrahospitalization transfer is defined in the *Glossary of Health Care Terms* as "a change in medical care unit, medical staff unit, or responsible physician, of an inpatient during hospitalization." The transfers are added to the information kept routinely. Much more information, e.g., sex and age group, may be added to the analysis of patients in a medical care unit if this is desired; but there should be a definite purpose for collecting this additional data to justify the time spent making the tabulation.

Example: An intensive care unit has 10 beds:

	Patients remaining midnight April 29	8
Plus	Patients admitted April 30	+ 1
Plus	Patients transferred to unit from another unit (intrahospital transfer)	+ 1
Minus	Patients discharged	- 0
Minus	Patients died	2
Minus	Patients transferred off unit to another unit	- 1
	MIDNIGHT INPATIENT CENSUS, April 30	7
Plus	Patients both admitted and discharged on April 30	+ 1
	ICU PATIENT SERVICE DAYS, April 30	8

Average Daily Inpatient Census (Average Daily Census) - Records the average number of inpatients present each day for a given period of time. To arrive at the average number of inpatients in the hospital, the total inpatient service days for the period are determined first. Every inpatient receives one inpatient service day each day hospitalized. A hospital renders as many inpatient service days on any one day as there are patients remaining in the hospital at midnight that day plus one inpatient service day for each patient both admitted and discharged the same day. The formula to obtain the average daily inpatient census for a hospital is:

$$\frac{\text{Total inpatient service days for a period}}{\text{Total number of days in the period}}$$

The average daily newborn inpatient census (average daily census) for newborn inpatients is generally reported separately. The following formula is used to determine the average daily inpatient census excluding newborn:

Total inpatient service days for a period (excluding newborn)
_____
Total number of days in the period

Example: A hospital rendered 3,650 inpatient service days to adults and children during April (the sum of adult and child inpatient service days for each day of April). April has 30 days. According to the formula, this 3,650 divided by 30 = 121.7. Therefore, the average daily inpatient census during April was 122 adult and child patients.

To determine the average daily newborn inpatient census the total newborn inpatient service days for a period is divided by total number of days in the period.

To determine the average daily inpatient census for a specific medical care unit the total inpatient service days for the medical care unit is divided by total number of days in the period.

Inpatient Bed Occupancy Rate (Percent of Occupancy) - This is the proportion of inpatient beds occupied. It is defined as the ratio of inpatient service days to inpatient bed-count days in a period under consideration. It is generally expressed as a percentage. The following terms and definitions taken from the *Glossary of Health Care Terms* will be helpful in this discussion:

Bed Count (bed complement) - the number of available facility inpatient/resident beds, both occupied and vacant, on a given day.

Bed Count Day - a unit of measure denoting the presence of one inpatient/resident bed (either occupied or vacant) set up and staffed for use in one 24-hour period.

Bed Count Days (Total) - the sum of inpatient/resident bed count days for each of the days in the period under consideration.

The inpatient beds counted are only those which are set up, staffed, and ready for patients. Beds in examining, therapy, labor, and recovery rooms, which are usually used by patients who have other beds, are not included in the count. Beds set up for temporary use (cots, beds in hall, beds on sun porch, etc.) are not included in the inpatient bed count.

The inpatient bed occupancy rate can be computed at any specified point in time or from any specified day. To compute the percentage for a specified day, the inpatient service days for that day are multiplied by 100 and divided by the inpatient bed count for that day. To obtain the inpatient bed occupancy rate as a daily average in a longer period, the formula is:

$$\frac{\text{Total inpatient service days for a period x 100}}{\text{Total inpatient bed count days in the period}}$$

The total inpatient bed count days in the period, simply stated, is the number of beds times the number of days in the period.

Example: A hospital has an inpatient bed count (bed complement) of 150. During April, the hospital rendered 3,650 inpatient service days to adults and children. April has 30 days. According to the formula, this is (3,650 x 100) divided by (150 x 30) or 365,000 divided by 4,500 = 81.11% Therefore, the inpatient bed occupancy rate for April was 81.1% or 81%.

Many times a hospital will not have the same bed complement for the entire period in which the bed occupancy rate must be calculated. To perform this calculation the inpatient bed count days must reflect the variation in bed complement.

Example: A hospital began the month of January with 200 beds. On the tenth, 5 beds were closed for remodeling. These beds were reopened with 5 additional beds on the twenty-fifth. The total inpatient service days was 5,950. To calculate the bed occupancy rate, 5,950 is divided by ([200 x 9] + [195 x 15] + [205 x 7]). The result is 5,950 divided by 6,160 = 96.6%, or 97%.

Bed Turnover Rate - This is another measure of hospital utilization. The bed turnover rate demonstrates the net effect of changes in occupancy rate and length of stay. There is no universal agreement on the most accurate formula, but the following two formulas yield basically the same results:

Direct formula:

$$\frac{\text{Number of discharges (including deaths) for a period}}{\text{Average bed count during the period}}$$

Indirect formula:

$$\frac{\text{Occupancy rate x Number of days in period}}{\text{Average length of stay}}$$

Example: A 200 bed hospital discharged 6,500 patients during the year. The average length of stay for these patients was 9 days and the bed occupancy rate was 80%. Using the direct formula, the bed turnover rate is computed as 6,500 divided by 200 = 32.5. Using the indirect formula, (.80 x 365) divided by 9

= 32.4. Thus during the year, each of the hospital's 200 beds changed occupants about thirty-two and a half times.

It is generally accepted practice to exclude newborn inpatients when figuring the average daily inpatient census (average daily census), the average length of stay, the inpatient bed occupancy rate (percentage of occupancy), and the bed turnover rate. When this procedure is followed, the newborn infant census, newborn average length of stay, and newborn inpatient bed occupancy rate, and bassinet turnover rate are computed separately to obtain a complete picture of the work of the hospital.

MEASURES OF CENTRAL TENDENCY AND VARIATION

When performing statistical analysis, an important step in some instances is to determine the one value from a group of related figures that best characterizes the entire group. This value is called the measure of central tendency. There are three measures of central tendency: the mean, median, and mode. Measures of variation or dispersion are also commonly used to describe the spread of data around its center. The health information practitioner should be familiar with the computation of these measures in order to use them in data collection and reporting systems.

MEASURES OF CENTRAL TENDENCY

Mean - The mean is the arithmetic average of values in a set and this chapter has already dealt with such mean values as the average length of stay and the average daily inpatient census. To obtain the mean, one sums all the available values and divides this sum by the number of values involved.

Median - The median is defined as the midpoint (center) of the distribution of values. It is the point above and below which 50% of the values lie. This measure is used to avoid one extreme value presenting a misleading picture. For example, if one patient in a group stays considerably longer than the others, a median length of stay would better reflect the center of the data than the mean.

Mode - The mode is defined as the most recurring or most frequent value in a set of scores.

Example: Suppose the following distribution of lengths of stay exists: 5, 1, 2, 3, 4, 5, 3, 1, 2, 1, 5, 1, 18, 8, 1. The total of these stays is 60. Dividing 60 by the number of patients, 15, the average length of stay, or mean, is 4 days.

Rearranging these values in descending order in one column and their frequency of occurrence in another column, one can readily visualize the median and mode.

STAY	FREQUENCY OF OCCURRENCE
18	1
8	1
5	3
4	1
3	2 – midpoint here so median is 3
2	2
1	5 – the most frequently recurring stay so mode is 1

Because most of the patients were short stay, a median of three is more reflective of the hospital length of stay than is the mean of four.

MEASURES OF VARIATION

Range - The range of a set of values is the difference between the largest and smallest values in the set. Sometimes the range is given by simply quoting the smallest and largest values. The range for the data in the preceding example may be expressed as 17 (the difference) or as 1 to 18.

The range is useful as a "rough" measure of variability. Because only two values are used in the calculation of range, however, it may give a misleading impression of the true variability of the data. More stable measures of the spread among the values in a set are the variance and standard deviation. The deviations of the individual numbers from the mean give an indication of how spread out the values are within the set. The larger the deviations, the more dispersed the values are from their center.

Variance - For a set of values, the variance is defined as the sum of squared deviations of individual values from the mean divided by the sample size reduced by one. The variance is denoted by the symbol s^2 The formula for variance is:

$$s^2 = \sum \frac{(x_i - \bar{x})^2}{n-1}$$

Example: For the length of stay example in the preceding section, the variance is computed as follows:

Patient (i)	Length of Stay (x)	$(x_i - \bar{x})$	$(x_i - \bar{x})^2$
1	5	1	1
2	1	- 3	9
3	2	- 2	4
4	3	- 1	1
5	4	0	0
6	5	1	1
7	3	- 1	1
8	1	- 3	9
9	2	- 2	4
10	1	- 3	9
11	5	1	1
12	1	- 3	9
13	18	14	196
14	8	4	16
15	1	- 3	9
$\sum$ n	60	0	270

$$s^2 = \frac{270}{15-1} = 19.29$$

Standard Deviation (S.D., or s) - This is used more frequently than the variance to express the variability of values in a set. It is derived from the variance, for the standard deviation is the square root of the variance. One standard deviation in both directions from the mean contains 68.26% of all values. Two standard deviations in both directions from the mean contains 95.44% of all values. Three standard deviations in both directions from the mean contains 99.74% of all observations. When the standard deviation is small, the data are close to the mean. The larger the standard deviation, the more spread out the values.

Example: In the preceding example, the variance was found to be 19.29. The standard deviation is the square root of 19.29, which is 4.4. This means that +1 standard deviation from the mean contains the values from 4.0 through 8.4. The values 8.4 through 12.8 are +2 standard deviations from the mean. The values 12.8 through 17.2 are +3 standard deviations from the mean. The values -0.4 through 4.0 are -1 standard deviation from the mean. Because the data in the example contains one value much greater than the rest (the one length of stay of 18 days), the standard deviation is fairly large, reflecting this spread. In addition to describing the variability in the data set, the standard deviation is also used to determine which if any, of the scores are so different from the others (i.e., those more than 3 standard deviations from the mean) that they should be discarded in presenting data. Figure 4 displays how the standard deviation is interpreted in graphic form.

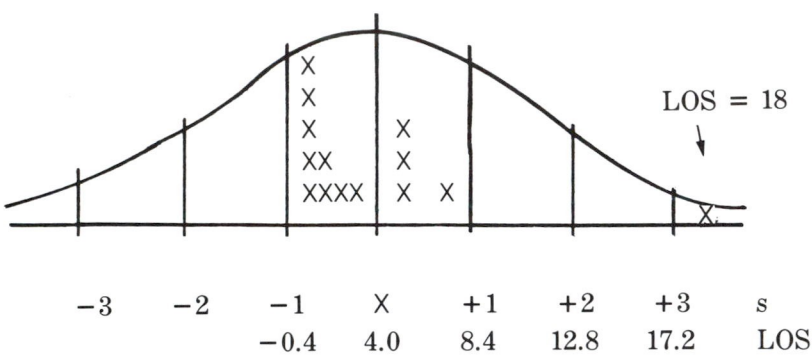

FIGURE 4. GRAPH OF STANDARD DEVIATION

PRESENTATION OF DATA

Statistical data should be presented in a manner which catches the reader's eye, entices interest, and makes the data easy to interpret and use. Presentation of data extends from simple tables to elaborate graphs.

In presenting data in any form, it is important to be very conscious of the users of the reports, their degree of sophistication in reading and interpreting data, and whether or not their interest needs to be stimulated by graphs or other pictorial presentations.

TABLES

Presenting data in the form of tables of figures needs little explanation. Tables are columns of figures, each labeled to identify its contents. The table should be titled, dated, and source identified. However, there are some rules governing frequency distribution tables in which there are ranges rather than simple numbers to enter in each column.

Frequency Distribution Tables

Grouping data into a number of classes with the corresponding number in each class constitutes a frequency distribution table. See Figure 5.

Age Distribution for Inpatients Excluding Newborn
DECEMBER, 19___

Ages	Number of Inpatients
Under 16	98
16-34	34
35-49	107
50-64	238
65 and over	393
Total	870

prepared by: Health Information Department from inpatient discharge analysis.

FIGURE 5. FREQUENCY DISTRIBUTION TABLE

The following are some basic rules for choosing the classes into which the data are to be grouped and the range of each.

1. Do not use fewer than five or more than fifteen classes as a general rule. This choice depends mostly on the number of values to be grouped.
2. Choose classes which cover the smallest and largest values and do not produce gaps between classes.
3. Make certain each item can go into only one class. Avoid successive classes which overlap or have common values.

Correct	Incorrect
Under 10	0 - 10
10 - 19	10 - 20
20 - 29	20 - 30
30 and Over	Over 30

4. Whenever feasible, classes should cover equal ranges of values. It is generally good to make these ranges (intervals) multiples of 5, 10, 100 or other value which facilitates tallying. This rule does not apply to the open classes at the beginning and end.

GRAPHS

Data presented graphically usually have more appeal than tables of numerical listings. The graph helps the reader obtain a quick overall grasp of the material presented. It should be simple in content and self-explanatory (correctly labeled). All graphs should be titled. When color or shading is used, a key is necessary; and when more than one variable is shown, each should be differentiated by means of a key(s).

Construction of a Graph

The graph proceeds from left to right (horizontal axis) and from bottom to top (vertical axis). Along the horizontal axis (referred to as the "x" axis) the independent variables are noted. These are the factors causing the results being graphed. They may be categories or classes of data, such as days of the week, medical staff units, DRGs, and so forth. They may also be ranges or mid-points of continuous data, such as groups of patient ages or numbers of days stay. The frequency divisions are placed along the vertical scale. The vertical scale (called the "y" axis) is thus used to record the dependent variables. The vertical scale should always start with zero. A misleading impression can be created by failing to show the total range of possibilities when one starts at a figure other than zero. If the zero line is omitted because the frequency spread is at the upper levels, the user should be alerted to this by the use of a device usually referred to as a "lightning mark." (See Figure 6.)

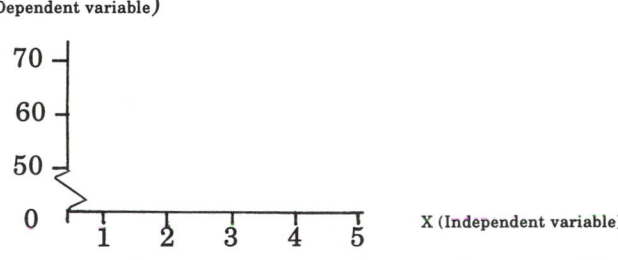

FIGURE 6. CHARACTERISTICS OF A GRAPH AND LIGHTENING MARK

If there is one extreme value which cannot be accommodated on the vertical axis, it must be indicated within the graph rectangle. (See Figure 7.)

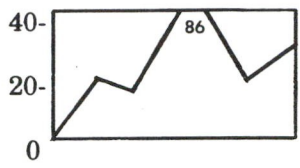

FIGURE 7. DISPLAY OF EXTREME VALUE ON A GRAPH

Different impressions are given by stretching or contracting the vertical and horizontal axes, easily accomplished by increasing or decreasing the number of subdivisions along either line. A general rule is that the vertical axis should be subdivided so the height of the maximum point is approximately equal to three quarters of the length of the horizontal axis. Figure 8 provides an example of proportional spacing.

Bar Graphs

Bar graphs are the simplest form of graph, used to present categories of data which are not continuous. Figure 8 is an example of a bar graph. Each independent variable (i.e., in the example the chronic activity limitation status) is unique, not

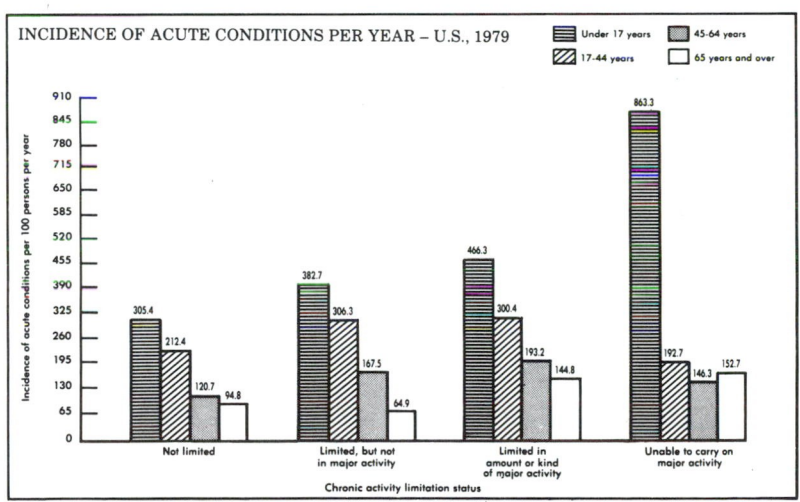

FIGURE 8. BAR GRAPH WITH PROPORTIONAL SPACING AND KEY

continuous. Bar graphs may be vertical or horizontal. A good rule to use in determining the direction is that if the "legend" describing each bar can be written under it when drawn vertically, the vertical graph should be used.

Histograms

A histogram is a graphic presentation of a frequency distribution. Histograms are constructed by representing class intervals (frequency groups) on the horizontal axis, the class frequencies on the vertical axis, and drawing rectangles whose bases equal the class interval and whose heights are determined by the respective class frequencies.

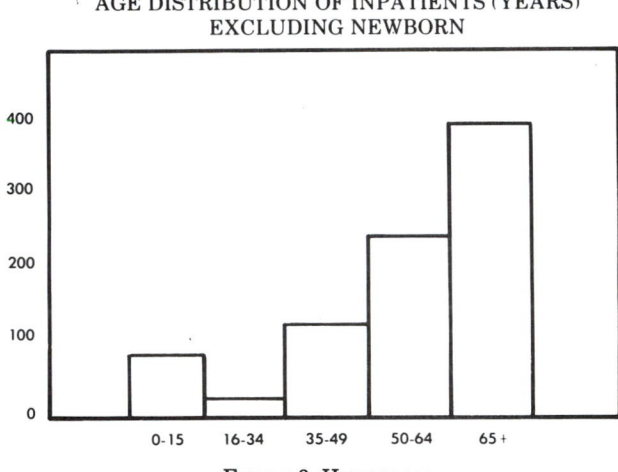

AGE DISTRIBUTION OF INPATIENTS (YEARS)
EXCLUDING NEWBORN

FIGURE 9. HISTOGRAM

A few rules for drawing histograms follow:

1. Establish between 5-15 classes (horizontal axis).
2. Form classes of equal width, if possible, to prevent distortion.
3. Draw bars the same width and distribute them evenly.
4. Always form nonoverlapping classes.

Line Graphs

A frequency distribution can also be represented graphically by a line graph (called a frequency polygon.) In a line graph, the midpoints of the classes are the points which connect the line. Figure 10 depicts the construction of a line graph from a histogram.

In a line graph, the assumption is made that one can read a value at any point along the line. For example, in the second quarter of 1987 the number of outpatient surgeries can be read off the graph to be 500.

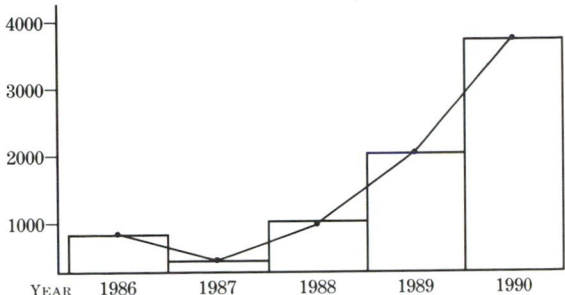

FIGURE 10. LINE GRAPH DRAWN FROM A HISTOGRAM

Pictorial Presentation

Just as the visual appeal of graphs exceeds that of tables, even more interest may be aroused by pictorial presentations. The ways in which data can be displayed pictorially are unlimited and depend on the imagination and artistic talent of the person preparing the presentation. A form sometimes seen is called the pictogram in which symbols are used (such as draw-

TOTAL DISCHARGES BY DRG
January–December 1984
4,800 Total Discharges

DRG		Number	% Dsch.
391	••	416	8.7
373	•••	398	8.3
430	•••••••••••••••••••••••••••••••••••	285	5.9
243	••••••••••••••••••	141	2.9
371	•••••••••••••••••	130	2.7
390	•••••••••••••••	93	1.9
60	•••••••••••••	84	1.8
389	•••••••••	76	1.5
55	•••••••••	74	1.5
355	•••••••••	74	1.5
225	•••••••••	73	1.5

FIGURE 11. PICTOGRAM

ings representing people, male and female symbols, or matchstick drawings) with each symbol representing a specified number. (See Figure 11.)

Pie Graph

The most common pictogram is a pie graph. A pie graph is a circle divided into pie-shaped wedges which are proportional in size to the frequencies of the categories. A pie graph always represents percentages so one must always convert the distribution into a percentage distribution. (Divide each frequency by the total number of items grouped and multiply by 100). Divide the 360 degree circumference according to the percentage of each category. See Figure 12. Pie graphs have added

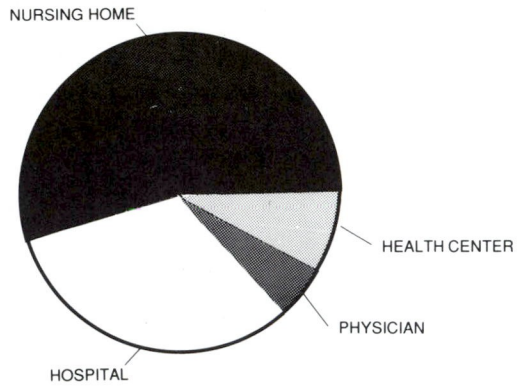

FIGURE 12. PIE GRAPH

visual appeal when sections are colored or shaded, or a piece of the pie is "cut out" to draw attention to a particular category.

Health information practitioners would be wise to take careful note of the manner in which graphs are presented by medical journals, newspapers, and advertisers for later application in their own departmental reports. Ads are clever and tell the stories efficiently.

Computer programs are available which will automatically convert data into graphic form given parameters specified by the user.

AMBULATORY CARE STATISTICS

With advances in medical technology and concern about the increased cost of health care, more care is being provided in an ambulatory care setting. When a hospital offers ambulatory care services in an outpatient department, statistics in terms of persons, tests, and treatments must be carefully tabulated and reported for good management decision-making and control. Outpatient statistics need to be gathered consistently, using standard definitions to permit uniform reporting and comparison among similar facilities. See Chapter 4 for further discussion of terms utilized to collect data on ambulatory patients.

The ambulatory care provided in free-standing facilities ranges from solo physician practice to group practice, outpatient surgery centers, emergency care centers, and neighborhood health centers. Many of the same types of statistics as hospital-based outpatient care centers may be calculated. Some free-standing ambulatory facilities (e.g. health maintenance organizations) emphasize preventive care in addition to curative care, so number of visits, encounters, and occasions of service may be calculated for each category to produce meaningful data for management decision-making and control.

LONG TERM CARE STATISTICS

Just as in short term hospitals, long term care facilities compile data needed by administration, medical staff, accreditation bodies, state health departments, federal and state government agencies, and others. Individual facility needs must be accommodated, but standard statistical compilations and computations should be used to permit uniform reporting and comparison among similar facilities.

Definitions for statistical terminology used in long term facilities are the same as for short term hospitals and are found in the *Glossary of Health Care Terms*. Long term care facilities frequently divide all statistical compilations into categories for patients over and under 65 years of age for reporting and managerial purposes. Additional age breakdowns may also be helpful.

It is also important to compile separate statistics for the different levels of care provided (e.g., hospice, skilled nursing, intermediate) and to carefully track transfers from one level of care to another. Separating statistics by level of care means patients must be discharged and readmitted on transfer to another level in order to obtain separate totals for each level. Leaves of absence are included as one continuous stay or separately tabulated in computing length of stay but are excluded, when compiling bed occupancy, counting inpatient service days, or preparing the patient census.

The health information practitioner needs to be alert to continuing changes in government and agency requests for statistical information needed from long term care facilities.

QUALITY CONTROL OF DATA
COLLECTION SYSTEMS

Inputting patient information into a computer for processing and storage does not diminish the health information department's responsibility for the accuracy and reliability of collected data. It is safe to assume that the computer can perform simple mathematical functions accurately. Quality control of data entered into the computer, however, remains the responsibility of the health information practitioner. Evaluation of the percentage of clerical error is an important consideration. Manual work sheets or computer abstracts should be randomly checked for errors. Other edit checks can be done by the computer, e.g., checking for male obstetric patients or deliveries in women over 50 years of age. Because items are released to many recipients, it is vital that data be reliable and accurately reflect the care rendered by the facility for a given period. Periodically, the format of the data collection sheets should be evaluated to determine if the most efficient method of collection is being used. Routine quality control studies in both manual and computerized systems can ensure that the necessary collection of statistical information is done in an effective and cost-efficient manner.

Criteria may be developed to determine if each item presently collected is necessary and justified by routine use. As agency and federal reporting requirements change, data elements can be altered or deleted to satisfy revised needs. It may also be discovered that several reports carry the same items if a cross-study is done with several other departments, such as the patient accounting department, admitting department, or the hospital administration. Duplication of effort may be avoided if one consolidated report satisfies everyone's needs.

VITAL RECORDS AND STATISTICS

Vital statistics refer to crucial events in life such as birth, marriage, death, and divorce. Birth and death certificates, and reports of fetal death often completed in hospitals or other health care facilities provide valuable information to private individuals, public health and welfare officials, lawyers, research persons, and social workers. A birth certificate is needed to establish citizenship or parentage, to obtain a passport, to show that a child is old enough to enter school, to register as a voter, to get a driver's license, or to obtain Social Security benefits. Statistics taken from birth certificates help in evaluating population changes and growth, evaluating birthrate trends, maternal and child health, and socioeconomic factors. Death certificates help in the settlement of life insurance claims and estates by showing proof of death. Statistics derived from death certificates help in evaluating underlying causes of death, multiple causes of death, and the frequency of certain conditions occurring together. All of this information is vital for basic research, epidemiological studies, and planning public health programs. It is, therefore, absolutely necessary that the data on these certificates be complete and accurate.

THE VITAL STATISTICS REGISTRATION SYSTEM OF THE UNITED STATES

The National Center for Health Statistics, Public Health Service, of the U.S. Department of Health and Human Services prepares standard certificates of live birth and death, and forms for reporting fetal death. These serve as models for use by the states. The purpose of the models is to develop uniform national statistics. The certificates used by most states conform to the standard ones. Some states modify the forms because of particular needs or because of special provisions in the state's vital statistics laws. Periodically the National Center for Health Statistics, in consultation with certain national and state health officers, evaluates and revises the standard certificates. This reevaluation assures that the data collected from the certificates are useful for certain legal, medical, registration, and research needs.

When a certificate is filed, the local registrar or vital statistics office keeps a record on file and forwards the original to the state registrar as the permanent reference. The state registrar is the source of certified copies. The State registrar also sends a copy to the National Center for Health Statistics. The National Center prepares special statistical reports from these certificates for the United States as a whole and in comparable form for each state. The National Center also sends certain information to the World Health Organization.

DEFINITIONS FOR REPORTING OF REPRODUCTIVE HEALTH STATISTICS

Committees of the World Health Organization formulated definitions of "fetal deaths" (stillbirths, abortions) and "premature infants." This was done so reports concerning these events would be uniformly comparable throughout the United States or the world. The terms were officially adopted by the Third World Health Assembly in June, 1950. Since that time, the terms "stillbirth" and "abortion" were replaced by "fetal death." "Premature infant" was replaced by "immature birth." Until all states amend their laws and/or health regulations to conform to the use of "fetal death" and "immature infant," hospital personnel must be familiar with all terms and use those terms adopted by agencies to which the hospital reports. The following definitions are recommended for reporting of reproductive health statistics in the United States:

Fetal Death - death prior to the complete expulsion or extraction from the mother of a product of human conception, fetus and placenta, irrespective of the duration of pregnancy; the death is indicated by the fact that, after such expulsion or extraction, the fetus does not breathe or show any other evidence of life, such as beating of the heart, pulsation of the umbilical cord, or definite movement of voluntary muscles. Heartbeats are to be distinguished from transient cardiac contractions; respirations are to be distinguished from fleeting respiratory efforts or gasps. This definition excludes induced termination of pregnancy.

Induced Termination of Pregnancy - the purposeful interruption of intrauterine pregnancy with the intention other than to produce a liveborn infant, and which does not result in a live birth. This definition excludes management of prolonged retention of products of conception following fetal death.

Live Birth - the complete expulsion or extraction from the mother of a product of human conception, irrespective of the duration of pregnancy, which, after such expulsion or extraction, breathes or shows any other evidence of life, such as beating of the heart, pulsation of the umbilical cord, or definite movement of voluntary muscles whether or not the umbilical cord has been cut or the placenta is attached. Heartbeats are to be distinguished from transient cardiac contractions; respirations are to be distinguished from fleeting respiratory efforts or gasps. Live births may be classified

Low Birthweight Neonate - any neonate, regardless of gestational age, whose weight at birth is less than 2,500 grams.

Preterm Neonate - any neonate whose birth occurs before the end of the last day of the 38th week (266th day), following onset of the last menstrual period.

Term Neonate - any neonate whose birth occurs from the beginning of the first day (267th day) of the 39th week, through the end of the last day of the 42nd week (294th day), following onset of the last menstrual period.

Postterm Neonate - any neonate whose birth occurs from the beginning of the first day (295th day) of the 43rd week following onset of the last menstrual period.

COMPLETION OF CERTIFICATES

The civil laws of every state provide for the registration of births and deaths and reporting of fetal deaths. In some states the hospital administrator is responsible for issuing birth certificates for those born in the hospital or enroute. The required information is gathered and filed with the local or state registrar. In other states, the attending physician is responsible.

The trend is to place final responsibility for completion of vital records in the health information department. One reason is that health information personnel are aware of the importance of accuracy and promptness in completing forms. Another reason is that information on these certificates may be needed later and will be readily available if there is a copy in the medical record. Also, the National Center for Health Statistics recommends the use of any recognized system of disease nomenclature in certifying causes of death; and health information personnel are most familiar with the terminology used in these publications.

To assure accurate and complete information in the medical record, a copy of the birth or death certificate should be included in the patient's record. A copy of the report of fetal death should be placed in the mother's record if a separate record is not prepared. (This will be impossible in those states in which the hospital is not responsible for reporting.) This copy may be carbon, snap-out form, stub, or multiple-copy form, depending on the type of certificates used.

Computerized or electronically generated birth certificates are common. Some states provide software to hospitals for birth certificate reporting.

RESEARCH STUDIES

In keeping current with health care delivery trends and advances in medical technology, health information practitioners will frequently read reports of research studies. It is important to understand the steps in the research process and to evaluate information collected in research projects and special studies. For example, in reading a research paper, the health information practitioner should understand why the researcher reports on a review of literature and why limitations on the research study are explained. The sample size and type should be evaluated; the appropriateness of the statistical tests should be determined; and the reliability and validity of the results should be considered. Health information practitioners may also be a part of a research team, collecting data from medical records or other sources. Studying health information practice issues may also be performed in a formal research manner.

Research is a systematic investigation of a subject designed to expand knowledge and generate new ideas, which implies a prior assessment, gathering of appropriate data, analyzing and synthesizing of data, and applying its results. Research is varied; it may be "pure," or "basic," in which the research is motivated solely by intellectual interest and directed toward the acquisition of knowledge for knowledge's sake, or it may be "applied," "behavioral," "clinical," or "social" implying that the research is directed at solving a specific practical problem.

STEPS IN RESEARCH

In any research, several distinct steps are taken:

1. The research topic is identified as the issue about which the researcher is seeking information.

2. A frame of reference is developed by reviewing literature related to the research topic.

3. The specific research problem is isolated by narrowing the topic to specific questions the research study will answer.

4. The success potential of the contemplated research is estimated.

5. An indepth review of literature is conducted to determine if there are related studies that have been performed and how they were conducted.

6. The research design is selected. The research may test a causal relationship, explore an issue, or describe the nature of an event. In testing causal relationships, study designs are considered to be either comparative (determining the difference between two things) or correlational (determining the degree or direction of difference between two things).

7. The research hypothesis is stated as a single, clear question and expected answer.

8. Data gathering methods, techniques, and instruments are selected. Observation, questioning, and measurement are the techniques available. The technique chosen depends on many factors including cost, time, researcher's abilities, and the nature of the data.

9. Data gathering instruments and procedures are developed, such as observation checklists, interview plans, questionnaires, or measuring devices.

10. Data analysis plan is designed to develop the specific sampling techniques and statistical analyses to be used.

11. A pilot study is conducted as a test of the research plan and modifications are made as necessary.

12. The data gathering and analysis plans are implemented—this is the formal conduct of the study.

13. The research report is prepared—the purpose of the research report is to recapitulate the researcher's actions and results, including any limitations related to the results; to suggest further research; and to propose changes or actions within the problem areas. The research report should be written at the level of the intended reader's understanding. For example, if the results are to be published in a scientific journal, the statistical measures may be used without further explanation. If the results

are to be summarized in a newsletter with a broader readership, the statistics may have to be summarized in a narrative description rather than left in numerical form.

14. The findings are disseminated. Applied research implies that the results are expected to be useful. The results, therefore should be communicated to those who would find use for the results.

NATURE OF DATA

To evaluate the results of a research study the statistical measures used to explain the significance of research findings should be understood. This requires knowing the nature of the data.

Data may be nominal, or dichotomous (e.g., true/false, male/female, Medicare/non-Medicare); ordinal (ordered categories or ranks, such as low/moderate/high, never/sometimes/often/always); interval (units of equal size, such as IQ results); or ratio (units of equal size which may be placed on a scale starting with zero and thus able to be manipulated mathematically, such as 0, 5, 10, 15, 20).

SAMPLE SIZE AND TYPE

Most research is conducted on a sample drawn from the population about which a conclusion can be made. The size of the sample should be such that the sample is representative of the population. A representative sample size can be determined knowing the level of confidence the researcher has in the results falling within a level of acceptable error. A standard formula may be used to approximate the sample size, or more sophisticated statistical measures may be used. The formula is:

$$\text{sample size} = 0.25 \left(\frac{\text{certainty factor}}{\text{acceptable error}} \right)^2$$

where the certainty factor for 97% certainty is 2.170, for 95% certainty is 1.960, for 90% certainty is 1.645, and for 80% certainty is 1.281; and the acceptable error is the percent of error the researcher can tolerate in the sample process, such as 95%, 90%, and so forth.

The type of sample must also be chosen. Non-probability sampling permits the selection of a sample that is somewhat typical, if not absolutely representative, of a known population. In non-probability sampling the researcher may select cases based on convenient sections of the population (convenience sampling), on cases known to have specific characteristics that relate to the purpose of the study (purposive sampling), or on quotas from defined classes (quota sampling). The probability sampling techniques are ones in which each case in the population has an equal and independent chance of being selected so that the sample may be representative of the entire population being studied. A simple random sample is one selected using a random number table so that every element in the population has an equal chance of being included. A stratified random sample is one in which the population is divided into groups on the basis of prior knowledge about shared characteristics, such as diagnoses or medical staff units; and random samples are taken from each group. Systematic sampling begins with the random selection of one case, then cases are chosen on a fixed interval after that, such as every third patient, or every tenth record.

MEASURES OF RELIABILITY & VALIDITY

Reliability - This is the accuracy of the data in the sense of their stability, repeatability, or precision. A perfectly reliable data-collection instrument is one which, if administered twice under the same circumstances, would provide identical data. The correlation, usually denoted by r is the basic statistic used to estimate reliability. It describes the degree, or strength, of association between two variables (such as first administration of questionnaire and second administration of questionnaire), and is always expressed as a decimal number between -1 and +1. A high positive score means that the two sets of variables are closely related in the same manner (e.g., as one gets larger, the other gets larger). A high negative score means that the two sets of variables are closely related in an opposing manner (e.g., as one gets larger the other gets smaller). Low scores mean there is less association, and thus less reliability. There are several kinds of correlation statistics that can be calculated based on the type of data being collected.

Validity - This deals with the relationship of the data obtained to the purpose for which it accomplishes or measures what it seeks to measure. Face validity is simply a review of the instrument and a statement made as to whether or not the instrument appears to measure what it is intended to measure. Content validity argues that the instrument measures what it purports to measure because there was a rational basis to the selection of the content (e.g., the instrument was previously used in studies of this type). Empirical studies which actually use a statistic to test validity are also available. There are a wide variety of such statistics, each chosen for the nature of the data in the study. The t-test is a commonly used statistic to test validity, although it is the weakest of the empirical methods. The t-test is a way of testing the statistical significance of the difference between the means of two groups. Statistics textbooks should be referenced to determine how the t-test and other tests of statistical significance are used and interpreted.

SUMMARY

The information presented in this chapter describes the basic statistical data needed by a facility's governing board, administration, and medical staff, and by outside agencies. The health information department may receive requests for non-routine information, which can be filled if data are kept in sufficient detail. Methods of presentation and evaluation of research studies are described. Tabulations for special studies should be maintained only as needed. All statistical compilations and reports should be reviewed on an annual basis to determine their use so those not needed may be discontinued. Requests should be reviewed and the administrative and medical staff consulted before a decision is made to discontinue data compilation. Data quality must also be evaluated regularly, for information is only valuable if the data used in compilation are accurate.

STUDY QUESTIONS

1. Describe how a health information practitioner determines the amount and type of data to be collected in a hospital data collection system.

2. Explain the purpose of a data set and list the data elements in the UHDDS.

3. Describe how data may be collected for and the reports obtained from inpatient discharge analysis.

4. Describe the manner in which patients should be assigned to a "service."

5. Perform percentage computations and round results.

6. Describe the importance of mortality and autopsy data and identify the reference for death rates relating to pregnancy.

7. Define the following terms and give the formulas for computing each:
    a. Hospital Death Rate
    b. Hospital Infection Rate
    c. Gross Autopsy Rate
    d. Hospital Autopsy Rate
    e. Net Autopsy Rate
    f. Average Length of Stay
    g. Inpatient Service Day
    h. Average Daily Inpatient Census
    i. Inpatient Bed Occupancy Ratio
    j. Bed Turnover Rate

8. Explain the importance of morbidity data.

9. Distinguish between mean, median, and mode as measures of central tendency; and between range, variance, and standard deviation as measures of variation.

10. Describe how a (1) bar graph, (2) histogram, and (3) line graph are constructed and how to best communicate data from statistical reports.

11. Describe the health information department's responsibility for quality control in data collection systems.

12. Describe the purpose of vital records and statistics.

13. Identify the factors to consider in evaluating a research study.

REFERENCES

American Hospital Association, *Guide to the Health Care Field,* (Chicago: AHA, published yearly).

American Medical Association, *Directory of Residency Training Programs,* (Chicago: AMA, 1980).

American Health Information Management Association, *Glossary of Health Care Terms,* (Chicago: AHIMA, 1994).

Armore, Sidney J., *Elementary Statistics and Decision Making,* (Columbus, Ohio: Charles E. Merrill Publishing Co., 1973).

Avery, Maurine and Bonnie Imdieke, *Medical Records in Ambulatory Care,* (Rockville, Maryland: Aspen Systems Corporation, 1984).

Berger, Elaine, et al., "Managing the Medical Record on a Concurrent Basis: Facts and Possibilities," *Journal of the American Medical Record Association,* (May 1988): 24-33 and (June 1988): 25-36.

Duncan, Robert C., Rebecca G. Knapp, and M. Clinton Miller III, *Introductory Biostatistics for the Health Sciences,* (New York: John Wiley & Sons, 1977).

Finnegan, Rita, *Data Quality and DRGs,* (Chicago: American Medical Record Association, 1986).

Fottler, Myron D., Donna T. Slovensky, and S. Jean Rogers, "Public Release of Hospital Specific Death Rates: Guidelines for Health Care Executives," *Journal of the American Medical Record Association,* (December 1987): 22-26.

Hospitals' and Physicians' Handbook on Birth Registration and Fetal Death Reporting, PHS Publication No. 87-1107, (Washington, D.C.: Public Health Service, U.S. Dept. of Health and Human Services, 1987).

Iownie, N. M. and A.R. Starry, *Descriptive and Inferential Statistics,* (New York: Harper and Row, 1977).

Joint Commission on Accreditation of Healthcare Organizations, *Accreditation Manual for Hospitals,* (Chicago: Joint Commission, 1994).

"Legislative Currents," *Journal of the American Medical Record Association* (May 1985): 17-19.

Long-Term Health Care Minimum Data Set, (Washington, D.C.: Public Health Service, U.S. Dept. of Health and Human Services, August 1980).

O'Gara, Sara, *Data Quality Issues for Statewide Patient Discharge Data Systems,* (Sacramento: Office of Statewide Planning & Development, 1988).

Physicians' Handbook on Medical Certification of Death, PHS Publication No. 87-1108, (Washington, D.C.: Public Health Service, U.S. Dept. of Health and Human Services, 1987).

Pierce, Patricia J., *Commonly Computed Rates and Percentages for Hospital Inpatients,* (Chicago: American Medical Record Association, 1987).

Rimm, Alfred, et al., *Basic Biostatistics in Medicine & Epidemiology,* (New York: Appleton-Century-Crofts, 1980).

Runyon, Richard P. and Audrey Haber, *Fundamentals of Behavioral Statistics,* (New York: Random House, 1988).

Shala, Thomas J., "HCFA Release of Hospital Specific Death Rates: Where Are We and Where Are We Going?," *Journal of the American Medical Record Association,* (Sept., 1988).

Welkowitz, Joan, Robert B. Ewen, and Jacob Cohen, *Introductory Statistics for the Behavioral Sciences,* 3rd Ed., (San Diego, CA: Harcourt Brace Jovanovich, Publishers, 1982).

chapter *12*

HEALTH INFORMATION IN REIMBURSEMENT

Obtaining payment for health care services is one of the most complex aspects of the health care delivery system, and certainly has had a major impact on health information department operations. While the primary function of the health information department is ensuring that an accurate and complete medical record is available for patient care, providing accurate and complete clinical data for billing is also very important if the facility is to survive financially. In addition to providing raw data for billing, the health information department also provides clinical information for planning the types of services the health care facility will offer. In this chapter a basic description of health care reimbursement is provided as a backdrop to the functions performed by the health information professional.

THE ISSUE

The cost of health care and how to pay for it is a major national issue. In 1993, health care costs accounted for 14 percent of the US gross national product (GNP), which is the total amount of money spent on all goods and services in a nation during a year. At issue, though, is not only the immense amount of money this represents, but the fact that the amount has been increasing at a drastic rate. In 1960, health care costs were 5.3 percent of GNP, in 1970 - 7.5 percent, and in 1980 - 9.5 percent. The increased rate of expenditure is believed to be due to improved access to health care, increased number of hospital beds, oversupply and maldistribution of physicians, increased number of people covered by health care insurance, advancements in medical technology, growth in population of those 65 years and over, aging of the population (longer lifespan), and increasing use of health care services by the aged.

As a result of the tremendous increase in health care costs, measures are being taken to contain costs. The federal government has taken the lead in cost containment, although private business and industry have recently followed suit. The federal government is concerned because it is a major payer for health care services. Private business and industry pays for the majority of the remainder of the expenditures through employee insurance benefits. Just like consumers of any product the federal government and industry are concerned about how much they are paying and the quality of the product - health care - they are purchasing.

HISTORY OF REIMBURSEMENT

The history of health care payment in the US is a history of charity, philanthropy, and retrospective fee-for-service payment. In the early years, persons who were ill and did not have the means to pay for care were treated to the extent possible through the efforts of religious and other charitable organizations who depended on the generous contributions of others. In some areas, local or state institutions were created to provide care for the poor. As a charitable, and "caring," business, health care workers were largely from religious orders with some wealthy volunteers. Many physicians contributed part of their time to care for the poor. Wages and salaries were at subsistence levels and more was not expected. As times changed and specialized workers were needed to manage the advances in health care technology, health care workers' demands for equitable pay necessarily contributed to increased costs.

Those who could pay were assured of access to health care services. Services were paid for on a retrospective fee-for-service basis. Health care providers charged patients for each service, determining the charge for the service after it was performed. Charges were sometimes based on the ability of the patient to pay, but also on the overall costs of providing the service plus the amount the provider wished to earn. Most hospitals were not-for-profit and attempted to cover their costs with only minimal earnings beyond actual costs for reserves. Physicians were more able than hospitals to alter their fees based on a patient's ability to pay, but also expected higher earnings in compensation for the skills they utilized in providing health care.

While health insurance was an important advancement, it also contributed to rising health care costs. Many believe that insurance removes the risk of financial hazard for the individual consumer by taking away the responsibility for paying many of the costs associated with health care, so the consumer is less likely to be appreciative of the enormity of the costs, less concerned about their accuracy, more inclined to use health care services, and ultimately more demanding of the health care system.

As health care became more accessible and technology more advanced, consumer expectations rose. Malpractice suits also rose when expectations were not met. The cost of malpractice insurance for physicians and hospitals skyrocketed.

Private health insurance also broadened the gap even further between those with access to health care and those who lacked access.

PRIVATE INDEMNITY INSURANCE

Health insurance was first conceived in the late 1930s. Basically, payment for health care under indemnity insurance was retrospective fee-for-service reimbursement of charges.

The dictionary defines reimbursement as a "paying back." Health care reimbursement, however, is more broadly defined as charging and receiving payment for services after they are rendered. In general, while a patient is responsible for paying some of the costs directly to the provider after services are rendered, and receives a copy of the bill for services, insurance for which the patient has paid premiums pays the bulk of the costs directly to the provider. Thus, the insurer is a third party acting for the patient in health care reimbursement.

Indemnity insurance is paid on a premium basis. The insured pays periodic (monthly, or other period) payments to the insurance company, which invests the money. When the insured requires health care, a claim is filed after services are rendered. The insured frequently has to pay a deductible, which is an amount payable by the insured to the provider before the insurance company makes reimbursement. The amount frequently is $100, $200, $500, or more depending on the insurance plan. The deductible may relate to each claim or to all claims within a one year period. The purpose of the deductible is to decrease the amount of small claims which are costly for an insurance company to handle. The insured may also pay a copayment, which is a percentage of the claim. Whether a copayment is required and the percentage (20 percent is a common amount) is dependent on the insurance plan. For example, many plans cover 100 percent of a hospital claim after the deductible, but cover only 80 percent of a physician's claim. Blue Cross/Blue Shield (BC/BS) is the largest third party payer. It is a nationwide federation of local, not-for-profit insurance organizations, known as Blue Cross and Blue Shield Plans, that contract with hospitals and other health care providers to pay for health care services provided their subscribers.

Insurance plans generally reimburse only "covered services." Covered services are those specific services and supplies for which the insurance plan has designated it will pay. For example, an insurance plan will generally cover room and board during hospitalization for medical care but will not pay telephone or television charges. Many insurance plans do not cover cosmetic surgery. The amount of the charge the insurance company will pay for covered services is also defined as "reasonable, necessary, and customary charges" which are one of: 1.) the lowest of the usual charge by a health care provider for the same or similar services or supplies, 2.) the usual charge of most other providers of similar training or experience in the same or a similar geographic area for the same or similar services or supplies, or 3.) the actual charge for the services or supplies.

FEDERAL INSURANCE

Until 1965, most of the poor and many of the aged in this country were completely without access to major health care.

As a result of public pressure calling for attention to this growing problem, Congress passed Public Law 89-97 as an Amendment to the Social Security Act. This included Title XVIII (Medicare) and Title XIX (Medicaid). The Health Care Financing Administration (HCFA) of the US Department of Health and Human Services is the federal agency which administers the Medicare program and certain aspects of the state/federal Medicaid program.

Medicare

Medicare - Health Insurance for the Aged - became effective July 1, 1966. The legislation was designed essentially to help pay for medical care for the elderly, that is, for persons 65 years of age and over and eligible for social security.

Medicare health insurance protection is available to eligible persons without regard to income. It is available under two separate but coordinated programs: hospital insurance (Part A) and medical insurance (Part B). Hospital insurance is financed by the federal government through payroll taxes on the working population. Initially it paid for hospitalization and home health care. Subsequently, coverage for "extended care," that is, nursing home care, was added. Coverage for those eligible for social security disability payments for over two years and those who need kidney transplantation or dialysis for end stage renal disease (ESRD) was also added.

Medical insurance (Part B) is optional and is financed by monthly premiums paid by eligible individuals, and by federal revenues. It helps pay for physicians' services, outpatient hospital care, services and supplies prescribed by attending physicians, and certain other medical costs not covered by Part A.

Medicaid

Medicaid is a medical assistance program designed to meet the needs of low income people. The program is funded partially by the federal government and partially by the states (and sometimes local governments). The federal government specifies certain required services which must be covered by every state, specifies the eligibility of individuals to receive benefits, and, in general, identifies the allowed rate of payment to providers. Benefits include inpatient hospital care; outpatient hospital care; laboratory and x-ray services; skilled nursing facility and home health services for persons over 21;

physician's services; family planning services; rural health clinic services; and early and periodic screening, diagnosis, and treatment services. The states may cover additional services as well.

Other Federal Insurance

Two other federal programs cover health services for specified populations. These are CHAMPUS and the Veteran's Administration.

The Civilian Health and Medical Program of the Uniformed Services (CHAMPUS) program is administered by the Department of Defense. It pays for care delivered by civilian health providers to retired members and to dependents of active and retired members of the seven uniformed services of the US. The Veteran's Administration (VA) was established in 1930 to provide hospital, nursing home, domiciliary, and outpatient medical and dental care to eligible veterans of military service in the Armed Forces. The VA operates over 150 medical centers and many other facilities, and provides benefits for veterans in non-VA operated facilities as well.

PROSPECTIVE PAYMENT SYSTEM

It should be obvious that retrospective fee-for-service reimbursement does not encourage cost containment. A provider's earnings increase as more services are provided. There may even be less incentive for quality care as complications extend the services required. While general medical ethics and the threat of malpractice suits limit the latter, there is no limiting factor on the former.

LEGISLATION

In early 1982, Congress recognized that the cost of health care had reached critical dimensions. The Medicare Trust Fund, which is the repository for payroll tax contributions to Medicare, was nearly depleted. Congress thus passed the Tax Equity and Fiscal Responsibility Act (TEFRA) which set overall limits on Medicare spending and imposed a deadline on itself to develop a prospective payment system (PPS) for inpatient hospitalizations by the end of 1982.

A plan was formalized into amendments to the Social Security Act by Congress. The plan described in general form a prospective payment system for acute inpatient hospitalization. Psychiatric, children's, rehabilitation, and long term care facilities, as well as such units in an acute care hospital, were excluded in the initial plan. An implementation schedule over a three year period was also included in the plan with the initial implementation effective October 1, 1983. Every year regulations with respect to the system are revised and updated. The regulations are printed in the *Federal Register.*

PAYMENT PER CASE

Medicare's prospective payment system for inpatient hospitalization establishes payment rates to hospitals before services are rendered. The payment rates are based on Diagnosis Related Groups (DRGs). DRGs were developed at Yale University as a classification system to describe the type of patients admitted to hospitals. A full description of the DRG classification system is provided in Chapter 9.

Payment rates for each DRG are determined from two basic sources. First, each DRG is assigned a relative weighting factor. The relative weighting factor represents the average resources required to care for cases in that particular DRG relative to the national average of resources used to treat all Medicare cases. The average Medicare case is assigned a relative weighting factor of 1.0000. Thus, cases in a DRG with a weight of 2.0000, on average, require twice as many resources as the average Medicare case; or cases in a DRG with a weight of 0.5000, on average, require half as many resources as the average Medicare case. Each year the DRGs' relative weighting factors are updated to reflect changes in treatment patterns, technology, and any other factors that may change the relative use of hospital resources.

The second source that determines the payment rate is the individual hospital's payment rate per case. This individual hospital rate is based on a regional or national adjusted standardized amount considering the type of hospital; designation of the hospital as large urban, other urban, or rural; and a wage index for the geographic area in which the hospital is located.

Thus, the actual amount the hospital is reimbursed for each Medicare inpatient is the hospital's individual payment rate multiplied by the relative weighting factor of the DRG, less any applicable deductible amount. For any given patient in a DRG, the hospital knows, in advance, the amount it will be reimbursed by Medicare. It is up to the hospital to ensure that its utilization of resources is in line with the payment it will receive.

In addition to the basic payment rate, Medicare also provides for an additional payment per case for outliers. These are cases in which patients require considerably more resources than average, reflected in their length of stay or cost of care. Once a threshold length of stay or cost is reached, an additional payment is made. For example, a patient admitted for a transurethral resection of prostate without any significant complications or comorbidities stays in the hospital, on average, 2.5 days. If the patient requires considerably more care, the hospital, with documentation supporting the necessity of the care, will be reimbursed an additional amount.

PAYMENT OF CLAIMS

Medicare claims are paid to providers through contract arrangements with a third party organization. The organization may be a Blue Cross Plan, private insurance company, or other public or private agency. A contractor that processes and pays provider claims on behalf of Medicare Part A hospital insurance is called a fiscal intermediary; a contractor that processes claims and performs other services under Medicare's Part B supplementary medical insurance program is called a carrier.

It is actually the fiscal intermediary which assigns the DRG to an inpatient hospital claim, based on the ICD-9-CM codes for the principal diagnosis, secondary diagnoses, and procedures attested to by the attending physician (see example of attestation statement form in Figure 1) and supplied by the hospital. Most hospitals, however, identify the DRG for their own records, so they may use the data in planning activities.

PEER REVIEW ORGANIZATION

To ensure that the government pays only for medically necessary, appropriate, and quality health care services, HCFA contracts with medical review organizations called Peer Review Organizations (PROs). PROs review services provided under the Medicare program for the purpose of determining:

- whether the services provided or proposed to be provided are reasonable and medically necessary.
- whether those services furnished or proposed to be furnished on an inpatient basis could be effectively and appropriately fur-

---

Clinical Data Editor
with DRG Assignment

Patient Name: Medical Record No:
Admit Date: 12/20/19   Discharge Date: 12/23/19
Optional:

Age: 38   Sex: Female   Discharge Disp: 1 Home
MDC: 8   Diseases & disorders of the digestive system
DRG: 174   G.I. hemorrhage age > 69 and or C.C.

Principal Diagnosis
5780 Hematemesis

Secondary Diagnosis
#29592   Schizophrenia NOS-chr   (DRG)
2800   Chr blood loss anemia   (CC)
7870   Nausea and vomiting
7890   Abdominal pain
7807   Malaise and fatigue

No procedures performed

No errors found

Primary Pay Source: 1 Medicare

Actual LOS: 3   Average LOS: 6.7
                                                Outlier LOS Threshold: 29
                                                # of Outlier Days:

Total Charges: $1,133.   DRG Payment: $ 2,269.
                                                Outlier Payment:
Cost Weight: 0.9185   Total Payment: $ 2,269.

Physician Certification

I certify that the narrative description of the principal and secondary diagnoses and the major procedures performed are acurate and complete to the best of my knowledge.

Physician Signature:_____   Date:_____

FIGURE 1. ATTESTATION STATEMENT

nished on an outpatient basis or in an inpatient health care facility of a different type.
- the medical necessity, reasonableness, and appropriateness of hospital admissions and discharges.

- whether a hospital has misrepresented admission or discharge information or has taken an action that results in an unnecessary admission or inappropriate practice.
- the validity of diagnostic and procedural information supplied by the provider.
- the completeness, adequacy, and quality of hospital care provided.
- whether the quality of services meets professionally recognized standards of health care.

AMBULATORY PROSPECTIVE PAYMENT SYSTEM

The number of patients receiving care in ambulatory surgery centers, emergency departments, hospital outpatient departments, health maintenance organizations, and physician group practices is increasing each year. To manage the Medicare reimbursement of these services, Congress has mandated HCFA to develop a prospective payment system for ambulatory care.

To initiate the database needed to implement an ambulatory prospective payment system, physician and hospitals treating outpatients must code diagnostic information on physician office or outpatient or claims. ICD-9-CM is used to code diagnoses and HCPCS is used to code procedures. At present, a type of DRG system is not being required by HCFA.

Frequently, encounter forms, or super bills as they may be called, are used to collect diagnostic and procedural data for billing purposes. An example of such a form is provided in Figure 2. When an encounter form is used, quality reviews are critical. Because the encounter form can only list a limited number of diagnoses and procedures, those which are not listed must be coded according to ICD-9-CM or HCPCS, as applicable.

RESOURCE BASED RELATIVE VALUE SYSTEM

Beginning in 1992, the federal government began paying physicians based on a prospective payment system called the resource based relative value system (RBRVS). RBRVS is the outcome of a law passed in 1989, the Omnibus Budget Reconciliation Act, which required the government to set up a system of physician payment reform. The government opted to use a system already developed by Harvard University.

The resource based relative value system was created to make doctors' payments reflect the time, skill, and resources required for each procedure or office visit. The government

---

Billing Area: _____ Location _____ IP _____ OP __X__ Other _____

Admission Date: _0_ _4_ _1_ _2_ _8_ _9_ Provider Code: _____

Patient Medical Record #
19-11-12

Notes: 80 year old patient brought in by wife because of his ongoing belligerent threatening behavior. Been fighting, wanting to go out, forgetful.
PE reveals no significant physical findings. Mental status poor. Patient does not know date, President but does know he is at ABC Clinic.
Prescribed Haldol 1 mg. three times a day. Nursing home placement may have to be considered for his Alzheimer's disease if medication doesn't control behavior.

Hal Jones

Patient Name:

Physician Signature: *J. Smith*

CODE	PROCEDURES	FEE	CODE	PROCEDURES	FEE	CODE	PROCEDURES	FEE
	OFFICE VISITS		90320	Comprehensive history		20610	Injection of bursa or tendon	
	NEW PATIENT			**SUBSEQUENT CARE**		90782	Injection intramuscular or soft tissue	
90000	Brief service		90340	Brief service				
90010	Limited service		90350	Limited service		20605	Joint aspiration	
90015	Intermediate service		90360	Intermediate service		62270	Lumbar puncture	
90017	Extended service		90370	Extended service		89190	Nasal smear for eosinophils	
90020	Comprehensive service			**PROCEDURES**		88150	Pap test preparation	
	ESTABLISHED PATIENT		90784	Administration I-V meds		49080	Paracentesis initial	
90030	Minimal service		92960	Arrhythmia reversion acute		45300	Proctosigmoidoscopy	
90040	Brief service		36600	Arterial puncture		50200	Renal biopsy	
90050	Limited service		10160	Aspiration abscess or cellulitis and culture smear		87205	Stool Gram stain for inflammatory cells	
90060	Intermediate service							
90070	Extended service		87040	Blood culture		82270	Stool test for occult blood	
90080	Comprehensive service		85095	Bone marrow aspiration		26100	Synovial biopsy	
	CONSULTATION		36010	Central venous pressure line		32000	Thoracentesis	
90600	Limited consultation		92950	CPR		47000	Liver biopsy	
90605	Intermediate consultation		93010	Electrocardiogram acute reading			**UNLISTED PROCEDURES**	
90610	Extensive consultation		78003	Endocrine stimulation or suppression tests				
90620	Comprehensive consultation							
90630	Complex consultation		88160	Examination of blood smear				
	NURSING HOME FACILITIES		81000	Examination of urine				
	INITIAL CARE		88312	Examination of Gram stain of sputum				
90300	Brief history							
90315	Intermediate history		87210	Examination of vaginal exudate				
				DIAGNOSES				
789.0	Abdominal pain		239.4	Bladder tumor		250.00	Diabetes mellitus	
724.5	Back pain		585	Chronic renal failure		252.0	Hyperparathyroidism	
786.5	Chest pain		595.9	Cystitis		242.9	Hyperthyroidism	
564.0	Constipation		590.8	Pyelonephritis		253.2	Hypopituitarism	
786.09	Dyspnea		590.2	Renoathiasis		244.9	Hypothyroidism	
780.6	Fever of unknown cause		239.5	Renal tumor		278.0	Obesity	
780.9	Generalized pain			**GENITAL TRACT**		241.0	Thyroid nodules	
784.0	Head pain		180	Carcinoma cervix			**HEMATOLOGIC**	
729.5	Upper extremity pain		183	Carcinoma ovary		283.9	Anemia hemolytic	
729.5	Lower extremity pain		185	Carcinoma prostate		280.9	Anemia iron deficiency	
723.1	Neck pain		182	Carcinoma uterus		281.2	Anemia due to folate deficiency	
780.2	Syncope		617.9	Endometriosis		281.0	Anemia pernicious	
	CIRCULATORY SYSTEM		604.90	Epididymitis		282.6	Anemia sickle cell	
427.9	Cardiac arrhythmias		302.72	Impotence		285.9	Anemia	
425	Cardiomyopathy		620.2	Ovarian cyst		288.0	Neutropenia	
414.0	Coronary heart disease		614.9	Pelvic inflammatory disease		287.5	Thrombocytopenia	
401	Hypertension		601.9	Prostatitis			**MENTAL DISORDERS**	
402	Hypertensive cardiac disease		633.0	Tubal pregnancy		311	Anxiety depression	
428.1	Left ventricular failure		597.80	Urethritis		300.81	Briquet's syndrome	
424.0	Mitral valve prolapse		616.10	Vaginitis		300.11	Conversion hysteria	
428.0	Right ventricular failure			**MUSCULOSKELETAL**		300.7	Hypochondriasis	
424.90	Valvular heart disease		716.90	Arthritis		296.00	Psychoses affective	
	DIGESTIVE SYSTEM		727.3	Bursitis		295.00	Psychosis schizophrenia	
153	Carcinoma colon		710.9	Collagen vascular disease		306.9	Somatization disorders	
155.0	Carcinoma liver		274.9	Gout			**NEUROLOGICAL**	
151	Carcinoma stomach		719.9	Leg joint disease		436	Cerebrovascular accident	
575.0	Cholecystitis		729.1	Myositis		290.0	Dementia	
535.5	Duodenitis gastritis		714.0	Rheumatoid arthritis		346.9	Migraine	
562	Diverticulitis		726.90	Tendonitis		332.0	Parkinson's disease	
564.2	Dumping syndrome			**INFECTIOUS DISEASES**		780.3	Seizure disorders	
530.1	Esophagitis		490	Bronchitis			**RESPIRATORY**	
565.1	Fistula in ano		009	Gastroenteritis		477.9	Allergic rhinitis	
573.3	Hepatitis due to virus or drugs		098	Gonorrhea		493.90	Asthma	
564	Inflammatory bowel disease		054.1	Herpes genitalis		239.1	Carcinoma of the lung	
577.0	Pancreatitis		462	Pharyngitis		496	Chronic obstructive pulmonary disease	
211.3	Polyp. colon		486	Pneumonitis		496	Chronic restrictive pulmonary disease	
532.9	Ulcer duodenum		473	Sinusitis		011.90	Pulmonary tuberculosis	
531.9	Ulcer gastric		097	Syphilis			**UNLISTED DIAGNOSES**	
	GI SYSTEM			**ENDOCRINE**		290.10		
584.9	Acute renal failure		255.0	Cushing's syndrome		331.0	*Alzheimers Disease*	

FIGURE 2. ENCOUNTER FORM

---

adapted the system to Medicare and made it the reimbursement method for physician claims beginning January 1, 1992.

The RBRVS payment formula is divided into these three parts:

RELATIVE VALUE UNITS (RVUs) AND RELATED INFORMATION

CODE	DESCRIPTION	WORK RVUs	PRACTICE EXPENSE RVUs	MALPRAC-TICE RVUs	TOTAL RVUS	GLOBAL FEE PERIOD
10040	Acne Surgery	1.41	0.33	0.03	1.77	010
10060	Drainage of Skin Abcess	1.17	0.46	0.04	1.67	010
10061	Drainage of Skin Abcess	2.61	0.68	0.06	3.35	010
10080	Drainage of Pilonial Cyst	1.71	0.54	0.05	2.30	010

FIGURE 3. RELATIVE VALUE UNITS (RVUs)

1. Each CPT code has three relative value units (RVUs). One is for the work involved in the procedure, one is for the cost of overhead, and one is for malpractice costs. Figure 3 shows an example of the information published in the Federal Register, updating RVU amounts for CPS codes.

2. Each geographic area is assigned work, practice, and malpractice indices and they are multiplied by the RVSs as in Figure 4.

work RVU x geographic work
plus
practice expense RVU x geographic practice expense
plus
malpractice RVU x geographic malpractice
Multiply the sum by the conversion factor (31.001)
for the total payment

FIGURE 4. RBRVS PAYMENT FORMULA

3. The total of the RVUs multiplied by their geographic indices is multiplied by a "conversion factor." The conversion factor can change each year, and it can make Medicare payments go up or down significantly. For example, in 1992, the conversion factor was $31.001 for all services, but in 1994, it was revised to $35.158 for surgical care, $33.718 for primary care, and $32.905 for nonsurgical care.

The RBRVS system makes CPT coding critical to doctors' Medicare incomes, just as the DRG system made ICD-9-CM coding critical to hospitals' Medicare reimbursement. If the office selects the wrong CPT code, the payment will be inaccurate. If the office is using out-of-date CPT books, it risks having claims denied.

PPS IMPACT AND EVOLVING REIMBURSEMENT REFORM

The impact of Medicare's prospective payment systems has been widespread. The most obvious impact has been the financial decline of some hospitals, to the point where a number of small and rural hospitals have closed. Because the DRG payment rate is based on an average, some hospitals may find they are consistently above or below the average with respect to their costs.

Hospitals have become very creative in their efforts to survive. Managing case mix information, as described later in this chapter, is a key to that survival. In addition, changes in hospital management have included hospital utilization of contracted services for some clinical functions; mergers into corporations; development of new services and specialties; new ways of delivering care, and sources for nonpatient care revenue.

RBRVS is having a similar effect on physicians' practices. Because it is being phased in however, the full impact of RBRVS may not be known for several years. Nonetheless, physicians whose Medicare income is cut back under RBRVS are looking for ways to manage their practices more effectively, to market their services to the right patients, and to join with other practices so they can offer a broad range of service.

HEALTH CARE REFORM

At the time this book went to print, the topic of health care reform is being debated widely. Congress is considering several bills that would restructure the way health care is reimbursed and who would pay for the care. The bills vary widely, and the coverage, payment, and reimbursement issues are far-reaching.

Even though any law that is ultimately passed may be very different from the bills proposed in 1994, it is important to understand some of the areas of debate and some of the terms.

The most discussed goal of health care reform is to make sure all citizens have basic health benefits. Covering everyone, regardless of risk or employment or income, is termed universal coverage.

The package of basic health benefits proposed to be part of universal coverage is called a standard health plan or accountable health plan.

The main plans under consideration in 1994 are all rooted in "managed competition." Under a managed competition type of health care coverage, the government would encourage bidding or competition among health care plans for the basic coverage, with the goal of holding down costs while enhancing quality.

MANAGED CARE

Managed care is not a new concept. However, due to both prospective payment's limitations on reimbursement and to discussions of health care reform, it is an increasingly popular model.

While managed care varies with the model adopted, the Joint Commission on Accreditation of Healthcare Organizations defines managed care as "the provision of health care services efficiently to a designated group of members by managing patient access to and across a spectrum of health care settings."

Managed care systems may be divided into two general categories: health maintenance organizations (HMOs) and preferred provider organizations (PPOs).

Health Maintenance Organizations

The Health Maintenance Organization Act was passed in 1973. It created an alternative to the traditional indemnity health care insurance plan. In the HMO plan, the HMO has management responsibility for providing comprehensive health care services on a prepayment basis to voluntarily enrolled persons (members) within a designated population. There are several models:

A staff model HMO is a multispecialty group of physicians practicing at a facility which is the HMO and whose physicians are salaried employees. Members receive nearly all services at this facility and pay only a small copayment for each visit. Except for emergencies, members must be referred by staff physicians before receiving services outside the facility if they expect the plan to pay for the service.

A group model HMO is similar to the staff model, but there is no specific facility called an HMO. Frequently, one or more multispecialty groups of physicians contract with the HMO to provide nearly all services to members. Reimbursement is usually capitated (a monthly payment set in advance and independent of the services actually used) and may include an arrangement in which the group assumes responsibility for referral services as well as primary services. Except for emergencies, members must be referred by physicians in the group before receiving covered services outside the facility.

An individual practice association (IPA) model HMO is one in which the HMO contracts with primary care physicians and specialists to provide services for members in their private offices. Members generally are required to select one primary care physician who provides the majority of care and refers members to contracting specialists for additional services. Reimbursement is most often capitated to the primary care physician and fee-for-service to specialists.

Preferred Provider Organizations

The Preferred Provider Organization (PPO), also known as Preferred Provider Arrangement (PPA), is the second type of managed care. It is a fee-for-service alternative to traditional health insurance. In a PPO there is a contractual relationship between a group of providers and a group of patients (typically with a third-party payer as an intermediary) in which discounted medical provider fees and restrictions on utilization are exchanged for incentives that direct patients to specific providers. PPOs can be organized by employers, governmental bodies, brokers, insurers, or providers, although hospitals and physicians have been the most active. This arrangement offers the freedom of choice of a fee-for-service system, while encouraging the use of cost-effective providers.

ROLE OF HEALTH INFORMATION DEPARTMENT

The health information department is the primary source for the clinical data required for reimbursement, whether by

Medicare, private insurance, or other payers. Clinical data abstracted from medical records and coded in the health information department are submitted to the business office for placement on the claim. Often this is accomplished via computer linkage of the medical record abstracting system with the billing system.

Uniform Bills

Hospital claims processing, in general, benefits from uniformity. As a result of this concern, representatives from insurance companies and the government gathered in 1975 to develop an acceptable uniform bill. This group called themselves the National Uniform Billing Committee. The committee estimated that each hospital had to deal with as many as ten different forms in submitting bills to third party payers. To make matters worse, in over one third of cases, two or more forms were involved for one patient. The advantages of a single, uniform bill are obvious: less staff time and training for billing personnel, fewer errors, less paperwork, speedier reimbursement, and better coordination among third party payers.

In 1982, the committee released the Uniform Bill-82, or UB-82 as it became known. A revised version, called the UB-92, went into effect for Medicare claims in 1993. The UB-92 is intended for use by the major third party payers and most hospitals for inpatient and outpatient billing. The data on the form (see Figure 5) can be divided into two types: a set of data basic to most payers generally available from the hospital's medical records, and certain other elements needed only by a few payers (for example, employment status information is needed by some commercial insurers but not Medicare). UB-92 has spaces for nine diagnosis codes, six procedure codes, and one E code.

The health information department must ensure that complete data is obtained from physicians on a timely basis and that its staff accurately code and abstract data needed for submission of claims and subsequent use in analysis.

Physician offices use a different form for submission of claims to Medicare and other federal insurers. This form is the HCFA-1500 Health Insurance Claim Form (Figure 6). Provisions of the Medicare Catastrophic Coverage Act require ICD-

9-CM codes to be recorded in the section on diagnoses, and HCPCS codes to be recorded in the section on procedures.

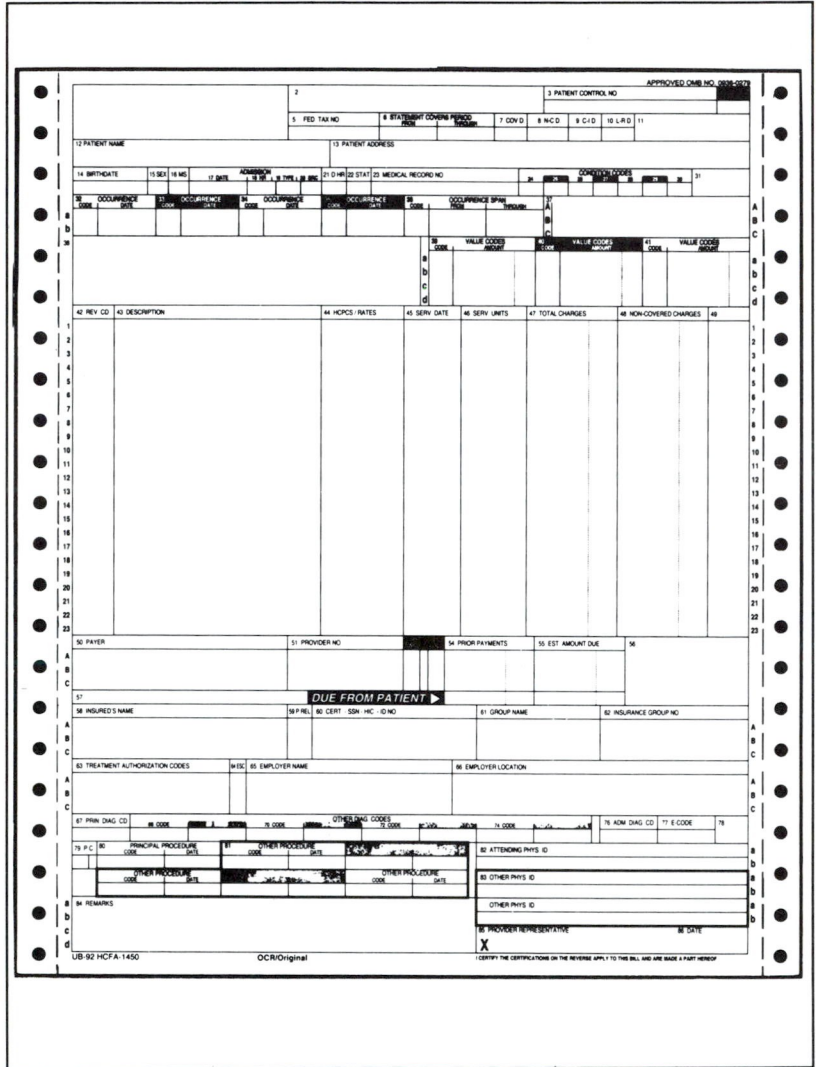

FIGURE 5. UB-92

DATA QUALITY

Health information professionals in hospitals or those providing services to physicians must be primarily concerned with data quality. There are eight basic components to data quality:

reliability, validity, completeness, timeliness, accessibility, confidentiality, security, and accountability.

Ensuring that data are reliable ensures consistency. Data must also be valid, that is, data which are abstracted and coded must accurately reflect the original data in the medical record.

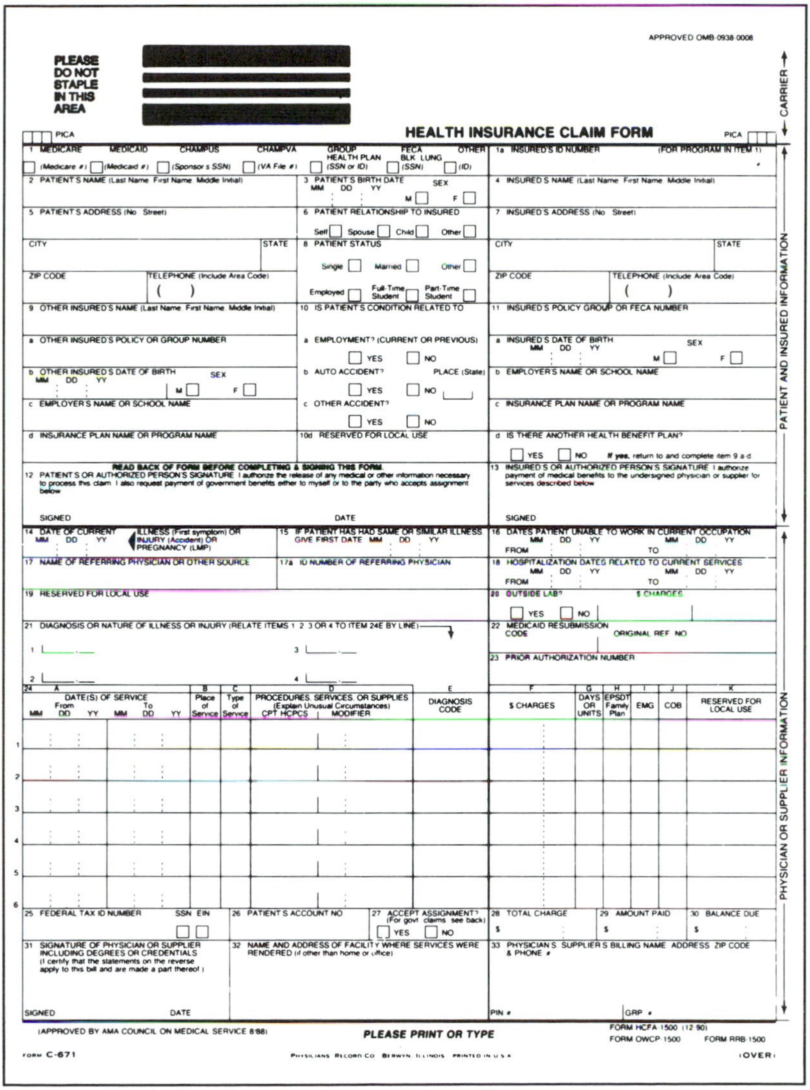
APPROVED OMB-0938-0008

PLEASE DO NOT STAPLE IN THIS AREA

CARRIER

PICA HEALTH INSURANCE CLAIM FORM PICA

1. MEDICARE (Medicare #) MEDICAID (Medicaid #) CHAMPUS (Sponsor's SSN) CHAMPVA (VA File #) GROUP HEALTH PLAN (SSN or ID) FECA BLK LUNG (SSN) OTHER (ID)
1a. INSURED'S ID NUMBER (FOR PROGRAM IN ITEM 1)
2. PATIENT'S NAME (Last Name, First Name, Middle Initial)
3. PATIENT'S BIRTH DATE MM DD YY SEX M F
4. INSURED'S NAME (Last Name, First Name, Middle Initial)
5. PATIENT'S ADDRESS (No., Street)
6. PATIENT RELATIONSHIP TO INSURED Self Spouse Child Other
7. INSURED'S ADDRESS (No., Street)
CITY STATE
8. PATIENT STATUS Single Married Other
CITY STATE
ZIP CODE TELEPHONE (Include Area Code) ( )
Employed Full-Time Student Part-Time Student
ZIP CODE TELEPHONE (Include Area Code) ( )
9. OTHER INSURED'S NAME (Last Name, First Name, Middle Initial)
10. IS PATIENT'S CONDITION RELATED TO:
11. INSURED'S POLICY GROUP OR FECA NUMBER
a. OTHER INSURED'S POLICY OR GROUP NUMBER
a. EMPLOYMENT? (CURRENT OR PREVIOUS) YES NO
a. INSURED'S DATE OF BIRTH MM DD YY SEX M F
b. OTHER INSURED'S DATE OF BIRTH MM DD YY SEX M F
b. AUTO ACCIDENT? PLACE (State) YES NO
b. EMPLOYER'S NAME OR SCHOOL NAME
c. EMPLOYER'S NAME OR SCHOOL NAME
c. OTHER ACCIDENT? YES NO
c. INSURANCE PLAN NAME OR PROGRAM NAME
d. INSURANCE PLAN NAME OR PROGRAM NAME
10d. RESERVED FOR LOCAL USE
d. IS THERE ANOTHER HEALTH BENEFIT PLAN? YES NO If yes, return to and complete item 9 a-d.
READ BACK OF FORM BEFORE COMPLETING & SIGNING THIS FORM.
12. PATIENT'S OR AUTHORIZED PERSON'S SIGNATURE I authorize the release of any medical or other information necessary to process this claim. I also request payment of government benefits either to myself or to the party who accepts assignment below.
SIGNED DATE
13. INSURED'S OR AUTHORIZED PERSON'S SIGNATURE I authorize payment of medical benefits to the undersigned physician or supplier for services described below.
SIGNED

PATIENT AND INSURED INFORMATION

14. DATE OF CURRENT: MM DD YY ILLNESS (First symptom) OR INJURY (Accident) OR PREGNANCY (LMP)
15. IF PATIENT HAS HAD SAME OR SIMILAR ILLNESS, GIVE FIRST DATE MM DD YY
16. DATES PATIENT UNABLE TO WORK IN CURRENT OCCUPATION MM DD YY FROM TO
17. NAME OF REFERRING PHYSICIAN OR OTHER SOURCE
17a. ID NUMBER OF REFERRING PHYSICIAN
18. HOSPITALIZATION DATES RELATED TO CURRENT SERVICES MM DD YY FROM TO
19. RESERVED FOR LOCAL USE
20. OUTSIDE LAB? YES NO $ CHARGES
21. DIAGNOSIS OR NATURE OF ILLNESS OR INJURY. (RELATE ITEMS 1, 2, 3 OR 4 TO ITEM 24E BY LINE)
1. 3.
2. 4.
22. MEDICAID RESUBMISSION CODE ORIGINAL REF. NO.
23. PRIOR AUTHORIZATION NUMBER

24 A DATE(S) OF SERVICE From MM DD YY To MM DD YY	B Place of Service	C Type of Service	D PROCEDURES, SERVICES, OR SUPPLIES (Explain Unusual Circumstances) CPT/HCPCS MODIFIER	E DIAGNOSIS CODE	F $ CHARGES	G DAYS OR UNITS	H EPSDT Family Plan	I EMG	J COB	K RESERVED FOR LOCAL USE
1										
2										
3										
4										
5										
6										

25. FEDERAL TAX I.D. NUMBER SSN EIN
26. PATIENT'S ACCOUNT NO.
27. ACCEPT ASSIGNMENT? (For govt. claims, see back) YES NO
28. TOTAL CHARGE $
29. AMOUNT PAID $
30. BALANCE DUE $
31. SIGNATURE OF PHYSICIAN OR SUPPLIER INCLUDING DEGREES OR CREDENTIALS (I certify that the statements on the reverse apply to this bill and are made a part thereof.)
SIGNED DATE
32. NAME AND ADDRESS OF FACILITY WHERE SERVICES WERE RENDERED (If other than home or office)
33. PHYSICIAN'S, SUPPLIER'S BILLING NAME, ADDRESS, ZIP CODE & PHONE #
PIN# GRP#

PHYSICIAN OR SUPPLIER INFORMATION

(APPROVED BY AMA COUNCIL ON MEDICAL SERVICE 8/88) PLEASE PRINT OR TYPE FORM HCFA-1500 (12-90) FORM OWCP-1500 FORM RRB-1500

FORM C-671 PHYSICIANS RECORD CO. BERWYN, ILLINOIS PRINTED IN U.S.A. (OVER)

Form courtesy of Physicians' Record Company

FIGURE 6. HCFA 1500 FORM

Data abstracted from the medical record form a database which is vital to management of the health care facility and the provision of information for many other purposes, including patient care, clinical research, medical education, and so forth. The health information department must take an active role, if not full responsibility, for the design and maintenance of this database whether it is in manual or computer form. The data supplied to the database must be complete and accessible.

The manager of the health information department may need to take an active role in ensuring that explicit content requirements for the medical record exist in order to ensure completeness. It may also be necessary to evaluate how patient care information is kept. Ideally, patient care information should be centralized so the entire record is available not only for patient care but also for processing.

The database should also permit access to the data contained therein. The database must permit retrieval of standard statistical reports and ad hoc information. The manager of the health information department must be able to access the database and design reports to meet any user's needs.

Data must also be collected and entered into the database on a timely basis. This is especially critical for data which must be submitted on a claim. Each day the health care facility is delayed in submitting a claim affects its cash flow and there is a potential for loss of revenue. Penalties may also be incurred by not submitting bills on time.

Health care financial managers generate daily reports on unbillable accounts (see example in Figure 7) and closely monitor the number of days' revenue in net accounts receivable. Net accounts receivable (often abbreviated "net A/R") is the total amount of money that is owed to the facility and expected to be received for patient services. (The total amount owed is generally greater than the amount expected to be received because of charity cases, discounts to third-party payers, and uncollectible accounts.) The number of days' revenue in net accounts receivable depends on many factors, including medical record completion by physicians, abstracting and coding of data for the claim, claims processing in the facility's business office, mailing of the claim to the insurance carrier, processing by the carrier (which may include request for additional information), and mailing the amount due to the facility. Typically, hospitals must wait 50 to 70 days to receive payment on an account. Anything that can be done to reduce the time means quicker access to funds and overall improved financial status for the facility.

UNBILLABLE MEDICARE ACCOUNT STATUS REPORT
(May 15, 198x)

Patient Identification	Admission Date	Discharge Date	Status Code*	Days Since Discharge	Total Hospital Charges	Outlier Cost	Physician Identification
321-10-0001	5- 7-8x	5- 9-8x	10	6	1,754	106	1234
432-20-0002	5- 2-8x	5-10-8x	10	5	3,794	542	2345
543-30-0003	4-12-8x	5-11-8x	30	4	12,490	2,452	3456
654-40-0004	4-29-8x	5-11-8x	68	4	7,640	271	4567
765-50-0005	5- 9-8x	5-13-8x	51	2	2,975	84	5678
etc.							
TOTAL	5	—	—	See below	—	28,653	3,075	5
AVERAGE	—	—	—	—	4.2	5,731	615	

Status Codes

	Total
00 (No problem)	0
10 (Awaiting M.D. certification)	2
20 (Awaiting PRO review)	0
30 (Day outlier pending)	1
31 (Day outlier approved)	0
32 (Day outlier denied—appeal?)	0
33 (Day outlier appealed)	0
34 (Day outlier denied)	0

Status Codes

	Total
40 (Cost outlier pending)	0
41 (Cost outlier approved)	0
42 (Cost outlier denied—appeal?)	0
43 (Cost outlier appealed)	0
44 (Cost outlier denied)	0
50 (Retrospective denial pending-DRG)	0
51 (Retrospective denial pending-Admission)	1
52 (Retrospective denial pending-Procedure)	0
53 (Retrospective denial pending-Other)	0
68 (DRG 468—hold for review)	1
90 (Hold for other administrative review)	0

FIGURE 7. UNBILLABLE MEDICARE ACCOUNT STATUS REPORT

The manager of the health information department must establish appropriate procedures for analyzing the medical record on a concurrent basis if necessary. A system must be in place which notifies physicians of incomplete records on a timely basis. Of course, to be effective these procedures must be supported by medical staff policies and procedures, and administration. Furthermore, the health information department manager must ensure timely and accurate coding and abstracting so that claims can be promptly submitted and so there are no errors which may results in insurance carrier delay of payment.

Confidentiality and security are also components of data quality. Data must be protected from unwarranted disclosure, loss, or damage.

Finally, accountability is an important management component of data quality. Accountability refers to the identification of the person or persons processing the data to ensure appropriate performance evaluations as well as to the controls placed upon data collection and processing.

Data must be traceable to their origin to ensure that corrective measures can be taken to improve all aspects of data quality. In the Medicare prospective payment system, accountability begins with the attending physician who ensures that the narrative description of the principal and secondary diagnoses and the major procedures performed are accurate and complete. Next, the person or persons who assign codes and abstract data from the medical record must be identifiable. If errors are being made, the manager of the health information department must be able to identify the type of errors and take corrective action. Corrective action may include additional training or education, or it may be disciplinary action. If the business office processes the data in any way after it receives it from the health information department, the person or persons entering data must also be identifiable and held accountable in the same manner as persons in the health information department. The person or persons who audit or evaluate the data and/or the database must also be held accountable for their actions. Finally, the manager of the health information department is accountable for establishing appropriate record processing and quality control procedures.

The quality control procedures that ensure data quality originate with national initiatives. For example, guidelines are promulgated by the federal government to describe sequencing and designation of the principal diagnosis. (These are described in the Uniform Hospital Discharge Data Set and Uniform Ambulatory Care Data Set.) The American Health Information Management Association has published essentials of accurate coding. The health information department staff should ensure that they select all diagnostic and procedural statements substantiated in the medical record and code and sequence them according to accepted definitions and coding principles to ensure the appropriate reimbursement category. A hospital must be cautioned against deliberately selecting and sequencing the diagnoses and procedures which will result in the highest reimbursement without concern for their substantiation in the medical record, accepted definitions, or coding principles.

Each facility must establish coding policies which incorporate national guidelines and address its own specific needs. Some hospitals, for example, may wish to capture more than the number of diagnoses and procedure codes allowed on the Medicare claim.

The health information department must establish standards of performance and measure productivity. Specific quality control techniques must be developed. For example, medical record audits should be performed on a regular basis from an appropriate sample of records.

The health information department should know precisely the level of coding accuracy of each of its coders and its overall coding accuracy. It should not wait for the PRO to determine this. Some hospitals hire independent consulting firms to evaluate coding accuracy; however, regular internal reviews can be very effective.

INSURANCE AUDITS

In addition to coding audits, many health care facilities have developed "insurance defense audits" in response to increasing requests from insurance companies and patients to reconcile the patient's bill to the medical record to ensure that all services rendered are charged accurately. In such an audit, physician orders are compared to the services rendered by matching the record item-for-item against the itemized bill. A hospital may wish to do such an audit for every patient, a sampling of patients, or upon request by an insurance carrier. Health information professionals or others experienced in both hospital operations and insurance regulations may perform insurance audits in hospitals.

CASE MIX MANAGEMENT IN HOSPITALS

The categories of patients (type and volume) treated by a hospital represent the complexity of the hospital's case load and are referred to as the hospital's "case mix." Case mix information is valuable to a hospital in order to predict its income and to evaluate any changes it may need to make to improve its financial position.

Case mix management reports can vary from the most elementary to the most sophisticated depending on the data elements collected. Basic data reported generally include the following:

> DRG
>
> Number of patients per DRG (in summary or detailed)
>
> Weight value
>
> National mean LOS per DRG
>
> Actual or average LOS
>
> Reimbursement per DRG
>
> Actual or average charges/costs
>
> Variance between mean LOS and actual or average LOS
>
> Variance between reimbursement and actual or average charges/costs

Other elements could include level of care, discharge status, outlier designation, special care days, financial category, clinical service per DRG, utilization profile, prepay source, and ancillary charges. The latter often play a major role in determining over-utilization or under-utilization as well as productivity indicators. Some hospitals have shown an interest in displaying the average daily cost per DRG, diagnosis codes, and DRG ranking. Many other variables may also be used by hospitals tailoring reports to their needs.

These data elements may be used to produce a variety of case mix reports. Basic reports may display information such as length of stay by DRG such as in Figure 8. Such case mix reports are used by hospital management, physicians, and governing boards to identify the high cost/low reimbursement factors in the provision of patient care. Careful study of these reports will determine areas of care which are cost effective versus those which may require modification to achieve a fi-

Length of Stay by DRG, 3rd Quarter, 19xx		
DRG	Our Length of Stay	Government Average Length of Stay
001	11.7 days	7.9 days
002	2.5 days	3.0 days
003	7.6 days	6.5 days
004	3.4 days	3.2 days

FIGURE 8. BASIC CASE MIX REPORT

nancial balance in the facility. For instance, in Figure 8 DRG 001 far exceeds the government's average length of stay, so may be a target for intensified review.

Cost reports provide a breakdown of cost by DRG and attending physician and, in addition, can be most helpful in establishing cost standards by DRG for monitoring of ancillary service utilization by physician or department. (Figure 9, provides an example). Comparisons among physician groups with similar case loads may prove useful, although the limitations of the data must be recognized.

Profit and Loss By Physician, 3rd Quarter, 19xx			
DRG 01			
Physician Number	Number of Patients Treated	Average Cost	DRG Rate
143	40	2006	2112
199	6	4796	2112
207	34	3672	2112
248	18	2985	2112
etc.			

FIGURE 9. CASE MIX REPORT BY PHYSICIAN

Case mix data on physician performance should be used with extreme caution, unless acuity or severity indexes are computed. A physician with above average charges per DRG may actually treat patients with more comorbid conditions. When case mix reports are analyzed, many questions may be identified which may be answered only by individual medical record review. The health information practitioner must ensure that the administrator and the medical staff use case mix data appropriately.

CASE MIX MANAGEMENT IN PHYSICIANS' OFFICES

Like hospitals, physicians offices must collect and analyze information on their patients. Such information is valuable for financial management of the practice, as well as assessing options such as merging with another practice, signing up with managed care organizations, or adding other specialties to the practice.

The following are basic data elements that physicians' practices are likely to need or to collect:

- The age and sex of patients.

- Patient origin.

- Employment status of patients.

- Patient utilization patterns.

- Payer mix.

SUMMARY

The health information department has achieved important status as the resource for the clinical data needed to manage a hospital under present financial constraints. It is critical that practitioners understand the financial aspects of reimbursement in order to meet the data needs of their institutions. With increased recognition comes increased responsibility. The manager of the health information department is accountable for the department's impact on revenue. This accountability must be demonstrated through systems and procedures which ensure smooth flow of accurate medical data. Health information practitioners may further enhance their importance to their institution through their ability to merge clinical and financial data and to anticipate questions to which answers may be provided through ad hoc reports. Health information practitioners must also keep constantly abreast of changes in reimbursement regulations and translate such changes into everyday practices.

STUDY QUESTIONS

1. Outline the history of reimbursement in the United States.

2. Distinguish between indemnity insurance, Medicare's prospective payment system, and managed care.

3. Explain why retrospective, fee-for-service reimbursement does not encourage cost containment.

4. Describe how payment is made to a hospital using DRGs.

5. State the purposes of peer review organizations.

6. Define data quality.

7. Explain the role of the health information department in the prospective payment environment.

8. Define case mix management and describe the types of reports which may be generated in a case mix management system.

REFERENCES

Aaronson, Peter, "Evolutionary Development of Systems," *Managed Care*, Vol. 9, No. 2, (February 1988).

Amatayakul, Margret K., *Finance Concepts for the Health Care Manager*, (Chicago: American Medical Record Association, 1985).

Bolms, Dale M., "A Professional Insurance Defense Audit Program," *Computers in Healthcare*, Vol. 7, No. 8, (August 1986).

Frith, Sandra and Janice Cannan, "Effective Internal Auditing," *Newsletter of CMRA*, (October 1987).

"Health care reform has a language all its own," *Medical Records Briefing*, (April 1993).

Health Insurance Association of America, *1988 Update—Source Book of Health Insurance Data*, (Washington, DC: HIAA, 1988).

Lichtig, Leo K., *Hospital Information Systems for Case Mix Management*, (New York: John Wiley & Sons, 1986).

"Medicare's 1994 rules effective January 1," *Briefings on Practice Management*, (January 1994).

"RBRVS regulations bring good and bad news," *Medical Records Briefing*, (January 1992).

Richards, Carol, "Managed Care—HMOs and PPOs as Alternative Health Care Systems," *The Professional Medical Assistant*, Vol. 21, No. 1, (January/February 1988).

Smith, Howard L. and Myron D. Fottler, *Prospective Payment—Managing for Operational Effectiveness*, (Rockville: Aspen Systems Corporation, 1985).

"Taking the risk out of managed care," *Briefings on Practice Management*, (March 1994).

chapter 13

COMPUTER SYSTEMS IN HEALTH CARE

INTRODUCTION

Approximately twenty-five years ago, Dr. John Kemeny of Dartmouth College said, "Knowing how to use a computer will be as important as reading and writing." Today, the validity of Dr. Kemeny's prediction is apparent. The health information professional now deals with both computerized and manual patient records as well as computerized systems in the health infotmation department. Health information practitioners must be skilled in the areas that this technology requires. The purpose of this chapter is to introduce basic computer and systems analysis concepts as they impact health care. The next chapter provides an overview of computer applications in health care facilities and describes health information department applications.

COMPUTER DYNAMICS

No other technology has developed as rapidly as that of the computer - and the future can be expected to see continued advances. An appreciation for the rate of growth in general and in medical applications in particular can prepare the health information practitioner for tomorrow.

COMPUTER GENERATIONS

The first practical forerunner to the electronic computer was a punched-card tabulating machine developed for the 1890 US. census. In 1946, as a result of the need for rapid, accurate scientific calculations in World War II, the first actual electronic computer - the Electronic Numerical Integrator and Calculator (ENIAC) - was developed. The first computers to become available commercially, the IBM 650 and UNIVAC I marked the start, in 1951, of what has been termed the generations of computer development. While various computer historians differ on the exact time frames, the following briefly describes the advancement of computer technology.

- First generation (1951-1958) was significant for computers being entirely electronic and able to store data and programs for reuse. These computers were immense pieces of equipment built of vacuum tubes which required special temperature and humidity controls.

- Second generation (1958-1964) saw immense changes with the development of transistors. Smaller computers could now be built that did not require such rigid environmental controls. They also had vastly superior logic, magnetic core memory, and magnetic disk storage.

- Third generation (1964-1970) computers replaced magnetic core memory with the integrated circuit. The integrated circuit placed what had been separate parts of an electronic circuit on a single "chip." Computers built on chip technology were smaller and faster, operating in nanoseconds (billionths of a second).

- Fourth generation (1970-1981?) began with a clear-cut technological advance - large-scale integration (LSI) which compresses not only the components of one circuit, but many integrated circuits on a single chip. LSI allowed the creation of the microprocessor. The microprocessor incorporates all the circuits needed to perform the basic functions of an entire computer and are now being put into microwave ovens, artificial limbs, touch-and-spell games for children, industrial robots, microcomputers, and so forth.

- Fifth generation (1976-?) and beyond is marked by small explosions of technological advances, making it harder to delineate time frames. The microcomputer made possible by the microprocessor certainly was a milestone. First available only in kit form to be assembled by the hobbyist-user the microcomputer revolution was forged when all components of a microcomputer were combined on a single circuit board. The fifth generation may technologically have started in the mid-'70s with a microcomputer from Apple Computers, Inc., but some would mark the beginning of the fifth generation with IBM's entrance into the microcomputer market. Apple products were at first directed to hobbyists, other home users, and schools, whereas IBM marketed its microcomputers (Personal Computer, or PC, became their trademark) primarily to the business community. Spreadsheet programs such as Visicalc and Lotus 1-2-3 were designed for use on IBM PCs to assist businesses in carrying out extensive profit-loss mathematical calculations. Microcomputers also became popular in hospitals. A study in 1985 reported that 75% of the nation's community hospitals were using microcomputers, with an average of seven in each hospital using them. The study also reported that microcomputer use was heaviest in health information applications - DRG assignment, abstracting, and word processing.

Client server processing has emerged in the 1990s. Client/server technology is a combination of mainframe (or host) computers and personal computers and workstations. A host computer or "server" provides data and services to the "client" workstations. The client handles as many functions as possible, thus reducing central processing unit time. The server handles functions that the client cannot handle efficiently, such as database management, security, and automated network management. The client handles the front end computing, organizing data into graphs and reports. The server supplies the data needs as well as any computing that requires extra machine needs.

FUTURE TECHNOLOGIES

The trend is toward networking microcomputers, rather than utilization of large-scale mainframes which require immense capital outlays and human resources to program and operate. The speed and capacity of the microcomputers can exceed those of mainframes. The sophistication and consistency of the human/computer interface of most "hospital information systems" has also lagged behind the easy to use technology of microcomputers. The emergence of simpler tools to access computerized data in microcomputers - such as the point and click mouse - provide more efficient methods for commanding computer operations than typing on a keyboard or even using touch-screens. Recent tools for incorporating images and drawings provide the flexibility of seeing actual radiology films, anatomical scans, laboratory slides, and so forth on the microcomputer.

Artificial intelligence, or expert systems as applications of artificial intelligence are often called in medicine, also depend on the ability to store and retrieve data from very large files and to network reliably. Optical disk storage technology is very new and already advances are being made in improving it. Standards are being developed to simplify the task of interfacing computer systems of different and even competitive vendors. Natural language programming will greatly impact computer use. This could result in knowledge systems with virtual intuitive capability.

Hardware will continue to reduce in size, increase in processing capabilities, and decrease in cost. Disk storage devices such as magnetic disk drives have been reduced to a fraction of their initial development size, while their capacity has increased. New disk technology includes lasers to record data. Entire computer systems can now be carried in a briefcase and have been termed "laptops" and even "palmtops." The benefits of the hardware miniaturization trends include increased use of bedside terminals in health care facilities. Such portable terminals allow the physician or nurse to enter new orders or review patient data.

Software is becoming more generic and is less often dependent on a particular brand of hardware to work. Systems will experience shorter life cycles because of the pace of development. Graphic user interfaces are front-end structures which allow information to be presented in a familiar format to allow a natural style of interaction without requiring a computer language. In other words, the user points to the area on a familiar icon and clicks the mouse to direct the computer.

DEFINITION OF TERMS

One of the major barriers in learning about computers is the unique vocabulary associated with them. Some basic conceptual terms are presented here.

DATA VS. INFORMATION

The terms data and information are often used synonymously. The term data refers to raw facts, figures, observations, etc. Information is defined as data which have been processed. Information is data that have been manipulated in a formal, intelligent way so the results are directly useful.

DATA PROCESSING

The distinction between data and information helps define data processing. Data processing is the collecting, recording, and manipulating of raw data which results in the generation of new, meaningful information. Unfortunately it is very easy to amass huge quantities of data which are never effectively transformed into information. This is not to suggest that data storage and transmission are inappropriate; the computer is highly effective in performing these functions. What too often happens is that data generated from a computer are considered information and no effort is made to pare down the data or make the data meaningful. Thus the full benefit is not derived from computerization.

As a first step in insuring that information will be produced by a computer and available when desired, all members of the health care team should understand the distinction between data and information and develop the computer expertise necessary to participate in planning data processing applications with the aid of a computer.

SYSTEM

Data processing does not occur by itself as a separate activity, but rather as a part of a system. A system is a group of interrelated elements which work together to accomplish something.

Elements include the physical parts or components of a system, such as pieces of computer equipment. Elements also include people with different types of expertise and expectations such as planner, creator, designer, operator, user, etc. Processes, functions, and procedures are also elements which make up a system.

Elements, however, cannot be arranged randomly. There must be specific relationships, dependencies, interfaces, and linkages between elements. A system implies order and organization. Thus, elements have specific, known relationships to one another.

In addition, the interrelated elements must work together. The mere presence of all the elements does not guarantee their cooperation or their ability to perform together.

Finally, all systems have a purpose. Goals are defined, and success of a system is determined by whether or not it meets its goals. The more specific the goals, the easier it is to determine the system's success.

With respect to computers, both "computer system" and "information system" can be described. A computer system is basically computer equipment working together to capture and process data. Computer system does not imply any particular type of data processing. An information system focuses on specific data processing applications. A "medical information system" may refer to the integration of all clinical data processing - the laboratory, physician order-entry, medication administration, and so forth. "Hospital information system" may refer to the integration of financial and operational data processing. Many other types of information systems exist.

DATA PROCESSING CYCLE

Data processing cycle refers to the fact that processing data into information is a series of cyclical steps. The steps include data origination, input, manipulation, output, and storage.

Data origination refers to the source of data. Sometimes intermediary documents (called source documents) are used to abstract data from their original place in preparation for input into the computer. For example, the medical record of a discharged patient may have data abstracted from it and placed on a paper source document, or "abstract."

Input refers to the transmission of data from the source to the computer's central processing unit. Sometimes preparatory steps are taken to input data, such as coding data into symbolic form or converting data from one medium to another. Some medical data are very commonly coded, such as narrative descriptions of diseases and procedures (using ICD-9-CM, CPT, or other classification system). Data abstracted from medical records of discharged patients are frequently input and stored on a computer disk until an entire month's data are collected before processing occurs. The goal of future technology is to make data origination and input as close to one step as possible and to make that step as efficient as possible.

Manipulation is the conversion of data into information. Manipulation involves three aspects. One is the production of information by classifying, sorting, sequencing, merging, matching, selecting, calculating, comparing, and summarizing data. A second aspect is controlling data accuracy, security, and assurance of computer system operation. Programs are written to check for logical errors, provide positive identification, and detect circuit breakage and other types of equipment malfunction. The third aspect of manipulation is file updating and maintenance. Because data processing is cyclical, data and information are continually added to and deleted from various files. Periodically, it is necessary to update master files and ensure that all data are organized properly. This regular file maintenance contributes to the speed with which data can be accessed from computers.

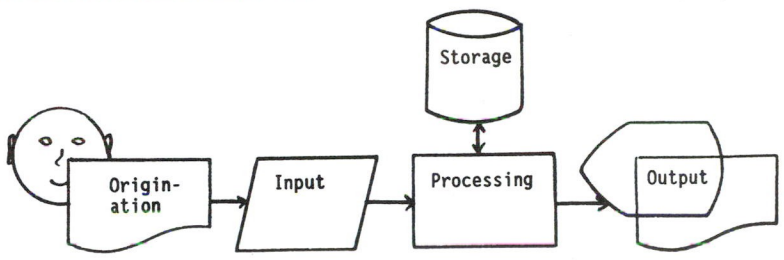

FIGURE 1. DATA PROCESSING CYCLE

Output refers to the provision of data and/or information to the user. The most common forms of output are displays and reports. Computers may also beep, produce tones or alarms, or even synthesize the human voice.

Storage is the final step in data processing. Both data and information may be stored for reuse. Many times the original data are not output, but only stored. Frequently, information is both output and stored. Storage consists of retaining data or information, organized in files, and in a form amenable to computer handling.

SYSTEMS ANALYSIS

Careful planning must be carried out to insure that all components exist in an information system and that the appropriate equipment and programs are available in a computer system. Such planning is generally encompassed in systems analysis.

Systems analysis is the structured approach to creating a computerized information system where none existed before or the modification of an old system to meet new information requirements and/or new equipment needs. Systems analysts direct the efforts and are responsible for the eventual design and implementation of systems. Although a data processing or information systems department is comprised of many specialists, the systems analyst generally has the most interface with the user.

SYSTEM DEVELOPMENT LIFE CYCLE

System development follows a logical sequence of steps. First, the present situation or existing system is analyzed. Alternative approaches to the design or redesign of the system are identified and evaluated to select the most appropriate. Then the new system is designed, details developed, and the new system implemented and evaluated.

Figure 2 displays a flowchart of the system development life cycle. It should be understood that in actual practice steps may be combined, performed simultaneously, or otherwise changed to meet the needs of the particular health care facility.

SYSTEMS ANALYSIS TECHNIQUES & TOOLS

The purpose of systems analysis is to ensure that user needs are met in the most efficient and effective manner in developing an information system. The health information professional must be knowledgeable about systems analysis techniques in order to formulate expectations for the tasks the persons involved are to accomplish and to participate in their development.

Over time different systems analysis techniques have been developed. The most common of these are the "traditional," HIPO, and "structured analysis." Differences in the techniques are most notable in the design phase of systems analysis.

In whatever systems analysis technique is used, a variety of tools are available to carry out the steps in systems development. Many of the tools used in systems analysis are also valuable for evaluating and implementing smaller-scale

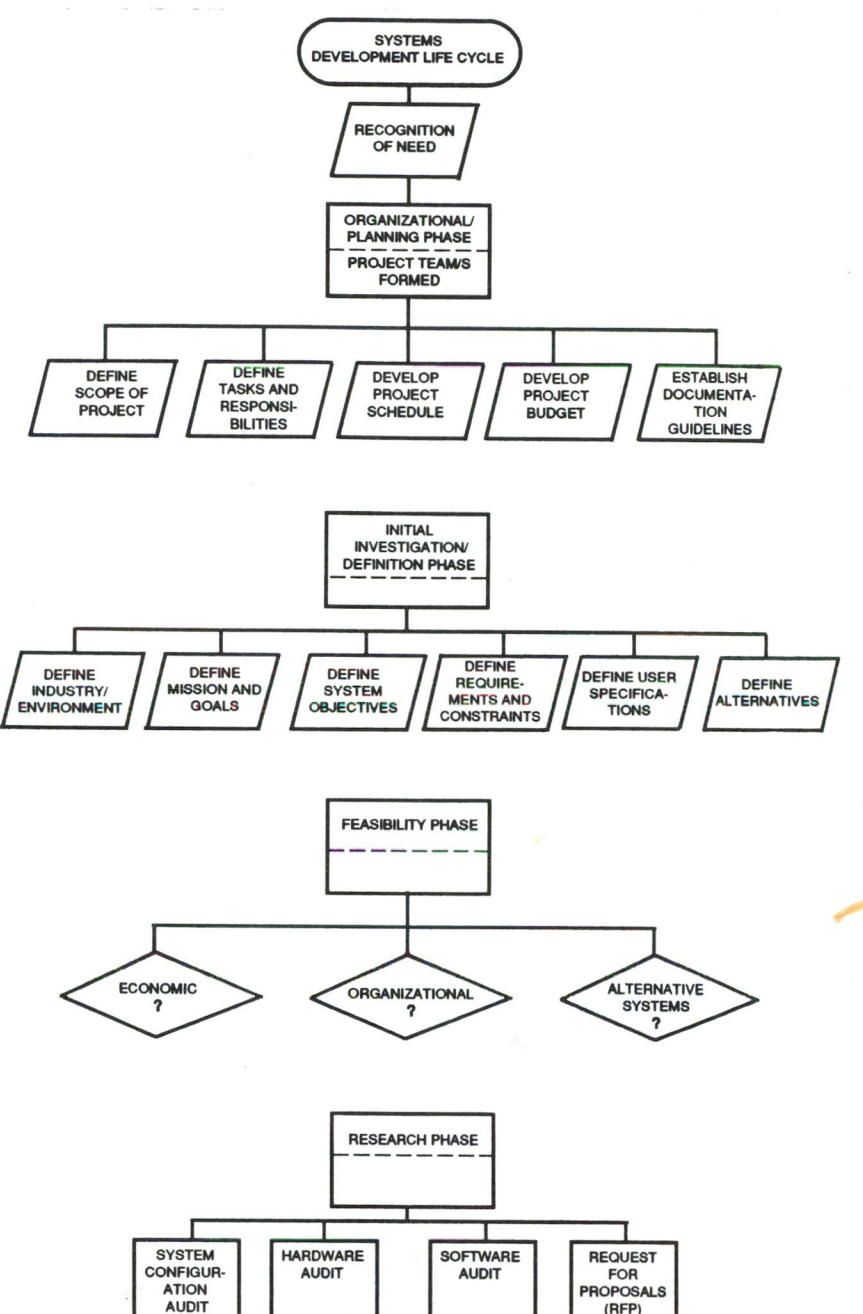

FIGURE 2. FLOWCHART OF SYSTEM DEVELOPMENT LIFE CYCLE

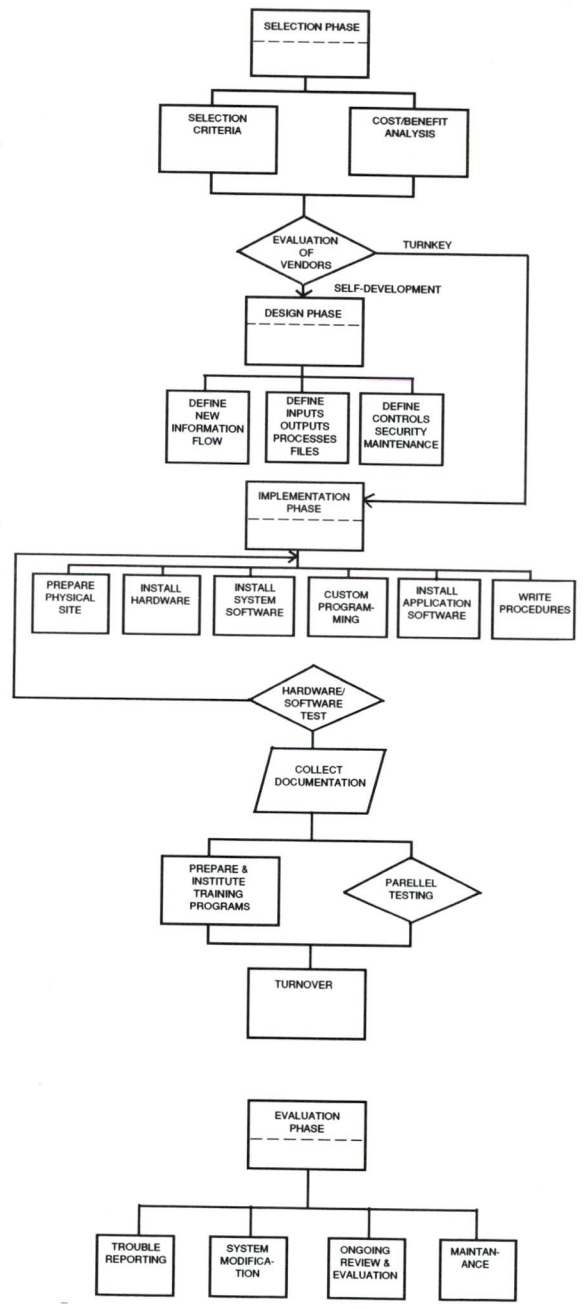

FIGURE 2. FLOWCHART OF SYSTEM DEVELOPMENT LIFE CYCLE

changes in departmental operations. Figure 3 lists some of the tools which may be used in each phase in the system development life cycle.

Organizational/Planning Phase
    Task List/Responsibility Matrix/Activity Diagram
    Gantt Chart/PERT Chart
    Project Budget/Manpower Usage Chart
Initial Investigation/Definition Phase
    Organization Chart
    Interview/Observation Checklists
    Questionnaires
    Forms File
    Resource Usage Sheets
    Procedure Manual
    Vendor Literature
    Systems Flowcharts
Feasibility Phase
    Report
    Oral Presentation
    Graphics and Pictorial Aids
Research Phase
    Configuration Chart
    Request for Proposal
Selection Phase
    Cash Flow Analysis
    Break Even Analysis
    Cost/Benefit (NPV, IRR, Payback) Analysis
    Weighted Candidate Matrix
Design Phase
    Traditional: Systems flowchart, decision trees and tables, program flow charts, equipment layouts, data descriptions, input/output sheets, etc.
    HIPO: Hierarchy chart, IPO worksheets
    Structured Analysis: Decision tables and trees, data dictionary, data flow diagrams, structured English
Implementation Phase: Training Manuals, System Test checklist,
    Test Results Logs
Evaluation Phase: Error Reports and Logs System Modification
    Request, Maintenance Schedules and Logs

FIGURE 3. TOOLS FOR SYSTEMS ANALYSIS

Organizational/Planning Phase

Groundwork for an information system's project begins by forming a project team consisting of representatives of management, key users, and systems analysts. The health information professional should be an active participant in project teams for the design of medical record systems. Software has been developed to help with this function. The scope of the project is defined and tasks and level of responsibility for each project team member are delineated (see Figure 4). An overall schedule and budget are developed.

It is also desirable to establish documentation standards early in systems analysis. In the course of creating an information system, a very large quantity of data are generated. These data would be worthless if not organized and standardized to facilitate communications. Documentation aids analysis, assists in design, provides control over system development progress and costs, ensures completeness, facilitates communication, and aids in training. It also facilitates the modification of systems designed in the past and allows systems to be modified for the future. Although the systems analyst is generally in charge of maintaining the documentation, as an expert in forms design, indexing, and filing systems, the health information professional may serve as a resource person in the design of documentation.

During the project three files are generally created. The project file contains the latest version of approved documents, and since it is a working file, also includes drafts, concepts, and preliminary documentation of work in progress. It represents the current state of the systems effort. Only one such file should be maintained, with one person responsible for seeing that it is appropriately updated.

A history file is also created to collect all final materials relating to the work performed. This is the permanent file usually maintained by the systems analyst.

A user file contains information derived from the content of the project file by reorganizing and rewriting as necessary to adapt it to specific user needs. Many files which may be exact duplicates or sections only may be maintained in the departments involved in the system. These files require updating if changes are made following implementation of the system.

Initial Investigation/Definition Phase

The initial investigation phase and the design phase are the points where most of the systems analysis tools are used. As a

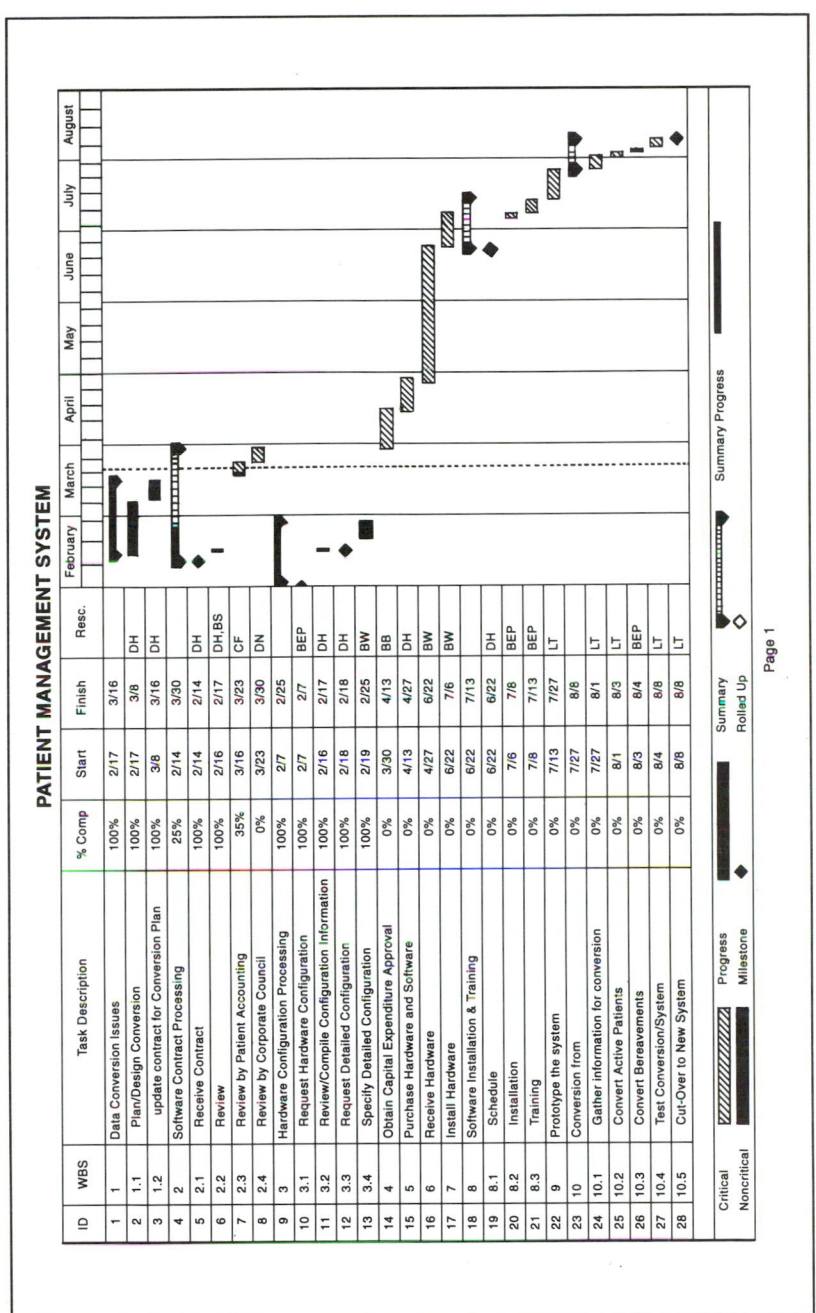

FIGURE 4. PATIENT MANAGEMENT SYSTEM

result, most of the documentation is generated at these two points.

During initial investigation all existing information about the environment in which the information system will exist and the objectives, requirements, constraints, and user specifications are collected. For example, if the health information professional was designing a record tracking system, the number of medical records in file, the number of locations where medical records may be used in the facility, the duration of time medical records may spend in one location and other factors relative to file area functions would describe the environment. The objectives of a record tracking system may be defined as generating a medical records pull list, determining current location of medical records, creating a report of overdue medical records, and so forth. The requirements might include instantaneous access to system data, two-hour ad hoc report generation, capacity to store 100,000 transactions, and others. Compatibility with existing computer equipment is an example of a constraint. User specifications are the outputs desired and data elements required to generate the outputs. The frequency of the outputs, their formats, distribution, and other factors should also be specified.

Information about alternative information system designs is also collected. This includes preliminary information from vendors selling turnkey products (i.e., systems installed as developed by the vendor) or packages (i.e., commercial systems that can be modified by the user). It includes information about in-house or consultant capabilities for self- or custom-development of systems. Consideration must also be given to whether the computer system will be in-house, shared, or used via a commercial service. Responsibility for maintenance and upgrading, flexibility in design, control over components and usage, and cost are all factors that must be considered. Process redesign must also be investigated as systems should not be installed to merely automate the current function, but to allow work to be done more efficiently.

Feasibility Phase

The feasibility phase is a decision-making point. Information from the investigation phase is completed and summarized. A formal report is developed and presented to administration.

The economics of implementing a new system, the organizational climate, and the existence of appropriate alternatives are considered in deciding whether to proceed.

Research Phase

The research phase is an extension of the investigation phase in which more detail is collected about the existing system and alternatives for system design are narrowed down. In the record tracking example, a system design that allows for key entry of record location may be one alternative and bar coding a second. In the research phase, the design may be narrowed down to several vendors of bar coding systems. The outcome is a formal request for proposal (RFP) that explains the existing environment and the requirements for the new system. The RFP seeks proposals, or bids, from vendors and/or system consultants.

Selection Phase

In the selection phase vendors and/or consultants' proposals are evaluated against selection criteria. Cost/benefit analyses for capital equipment purchases are also prepared in order to select the vendor or vendors who will supply hardware. Once again this is a decision point for management.

Design Phase

If a turnkey system is purchased, the design phase may be minimal or non-existent. Self-developed or custom-designed systems, however, must be developed in every detail.

Traditional design techniques include the development of a systems flow-chart (such as used to describe the steps in the systems development life cycle in Figure 2). From that detailed data descriptions, input/output sheets, file/record sheets, and logic descriptions are developed to aid in creating input formats, programs, file structures, report formats, controls, and so forth. Examples are provided in Figure 5.

As systems have become much more free-form and integrated, the traditional tools have been somewhat limited in their usefulness because they present the physical system or what is happening, rather than the logical system of how things happen. HIPO (Hierarchical Input/Process/Output) is a technique developed by IBM to aid in the design of a modular system, where a hierarchy diagram and an associated set of Input/Process/Output (IPO) charts provide visualization of functional structure. Figure 6 provides an example.

Printer spacing chart

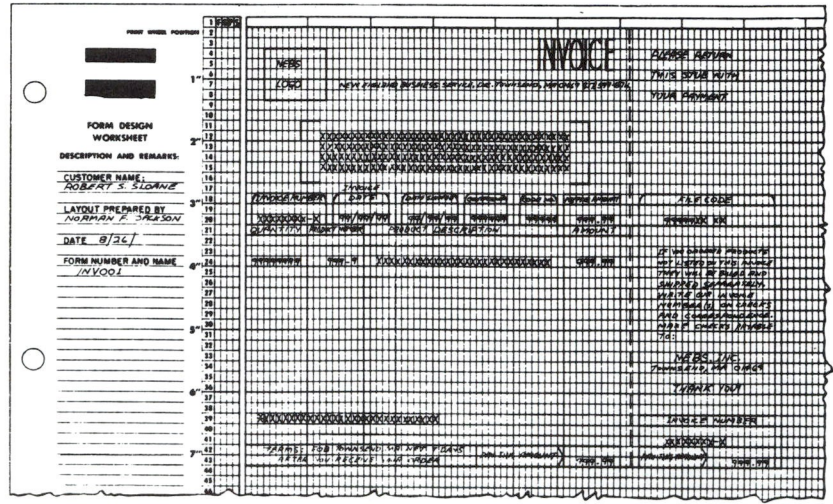

Title: RELEASE OF INFORMATION Rules:	1	2	3	4	5
Conditions:					
1. Confidential information?	N	Y	Y	Y	Y
2. Patient authorization?		N	N	Y	Y
3. Legitimate subpoena?		N	Y		
4. To pay hospital bill?				Y	N
5. For reason other than bill?					Y
Actions:					
a. Release information	X			X	
b. Charge fee and release information			X		X
c. Do not release information		X			

Decision Table

FIGURE 5. PRINTER SPACING CHART, DECISION TABLE, AND DATA DESCRIPTIONS

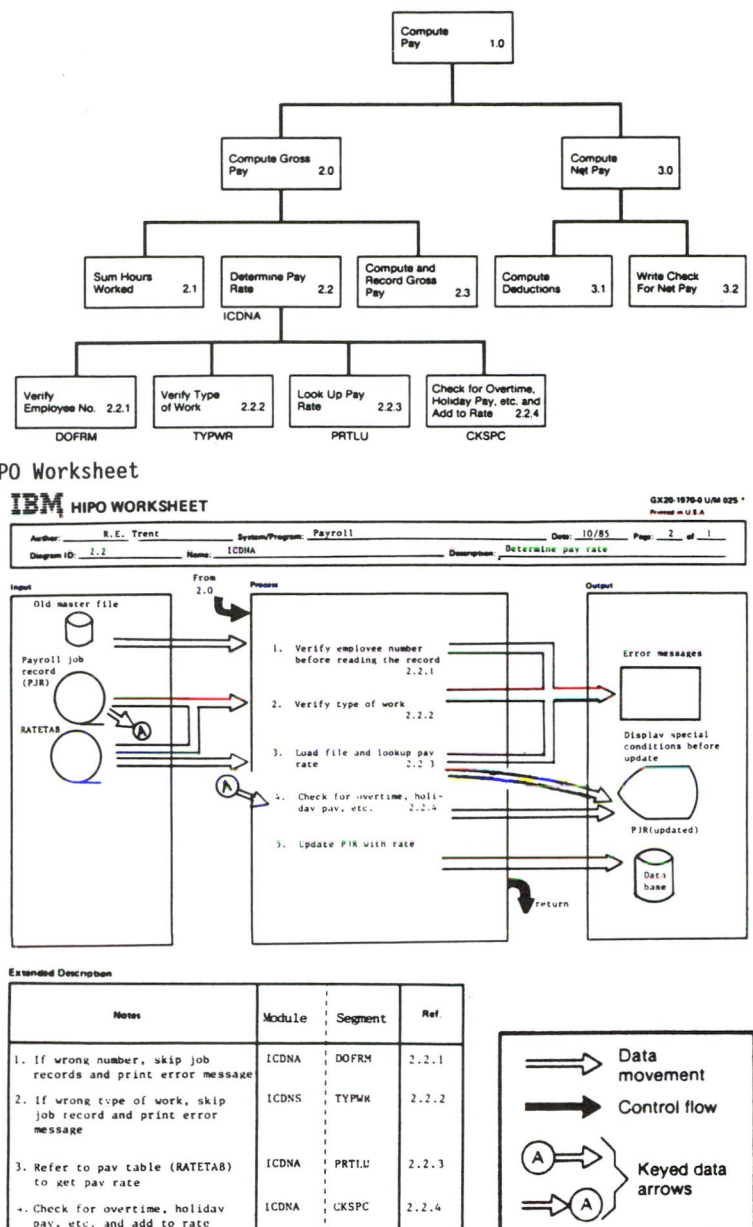

FIGURE 6. EXAMPLES OF HIPO TECHNIQUE DOCUMENTS

Structured analysis is yet another set of techniques and graphical tools for systems analysis. It uses the traditional decision tables and decision trees. It uses a data dictionary to define data elements and their relationships to other data elements; structured English for programming to differentiate between physical and logical systems; and data flow diagrams (DFD) to depict data sources, flow, and processes. Figure 7 explains the basic symbols and provides an example of the DFD.

Basic Symbols

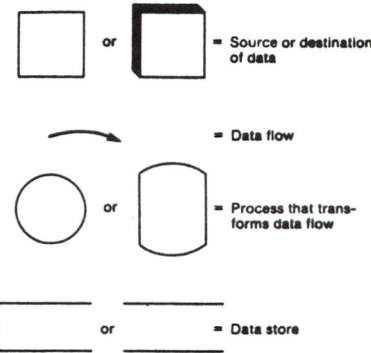

Example of Diagram

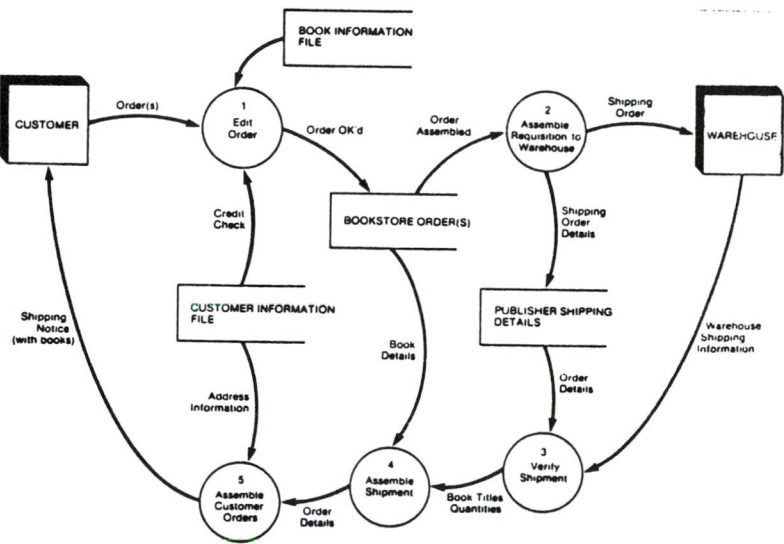

FIGURE 7. DATA FLOW DIAGRAM TECHNIQUE

Implementation Phase

Once a system is designed implementation takes place. Two substeps are often recognized - installation and conversion. The documentation created in the design phase or provided by the vendor is critical in directing the site preparation, installing of hardware and software, custom programming, writing procedures, and conducting the initial system testing (using vendor supplied test data - this may be called "alpha" testing). Once completed, conversion takes place. This involves detailed user training; parallel, or "beta" testing (using user supplied data); and turnover of the system to the user.

One of four different turnover methods may be used. Direct, or straight, turnover means that all operations are converted to the new system at once and all manual processing ceases. Parallel processing is the turnover method in which the new system is operated side-by-side with the old system for a period of time. In phased turnover, parts of the system are converted either directly or in parallel over a period of time. Finally in history processing the old and new systems operate simultaneously for a period of time (as in parallel processing) AND data existing prior to installing the new system are also entered. There are obviously advantages and disadvantages to each method which the health care facility must evaluate.

Evaluation Phase

The final phase of evaluation should be a continual one of solving any unforeseen problems, implementing modifications based on changes in regulations or other factors impacting the information system, and refining subsets based on new technology. Regular ongoing maintenance must also occur to reduce the risk of unscheduled downtime. All systems should follow the plan, do, check, act cycle to continually improve the process.

COMPUTER SYSTEMS

User involvement in systems analysis is critical. The user, however, must have some fundamental understanding of the nature of computer systems. As health information managers, health information practitioners must be well versed in computer technology.

As a system, the computer is comprised of several elements which work together to process data. These include hardware, software, and "peopleware."

HARDWARE

Hardware refers to the equipment in a computer system - the central processing unit and peripheral equipment including input, output, and storage devices. While all computer systems include at least one of each of these hardware components, systems vary according to the size of the central processing unit and the number and type of peripheral devices.

Computer System Configurations

Computer system configurations may be categorized as supercomputer, mainframe, minicomputer, and microcomputer. Supercomputers have enormous capacity and speed; the most recent advances include use of the pentium chip All other computer configurations may be found in health care facilities.

A mainframe computer refers to the one main computer in an organization. A wide variety of peripheral equipment and even microcomputers are directly (via cable) or indirectly (via telephone) connected to this one main computer. In order to accommodate such a variety of peripherals, the mainframe is usually a large-scale computer, that is, its central processing unit has a very large capacity for processing data.

A minicomputer is smaller than a large-scale computer, and thus not able to have as many peripheral devices connected to it. A minicomputer, however, may act as a mainframe, if it is the facility's one main computer. A microcomputer is an even smaller computer yet still fully functional. As its alternate name, personal computer, suggests, it is small enough (both in size and price) to be purchased and used by one person. A health care facility may have many microcomputers, which may or may not be connected (in a network) to one another and/or to a mainframe computer.

Most hospitals have been wired with twisted pair wiring; however fiber optic cables are being installed in many health care networks because fiber gives the capability to move large volumes of data quickly. Speed, image clarity, and cost savings are all benefits to fiber optic cabling.

Central Processing Unit

The heart of the computer system is the central processing unit (CPU). The CPU is made up of three sections: the control unit, the arithmetic-logic unit, and primary storage unit, or memory. The primary storage unit is often called the computer's memory. It temporarily holds the set of instructions (software) used to process data and all or a portion of the data being processed. Instructions and data are constantly shifted from memory into the control unit and arithmetic-logic unit respectively during processing. The control unit directs the operation of other central processing unit sections and all computer components (such as input devices, etc.). The control unit controls the flow of data via the program instruction it contains at any instance of processing. The arithmetic-logic unit adds, subtracts, multiplies, divides, compares, shifts, and tests the elements of data it contains at any instance.

In microcomputers, the system board contains microprocessor chips which house the CPU and other processors that drive the peripheral devices. In order for the control unit and arithmetic logic unit to perform their functions, they contain circuitry with read-only memory (ROM). This memory contains software that has been permanently stored during the manufacturing process. The chips which contain primary storage circuitry are comprised of random-access memory (RAM). RAM chips are those which can have data retrieved directly from their addresses, independent of the order in which they are stored. Data and programs stored on RAM chips are not permanently stored, but are transferred into memory when needed and out of memory when processing is completed.

Binary Data Representation

All computational devices ever invented are based on the concept of representing numbers via two states: by the presence or absence of a bead or hole, or the direction of a charge in a given position on the device's parts. Today the passage of electrons in one direction or another is used to represent numbers. This system of representing data in a computer via two states is called the binary number system. In the binary system, there are only two digits, usually represented as 0 and 1. To represent larger numbers, the binary digits, or bits as they are called, are grouped with each bit holding a position representing a multiple of two:

1 = one

10 = two (one times two)

100 = four (two times two)

1000 = eight (four times two)

10000 = sixteen (eight times two) etc.

To form any number in binary, each position is "filled" with either a one or a zero to indicate the value of the place. For example, the binary representation of 13 is 1101 (8+4+0+1=13).

The binary system can also be used as a code to represent alphabetic characters. For example "A" may be represented by the following code: 100 0001.

While health information practitioners do not need to become skilled in binary arithmetic or alphabetic representation, they should be aware that it is the system used by computers because when using a computer, the size of the storage devices and central processing unit are described in "bytes." A byte is a grouping of bits, representing either a number or character. One common grouping scheme used in microcomputers is the American Standard Code for Information Interchange (AS-CII).

Computer space is usually measured in kilobytes (one K = 1024 bytes) or megabytes (MB; MB = approximately 1 million bytes) so that a "640 K computer" would have a central processing unit capable of holding approximately 640,000 bytes (or characters), and a 5 MB magnetic disk would hold approximately 5,000,000 bytes (or characters). A typewritten, single-spaced page of text generally contains 2 K bytes.

Input Devices

Input devices feed data into the computer. Some common input devices in health care facilities include terminals, optical scanning devices, voice recognition devices, punch card readers, keyboards, and "mouses."

The most common input device for a mainframe computer is a terminal. Many different types of terminals exist. The most common type is composed of a typewriter-like keyboard and a visual display device (cathode ray tube [CRT]), or screen. Data are input into the computer system by keying the data on the keyboard, verifying the data visually on the display screen, and entering the data into the central processing unit by striking an enter key. Data may also be entered by touching heat-sensitive spots on the screen, or directing a light pen at light-sensitive spots on the screen. Handheld terminals, termed bedside terminals or point of care terminals in the health care industry, are another one of the many different types of terminals available.

Optical scanning devices operate by optically sensing marks on specially-designed forms or other items and comparing them to predetermined patterns. Some examples of these devices include:

- Optical scanners which read marks on specially treated paper. Examples of use may be in discharge abstracts or patient-completed questionnaires.
- Optical character recognition (OCR) devices which read specially formed characters may also be used for abstracting data, although the special formation of the characters limits use.
- Bar code readers that read bar codes from labels applied to medical records, test tubes, patient identifying bands, and so forth.
- Pattern recognition devices that read handwriting, thumb prints, and so forth, previously stored in the computer - offering positive identification in accessing computer-stored data.

Another type of input device, similar in concept to optical scanning is voice recognition in which sounds rather than marks are captured. Health care facilities are beginning to use this technology for physician dictation.

Punched card readers were the forerunners to optical scanning. There may still be a few applications that use punched cards, although for the most part new technology has replaced them.

In microcomputers, the primary input device is the keyboard, and the monitor may be used for verification of input accuracy. In addition, pointing devices such as a mouse may be used as an adjunct to the keyboard.

Before leaving the discussion of input devices, there are three concepts relating to the devices that are important.

In a mainframe computer system where there are many input and output devices, control units and data channels are used between the CPU and the devices to temporarily store and sequence transmission of data to and from the CPU. This equipment acts as a traffic cop.

The second concept is that data may be input in batch or real time modes. Collecting data and entering an entire batch at one time is called batch processing. Inputting data as it originates is called real-time processing.

The final concept is data communications, sometimes called telecommunications. Within a health care facility input/output devices are generally connected to the CPU via cable. But cable is expensive, so computer equipment may be connected by telephone wires or other communications media. This requires special equipment, such as a modem connected to a telephone that converts data at the terminal or micro-computer into a form able to be transmitted across telephone lines. Then, a modem at the central computer site converts the data back to machine-readable form. The communication control unit acts much like the control unit and data channel in a cable input system to control the flow of data. See Figure 8 for a diagram of the equipment.

A data communication system captures data at the point of origin and disseminates information rapidly to remote areas. There are many applications of data communications:

- Source data collection allows input and storage of data at a remote terminal for later transmission to a central computer. Many medical record abstracting services have users enter all data for a month onto a magnetic disk, then transmit the contents of the disk at one time.

- Remote job entry is also a batch processing application where data are entered at a remote terminal and output returned to a remote printer at a later time. Medical record abstracting companies also use this procedure where data are sent directly to the main computer as they are entered, but results are not received until all data in the batch have been transmitted.

- Message switching permits the sending of a message from one terminal to another. An example is electronic mail in which messages are entered into a computer system where they are batched and ready for the recipient to access whenever the mail service is accessed.

- Online inquiry makes information available in real time to a user who has keyed in a request at a terminal. This application is used extensively by retailers to check the credit status of credit card customers. Hospitals may use it to link to insurance carriers to check on coverage and process claims.

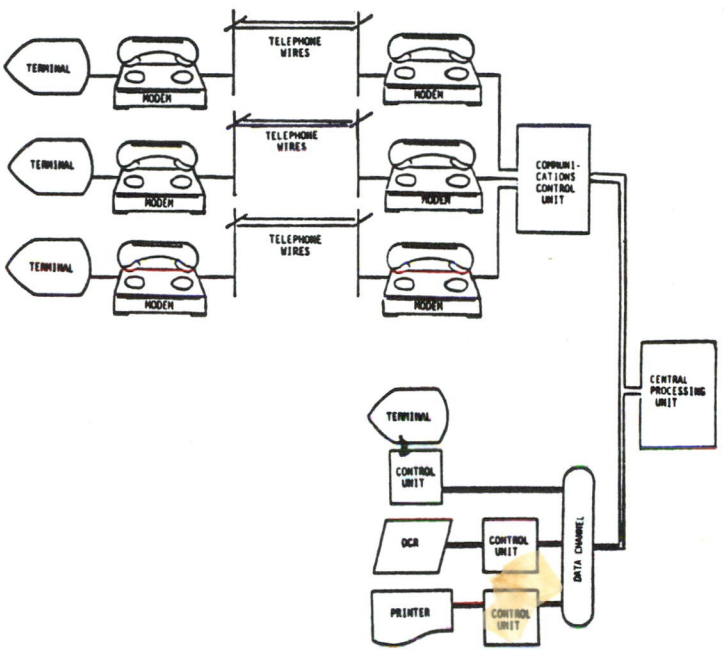

FIGURE 8. INPUT/OUTPUT DEVICES AND RELATIONSHIP TO CPU

- Time sharing refers to sharing of a computer's CPU by multiple users. Frequently, small facilities time share the use of a large computer at perhaps a local bank or school. Each access is billed to the user. The user may use the computer in a batch or real time mode.
- Networking is one of the most complex and important data communications applications. In this situation several whole computer systems are linked together allowing for real time processing. There are several different configurations of networks.

Networks with a mainframe and two minicomputers provide a central database and also allow additional modules to be added as needed by adding other smaller computers to the system (Figure 9). Here, subsystems such as pharmacy and

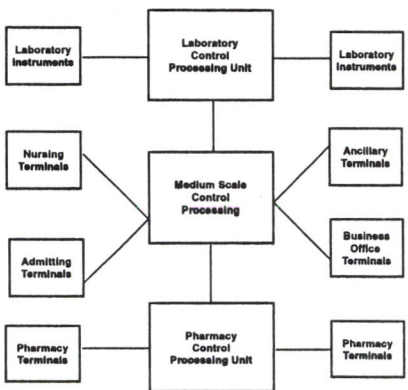

FIGURE 9. NETWORK USING MEDIUM SIZE HOST

laboratory have their own CPUs. These smaller CPUs are connected by cable to the mainframe CPU. The small CPUs communicate only with the central CPU and not with each other. All communications with terminals throughout the facility, other than within the laboratory or pharmacy systems, must go through the central CPU.

Minicomputer networks are composed of two or more computers linked to each other and attached to several types of output and input devices. A star network consists of a central host minicomputer and terminals and/or personal computers connected together to form a star. The star network may consist of dedicated subsystems such as the admitting, laboratory, and pharmacy systems shown in Figure 10. The central host computer provides the linkage to all the subsystems located on the arms of the star. In this configuration, if the central CPU goes down, the subsystems with their own dedicated processors continue to operate but communication throughout the entire system is not possible. A ring network uses a series of computers which communicate with each other directly without passing through a central host CPU. Each computer can perform all the functions of the network. If one CPU goes down, the others take over its functions until it starts to operate again.

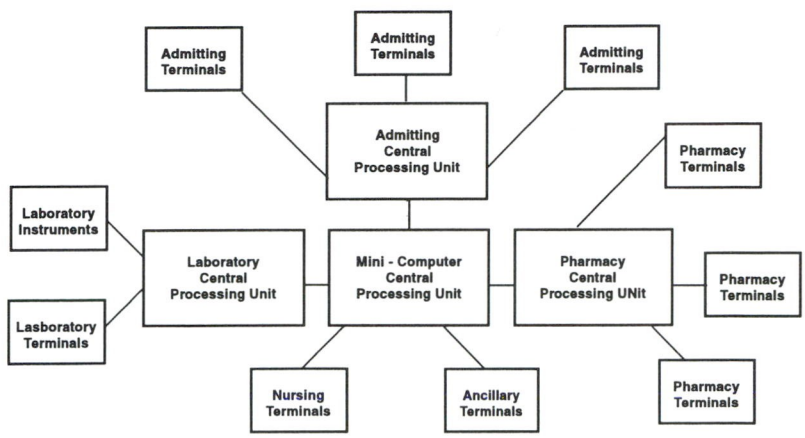

FIGURE 10. COMMUNICATING STAR NETWORK

Networks

Most networks fall into two categories: LAN and WAN. A LAN, or local area network, supports a geographically-contained group of users, perhaps a single floor of a building. (See Figure 11.) WAN, or wide area network, supports a geographically disbursed group of users, perhaps even a global usership. It is most often the case that a WAN is created by linking together many LANs.

LANs have different topologies, that is, different patterns for wiring users together and different computer programs that manage the electronic address book of users. Two common topologies are Token-ring and Ethernet. Similarly, the LAN may be composed of different types of physical cable wire: twisted-pair, coaxial, or fiber optic. Topology and physical cable characteristics work together to determine the speed at which the network will run.

LANs link microcomputers within a limited geographic area such as a single building or group of buildings. LANs were developed to allow the growing numbers of microcomputers to communicate with each other through electronic mail and text transmission, share hardware resources such as letter quality printers, and to share data. The computers are connected to each other through cables in a single line, a star formation, or a ring formation. LANs are expected to be established in increasing numbers in the health care environment and have important implications for health information professionals. Health information professionals must become assertive part-

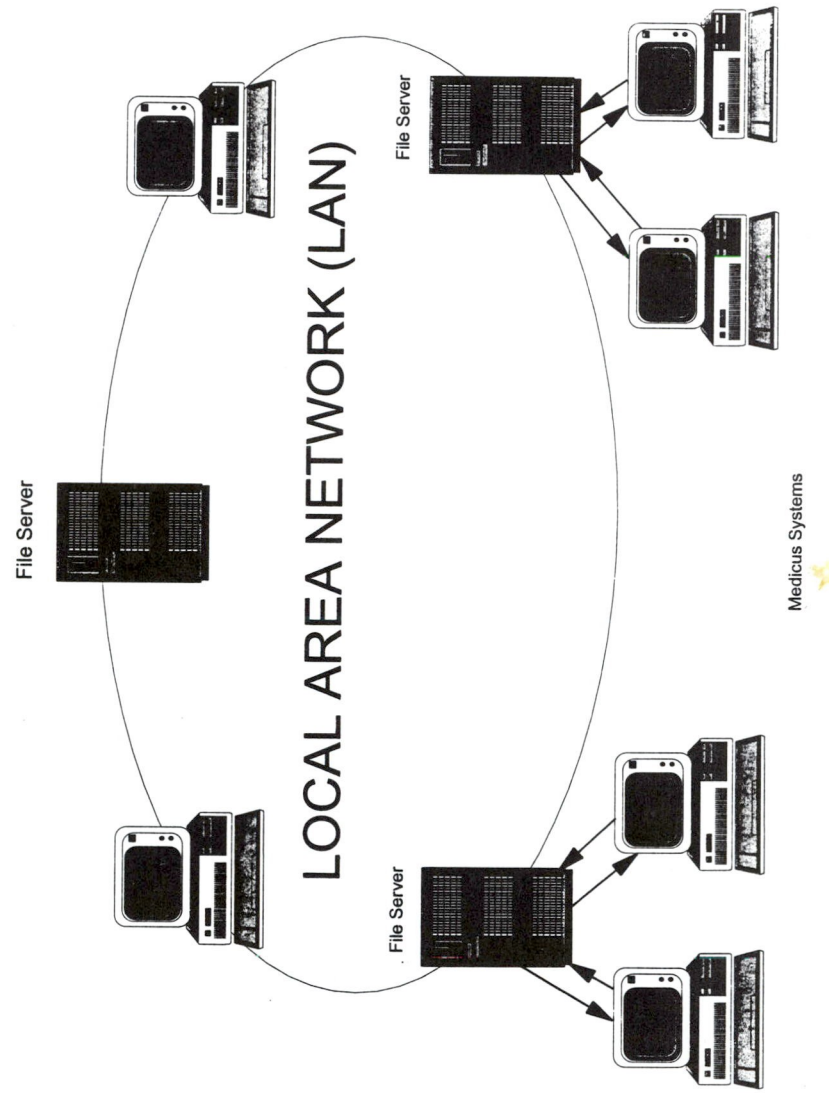

Source: Medicus Systems

FIGURE 11. LOCAL AREA NETWORK (LAN)

ners in the development of these systems through interaction with data processing departments and other health professionals.

Output Devices

Output devices communicate the results of the computer's processing to humans or to other computers. Among the common output devices are printers, visual display devices, audio response devices, digital plotters, and microfilm units.

Other than visual display devices, printers are by far the most common output device. Printers come in many sizes, speeds, and qualities. One of the most important distinguishing characteristics is whether the printing occurs by impact (of a mechanical part onto paper) or nonimpact. Impact printers are still the major type of printer for most computer centers as they are relatively inexpensive to purchase and operate, and they print at high speeds. Serial impact printers print one character at a time, using a type-bar, "golf-ball" type element, or daisy wheel type element. Line impact printers print a whole line at a time. Dot matrix printing does not utilize a type element but rather small rods that construct each character from rows and columns of dots (the matrix). The more dots included in the matrix, the sharper will be the appearance of the resulting print.

There are four types of nonimpact printers. These are typically found in user areas, such as nursing units and health infotmation departments, where printing noise must be minimized. Thermal printers use heating elements to construct characters on special heat-sensitive paper. Electrostatic printers use small pins that charge specially treated paper with electricity. Laser printers use a laser beam to create an image of a character. These printers produce very high quality output on regular paper. They also have the ability to print in various type styles simultaneously using different type fonts. Ink-jet printers are the fastest nonimpact printers. They employ an array of tiny nozzles to spray ink that forms images onto a page or another type of object. Ink-jet printers may also print in various colors and plot graphs.

Storage Devices

A final major type of peripheral equipment in computer systems is the storage device. These devices are capable of storing vast quantities of data or information on various types of media. Storage devices include magnetic tape units, magnetic disk units, optical disk units, and other less common devices. Storage devices are usually connected directly to the central processing unit by cable. All are basically housing and/or transmission devices for the magnetic tapes, magnetic disks, optical disks, or smart cards on which data are stored. There are advantages and disadvantages to each type of storage device.

Magnetic tape contains data that have been entered, via an input device, in a sequential manner. Any additions made to data on the tape must be made at the physical end of the tape. If there are many additions all of which will not fit on the end of one tape, a second tape must be used. Periodically these detail tapes must be merged within the CPU to create new tapes that are better organized. The sequential nature of the tape helps the central processing unit sort data. But because all data must be read in sequence in order to access data from it, the tape device is relatively slow.

Data may be stored on magnetic disk in a random fashion. The magnetic disk units, some of which can house several disks at a time, have read heads which pass over tracks within segments on the disks to directly access data rapidly. They can also store additional data in a random fashion for quick access.

Smart cards are also a new technology, more popular in Europe than the US. These are plastic cards the size of a credit card in which a microprocessor is implemented that can hold a small amount of data. One application of smart cards is to store portions of medical records so medical personnel with a smart card reader may have instant access to data needed in an emergency.

One other concept of storage is its relation to the CPU. When a storage medium, such as a reel of magnetic tape, magnetic disk, optical disk, or smart card is placed into the storage unit connected to the CPU, it is said to be online, i.e., immediately accessible to the CPU. When the storage medium is housed away from the storage unit, such as in a vault or on someone's desk, it is said to be offline. Offline storage is not immediately accessible to the CPU.

In concluding the description of storage devices, it should be noted that data are stored on any storage medium in files. Traditional file organization in a computer system is quite similar to a manual file system. The problem with traditional file organization is that the same data are often stored in many different places. This is referred to as data redundancy. Data base file organization solves this problem. A database is a collection of related data items that are stored together for multiple applications. Figure 12 is a diagram of the concept of a database.

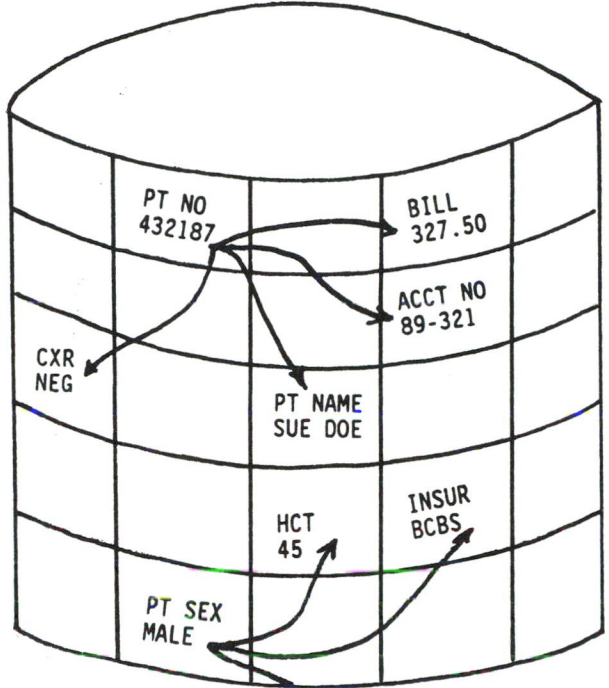

FIGURE 12. CONCEPT OF A DATABASE

Although a database solves many problems of data redundancy, creating a database is not nearly as easy as creating traditional files. Database management system (DBMS) software is required. Data security is also of greater concern, as more data are potentially available to more users. Data must be coded according to who may have access and controlled by passwords or other techniques. A database should be considered for storage of data that needs to be regularly integrated and quickly accessed.

Optical Disk-based Storage Systems

As mentioned in chapter 8, optical disk storage is an increasingly popular way to store medical records and related medical information. An optical disk based image/data management system is a networked computer system that uses optical disks as the means of storing large amounts of information. (See Figure 13.)

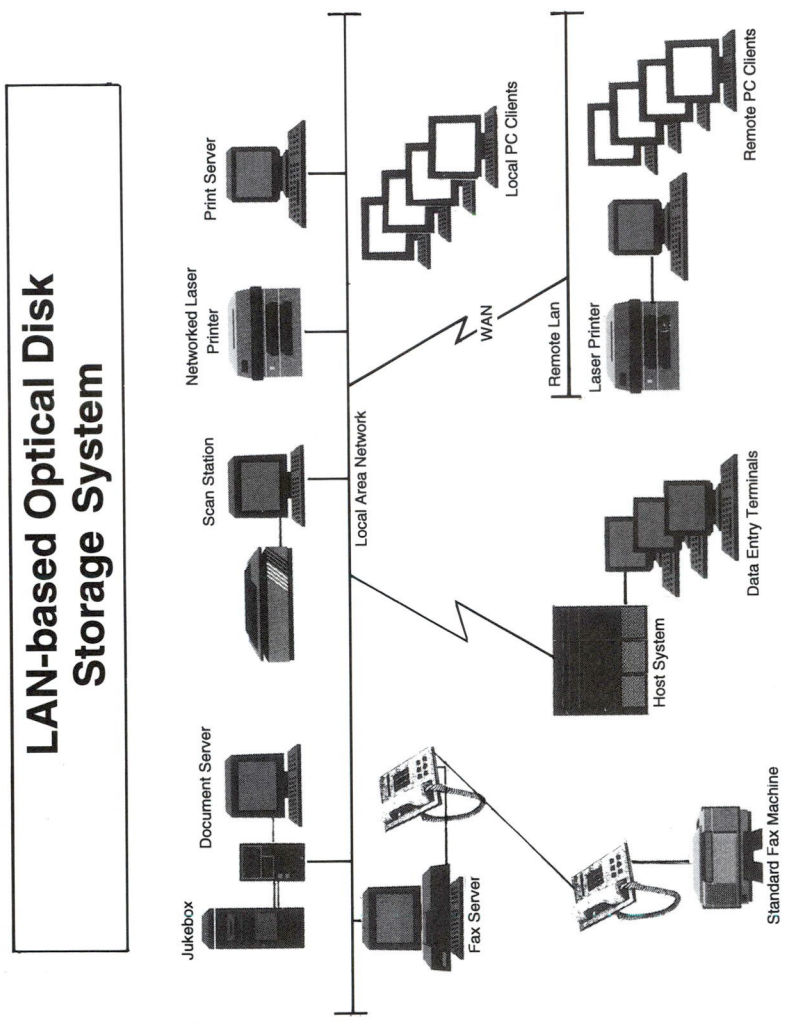

FIGURE 13. LAN-BASED OPTICAL DISK STORAGE SYSTEM

There are many different systems available on the commercial market, and they are very different in the way they operate and the applications for which they are used. The commonality is the ability to store and deliver representations of documents from paper as well as the ability to store data.

For health care facilities, this means that an optical disk system can store the entire patient record, including all its documents, as well as downloaded information from other computers, transcribed text, and even diagnostic images and records. Facilities using optical disk based systems report many benefits, including reduced storage space and quick access to medical information.

Some facilities add software to their optical disk systems that allows analysts to review incomplete records online, physicians to complete records online, and coders to review documents and code online. Such additions to optical disk systems increase its use beyond storage and retrieval.

Medical information is input into optical disk systems by several means. Paper scanners are the most common, and they work somewhat like photocopiers. Information can also be downloaded from other computer systems in the hospital, such as laboratory results reporting systems, or uploaded from word processors, thus eliminating the need to scan certain portions of the paper medical record.

The physical repository is the optical disk platter. Platters come in different sizes, shapes, and abilities; compact disks containing music are one example. Most facilities use write-once-read-many (WORM) platters in which information is permanently stored without the ability to modify. Even though a larger platter can store up to 150,000 scanned document pages, a facility will likely need several platters to store medical information. Jukeboxes, or libraries, store the platters and electronically retrieve disks when a user requests medical information.

SOFTWARE

Software is the collective term used to describe the various types of instructions required for computer hardware to process data. There are two major types of software: operating system software and application programs.

Operating System Software

Operating system software is a group of programs that allows a computer to manage its operations. Different types of operating system software are used with different brands and models of computers. Thus, the operating system software used on a large IBM mainframe is different than that used on an Apple microcomputer.

In general, operating system software causes programs and data to be loaded from an input device and/or online storage into the central processing unit (CPU). It causes the parts of the CPU to process instructions necessary to manipulate data. Operating system software also causes information to be output to an output device and/or online storage.

In large computer systems, operating system software also manages efficiency of computer use. It keeps track of all jobs that users want run on the computer. It monitors input/output so flow of data is smooth. It also monitors real-time processing response time, using a priority system so critical jobs are handled first. Information on system efficiency may be reported to the user from the operating system. The user can then make policy changes within the organization to increase efficiency. For instance, too many routine or low-priority administrative jobs may be run during the day. This can slow the response time for the medical information system. Users can be required to run these jobs at night. Operating system software may also keep track of and report charges for running jobs. In this way, each department using the computer is billed for the time it uses. In addition to running application programs, operating system software helps programmers write application programs.

Application Programs

As the operating system is specific to the computer hardware, the application programs are specific to particular data processing applications. One application program processes data for one purpose. For example, one program is required to process budget data while another is needed to run a master patient index.

Different levels of programming languages have evolved throughout the generations of computers. Level means how close to binary the program represents characters, the program's sophistication for processing data, and its ease of use. There are four levels of programming language. The lowest level programming language is machine language. It consists of instructions expressed in binary and is the only language a computer understands. While every program must be converted to machine language, it should be obvious that writing in this language is very time-consuming and prone to error.

To solve the problem of writing in machine language, yet still retain the desired precision, assembly level languages were created. Assembly languages use mnemonic codes in place of binary and are translated into machine language by an operating system program called an assembler. Thus, programming in an assembly language is not quite so tedious as programming in machine language. Assembly level languages are commonly used to write operating system software.

High level languages are used almost exclusively for writing application programs. They are much more English-like and thus easier to learn and use. High level languages are translated into machine language by operating system programs called compilers or interpreters. Thus, the number of high level languages which a computer can use is limited only by the existence of such control programs. While there are hundreds of high level languages, and as many different kinds of programs as applications, all high level languages use similar characteristics for writing application programs. All have:

- statements to describe variables
- statements which direct input/output control
- statements that alter the flow of processing such as for performing repetitive operations
- arithmetic statements which process data
- termination statements

Some examples of high level languages are FORTRAN, COBOL, PASCAL, MUMPS and BASIC. In the introduction to the computer generations BASIC was described as a training language, and is commonly used to program microcomputers. MUMPS, which stands for Massachusetts General Hospital Utility Multi-Programming System was developed in the late 1960s to provide interactive support specifically for medical database applications. Although standard MUMPS has many features in common with the more complete versions of BASIC, the syntaxes used in the two languages are different, as MUMPS was designed especially for handling data structures commonly encountered in medical applications.

Fourth generation languages are the closest to free-form conversation currently possible in a programming language. Two characteristics make fourth generation, or "very high level" languages, different than the first three levels. They are non-procedural so the programmer does not tell the computer how to do something, just what to do. A second characteristic is that fourth generation languages are generally linked to a database giving users access to predefined data.

There are three types of fourth generation languages. Database query languages allow a record stored in a database to be output in response to a query. Report generators make it possible to extract data from a database and create any type of report the user would like. With high level languages, users were limited to report formats that were pre-programmed. Many medical record abstracting systems use these programming languages, allowing the health information practitioner to instantly produce ad hoc reports in response to virtually any query. Application generators are the third type. They enable a programmer to create an application program with preprogrammed routine functions. Some individualized programming is required, but common tasks such as editing, inputting, sorting, and so forth already exist and can be incorporated into the program.

Writing an application program (in any language) consists of a series of steps in which the specific computer instructions are developed from the broad application itself. The steps include problem definition, program planning, coding, debugging and testing, and documentation. Every health information practitioner should be familiar with these steps. Health information practitioners frequently require an application within the department to be programmed for computer use. While the health information practitioner is the user and will not actually write the program, involvement in all steps ensures a better program.

PEOPLEWARE

The third major computer system component is "peopleware." While often the forgotten component in the world of "high tech," people are still necessary to design and build computers (engineers), create systems (systems analysts), write programs (programmers), enter data (data entry technicians), and use the information generated (users). Each person is a specialist, yet no one individual can operate alone.

COMPUTERIZED PATIENT RECORDS

A 1991 report from the Institute of Medicine defined a computer-based patient record (CPR) as an electronic patient health record that resides in a system specially designed to support users by providing accessibility to complete and accurate data, alerts, reminds, clinical decision support systems, links to medical knowledge, and other aids.

Several groups are working to educate persons, set standards, and remove obstacles to the computerized patient record. Among them is the Computer-based Patient Record Institute (CPRI), begun in 1992, whose mission is to initiate and coordinate urgently needed activities to facilitate and promote the routine use of computer-based patient records throughout health care. Others, including the American National Standards Institute and the American Society for Testing and Materials, are developing standards for characteristics and performance of computer systems.

As this book is published, there is not a computer system currently capable of fulfilling that definition, even though many facilities, health information professionals, and vendors are eager to move from paper records to computerized ones. The ultimate solution will likely require integrated systems, transitional plans, and open design. The health information professional's expertise in data collection, data accuracy and security, and current requirements for documentation will be critical to the development of CPR.

SUMMARY

An understanding of systems theory and computer technology is critical for anyone to survive in the Information Age. Health information practitioners must be a part of any project team designing medical record systems or computerizing the patient record. To be a part of that team requires not only knowledge of existing medical record content, data sources, systems analysis techniques, and components of computer systems, but an open attitude and ability to think creatively. The computer can open many doors - not only to improved data communications and ultimately financial viability and better patient care in the health care facility, but an improved image and expanded opportunities for health information practitioners.

STUDY QUESTIONS

1. Identify the major characteristics of each of the five generations of computers.
2. Define conceptual terms associated with data processing and systems analysis.
3. Describe the steps in systems analysis and the techniques which may be used to aid each.
4. Explain the three major types of computer configurations.
5. List the components of the central processing unit.
6. Explain how the binary number system represents data and calculate storage requirements for given applications.
7. List and describe the major features of input, output, and storage devices used in health care facilities.
8. Identify applications of data communications in the health care industry, especially networking.
9. Distinguish between operating system software and applications programs, and describe the features of the four levels of application programs.
10. Describe the importance of "peopleware."

REFERENCES

Awad, Elias M., *Systems Analysis and Design*, (Homewood: Richard D. Irwin, Inc., 1985).

Brousell, David R., "Industry Outlook," *Datamation*, January 1, 1991.

"Computerized Record is 'combination of technologies,'" *Medical Records Briefing*, April 1993.

Dick, Richard S. and Steen Elaine B., *The Computer-Based Patient Record: An Essential Technology for Health Care*, (Washington, DC: National Academy Press, 1991).

Dorenfest, Sheldon I., "Microcomputers and Software—Hospital Computer Use Soars," *Modern Healthcare,* (June 21, 1985).

Dykeman, John B., "Managing Records in a Rightsized Environment," *Datamation*, January 1, 1991.

Frankenfeld, Frederick M., "Trends in Computer Hardware and Software," *American Journal of Hospital Pharmacy*, April 1993, Vol. 50.

Hausam, Robert R., MD, E. Andrew Balas, MD PhD, "Computerized Medical Records: Dream or Reality?", *Missouri Medicine*, (October 1993), Vol. 90, No.10.

Information Packet, Computer-based Patient Record Institute, Inc., (Chicago: 1994).

Inguanzo, PhD., Joseph Louis Pol, PhD, "Building the Data Intensive Hospital," *Hospitals and Health Networks*, (October 5, 1993), page 80.

Lindberg, Donald A.B., *The Growth of Medical Information Systems in the United States*, (Lexington, MA: Lexington Books, 1979).

Little, MS, RRA, Eunice K., "Patient Health Record Imaging Systems and the Computer-based Patient Record," *Journal of AHIMA*, (April 1993), Vol. 64, No. 4.

Lumsdon, Kevin, "The Clinical Connection," *Hospitals*, (May 5, 1993), page 16.

McBride, John S., "A Case for Enterprise-wide Optical Disk Archiving and Work Process Redesign," *Healthcare Informatics*, (October 1992).

Miller, Cynthia, RRA, "The Electronic Medical Record: A Definition and Discussion," *Topics in Health Record Management*, (Aspen Publishers, 1993).

Rizzo, John, "CD-ROM Drives," *MacUser*, October, 1993.

Roach, William H., "Legal Review: The Case For and against Optical Disk Storage," *Topics in Health Record Management*, (Aspen Publishers, March 1989).

Shelly, Gary B. and Thomas J. Cashman, *Computer Fundamentals for an Information Age*, (Brea, CA: Anaheim Publishing Company, Inc., 1984).

Simpson, Roy, "Client/Server technology: A New Way to Manage Information," *Nursing Management*, Vol.24, No.5.

Sneider, Richard M., *Management Guide to Health Care Information Systems*, (Rockville, MD: Aspen Publishers, Inc., 1987).

Sumner, Mary, *Computers-Concepts and Uses*, (Englewood Cliffs: Prentice-Hall, Inc., 1985).

"The watchword for imaging systems: Know what you want to accomplish," *Medical Records Briefing*, (June 1993).

Waters, Kathleen A. and Gretchen F. Murphy, *Systems Analysis and Computer Applications in Medical Record Management*, (Rockville, MD: Aspen Systems Corporation, 1983).

Weber, Joe, "Power of the Computer-based Patient Record," *Journal of the American Medical Record Management Association*, (February 1993), Vol.64, Issue 2.

chapter ***14***

INFORMATION SYSTEMS IN HEALTH CARE

INTRODUCTION

Computer applications in health care have closely followed the development of computers generally. Computers were initially designed to perform arithmetic operations quickly and reliably. The first major application area, then, was accounting. In hospitals, and other health care facilities, computers were first used for billing, payroll, accounts management, and so forth. The first health related applications were those requiring arithmetic operations and which related to the accounting functions: registration-admission, discharge, and transfer (R-ADT); census; hospital statistics; abstracting of medical records; and indexing.

As database programming capabilities and mass storage grew, computers came to be used for storage and retrieval functions as well. "Total hospital information systems" were designed to automate laboratory results reporting; physician order-entry; medication administration; and inventory control in the pharmacy, central supply, and dietary areas.

Today, the emphasis is less on "total" hospital information systems comprised of modules all feeding into one central processing area. Rather, the focus is on developing interactive systems - administrative and clinical information systems which may operate independently and have interfaces with other existing systems through networking.

These types of systems can be developed when vendors use an open system strategy. Where computer systems of different types and different vendors work together because standards for operating systems, interfaces, and programming languages allow communication across the boundaries of a wide spectrum of vendors. Adhering to the standards allows this linking of information technology.

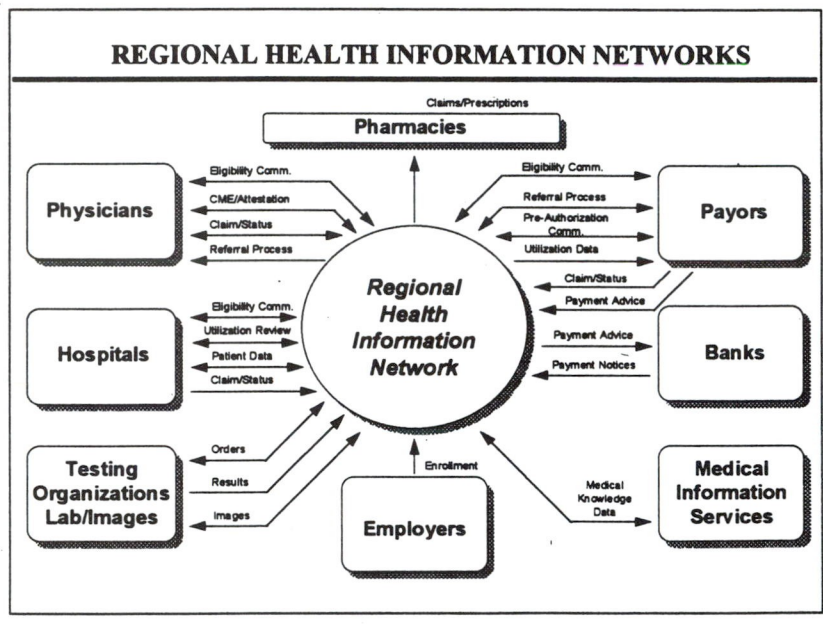

Source: Ameritech

FIGURE 1. REGIONAL HEALTH INFORMATION NETWORKS

In addition, health care systems realizing a need to streamline and share information, reduce data redundancy, and improve the overall community health status, have started forming Community Health Information Networks (CHIN) and Regional Health Information Networks (RHIN). These systems link hospitals, insurance companies, and physicians' offices, allowing data sharing. Figure 1 illustrates such a network.

NEW INFORMATION SYSTEMS

A detailed analysis of object-oriented technology is beyond the scope of this textbook. However, a few highlights can illustrate the principles behind it and the benefits of using it. Computer-based information systems can be comprised of literally dozens of software programs. These programs are linked and work together to provide all of the data processing functions of the system to the user. For example, major functions of a medical record system might include a master patient index, medical record number assignment, coding and abstracting, chart completion tracking, transcription, and so on. All of these are pieces of a large and complex information system.

In this technology, "objects" and the communications between them are the basic building blocks of the software product. Just as in common usage or as defined in a typical dictionary, objects can be thought of simply and non technically, as person, places, or things. In the domain of a medical records system, objects could exist for a patient, physician, and coder (persons); for a hospital, clinic, and nursing home (places); and for a chart, card embosser, optical scanner, the billing system, and ICD-9-CM codes (things).

Current developments in input devices have enabled considerable progress to be made in the concept of a clinical workstation. For example, image scanning has improved radiology reporting. Bar coding has improved inventory control and tracking applications.

The actual processing performed by computers also continues to be improved in many ways. Increasing memory and storage capacity, as well as miniaturization of processing hardware have greatly enhanced processing capability and speed. For example, encoding, wherein the computer prompts the coder with a series of questions about the diagnosis entered and quickly assigns the correct code from thousands of possibilities, has been made possible through computer technology.

Miniaturization has brought computer power to many people via microprocessors in specialized equipment and microcomputers; and, advanced data communications capabilities between microcomputers and other computers provide linkages never possible before. Patients can receive improved care with small bedside terminals linked to a mainframe. Billing can be accomplished on a more timely basis with direct transfer of claims to insurance companies.

Artificial intelligence is the most sophisticated application of computers to date. Artificial intelligence is a special type of computer programming in which researchers develop models that enable computers to handle functions that would require the intellectual capabilities of humans. Artificial intelligence has been used to develop simulations of events for training and analysis. For example, flight simulations are used to train pilots. In health care, artificial intelligence is being used in "expert systems." These are computer-based systems that capture the rules of thumb, unwritten procedures, and intuitive judgments of experts in a field. Medical diagnosis and treatment planning systems are currently under development.

SUMMARY OF INSTALLED SYSTEMS, 1987-1992						
SYSTEM TYPE	1987	1988	1989	1990	1991	1992
Financial System	5,579	5,622	5,557	5,618	5,698	5,732
Patient Care System	2,451	2,670	2,765	2,870	3,210	3,253
Laboratory System	2,387	2,646	2,472	2,742	3,028	3,456
Radiology System	457	728	939	1,218	1,383	1,625
Pharmacy System	1,561	1,903	2,597	3,037	3,507	3,895
Non-Hosp Laboratory	-	-	806	794	927	988
Non-Hosp Radiology	-	-	129	186	216	224

Source: R. Johnson, Danville, Ca.,"Computer Trends for Health Care — A Vendor Review," *Proceedings,* 1994 HIMSS, Chicago, Il

FIGURE 2. COMPUTER APPLICATIONS IN COMMUNITY HOSPITALS 100+BEDS

Computer usage in health care is very widespread. Figure 2 summarizes the extent of computer use in community hospitals of over 100 beds. The application of "medical records" refers to medical record coding, abstracting, and so forth. It does not refer to the content of the medical record.

As Figure 2 indicates, nearly every community hospital has a computer system. Many hospitals also own several microcomputers, and may share the use of still other computers, or use commercial computer service bureaus as well. Other types of health care facilities also use computers. In general, computer use in health care may be categorized into three types: financial, administrative, and clinical.

FINANCIAL APPLICATIONS

Financial applications include those related primarily to billing and accounts management. Although most hospitals have had these functions automated for many years, they continue to receive significant attention from system developers. Financial stability of a health care facility is critical, thus better methods for improving the capture of charges, processing and transmitting claims, managing accounts receivable, and so forth are extremely important.

Linking financial data with clinical data provides health care systems with the ability to trend utilization of services by practitioner to assist with managing resources. Discussions of health care reform are moving toward capitated payments, so this information may be more critical in the future.

CHARGE CAPTURING

Third-party payers are very concerned that they pay only for medically necessary services the patient actually received. Computerized charge systems can produce more accurate bills. In a totally automated system, every medication provided, laboratory test performed, meal served, and so forth can be entered into the patient's medical record, with the appropriate charge recorded on the bill.

COST ACCOUNTING AND CASE MIX MANAGEMENT

The charge system is enhanced by automated cost accounting and case mix management. Capturing actual costs for each service has been difficult for facilities, as each service is a collection of many elements. Computerized cost accounting can make cost determination somewhat easier. It is important for facilities to know actual costs because payers of hospital claims impose many restrictions on what they will pay and how much they will pay. Determining actual costs helps a facility set reasonable charges and demonstrates to any payer how those charges were determined.

If the facility also knows its case mix it can identify the services it should focus on providing and the services it may wish to discontinue. Case mix is the categorization of patients (by type and number) treated by a facility. The assignment of each patient to a case type, either a DRG, severity of illness index, or other system is best performed in the health information department aided by a computerized "DRG grouper," severity of illness, or other system.

CLAIMS PROCESSING

Transmitting claims to payers in a timely manner is as important as accuracy of charge information. The faster the facility gets a claim to a payer, the sooner the facility is reimbursed. The process of transmitting claims via data communications is called electronic medical claims submission (EMCS). EMCS has been made possible by the implementation of the HCFA Uniform Bill 82 (UB-82) and by the National Electronic Information Corporation (NEIC). NEIC is a cooperative effort of the nation's largest private health insurance carriers to establish a national clearinghouse for electronic submission of claims.

The process of medical record coding has also been automated and is often considered a financial application. Encoders are computer programs that allow a coder to enter a diagnosis and be prompted to promote additional information from the medical record pertinent to the coding process. Ultimately, the computer provides a code. Encoders improve the consistency of coding. The accuracy of encoders depends upon the ability of the coder to provide the correct information, especially its principal diagnosis. The degree to which encoders improve coding accuracy and productivity has not been fully researched.

Another computer innovation - the smart card - is being evaluated to assist claims processing. A smart card is a piece of plastic the size of a credit card on which there may be up to four types of data storage. The smart card can be embossed with the patient's name and other identifying data. A magnetic strip on the back stores a small amount of additional data. In addition, these cards may also contain a microprocessor chip and/or laser storage area. The smart card can be read by a computer to verify insurance information and be updated with the latest claims information. Funds can also be transferred electronically. It is envisioned that clinical information needed to treat a patient in an emergency could be stored on a smart card. The cards contain their own operating system and support on-card programming. Individuals are identified and authenticated through use of a patient identification number. The future of smart cards depends upon the willingness of all providers to invest in card readers (attachments to personal computers), the development of standardized patient care data requirements, and improvements in data security.

OTHER FINANCIAL USES OF COMPUTERS

In a health care facility, accounts receivable represent money third party payers owe the health care facility. Even when claims are submitted promptly and accurately facilities must wait for payment. Computer generated information on the amount of accounts receivable and their age helps the facility collect these accounts. Payroll, accounts payable, general ledger, budget management, inventory control, and investment analysis are frequently computerized or computer aided.

Recently, hospitals have begun to link parts of their administrative computer systems with physician's offices. Such a system provides a physician with laboratory test results as soon as they are available in the hospital laboratory, enables the physician to preadmit patients, performs general financial functions for the physician, provides electronic mail communication, and provides the physician with practice analysis reports.

ADMINISTRATIVE APPLICATIONS

Administrative applications of computers include those related to departmental activities. Some of the most advanced administrative applications are found in the dietary, laboratory, materials management, pharmacy, and radiology departments. Many health information departments also benefit from computerization of various functions.

Many departmental systems will be able to easily interface and share data with other systems through use of an "interface engine." An interface engine is a machine that manages the multiple data exchange interfaces required between different health care systems. All departmental systems will interface the engine and the engine will pass the data to other systems. (See Figure 3.)

DIETARY

Computerization of dietary operations greatly reduces the time spent on paperwork leaving the dietitian available to work directly with patients. A computerized dietary system is based on a database of several files. The food item file stores data on the cost and usage of food items. The nutrient file is comprised of food composition tables. A recipe file manages food production and ingredient control. The patient information file contains demographic data, medical histories, diagnostic information, and dietary histories. Several applications are possible from these files. Computers can calculate nutrient analyses for menus, patient food consumption, metabolic diets, epidemiologic studies, nutritional surveys, and nutritional histories. Sophisticated mathematical techniques assist menu planning which considers food texture, flavor, and color in

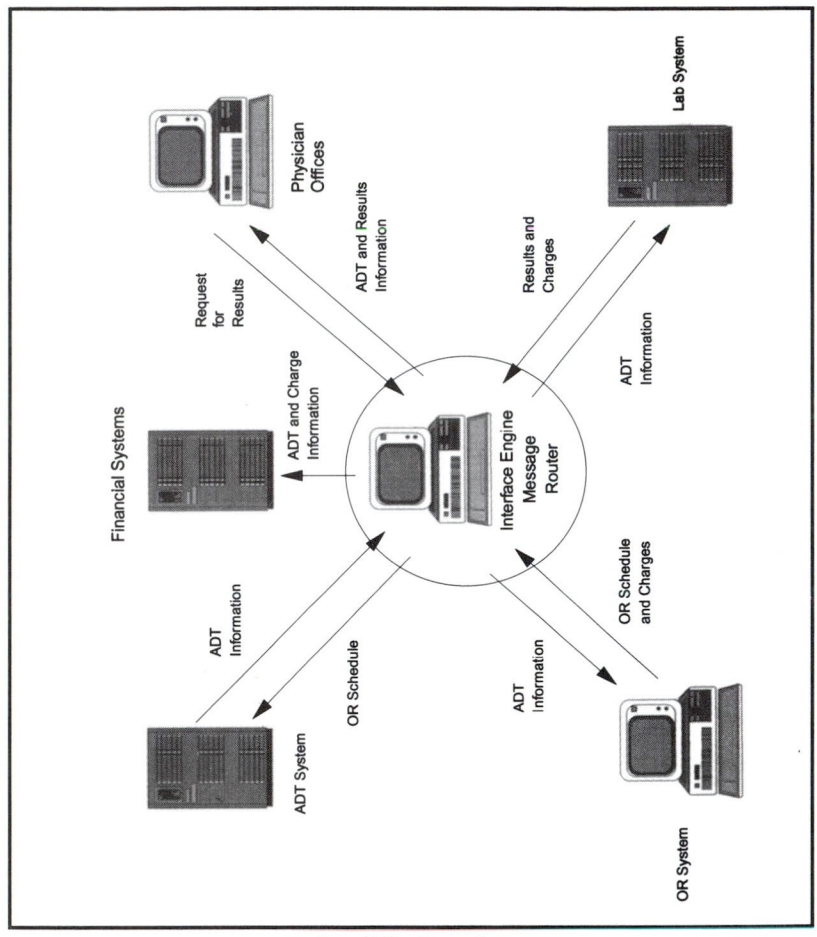

Source: Medicus Systems, Inc.

FIGURE 3. INTERFACE ENGINE SAMPLE HOSPITAL ENVIRONMENT

addition to nutrition, while producing a cost-optimized menu. Inventory control, production control, and cost accounting are also computerized.

LABORATORY

The laboratory is an area where functions have been computerized for a number of years in many hospitals. Patient billing, inventory of laboratory test materials and equipment, and department financial status reports are common administrative applications of computers in the laboratory. Laboratories are also aided by a "distribution and information" system. Computers provide specimen collection lists, labels for specimen containers, results sheets for technicians, and test results status reports. Quality control procedures have been simplified and are more accurate because of continual updating by the computer. Laboratory tests can also be ordered via computer and results charted via computer. Laboratory reporting in graphic form enhances visualization and further improves patient care.

Information systems are not the only automated aspect of the laboratory. Many laboratory tests are totally computerized. Many laboratory systems have expert systems designed for sequential laboratory testing and interpretation that can aid in diagnosing transfusion reactions and help facilitate quality monitoring.

PHARMACY

In many respects computerization of the pharmacy is similar to computerization of the laboratory. Medication administration systems improve patient care. More accurate control of pharmacy inventories result in greater control over drugs. More accurate medication charges result in increased revenue collection for the hospital.

A. Administrative	C. Drug distribution and information
1. Patient billing	1. Formulary and drug list
2. Inventory status	2. Drug information
3. Purchasing information	3. Prescription labels
a. Reorder notices	4. Dispensing of drugs
b. Purchase order	5. Poison control information
c. Vendor analysis	6. Parenteral compatibility control
B. Drug control	D. Medication ordering
1. Narcotics	1. Medication system
2. Investigational drugs	2. Medication listing
3. Dated drugs	3. Charting of drugs administered
4. Barbiturates and amphetamines	4. Preparation of histories and profiles

FIGURE 4. COMPUTER APPLICATIONS IN THE HOSPITAL PHARMACY

Pharmacy automation has taken one of two routes: Many pharmacists have developed standalone systems to improve operations in the pharmacy department itself. Systems analysts have also developed integrated medication ordering systems. Pharmacy software development has expanded to include electronic data interchange between pharmacies, on-line computer-based drug information, and computerized quality management programs that combine data from multiple sources for analysis and reporting. Figure 4 outlines the various computer applications in a hospital pharmacy.

MATERIALS MANAGEMENT

Materials management is obtaining patient care supplies at the best possible prices, storing them, and maintaining control over their distribution. This is basically an inventory management function. Since patient care supplies account for 20 percent of a hospital's operating budget, it is an important function for computerization. Recent innovations in bar coding have made keeping track of stock levels and distribution easier.

Bar coding is used in a number of areas of the hospital in addition to materials management. The pharmacy and laboratory benefit by labeling medications and test tubes with bar codes. Nursing services may use bar codes on patient identifying bands to ensure positive identification and to log in care services provided such as medication administration, taking of vital signs, and so forth. Health information departments may apply bar code labels to medical records for record tracking systems.

RADIOLOGY

One of the major components of any hospital information system is automation of the radiology department. Patient scheduling is often the first operation to be computerized - aiding both staff and patient scheduling as well as patient transportation. The film library may also benefit from computerization. Much like the health information department, the radiology department must manage storage, retention, and distribution of films. Picture archiving and communication systems (PACS) are being used in radiology departments to facilitate the storage, retrieval, and display of diagnostic images in an all-digital format. The systems provide immediate access to images and related patient information, improve productivity, and provide better patient care. PACS eliminate the need for offsite film storage facilities.

Another relatively new addition is computer-based dictation. Rapid Telephone Access System is an example of a system in which dictation equipment captures the dictation and stores it in a computer. A physician requiring the results can obtain them by telephone. Results are later transcribed for hard copy output. Voice recognition systems where the dictation does not have to be transcribed are also being utilized in some radiology departments. Radiology departments use computers for administrative processing like the other departments described.

PATIENT REGISTRATION

Some facilities consider computerization of patient registration a function separate from accounting or medical records. Patient registration systems are also called R-ADT systems (for registration-admission, discharge, and transfer). They capture demographic and payment source information, assign patient numbers, produce registration/admission forms and admission lists, update bed status, maintain census data, produce discharge lists, and generate statistical data on patient length of stay, hospital occupancy, etc. These functions are typically under the control of the admissions department and form the basis for patient accounting. In fact, a patient accounting system rarely exists without a patient registration system.

NURSING SYSTEMS

Nursing information systems provide for both administrative and clinical functions. Nursing management systems are described here and patient care information processing is described in the section on clinical applications.

Because nursing work load fluctuates from one shift to another, it is essential that nursing supervisors have information concerning patient needs in order to allocate nursing resources. Such a system may consist of five major components: patient database, automated acuity system, personnel database, automated scheduling system, and report generator. The hospital's R-ADT system links the nursing patient database with the patient acuity database to generate current listings of patients, their bed locations, patient information, and care hours each patient requires. The acuity system classifies patients according to the degree of assistance needed in activities of daily living (ADL), the complexity of administering medications and treatments, the extent of emotional and teaching support required, the frequency of observations, and the possibility of nursing intervention in critical care situations. These data are aggregated based on discharge diagnosis criteria and uploaded to the hospital's cost accounting system to evaluate costs associated with treating patients in various DRGs. (See Figure 5.)

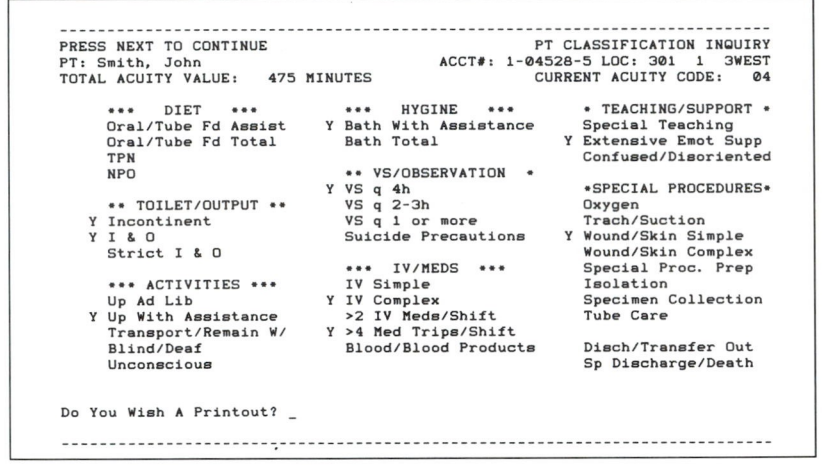

```
---------------------------------------------------------------------------
PRESS NEXT TO CONTINUE                                 PT CLASSIFICATION INQUIRY
PT: Smith, John                       ACCT#: 1-04528-5 LOC: 301  1  3WEST
TOTAL ACUITY VALUE:    475 MINUTES                    CURRENT ACUITY CODE:   04

       ***   DIET   ***         ***   HYGINE   ***       * TEACHING/SUPPORT *
       Oral/Tube Fd Assist    Y Bath With Assistance     Special Teaching
       Oral/Tube Fd Total       Bath Total             Y Extensive Emot Supp
       TPN                                                Confused/Disoriented
       NPO                      ** VS/OBSERVATION  *
                             Y VS q 4h                   *SPECIAL PROCEDURES*
       ** TOILET/OUTPUT **       VS q 2-3h                Oxygen
     Y Incontinent              VS q 1 or more           Trach/Suction
     Y I & O                    Suicide Precautions     Y Wound/Skin Simple
       Strict I & O                                       Wound/Skin Complex
                                ***  IV/MEDS   ***        Special Proc. Prep
       *** ACTIVITIES ***       IV Simple                Isolation
       Up Ad Lib              Y IV Complex               Specimen Collection
     Y Up With Assistance       >2 IV Meds/Shift         Tube Care
       Transport/Remain W/    Y >4 Med Trips/Shift
       Blind/Deaf               Blood/Blood Products     Disch/Transfer Out
       Unconscious                                       Sp Discharge/Death


Do You Wish A Printout? _
---------------------------------------------------------------------------
```

FIGURE 5. DETERMINATION OF PATIENT ACUITY

A nursing personnel database maintains nurses' employment records. Using this database prospective schedules based on skill level, shift assignments, and scheduling policies may be developed. Prior to the beginning of a shift, acuity data may be input to calculate the required staffing level. Actual staffing on a unit can then be compared with required staffing to determine if management action is needed. Schedules maintained on the system can be updated to reflect any movement of personnel from one unit to another as changes occur. The scheduling process facilitates generation of timely productivity and financial reports used by nursing administration. These reports convey information on staff utilization (productivity), budget utilization, and budget adequacy. The database created during the scheduling process may also be used to automate the production of time accounting forms.

Automation of practice guidelines or critical paths (tasks or steps to follow when caring for similar patients with similar diagnoses) has occurred in the 1990s. In addition, automation of exception charting, or only charting variations from the paths is also under development.

OTHER AND ANCILLARY DEPARTMENTS

Other departments or units of health care facilities are also using computers successfully. For example the surgery suite may be effectively managed with the aid of a computer. Scheduling is critical in this area. Instrument and supply needs can be managed with an automatic inventory control. A posting and log system which monitors surgeon and staff activities and performance improves productivity and enhances revenues.

Executive information systems (EIS) are being used at many health care facilities. These systems allow top level decision makers to access summary information about their operations from personal computers located at their desks. These systems allow executives to become direct users of information rather than relying on planning or finance departments to supply data upon request. These systems facilitate strategic planning, market analysis, financial modeling, and productivity management by integrating financial and clinical databases as well as external databases. Decision support systems (DDS) which merge medical records systems and billing systems to measure clinical outcomes and track resource utilization are continuing to be developed.

MEDICAL RECORD DEPARTMENT

As already noted, health information department activities are tied closely to a number of other financial administrative and clinical computer applications. For example, case mix management, DRG grouping, severity of illness indexing, encoding, patient registration, abstracting, and master patient index are all health information department functions that support financial and administrative activities. Computerization of these functions has already been described in various chapters. Utilization management, quality assurance, risk management, and registries are functions related to clinical activities and computerization of these has also been described in other chapters.

Within the health information department itself, several operations are aided by computerization.

RECORD LOCATION/TRACKING

Record location/tracking systems may be implemented as standalone microcomputer systems or may interface with the facility's mainframe information system or the facility's medi-

```
+-----------------------------------------------------------------------+
|                       CHART LOCATION INQUIRY                          |
|-----------------------------------------------------------------------|
|History Id: 33-33-33     Patient Name: Fulton, Paul R.    Volume 1  |
|-----------------------------------------------------------------------|
|                        Current Location                               |
|    Requestor          Date      Time     Location  Phone     Reason   |
|Code          Name                                                     |
|Nor 1     1 North Nursin 10/13/86  11:18 AM  NOR 1                     |
|-----------------------------------------------------------------------|
|                        Previous Locations                             |
|    Requestor          Date      Time     Location  Phone     Reason|
|Code          Name                                                     |
|ER       Emergency Room  10/11/86  12:00 PM  ER       3456       1   |
|ER       Emergency Room  10/10/86   2:48 PM  ER       3456       1   |
|FILE     Chart Returned  10/09/86  11:26 AM  CENTRAL           16    |
|QA       Quality Assura  10/09/86  11:22 AM  QA       3211      14   |
|55555    Lewis, M.D. Do  10/09/86  11:07 AM  ER       374-7676   6   |
|DIR      Medical Record  10/06/86   4:23 PM  ENTRAL   3211       9   |
|PMB      Boyle, RPh. Pa  10/06/86   4:20 PM  MICROFILM 253       4   |
|                                            HELP SCREEN AVAILABLE    |
|-----------------------------------------------------------------------|
|        f5-TRANSFER    f6-PENDING     f7-DEFICIENCY                     |
+-----------------------------------------------------------------------+
```

FIGURE 6. RECORD LOCATION SCREEN

cal record abstracting/analysis system. Systems usually use bar codes as input. They provide information about the location of a record at any given point in time and usually also provide

```
                        Search Card
                   Demonstration Hospital
    -----------------------------------------------------------
    Patient Name              Birth        Volume     History

    Carlisle, Mary J.         06/25/09     01         20-20-20

    -----------------------------------------------------------
    Date       Old       New       Requestor   Telephone   Reason
    Pulled     Location  Location
    -----------------------------------------------------------

    11/18/86   XRAY      QA        QA          3211        14

    -----------------------------------------------------------
    Pulled     Comments        Date        Time         Time
    By                         Requested   Requested    Pulled
                               11/18/86    10:39 AM
```

FIGURE 7. COMPUTER GENERATED SIGN-OUT SLIP

historical information about the record's past movement (Figure 6). In addition, these systems generate sign-out slips for outguides (Figure 7), pull lists based on pending record requests, and return reminder lists and/or letters (Figure 8).

Computerized record location/tracking systems thus may improve record access, facilitate record retrieval, and reduce the incidence of misplaced records. Most systems also generate a

```
                    Demonstration Hospital          RUN DATE:11/18/86
           CHART DELINQUENCY REPORT BY REQUESTOR    PAGE:      1
                    TERMINAL DIGIT ORDER

CHART DELINQUENCIES FOR:  Quality Assurance

PATIENT                    HISTORY     VOLUME    DUE            REASON
NAME                       NUMBER                DATE

Kinsey, Ralph A.           11-11-11    01        10/15/86       14
Barnett, Arthur L.         22-22-22    01        10/16/86       14
Barnett, Arthur L.         22-22-22    04        10/16/86       14
Lawson, Kevin P.           35-35-35    01        10/16/86       14
Carter, William O.         37-37-37    01        10/16/86       14
Hamel, Gary R.             40-40-40    01        10/16/86       14
Mitchell, Mary J.          41-41-41    01        10/16/86       14
Powell, Blair A.           46-46-46    01        10/16/86       14
```

FIGURE 8. COMPUTER GENERATED RETURN REMINDER LIST

variety of reports on chart activity and staff workload which assist the management staff in departmental management functions as well as record control activities.

RECORD COMPLETION SYSTEMS

Automated record completion systems provide a tool for monitoring record completion status. Based on the definition of medical record deficiencies in the medical staff bylaws, defi-

```
                        CHART DEFICIENCY
_____
MEDICAL RECORD NO    123456      Peters, Karen L.    DISCHARGE DATE 10/20/89
PHYSICIAN ID         98765       Carson, MD   David
OFFICE TELEPHONE                 555-1234
HOSPITAL PAGE                    1357
STATUS               P                               ASSIGNED DATE   10/21/89
                                                     COMPLETE DATE
- - - - - - - - - - - - - - - - - - - - - - - - - - - - - - - - -
DEFICIENCIES             SIGN    DICT/COMP    MORE    COMMENTS

Attestation              Y       N
Discharge Summary        N       N
History & Physical       Y       N
Operative Report         Y       Y
Consultation             N       N
Progress Notes           Y       N           10/18-2
Progress Notes           Y       N           10/19-1
Orders                   N       N
Other                    N       N
_____
            F1=INQUIRY  F2=UPDATE   F3=PRINT   F4=SAVE
```

FIGURE 9. RECORD DEFICIENCY ENTRY SCREEN DEFICIENCIES

ciencies are identified by the health information department staff as records are analyzed, and entered into the system (Figure 9). Deficiency information can also be entered onto

```
                       CHART DEFICIENCY REPORT
_____
DEFICIENCIES FOR      Carson, MD  David        SERVICE   Surgery
DATE                  11/1/89                   PAGE  1  OF  1
                  * S = SIGNATURE, D = DICTATE/COMPLETE
-----------------------------------------------------------------------
PATIENT      MEDICAL      DISCHARGE   ASSIGNED   TYPE   DEFICIENCY
             RECORD NO    DATE        DATE

Bacon, L.    235689       10/17/89    10/18/89    S     Attestation
                                                  S     Discharge Summary
                                                  S     Order
                                                  S     Order

Peters, K.   123456       10/20/89    10/21/89    S     Attestation
                                                  S     History & Physical
                                                  D     Operative Report
                                                  S     Operative Report
                                                  S     Progress Notes
CHARTS 10 DAYS OR LESS       2                    S     Progress Notes
CHARTS 11 DAYS OR MORE       0
TOTAL DEFICIENT CHARTS       2
```

FIGURE 10. COMPUTER GENERATED LISTING OF INCOMPLETE RECORDS

```
                    CHART DEFICIENCY SUMMARY REPORT
_____
DATE          11/1/89                                  PAGE   1   OF   1
DEPARTMENT    Medicine
NAME                     1 - 10    11 - 20   21 - 30   31 - 60   61 +
                         DAYS      DAYS      DAYS      DAYS      DAYS

Dr. Donald Barker        3         2         3         5         1
Dr. Edward Smith         2         12        6         1         0

          TOTALS         5         14        9         6         1
DEPARTMENT    Surgery
NAME                     1 - 10    11 - 20   21 - 30   31 - 60   61 +
                         DAYS      DAYS      DAYS      DAYS      DAYS

Dr. David Carson         2         0         0         0         0
Dr. Peter Daniels        0         0         18        22        11
Dr. George Forman        0         1         0         0         0
Dr. Mary Handman         4         6         1         0         1

          TOTALS         6         7         19        22        12
```

FIGURE 11. COMPUTER GENERATED SUMMARY OF RECORD DEFICIENCIES

```
                       CHART DEFICIENCY LETTER
_____
DATE          11/1/89

DOCTOR        Donald Barker, MD

You have      2      charts at least 11 days old.
You have      3      charts at least 21 days old.
You have      5      charts at least 31 days old.
You have      1      charts at least 61 days old.

Please stop by the Medical Record Department at your earliest convenience
to complete these charts.

If you have any questions, please call 555-0001.  Thank you.

                              Susan James, RRA
                              Medical Record Director
```

FIGURE 12. COMPUTER GENERATED WARNING LETTER

abstracts for batch processing or directly into the medical record analysis system. A number of useful reports may be generated, including listings of incomplete records by physician (Figure 10), listings of incomplete records by department or service, and summary chart deficiency statistical reports (Figure 11). Some systems also calculate the age of deficiencies based on defined time parameters and print physician warning letters (Figure 12) and suspension notices.

CORRESPONDENCE CONTROL

Correspondence control software allows the automation of various correspondence control functions, such as logging and monitoring requests for patient information, generating requisitions for needed patient records, and maintaining information on copying fees billed and received. Valuable management reports can be generated to help department managers assess the efficiency of correspondence activities.

TUMOR REGISTRY

Automated tumor registry systems allow clinical information on the treatment and diagnostic testing of cancer patients to be abstracted and collected in a database. These systems have ad hoc query capabilities to allow for report writing and trending of data.

The systems also have automatic follow-up letter generation so that the status of all cancer patients in the registry can be followed through letters to the patient's physicians or the patient at 15 month intervals, as required by the American College of Surgeons.

DEPARTMENT MANAGEMENT

A variety of software packages designed for general business applications for use on a microcomputer can facilitate health information department management activities such as budgeting, staff scheduling, statistical calculations, cost analysis, and report preparation.

Software packages that provide database management capabilities, for example, allow the health information manager to capture and manipulate data quickly and easily. Address files, small incomplete chart control systems, productivity logs, and other types of files can easily be created and maintained by the health information practitioner. Data within these files can be sorted, ranked, merged, deleted, and reported without the need to request such services from the data processing department. Some database systems also allow simple mathematical calculations to be performed. Reports may be formatted by the user, and many systems make graphic displays of data possible.

Software packages that provide electronic spreadsheet capabilities also can be valuable management tools. These packages greatly reduce the amount of time needed to perform repeated calculations and therefore are particularly useful for budgeting purposes. The health information practitioner may be able to download budget data from the hospital's mainframe to a microcomputer, then manipulate the data until a satisfactory budget is developed. Subsequent monitoring of actual expenditures and variance analysis can be performed. In addition, spreadsheets facilitate management decision-making by enabling quick and easy assessment of the impact of alternative situations, such as the effect of staffing variations on productivity. Spreadsheets make assessment of alternative situations feasible even when a large number of variables are involved, as is the case with a complex budget. One or more variables can be altered and an entire series of data elements recalculated quickly to determine the impact of the alteration.

Statistical packages are a third type of general purpose software that may be useful to the health information department which prepares many reports for clinical research, market research, and planning. Such packages enable the user to perform statistical calculations, create tables and graphs, manage data, and generate reports. Statistical routines range from simple descriptive measures and cross-tabulations to regression analysis and more sophisticated analyses. Data management capabilities allow the user to select, sort, and weight data, merge files, and aggregate data. Reports, tables, and graphs can be custom formatted; text only, graphics, and organizational charts created; and user-defined edits and data entry formats specified.

Some software packages combine database management, spreadsheet, word processing, graphics, and mathematical and other capabilities. These management information systems exist for a variety of purposes. Some are primarily designed for creating standard reports and designing ad hoc reports. Some are desk organizers which serve as a clock, calendar, calculator, notepad, filing system, and telephone dialer. Appointments can be scheduled into a "notepad," and an alarm sounds when it is time for an appointment. The phone dialer can locate phone numbers entered into the notepad. These systems often reside in the memory of a microcomputer and are available through a "window" on the screen while other programs are running.

Software specific to scheduling also exists which facilitates staff scheduling. Staff information includes employee skills, wages, vacation dates, and other data. Subsequently, the system produces schedules to coincide with departmental needs. Project schedulers aid in the planning of projects, including personnel, time, and resources. Cost analyses, time studies, Gantt charts, and multi-task referencing are available.

Desktop publishing is another type of software which imports text typed with a word processing package and converts it to typeset print. Text and images may also be scanned and imported into the document via the desktop publishing software. A very high quality laser printer is required to generate output, but the result is professional-looking forms, newsletters, promotional materials, and so forth.

Many individual software packages can also be enhanced by using other packages in conjunction with them. For example, a report generator may be added to a pure database package, a word processing package added to a spreadsheet package, or a graphics package added to a statistics package.

MEDICAL DICTATION AND TRANSCRIPTION

Comprehensive central dictation and medical transcription systems provide improved access to dictation systems and management control.

A computerized central dictation system translates analog voice input into digital computer code and stores it on hard disk, thus allowing instantaneous random access. The systems accommodate a large number of simultaneous dictators and transcriptionists. A report may be accessed not only by transcriptionists but also by physicians, via telephone, from the moment it is completed. Previous reports and other recent reports regarding the same patient may also be accessed via telephone. A computerized transcription management system facilitates assignment of work to transcriptionists, provides information on priority jobs and backlogs, and makes available detailed data on dictation and transcription work flow, transcriptionist productivity, and system activity by physician, transcriptionist, department, job status, etc.

WORD PROCESSING

Although not one of the three major categories of health information systems, word processing is a significant administrative use of computer technology, not only in the health information department but in other areas as well.

In the simplest context, word processing is the use of electronic equipment to type, change, print, and permanently store information. The development of sophisticated equipment for word processing has greatly increased the health information department's ability to handle the increased volume of patient care data received in the department. Standard repetitive letters, final reports of patient care studies, error-free medical transcription, procedure manuals; tumor registry correspondence, proposal development, and many other functions can benefit from automated word processing assistance.

EQUIPMENT

Word processing may be performed on an electronic device known as a word processor, or on a computer of any size using word processing software.

Word processors must be distinguished from electronic typewriters. Electronic typewriters are single units, similar in appearance to standard typewriters. They generally have a small visual display screen to view material being typed. A small memory component allows minimal editing of text just typed.

Some electronic typewriters have enough memory to store a few pages of text. In this way standard paragraphs for use in routine correspondence may be saved. For many typing applications an electronic typewriter may be adequate. If large amounts of text will not be stored, transmitted elsewhere, or manipulated into other forms at some future time, an electronic typewriter serves to produce high quality documents at reasonable cost.

Word processors look very much like computer terminals. Every unit has a screen and keyboard. Each stand alone word

processor has a storage device. Frequently, such word processing equipment is referred to as a dedicated word processor,
signifying that the equipment is dedicated to performing only
word processing.

Clustered or shared logic word processing systems allow
several persons at individual word processors to share one
computerized storage device and one printer. This allows a
department to obtain the benefits of word processing without
incurring the cost of individual peripheral devices.

In evaluating the applicability of using a word processor the
manager must consider the amount of formatting typed documents require, the frequency with which typed documents are
changed, and other aspects relating to the nature of the material to be typed.

Word processing software for use on a microcomputer or
mainframe also exists. Word processing software packages
available on mainframe systems are often rather limited in the
functions they perform. Since the primary function of the mainframe is data processing, not word processing, these systems
often have been created simply as adjuncts to satisfy minimum
word processing needs.

Word processing software available for microcomputers is
very sophisticated and as functional as dedicated word processors. Consideration must be given, however, to whether the
data processing features of a microcomputer are needed in
addition to word processing. If database, spreadsheet, statistical, or other functions are to be performed and possibly incorporated into the word processing function, then the
microcomputer is worth the additional cost.

FEASIBILITY STUDY

In evaluating word processing needs it may be necessary to
conduct a full feasibility study in which the economics, organizational factors, and all alternatives are evaluated.

Economic Factors

A feasibility study must consider the costs and benefits of
word processing. A full description of a cost/benefit study is
described in Chapter 17. In evaluating the costs and benefits of
word processing, typists' productivity is a major economic consideration. In addition to the direct cost of the equipment and

supplies most experts agree that word processing can increase a typist's output by 25-30 percent even before the merits and uses of general text editing and formatting are considered. However, the extent to which those other features will actually be utilized must be evaluated. In the health information department each application will vary. Furthermore if more paper is generated, staffing the separating, processing, and distribution of the increased paper must be considered. Often the clerical duties added to the word processing operation are underestimated.

Other economic considerations include the structure of the wage and benefit plan. Because word processing is a higher skill level than typing alone, word processing specialists may demand greater compensation. Perhaps an incentive pay program can be implemented. Word processing allows equitable and efficient measurement of quantity and quality of work produced. The following components should be included in the design of any pay incentive system:

- Equitable measurements of quantity of work produced
  - line counts defined
  - reliable methods of counting
  - procedures for recording production
- Equitable allocation/allowance for legitimate nonproductive time (in-service, department meetings, staff development, equipment down time, other employer demands)
  - adjust production up if nonproductive time is to be converted to equivalents of production
  - adjust work time down if nonproductive time is not to be credited
  - calculate production over longer periods of time where nonproductive time is spread evenly for all
- Competitive and reasonable pay policies
  - Quality standards to counter speed problems proofreading policies
  - standards for errors and error measurement
- Incentive pay schemes can be organized to pay each employee in one of many ways:
  - strictly by the unit of measure (line, minute, page, etc.)
  - a premium for units of measure over a minimum
  - utilizing a calculated average over a specified time period as a basis for determining an hourly rate

In an incentive pay scheme, using lines as the unit of measure, a transcriptionist would earn pay directly related to the
work produced. When a premium is paid, a minimum pay is
guaranteed. Both of these methods offer immediate payoff. The
first is most often found in independent transcription services,
and the second is found in health care facilities. The nonproductive allocation allowance plus the necessity for daily bookkeeping are a few of the disadvantages of these two methods. A
merit pay approach, where production totals are logged but
averaged over longer periods of time, requires less bookkeeping
and puts less pressure on the typist for a bad day or week. If
the merit system is tied into annual or periodic hourly wage
increases, the employee is rewarded for production but not
penalized for every reduction in output. For a merit system, the
production targets are defined and correlated to step increases
where the employee will merit a higher step increase depending
upon average production. This third system is less threatening,
requires less bookkeeping, and rewards an employee for past
work without the daily logging of non-productive time. If productivity increases are significant using word processing, consideration must also be given to changes in staffing and service
activity levels. It may be possible to reduce the number of full
time equivalent personnel or time may be available to produce
other work.

In areas where skilled medical transcriptionists are difficult
to recruit or retain, word processing systems that increase
productivity and possibly even allow for networking from home
may be a solution. Where other typing needs in the facility are
unmet or met inadequately the additional work may be appropriate.

When the definition of a line has been established (see next
section) and an equitable method of keeping track of production
is developed, gross staffing requirements are estimated by
dividing what has to be done by what one person can reasonably
be expected to do. There are many published standards on
minimum daily production targets for medical transcriptionists. Most, however, do not define the line equivalent; and
because of this, comparisons are difficult. The most often mentioned are 800-1,000 lines per day on an IBM Selectric Typewriter and 1,000-1,500 lines per day on word processing
equipment. Other measurements which may be used are word

counts, words per minute, cassettes typed, and number of reports or pages typed.

The following is an estimate of gross staffing for one transcription department.

ESTIMATE OF GROSS STAFFING

Community Hospital

Bed capacity - 200 beds

Average Occupancy - 82%

Dictation Transcribed:
   History and Physical
   Operating Room Summaries
   Labor & Delivery Summaries
   Industrial Clinic Notes
   EKSs/Consultations Other Reports

Average Lines per Month - 160,000

Daily Production Minimum Set - 1000 lines

Minimum workdays for volume - 160 $\frac{160,000}{1,000}$

Number of Workdays in Month - 20

Minimum Number of Full- time Equivalents (FTEs) to Handle Work - 8 $\frac{160}{20}$

The gross estimate of full-time equivalents must be qualified by turnaround expectations and paid time off before staffing patterns can be established. Tracking volumes by type of report, actual turnaround time (average but also worst examples), and dictation patterns will be necessary so staffing is organized for the best return. For example, dictation of history and physicals is often heavier on Sundays and late in the afternoons; emergency department dictation is heaviest on afternoons and weekends; operative reports are usually dictated during the day, as are discharge summaries. More dictation with 24-hour turnaround is available for afternoon-shift production; consults may be evenly distributed throughout the seven days of the week.

Profiling dictation patterns in light of turnaround times will be necessary if limited staffing resources are to be used properly. There is staff resistance to weekend, evening, midnight and holiday scheduling, especially if it represents a change from current scheduling. But as faster service is demanded, more complex personnel scheduling is necessary.

The conclusion drawn from the example hospital reflects production in terms of working days. Paid days off are not accounted for in this example. Employees on vacation or using sick time and personal days are not contributing a workday of 1,000 lines when they are not there.

To best estimate staffing requirements, a 15 percent adjustment factor should be added. In that case 9.2 FTEs would be a solid staffing target for the Community Hospital, provided 160,000 lines represent the average volume of transcription.

Organizational Factors

In addition to economic factors, organizational factors to consider include environment and dictation systems.

Environmental factors to consider include space, furnishings, and other related equipment. Health care facility policies on capital equipment purchases in general and computer systems in particular must also be considered.

Dictation equipment must be considered when word processing equipment is introduced into medical transcription because the input methods have an effect on the manner in which output plans are made. Convenience and proximity to nursing units, operating rooms, emergency rooms, clinics, and general patient intake areas enhance the timeliness of dictation by physicians. If certain types of reports are to be transcribed centrally, the proximity of dictating equipment to work stations for radiologists, pathologists, etc. is essential. Dictation formats guiding physicians through basic identifying information and report outline headings assists in producing complete reports and saves time for the transcriptionists in looking up patient medical records numbers and room numbers. The ability to download identifying data from the mainframe should be investigated. Physician dictation patterns and required turnaround time must also be considered.

The media on which medical transcription is recorded will be either self-contained or discrete. Discrete media include cassettes, minicassettes, microcassettes, and belts or disks which can be removed from the dictation equipment for transcription. Self-contained media such as endless loop, tape, or tanks are not physically handled by the operator. The advantages to discrete media are that they are all tangible, can be distributed quickly, have a visually measurable end, and can be counted. The disadvantages are that they can be more easily lost or misplaced, and forethought must be used to insure that ample supplies are available for dictation peaks and low staffed times.

The advantages of self-contained media are that there is no media handling, input priorities are well controlled, and lost dictation is minimal. Disadvantages include difficult access to stat work buried in a tank, volume recording cannot be distributed easily, and rerecording is necessary for some work distribution needs (particularly if certain work is being sent out to a service).

Alternatives

Factors to consider in evaluating alternative word processing systems include:

- Type of equipment - electronic typewriter, dedicated word processor, or word processing on a microcomputer or mainframe.
- Functions performed - see next section.
- Word measurement - Various techniques are used by systems to produce productivity data. Some word processors produce a count of bytes (see Chapter 13), others produce a count of words or lines. A line may be designated to contain a variety of different numbers of keystrokes, i.e., 50, 55, 60, 78, 84, etc. If word processing is being considered for medical transcription, volumes may be measured in terms of input as well. Input techniques count minutes of dictation, through the dictation equipment, and then utilize conversion formulas to represent work produced. Input conversion factors of 1:10, 11, or 12 (one minute of dictation equals 10, 11, or 12 lines) are commonly used.
- Service and maintenance agreements.
- Training, support services, and upgrades to software.
- Equipment compatibility, versatility, and potential for expansion.
- Outside transcription service - If word processing is being evaluated to increase medical transcription production, the alternative of contracting with an outside service should also be investigated. In many areas, well-managed

transcription companies which pick up the work or have it wired directly to their off-site offices are a viable and cost-effective option. Some of the advantages of off-site contracting are very attractive. The problems of personnel recruitment and retention are eliminated entirely, as are job orientation, training, and scheduling demands. Equipment purchase, maintenance, upgrading, downtime, and training are also eliminated. Because the service agency has a vested interest in ease of dictation, equipment purchase and maintenance of dictating equipment becomes a shared responsibility.

Problems with peak work are also eased. The contract with the service will specify turnaround times, and a well-negotiated contract should have financial or other consequences built in should turnaround times become a problem. A hospital which contracts all its work out will receive production priority over a hospital using the service periodically, so a full-contract hospital usually gets the best service by the most experienced transcriptionists.

The quality of reports completed by an outside company must be high in order to keep the customer happy, whereas the quality of in-house work often varies because of personnel, equipment and environmental pressures.

Facsimile and networking capabilities make it possible to receive instant printouts of work produced miles away. If the hospital wishes to limit its dictation equipment to in-house wiring, new speed recording devices allow for fast-forward recording from dictation equipment over telephone lines, thus eliminating the delivery and pickup delays. There are advantages to in-house transcription such as internal control, management experience and expertise, equipment availability for other word processing applications; responding to special requests, person to person contact for physicians, and confidentiality of in-house production, but space allocations and capital expenditure limitations often provide convincing reasons to investigate outside services.

Some contract services are interested in utilizing existing equipment (buying or leasing) and of staffing the allocated space rather than sending the work to off-site offices if the hospital has some capital invested in transcription equipment, or there is significant objection to removing the work from the premises.

Many transcription services solicit business through direct mail campaigns, although a recommendation from another user is a much more reliable method of initial company identification. The company's reputation, user satisfaction, and financial stability are of primary concern. After the field has been narrowed the one or two companies in the running should be visited. Billing procedures, workflow, quality of reports, and employee morale can be observed. The company will become a direct extension of the health information department, and it should exhibit a flexible and cooperative attitude in meeting the needs of the hospital.

Finally, a short term initial contract (three to six months) provides the best opportunity to evaluate an outside service's ability to provide timely, quality transcription for the hospital.

FUNCTIONS

Word processing accomplishes special functions through the use of codes that direct the operations in the central processing unit. Many of these codes are initiated through the use of function keys on the keyboard and/or by use of one or more special keys in combination with alphabetic keys. Functions that characterize word processing and distinguish it from typing include:

- Back-up
- Block move and copy
- Calculating totals and formulas
- Columns
- Creation of table of contents, lists, indexes, headers, foot-notes, end-notes, page numbering
- Dictionary and thesaurus
- Editing
- Error messages
- File maintenance
- Formatting (e.g., margins, tabs, indenting)
- Importing files in ASCII (computer code)

- Line drawing
- Merging documents
- Printing
- Searching and replacing text
- Sorting and selecting text
- Special effects (e.g., italics, pitch and font changes, proportional spacing, underline, bold, special characters, subscript, superscript, strikeout)
- Storing
- Text insertion
- Windowing (typing two documents simultaneously)

CLINICAL APPLICATIONS

Clinical applications of computers are those pertaining specifically to data used to diagnose and treat patients. While many of the administrative applications previously discussed supply data for use in diagnosis and treatment, they are designed primarily to improve productivity and decrease costs or increase revenues.

COMPUTERIZED MEDICAL RECORD

Clinical applications produce computerized medical record documentation. A computerized medical record is one that is interactive with the health care providers - physicians, nurses, therapists, technologists, etc. Providers make medical record entries into a computer and receive information from others' entries. Computerized medical devices may transmit data directly to a computerized medical record. Although a totally paperless medical record system does not exist, significant advances have been made. Facilities in which computerized medical record systems are the most advanced often print out medical record data for permanent storage, and frequently print out parts of the medical record for physician or others' use during patient care.

ORDER ENTRY AND RESULTS REPORTING

A computerized medical record is one in which all clinical documentation is entered into the computer and retrieved from it. Initial steps in computerization of the medical record often include physician order entry and results reporting.

At a minimum, physician order entry entails the physician entering orders into the computer which are transmitted to and initiate various services (i.e., pharmacy, laboratory, radiology, etc.) (Figure 13). A copy of the orders is maintained in the medical record system (Figure 14). Each point of service obtains orders pertaining to its area.

Results reporting refers to the results of all orders being reported to the computerized medical record and available for review by those treating the patient. Laboratory results, radiology reports, medication administration, vital signs, and so forth are entered into the computer and are available in a neat, legible, and organized manner. Data may be presented in graphic format so that a wealth of information is available at a glance (Figure 15).

NURSING SYSTEMS

Recent advances in basic patient care applications have brought the computer to the bedside. Clinical information systems originally included terminals located only at nursing stations. This often meant that intermediate paper documents were used for recording data on care given at the bedside until it was charted at the nursing station. Hand-held microcomputers, however, are bringing computers directly to the bedside. Called point-of-care information systems, these microcomputers are used to record vital signs, intake and output, medication and blood administration, etc. This information can then be transmitted to the main computer system and available for review by all providers.

Computerized bedside-based nursing assessment uses the computer to record specific data relevant for a particular patient. Using a branched-logic approach in which nonproblematic areas are addressed in outline and problematic areas are addressed in detail, the nurse can be assured that no important topics are missed. With use of simple menu-entry techniques, the assessment is completed in virtually the time required to carry out the dialogue with the patient. At the completion of the computerized assessment phase, all data are immediately available to all levels of health care providers.

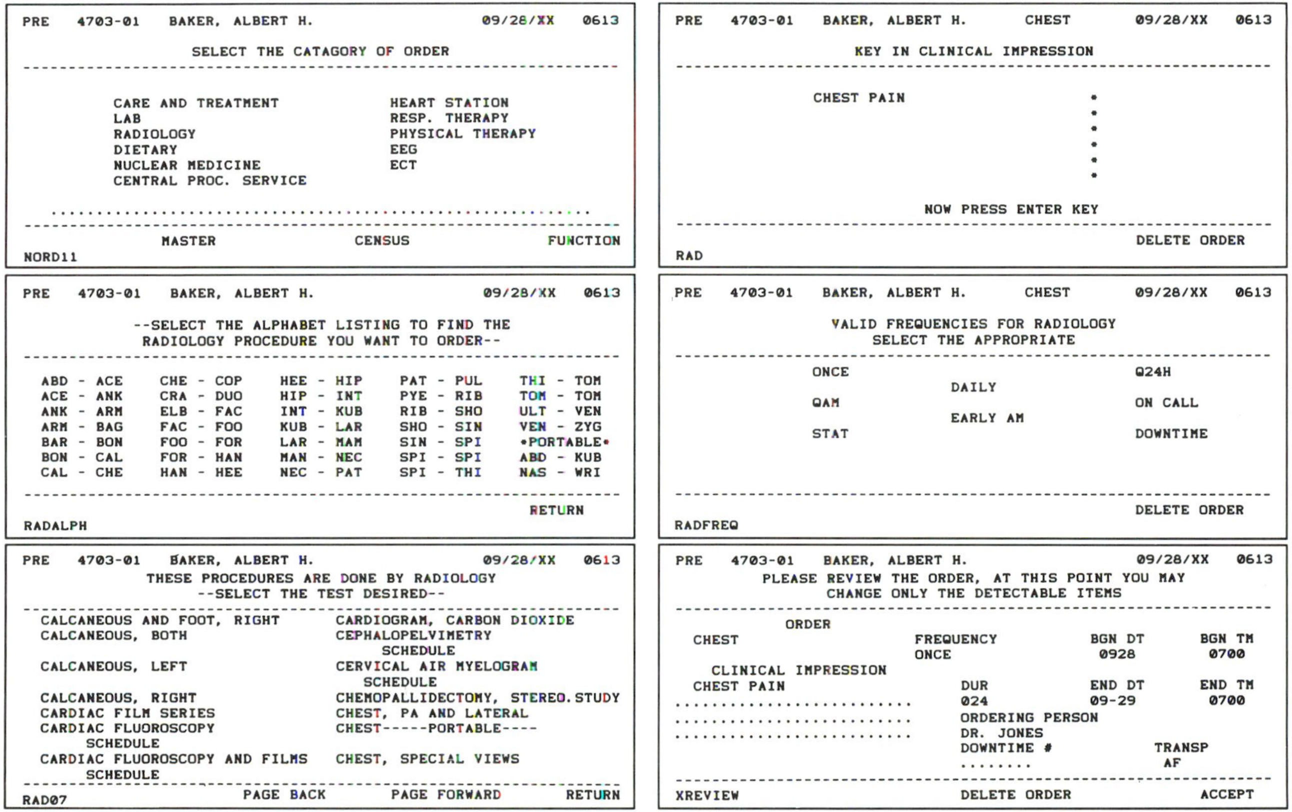

```
PRE  4703-01  BAKER, ALBERT H.                      09/28/XX   0613

                  SELECT THE CATAGORY OF ORDER

        CARE AND TREATMENT          HEART STATION
        LAB                         RESP. THERAPY
        RADIOLOGY                   PHYSICAL THERAPY
        DIETARY                     EEG
        NUCLEAR MEDICINE            ECT
        CENTRAL PROC. SERVICE

        MASTER          CENSUS                    FUNCTION
NORD11
```

```
PRE  4703-01  BAKER, ALBERT H.                      09/28/XX   0613

      --SELECT THE ALPHABET LISTING TO FIND THE
        RADIOLOGY PROCEDURE YOU WANT TO ORDER--

   ABD - ACE   CHE - COP   HEE - HIP   PAT - PUL   THI - TOM
   ACE - ANK   CRA - DUO   HIP - INT   PYE - RIB   TOM - TOM
   ANK - ARM   ELB - FAC   INT - KUB   RIB - SHO   ULT - VEN
   ARM - BAG   FAC - FOO   KUB - LAR   SHO - SIN   VEN - ZYG
   BAR - BON   FOO - FOR   LAR - MAM   SIN - SPI   *PORTABLE*
   BON - CAL   FOR - HAN   MAM - NEC   SPI - SPI   ABD - KUB
   CAL - CHE   HAN - HEE   NEC - PAT   SPI - THI   NAS - WRI

                                                   RETURN
RADALPH
```

```
PRE  4703-01  BAKER, ALBERT H.                      09/28/XX   0613

      THESE PROCEDURES ARE DONE BY RADIOLOGY
          --SELECT THE TEST DESIRED--

   CALCANEOUS AND FOOT, RIGHT    CARDIOGRAM, CARBON DIOXIDE
   CALCANEOUS, BOTH              CEPHALOPELVIMETRY
                                     SCHEDULE
   CALCANEOUS, LEFT              CERVICAL AIR MYELOGRAM
                                     SCHEDULE
   CALCANEOUS, RIGHT             CHEMOPALLIDECTOMY, STEREO.STUDY
   CARDIAC FILM SERIES           CHEST, PA AND LATERAL
   CARDIAC FLUOROSCOPY           CHEST----PORTABLE----
        SCHEDULE
   CARDIAC FLUOROSCOPY AND FILMS  CHEST, SPECIAL VIEWS
        SCHEDULE
            PAGE BACK    PAGE FORWARD             RETURN
RAD07
```

```
PRE  4703-01  BAKER, ALBERT H.    CHEST            09/28/XX   0613

                  KEY IN CLINICAL IMPRESSION

        CHEST PAIN

                . . . . . .

                  NOW PRESS ENTER KEY

                                              DELETE ORDER
RAD
```

```
PRE  4703-01  BAKER, ALBERT H.    CHEST            09/28/XX   0613

              VALID FREQUENCIES FOR RADIOLOGY
                 SELECT THE APPROPRIATE

        ONCE          DAILY          Q24H
        QAM           EARLY AM       ON CALL
        STAT                         DOWNTIME

                                              DELETE ORDER
RADFREQ
```

```
PRE  4703-01  BAKER, ALBERT H.                     09/28/XX   0613
      PLEASE REVIEW THE ORDER, AT THIS POINT YOU MAY
           CHANGE ONLY THE DETECTABLE ITEMS

   CHEST       ORDER       FREQUENCY     BGN DT    BGN TM
                           ONCE          0928      0700
         CLINICAL IMPRESSION      DUR    END DT    END TM
   CHEST PAIN                     Q24    09-29     0700
   . . . . . .       ORDERING PERSON
   . . . . . .       DR. JONES
                     DOWNTIME #            TRANSP
                     . . . . . .           AF
XREVIEW                 DELETE ORDER              ACCEPT
```

FIGURE 13. PHYSICIAN ORDER-ENTRY SCREENS

Computer systems also can create an automated Kardex. As each physician order is entered into the system and as each nursing intervention is created as part of the assessment and care planning process, the required observations and treatments are all automatically and immediately entered into an automated patient Kardex and care schedule (Figure 16).

```
1WEST-8694              TECHNICON HOSPITAL
                          PAGE 001                   ooo   oooo  oooo
                                                    o   o  o   o o  o
                                                    o   o  oooo  o  o
                                                    o   o  o o   o  o
===================================               ooo   o  o  oooo
MOSS NANCY C              F 32 208                ========================
 357078       ADM: 03/05/XX
===================================               ========================

      ORDERS CURRENT AS OF:                               9:02 am  4/19
==================================================================================

      MEDICATIONS:
R  3/10   124.   VALIUM INJ: DIAZEPAM-10 MG., IM, QHS, (03/10 09PM-..),
                 (HJK)
R  3/31   249.   MEPERIDINE-50 MG., IM, Q3H, PRN PAIN, (HJK).
R  4/6    272.   AMPICILLIN LIQ 250 MG./5ML., 2 TSP(10 ML.), PO, Q6H, (04/06
                 12NN-..), (HJK)
   4/13   289.   TIGAN, SUPP-200 MG., #1, PR, Q4H, PRN NAUSEA, (HJK)
   4/14   298.   PHENERGAN-INJ: PROMETHAZINE-50 MG., IM, Q4H, PRN NAUSEA,
                 (RJS)
                 R=TIME TO RENEW

      IV-S:
   3/15   180.   IV LINE-FOLLOW PRESENT IV W FREAMINE 4.25% IN 25%/D,
                 1000 ML W, SODIUM 30 MEQ (AS CHLORIDE), POTASS 30 MEQ (AS
                 CHLORIDE), POTASS 10 MEQ (AS PHOSPHATE), CALCIUM 5 MEQ (AS
                 GLUCONATE), MAGNES 8 MEQ (AS SULFATE), MVI CONC. 5 ML, REG
                 INSULIN 10 U, X1BTL, 125 ML/HR (31/125GTT), (HJK).
   3/15   181.   IV LINE-, ALTERNATE W FREAMINE 4.25% IN 25%/D, 1000 ML W,
                 SODIUM 30 MEQ (AS CHLORIDE), POTASS 30 MEQ (AS CHLORIDE),
                 POTASS 10 MEQ (AS PHOSPHATE), CALCIUM 5 MEQ (AS
                 GLUCONATE), MAGNES 8 MEQ (AS SULFATE), REG INSULIN 10 U,
                 X1BTL, 125 ML/HR (31/125GTT)....OTHER MISC--(INSULIN IN Q
                 BOTTLE AND MV1 IN Q OTHER BOTTLE), (HJK)

      TESTS AND SERVICES:
   3/10   115.   UNIT TESTS: URINE FOR GLUCOSE & ACETONE (DOUBLE
                 VOIDING), QID--IF SUGAR GREATER THAN 2% CALL MD. FOR
                 INSULIN ORDER., (HJK).
   3/10   138.   UNIT TESTS SPECIFIC GRAVITY, QID
   4/18   309.   (IN PROCESS) SMA-18 (PREP #1), TOM'RO, (04/19), (HJK).
   4/18   310.   (IN PROCESS) CBC, TOM'RO, (04/19), (HJK).

      PATIENT STATUS:
   3/6    36.    POSITIONING: ELEVATE FT OF BED-- 15 DEG X 15 MIN Q8H
                 TILL FULLY AMB., (HJK).
   3/6    37.    ACTIVITY, AMBULATE AS TOL, (HJK).
   3/11   142.   VITAL SIGNS, QID, (HJK).
   3/10   117.   WEIGH PATIENT DAILY, (HJK).
   3/10   134.   *IV DRUGS ARE TO BE GIVEN THRU CVP-HYPERAL'N LINE WHEN
                 PERIPHERAL LINE IS DC'D., (HJK).
   4/18   312.   DIET: FULL LIQUID, (HJK).
                          LAST PAGE
 -*-
```

Technicon Medical Information System (TMIS) printed report. Sample order report. ©1985, an unpublished work by TECHNICON DATA SYSTEMS CORP. All names are fictional.

FIGURE 14. COMPUTER GENERATED PHYSICIAN ORDERS

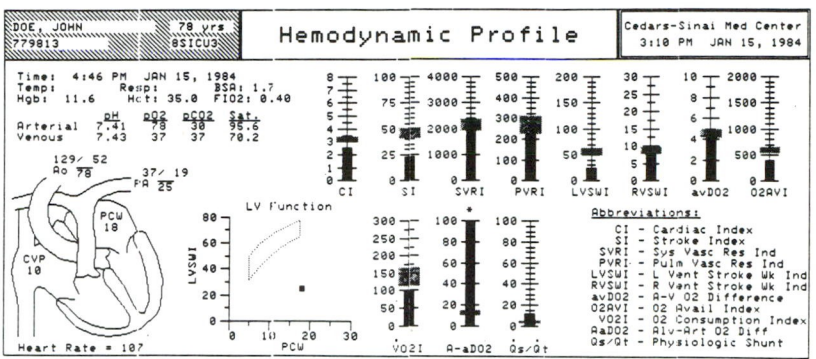

FIGURE 15. GRAPHIC DISPLAY OF DATA

```
--------------------------------------------------------------------------
PRESS NEXT TO CONTINUE                              NURSING CARE PLAN INQUIRY
Pt: SMITH, JOHN                      ACCT #: 0-00000-0 LOC: PRE

Problem:                                          Start    Stop      Sts
PROLONGED INACTIVITY/IMMOBILITY                   02/20/88           IN PR

Etiologies:
Due To Restrictions Of Traction                   02/20/88           IN PR
Due To Prolonged Bedrest                          02/20/88           IN PR

Goals:
Prevention Of Muscle Atrophy                      02/20/88 02/28/88 IN PR
Prevention Of Orthostatic Hypotension             02/20/88 02/28/88 IN PR

Interventions:
Frequent Position Changes                         02/20/88           IN PR
Lift Patient When Moving - Avoid 'PULLING' Up In Bed 02/20/88        IN PR
Frequently Observe Skin For Signs Of Breakdown    02/20/88           IN PR
Encourge Cranberry, Grape, Plum and Apricot Juices 02/21/88 02/23/88 COMPL
Push Fluids                                       02/22/88           IN PR
--------------------------------------------------------------------------
```

FIGURE 16. SAMPLE SCREEN OF NURSING CARE PLAN

AMBULATORY CARE SYSTEMS

While computerized medical records have many benefits, a totally computerized inpatient medical record is not yet available. With each advance, forecasters see the totally computerized medical record coming closer and closer in time.

Perhaps the closest to a totally computerized medical record exists in ambulatory care. Reasons for this are many. Compared to a hospital, ambulatory settings see a large number of patients for a very short time. Linkage of data between visits is essential for both medical and billing purposes, but the costs for services are low. There is no great demand for timely communication with other services, and where the need exists the patient can act as courier. Thus, ambulatory care systems are less expensive, designed primarily to impact patient care, and do not need to be as complete as hospital information systems with respect to communication functions.

A typical ambulatory medical record system which integrates administrative and clinical applications is outlined in Figure 17. The medical record plays a key role in the system. In the

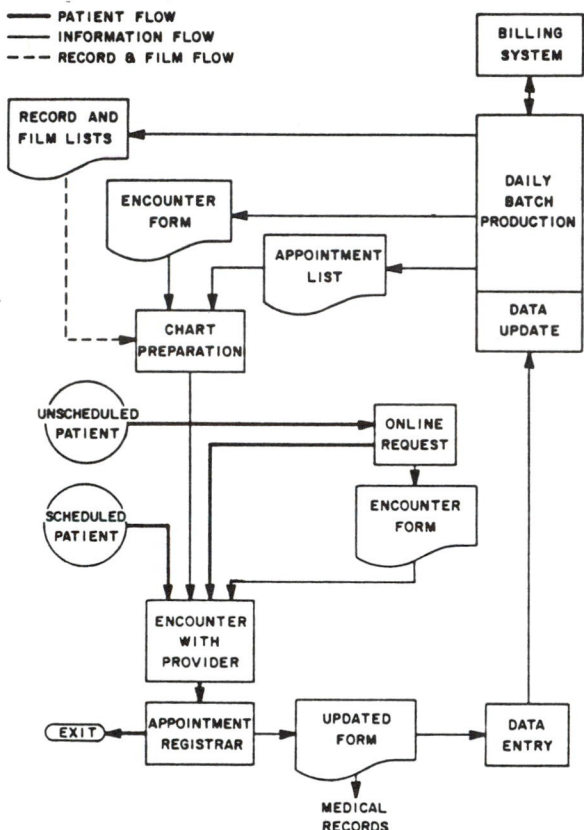

FIGURE 17. COMPONENTS OF AN AMBULATORY MEDICAL RECORD SYSTEM

ambulatory setting, computerization results in a medical record which is neither sequentially or physically constrained. Portions may be accessed directly or combined in alternative formats. The automated medical record is accessed from many different locations concurrently, always available, consistent in format and legible, and easily integrated with other data sources.

Several ambulatory care organizations have been instrumental in developing ambulatory medical record systems. The most widely used or most developed are COSTAR (Computer Stored Ambulatory Record), RMRS (Regenstrief Medical Record System), STOR (Summary Time Oriented Record), and TMR (The Medical Record).

COSTAR is an example of an ambulatory medical record system. It is comprised of six modules:

- *Security and Integrity Module* provides for user identification and access. It also provides routines to monitor system performance and prevent data loss.
- *Registration Module* allows for the entry, service, and modification of the patient registration data - identification, demographic, insurance, and administrative information.
- *Scheduling Module* supports an appointment system.
- *Medical Record Module* processes the medical data by accepting inputs from encounter forms and providing access to the complete medical and administrative database.
- *Billing and Accounts Receivable Module* uses the data captured during the registration and encounter form processing to prepare bills and optionally to support other financial processing.
- *Management Reporting Module* prepares preprogrammed standardized reports and also includes tools for searching and query.

COSTAR uses an encounter form to collect administrative information and medical data. There are fields for entering the vital signs and checking problems. Problems may be classified as major (M), minor (a check), status/post (S/P), and so on. Short comments may also be added. The problem codes are used for data entry and internal linkage.

Once data are entered, they may be retrieved in the form of an encounter report containing all data recorded for a single encounter, a case summary that includes current problems in a short format, a status report containing a more complete medical record, or a variety of special flow sheets. In addition to the modules and standard reports, COSTAR includes a Medical Query Language (MQL) which permits users with no programming background to search the database for ad hoc information needs.

Data communications advances have also made the clinical record available to the physician at the office or at home at nights and on weekends for emergency services. Record linkage beyond the scope of one facility is expected soon. Record linkage is the ability for persons at all care levels to access a patient's medical record and to input documentation regarding services. Thus, one record would serve a patient in the physician's office, hospital, nursing home, home health service, etc. Even beyond that, we may one day expect to see medical records available to health care providers across the country.

TEXT-BASED SYSTEMS

Text-based systems are systems that import text into a database and allow analysis of free text. Normally, free text is difficult for a computer to read; however, a text system automatically indexes each word so users can search for information buried in progress notes or other transcribed documents, such as operative reports, consultations, or radiology reports. Facilities may find a text database to be the beginning of a computerized patient record.

EXPERT SYSTEMS

A final application of computers in the area of clinical application is the advancing technology of expert systems. Expert systems, or artificial intelligence applied to medicine, are computer-based repositories of the knowledge of experts in a field. The programming structures of expert systems are such that information can be cross-referenced to such a degree that the expert system can draw inferences the way experts do. There are basically two parts to expert systems: online searching for medical information and computer-aided diagnosis and treatment.

Online Searching for Medical Information

The basic premise of the expert system is the compilation of a large body of information. Thus, an expert system must have access to the latest medical literature. Several systems have now been developed to index medical literature and make titles, key words, and even entire text available via data communications networking (see Chapter 13). These systems are available to subscribers whether they are developing an expert system or not. Thus, access to online medical information benefits all.

Computer-Aided Diagnosis and Treatment

Computer-aided diagnosis and treatment goes beyond simply compiling information about diagnoses and procedures. Expert systems designed for diagnosis and treatment assistance incorporate the knowledge and practice patterns of expert physicians in a field. They combine statistical algorithms with heuristics, which are simple qualitative rules of thumb. For example, "if the patient has anginal chest pain at rest, and the patient had a myocardial infarction in the past week, then perform a low level bicycle exercise test instead of a treadmill test" is an example of heuristic thinking that can be incorporated into an expert system. Coupled with a computerized medical record in which basic data about each individual patient exists, such expert systems provide:

- patient care plan suggestions to optimize quality and cost
- clinical findings to prevent oversight
- suggestions of possible diagnoses and procedures
- warnings or alerts
- standing order initiation
- identification of potential allergic reactions and contraindications
- protocol implementation
- scheduling conflict resolution
- options for lower cost drugs and test alternatives

One example of an expert system is CorSage. It was developed as a computerized decision aid for the management of patients admitted to the Coronary Care Unit (CCU). The system performs two functions. The first is to estimate the risk of the patient having another myocardial infarction in the year following admission to the CCU. This statistical risk assessment is calculated by combining the results of the patient's laboratory tests and the physical examination. The assessment forms the basis for deciding whether the patient can be discharged from the CCU into a less expensive regular hospital bed. The second function of the expert system is to ask the physician about plans to perform additional diagnostic or therapeutic procedures for a patient. CorSage generates a complete critique of the physician's plan in the form of a narrative report. Contraindications for particular procedures are noted as well as confirmations of correct plans.

Expert systems are potentially more accurate than the experts who programmed them, as they do not suffer loss of memory from a busy schedule or lack information because of failure to read the latest medical literature. They automatically provide a "second opinion" or consultation. Although some physicians question the wisdom of using such systems to assist in medical decision making, a well-designed expert system can be a valuable aid in the management of patients. This is true as long as the knowledge, rules, statistical routines, and decision-making components that are programmed into it are accurate and clearly understandable to the physician using it. Expert systems have the potential to augment other diagnostic tools by formalizing, encoding, and dispersing knowledge already accepted by the medical community.

Expert systems are in their infancy. They are generally being created at major universities and may not be available for general distribution to every physician nor for every field of medicine. Although once they required large-scale computers, today expert systems can be developed on microcomputers. Special programming languages have also been developed to aid in writing expert system programs.

DATA ACCURACY

While computers can do marvelous things for hospital finance, administration, and clinical care, the computer adage "garbage in - garbage out" must always be consistent by planning data accuracy controls. The information that results from a computer system is only as good as the data that was processed. Today, the computer is very sophisticated and can assist in managing data accuracy. However, all data accuracy controls must be specified by the user and programmed when a computer system is first developed.

Factors to consider in developing data accuracy controls include legal considerations relating to data accuracy, purpose of the controls, identification of areas within a computerized medical record where error can occur, and decisions about correction of errors.

LEGAL CONSIDERATIONS

When a medical record is computerized, it is necessarily a part of an integrated system. This integrated system also contains data on many financial and administrative aspects of the health care facility. For example, when a medication is ordered and supplied by the pharmacy, inventory levels are adjusted in the computer system at the same time as the medication administration is being charted. A legal consideration is the extent to which the financial and administrative applications become a part of the medical record. If a subpoena was issued to bring the medical record to court in a case where the patient is suing another party over an injury, the computer system must be able to separate the "medical record" from all other parts.

The format of the record which can be brought to court is another legal consideration. Obviously, a paper copy of the documentation can be produced. However, when the computer aids in decision-making, the physician is presented with a series of screens to which responses are made before the final documentation is developed. If a physician is being sued for malpractice, one issue is whether the decision screens are considered a part of the defense.

Authentication is also a legal consideration. Although it is generally accepted that the use of computer passwords, keys, and so forth are equivalent to a signature, the degree of care taken in securing these alternative forms of authentication may have to be proved. (Recent advances in voice and image recognition are making voiceprints and fingerprints more secure and reliable forms of right to access computerized data and authentication - see also below.)

CONTROLS

There are three major purposes of controls that must be considered in ensuring data accuracy in a computer system. Controls must detect the existence of an error, must locate the error, and must provide for the correction of the error. A very simple example is one in which the patient's birthdate entered at the time of patient registration does not match the patient's age entered by the physician on history taking. Should the system detect such an error? (Some errors such as this one may not be of great significance while others are. For example, the difference between cancer in the left breast and in the right breast could mean - and has meant - a mastectomy performed in error.) If the error is detected, which part of the discrepancy is in error - the birthdate or the age/right or left? The system should be able to identify all places where potential error exists and make them available for correction as appropriate. Computer systems can be programmed to make corrections, but this can be dangerous. For example, the computer can be programmed to assume that an initial entry is correct and any subsequent entry that is different is in error; or that two out of three occurrences is the correct occurrence. However, such assumptions may not always be valid.

Error Detection

Errors in computerized medical records are generally of three types: erroneous entries, omissions, and incorrect or inadequate record linkage. The key to detecting error is redundancy. If the same information is represented in two or more places or in two or more ways, then a comparison can be made among these representations. It is possible to construct checks based on these regularities and relationships.

There are two types of checks that can be programmed into a health information system to aid in detection of errors: validity and reasonableness. Validity checking is the determination that the value of a data item is a member of the set of valid values for that item. A great many items of medical data lend themselves to validity checking. In particular, any item that is represented as a code can be checked for validity. The fact that an item is a member of the code set does not mean it is "right," but an item which is not a member of the code set is by definition wrong.

In addition to formal coding schemes like diagnosis or procedure codes, many other types of information have well-defined sets of valid values. For example, it can be verified that a recorded admission date is not later than the recorded discharge date for the same episode of care. When two or more related measurements are made, a validity check can be constructed based on the nature of their relationship; e.g., systolic arterial blood pressure can never be less than diastolic pressure.

Reasonableness checking is the determination that the value of a data item is reasonable in the context in which it occurs. Reasonableness tests are divided into three subtypes. The first is a check for static values which are generally applicable. For example, a potassium level of 7.0 is "unreasonable" regardless of who the patient is. The second type takes into consideration the patient population. A reported age of 87 would be viewed differently in the records of a sports-medicine clinic than in a study of Medicare patients. At the third level, trends in an individual patient are considered in light of the body's capacity to support such changes. If a patient's daily weights were reported as 152, 153, 125, and 152, they would be rejected as unreasonable even though any one of the values taken out of context might be reasonable. Defining dates for reasonableness checks is easy; setting the limits for those checks is less easy. In many cases, it will be possible to establish limits through the exercise of medical judgment. In other cases, it may be more appropriate to use statistical methods to set limits. This is particularly true in population-based checks.

Error Location

All areas within a computerized medical record system where error can occur must also be identified. For each place there should be a plan for detection, location, and correction of errors. Errors can occur in data preparation, data recording, data transmission, input, processing, files, programs, output, distribution of output, and use of output.

Error Correction

Decisions to be made about correction of errors should consider the cost of making the correction and the risks of not making the correction. Control of data accuracy should consider the following points:

- Data can be more accurate in a computer system because of the ability to program decision pathways which must be completed.
- Inaccurate data are more apparent in a computer system than in a manual system, though possibly no more prevalent because error detection programs apply to all data.

Some factors to think about in deciding on correction of errors are patient care consequences, monetary consequences, frequency of error, cost of error control, later detection chance, consequences of late detection, and legal consequences.

Insuring that data accuracy is planned for and carried out in a computerized medical record system is an important function of the health information practitioner.

DATA SECURITY, PRIVACY, AND CONFIDENTIALITY

Concerns regarding data security, privacy, and confidentiality may have slowed the development of a computerized medical record. Data security refers to two issues: data loss and data misuse.

DATA LOSS

Data loss refers to the actual physical loss of data from the computer or from offline storage via theft, natural disaster (fire, flood, etc.), or other power failure. Security relating to data loss is generally the responsibility of the data processing department or company from which commercial services are purchased. The health information practitioner, however, should be concerned about the following four aspects of data loss:

- Contract (with commercial service) which spells out the various protections which are in existence, remuneration for loss, etc.

- Back-up systems that exist, including computer (e.g., alternate power source, data stored offline in a vault) and paper.

- Maintenance procedures and requirements that monitor the extent to which maintenance is performed. Instructions to users as to what to do if the system goes "down."

- Recovery procedures - the extent to which data will be lost from a system, how data can be retrieved, and so forth.

DATA MISUSE

Data misuse is the area of most concern to health information practitioners. Controls must exist over access to the system's inputs and outputs to ensure that patients' privacy is not violated and that data are maintained confidentially. Controls over data misuse include:

- Limit the number of employees who have access to the data stored by the computer.
- Use secret and unique passwords, fingerprints, or voice-prints to access data segments.
- Limit the number of times a password can be entered into the system.
- Change passwords frequently.
- Adopt log-in procedures.
- Limit the functions available to users.
- Provide for detailed accounting of computer usage.
- Monitor computer transactions at random.
- Use special coding algorithms to make highly sensitive stored data unintelligible to those who do not know the code.

PRIVACY AND CONFIDENTIALITY

Issues of privacy (where terminals are located, who enters data for the patient, etc.) and confidentiality (access to data and information by authorized users only) are extremely important. Many health information departments routinely participate in monitoring procedures relating to privacy and confidentiality. For example, health information department personnel who have been instructed in confidentiality, may be assigned to attempt to access data they are ordinarily not authorized to obtain. They may visit patient care areas and observe whether they can obtain confidential data.

Other inadvertent "leaks" of data should be monitored as well. When systems are being developed or repaired, data are often tested by personnel who are not health care professionals and who have not been oriented to the confidential nature of the data. Everyone who has any access to the computer system should be properly oriented. It is not too much to spend a few minutes to provide this orientation and to have the person sign a confidentiality statement indicating that dismissal from the job or discontinuance of the (service) contract will occur in the event of a breach of confidentiality.

SUMMARY

Computer use in health care includes financial, administrative and clinical applications. Financial systems are the oldest, although due to their importance continue to be upgraded. Administrative computer systems contribute to enhanced productivity. Clinical systems are those which computerize the medical record and patient care. Although physicians have been somewhat reluctant to utilize an automated medical record or expert systems, strides are being made to improve human/computer interfaces, integrate knowledge with data, and make systems more adaptable to the needs of the field of medicine. Finally, issues of data accuracy, security, privacy, and confidentiality are critical ones for health information practitioner involvement in computerized health care applications.

STUDY QUESTIONS

1. Describe the extent of information systems in health care facilities.

2. Distinguish between financial, administrative, and clinical applications of computers in health care facilities.

3. Describe the manner in which health information departments interface with charge capture, claims processing, and accounts receivable computer systems.

4. Outline the types of computer applications found in various hospital operations.

5. Describe the computer applications in use in the health information department.

6. Define word processing, identify word processing alternatives, and list word processing functions.

7. Define a computerized medical record and the basic components of clinical information systems.

8. Define expert systems and discuss their use in clinical information systems.

9. Identify steps to take in ensuring data accuracy in a computer environment.

10. Identify issues relating to data security, privacy, and confidentiality in a computer environment.

REFERENCES

Abdelhak, Mervat, Patricia Anania Firouzan, and Lynn Ullman: "Hospital Information Systems Applications and Potential: A literature review revisited, 1982-1992," *Topics in Health Information Management*, (May 1993, Vol. 13, No. 4).

Austin, Hubert, Harold Laufman and Lawrence Zelner, "Strategic Automation for Surgery," *Computers in Healthcare*, (September 1987).

Bertolli, Jeanne, "Computer-Aided Diagnosis; Views on Future Prospects," *Software in Healthcare*, (February/March 1985).

Blum, Bruce I., *Clinical Information Systems*, (New York: Springer-Verlag, 1986).

Bolms, Dale M., "A Professional Insurance Defense Audit Program," *Computers in Healthcare*, (August 1986).

Brown, Bob and Bob Harbort, "Automatic Validation of Medical Data," *Software in Healthcare,* (April/May 1985).

Camp, Blaine R., "Bar Coding Leads the Way," *Computers in Healthcare*, (September 1987).

Carter, Kim, "Information Systems," Special Section, *Modern Healthcare*, (September 11, 1987).

Chausmer, Arthur B. and Douglas R. Mackintosh, "On-Line Medical Software Exchange: Opportunities and Problems," *Software in Healthcare*, (April/May, 1985).

Chowning, Irene M., "Wrestling a Paper Tiger? Look into Paperless Claims," *Software in Healthcare,* (December/January 1984-85).

Davis, Michael W., "The Reality of Integration," *Computers in Healthcare*, (July 1987).

Derschowitz, Linda, "Computerizing the Dietary Department," *Computers in Healthcare*, (September 1986).

Dorenfest, Sheldon I., "The Dorenfest 3000+ Database," *Computers in Healthcare*, (September 1987).

Dowling PhD, Alan F. "Health Care Reform and Information Systems", *1994 HIMSS Proceedings*, Vol. 3.

Earle, Donald V., "An Overview of Automation in Radiology; Nodules of a Prototype System," *Software in Healthcare,* (October/November 1984).

Goldblatt, Sidney A., Terry Frederichsen, Bob Morrison, "The Implications of Open Systems in a Clinical Information Systems Environment," *1994 HIMSS Proceedings*, Volume 4.

Johnson, Chuck, 'Promoting Common Goals; A Hospital-Supplied Practice Management System," *Software in Healthcare*, (April/May 1985).

Keen, Cynthia, E., Margaret Anleitner, James Moss, Gail Penington, "Planning for PACS and Digital Image Management: A Primer," *1994 HIMSS Proceedings*, Volume 4.

King, Hugh, "Case Mix Management in Context," *Computers in Healthcare*, (February 1988).

Korpman, Ralph A., "Patient Care Information Systems: Looking to the Future - Part 4. The Changing Role of Computers in Nursing," *Software in Healthcare*, (October/November 1984).

Kralovec, O. John, Kathleen Adelman, Patricia Kelly Lee, "Reengineering the Delivery of Health Care", *Proceedings of the 1994 Annual HIMSS Conference*, Volume 1.

Lach, Jane and Karen M. Longe, "Bar Coding and the Medical Record Manager," *JAMRA*, (November 1987).

Lazarus, Carl, "Electronic Medical Records - The Why and How," *Computers in Healthcare*, Medical Records Special Edition, (April 1987).

Ledford, Cathe and Maureen Mikuleky, "Use of a Patient Classification System for Allocating Nursing Staff," *Software in Healthcare,* (April/May 1985).

Mahachek, Arnold R., "Computer Simulation; Supporting Management Decisions," *Software in Healthcare*, (April/May 1985).

Mathis, Bill W., "Technology and Human Values: Invitation to Dialogue," *Computers in Healthcare*, (June 1985).

McKnight, Wanda G., "Voice Recognition Technology," *JAMRA*, (December 1987).

Minard, Bernie, "Full-Time, Real-Time System Security," *Computers in Healthcare*, (October 1987).

Morgan, John and Scott Slivka, "Benefiting from Expert Systems," *Computers in Healthcare*, (January 1988).

Partridge, Tim and Dennis R. Tribble, "Anatomy of a Pharmacy Management Information System," *Software in Healthcare*, (October/November 1984).

Phillips, Joan, "Functional Aspects of a Tumor Registry Information Center," *Software in Healthcare*, (April/May 1985).

Reep, James, "The Community Health Information Network: Where Is It Now? Where Is It Going?", *1994 HIMSS Proceedings*, Volume 4.

Schraffenberger, Lou Ann, "Practice Bulletin, Data Security," *JAMRA*, (December 1988).

Singleton, Kathryn T., "Portable Information Technology," *JAMRA*, (September 1987).

Stachura, Cheryl Tabatabai, "Software Reference Guide," series, *JAMRA*, (September 1986 - August 1987).

Stefanchik, Michael F., "Patient Care Information Systems: Views from the Industry," *Computers in Healthcare*, (March 1987).

Walker, Deborah K., "Computers and Computerization: Trends in Hospital Pharmacies," *Computers in Healthcare*, Pharmacy Special Edition.

Wang, Frederick A., "The Promise and Perils of Information Integration," *Computers in Healthcare*, (December 1987).

Withers, Cathryn B., "Electronic Voicemail: One Hospital's Experience," *Computers in Healthcare*, (January 1988).

Yero, Mary, "Successfully Implementing a Point-of-Care System," *Computers in Healthcare*, (February 1988).

Zinn, Tim K., William Bria, MD, Mychelle Mowry, RN, MSN, "Emerging Technologies...Riding the Wave, Avoiding the Undertow," *1994 HIMSS Proceedings*, Vol. 4.

chapter **15**

THE LEGAL ASPECTS OF MEDICAL RECORD INFORMATION

OVERVIEW

This chapter focuses on the medical record as a legal document. Kept primarily for patient care purposes, the medical record serves a secondary and important purpose as a legal document. The legal aspects encompass requirements and principles related to creating the medical record, which includes its content and data extracted from it; using and controlling the record; maintaining it; securing it; and releasing information from it.

There are several sources for the rules and regulations which define the legal aspects of medical records. These include laws, regulations from governmental and non-governmental agencies, and institutional policy.

The health information practitioner plays a key role in assuring that legal requirements regarding the medical record are met by the health care institution. This responsibility includes seeing that policies and procedures concerning the medical record as a legal document are formulated and updated when necessary, and that they are appropriately disseminated, understood, and followed.

SOURCES OF LEGAL REQUIREMENTS

LAWS

The phrase "legal aspects" implies circumstances relating to the law. Law is a broad term that covers common law, statutory law, and regulations of administrative agencies.

Common law is the oldest body of law, derived from the common law of England and applied by courts in the United States. It consists of principles that have evolved over time from court decisions. Often called case law or judge-made law, these principles, once articulated by a court, establish precedent. Thus previous court decisions are used in the resolution of subsequent cases when a substantially similar set of facts is involved. This is known as the doctrine of *"stare decisis."*

Literally translated it means to abide by decided cases. This application of common law results in uniformity of decisions and stability in the legal system. *Stare decisis* is applicable within a system of courts in a vertical manner, but not horizontally. This means that a state trial court would be bound by the decision of the same state's appellate or supreme court, but not by other trial courts within the state, nor by courts in other states.

Statutory law consists of the rules and principles determined by legislative bodies. Statutes are written laws enacted by the United States Congress, a state legislature, or a local governmental unit, such as a city council. There is a hierarchical order which prevails, with the Constitution and federal law taking precedence over state constitutions and laws. States may enact laws which do not conflict with federal laws, and local jurisdictions may enact laws which do not conflict with state or federal laws. Statutes also take precedence over conflicting case law. Judges, however, often must interpret statutes, particularly when the wording of the statutory law is vague.

A third source of significant legal requirements for health care institutions is enacted by federal and state administrative agencies. Legislatures have neither the time nor expertise to enact all laws needed in specific areas or situations. Therefore, federal, state, and local legislative bodies enact fairly broad laws and empower their respective federal, state, or local administrative agencies to detail the laws in the form of administrative rules and regulations. The administrative agencies have both the power and the responsibility of carrying laws into effect. By delegation from their respective legislative bodies, governmental agencies also have law-making and judicial or quasi-judicial powers. The laws they enact are called rules and regulations. The primary or broad legislation usually stipulates what regulations an administrative body is empowered to make. The legislative body retains the power to change regulations issued by an administrative agency.

A powerful federal administrative agency of importance to the health care industry is the Health Care Financing Administration (HCFA). An agency of the Department of Health and Human Services (HHS), which is a part of the executive branch of the federal government, it is empowered to implement the laws governing Medicare and Medicaid. Regulations abound to carry out this duty. Examples of important HCFA regulations with which health information practitioners should be familiar are the *Conditions of Participation for Hospitals* in the Medicare and Medicaid program, the inpatient hospital prospective payment system, and the Medicare and Medicaid requirements for long term care facilities.

States also have administrative agencies whose responsibilities bring their staff in contact with the health information department. A state Workers' Compensation Commission is an example.

RESOURCES

Health information practitioners have a variety of ways to obtain information about state and federal statutes and regulations. The *Journal of the American Health Information Management Association,* and other publications, provide up-to-date information on these topics. State associations' legislative committees are active in tracking and influencing appropriate legislation and reporting to members. Most of the component state associations have legal manuals which supply state-related information on a variety of laws and regulations.

Health information practitioners should be familiar with where laws and regulations can be found and the meaning of notations used in conjunction with them so it is possible to correctly cite a law or regulation, obtain a copy of recent legislative action, or provide a library reference.

Generally, statutes are collected into volumes or "codes," which are groupings of laws by subject. These groupings allow laws to be presented in a concise and usable form without requiring review of many volumes.

For example, federal regulations are printed as the *Code of Federal Regulations* (C.F.R.). The C.F.R. is divided into 50 subjects, or titles. For example, the Medicare and Medicaid regulations are found in Title 42, C.F.R. The *Code of Federal Regulations* is revised annually, and only regulations in effect at the time of publication are included. There is a system for updating between issues of the C.F.R.

Copies of the text of recently passed federal laws and amendments to existing laws can be obtained from the Superintendent of Documents at the U.S. Government Printing Office. Copies of state legislation can generally be obtained from a Legislative or Bill Documents Room in each state capital shortly after passage, often free of charge. Many states also have toll free numbers which provide information during legislative sessions on the status of bills. Another source for copies of recent legislation is the local office of a U.S. or state legislator.

Although common law is referred to as unwritten law to distinguish it from written statutes, the case law of certain courts is written and available for reference. There are no written records of every case tried in every court because of the volume of cases and because the lower courts usually render decisions without offering further information about the basis of the decision. However, federal and state appellate courts as well as the U.S. Supreme Court and state supreme courts do render interpretations or opinions as an outcome of their deliberations. These opinions constitute the record of the court. They are reproduced in "reporters," which are volumes or sets of volumes in which a description of the case and the judicial opinions are printed. They are numbered for reference purposes. The citations of case law are uniform in format and sufficient to locate the case. A citation consists of the names of the litigant parties, followed by the name of the reporter in which the case is printed. A case may be printed in more than one reporter, and both are listed when this occurs. Next is the name of the court and jurisdiction of the court deciding the case in the form it is listed in the reporter. The final notation is the date of the decision.

Example: the citation, "Carter v. Cangello, 164 Cal. Rptr. 361 (Cal. Appl 1980)" provides the names of the two litigants (with the plaintiff - or person who initiates the suit - listed first, and the defendant listed second). The description of the case and opinions rendered can be found in volume 164 of the *California Reporter,* on page 361. The court in which the case was heard (in the form listed in the reporter) was the California Court of Appeal, and the decision was rendered in 1980.

Federal regulations can be found in the *Federal Register,* a daily government publication. The procedure used is to publish a proposed regulation or proposed changes to existing regulations and allow a specified period of time for interested persons to submit written comments. The comments received by the agency are considered and often result in changes to the originally proposed rules. The final regulations, with an effective date, are eventually printed in the *Federal Register.*

LEGAL ASPECTS OF MEDICAL RECORDS

REQUIREMENTS FOR KEEPING MEDICAL RECORDS

State laws and regulations specify that medical records must be kept by health care institutions. There are no federal laws or regulations which apply to every type of health care institution requiring them to maintain medical records on patients. Requirements of the federal government which address medical records are limited to specific types of institutions or circumstances. However, in the absence of federal and even state requirements, hospitals and other health care institutions would keep medical records because of their importance as patient care and legal documents.

State licensing laws usually address at least the minimum content. For example, the Indiana state law mandates in part, "an inpatient hospital record shall include identification data, chief complaint, present illness, past history, family history, physical examination progress notes, reports on consultations, copy of transfer forms, reports on laboratory, x-ray and operative procedures, special reports, doctor's orders (signed and dated), notes and observations, treatment records of nurses, dietitian, therapists, and other personnel, reports on vital signs, final discharge summary, and summary sheet giving final diagnosis, complications, operative procedures, and signature of the attending physician."

Specificity as to content may vary depending on the type of health care facility. Mental health codes, for example, often contain more detailed requirements than those specified for general hospitals.

In addition to state regulations and statutes, there are federal laws and regulations which apply in certain circumstances. Institutions seeking reimbursement for the treatment of Medicare and Medicaid patients must meet the federal regulations for keeping medical records, as specified in the *Conditions of Participation*. Federal laws also exist for facilities with alcohol or drug abuse treatment programs.

Non-governmental organizations which accredit hospitals and other health care facilities also have regulations about keeping medical records. The Joint Commission on Accreditation of Healthcare Organizations and the American Osteopathic Association (AOA) are examples of such organizations. The Joint Commission standards state that: "The medical record contains sufficient information to identify the patient, support the diagnosis, justify the treatment, document the course and results accurately, and facilitate continuity of care among health care providers." Health care institutions which voluntarily apply for recognition by such organizations must meet their requirements for keeping medical records, and health information practitioners must be familiar with these requirements.

OWNERSHIP OF THE MEDICAL RECORD

It is a generally accepted principle that the medical record is the physical property of the health care institution. In many states legislation addresses this ownership right. However, the medical record is an unusual type of property because the content of the record is generally conceded to be the property of the patient. This principle implies that the health care institution owns the medium on which the record is contained (paper, computer tape, etc.) and thus the patient cannot take possession of the original record. However, the patient has control over the information in the record, except in those instances where this is limited by law or in circumstances where the health care institution must defend its interests or the best interests of the patient. The ownership rights of the patient to the content of the medical record are not widely understood. Despite the fact that health care providers are held responsible for generating the information contained in the record, they do not have the primary right to control the release of the contents. This right is the prerogative of the subject of the record - the patient, or the patient's legal representative.

CONTENT OF THE MEDICAL RECORD

Health care facilities should identify with clarity the types of documents which constitute the official, permanent medical record. Each facility must include in the definition of the medical record those contents required by law or regulation. The inclusion of additional documents should be specified in the institution's approved policy, if they are to be considered a part of the record. These policies should be reviewed by the institution's legal counsel and approved by both administration and the medical staff.

In general, only information which is necessary for the current and future care of the patient should be a part of the record. However, consideration must also be given to maintaining information which will provide proof that adequate care was rendered. Information in addition to this core data should not be considered a part of the official medical record.

Institutional policies and procedures should also address with sufficient specificity the data that must be recorded on these documents, who is responsible for recording it, and when.

Some documents, not specified as part of the official record, may be filed in the medial record folder for convenience. Included in this category are copies of records from other facilities, as well as miscellaneous correspondence related to the patient. A definition of the content of the medical record clarifies what information can be authorized by the patient for release and what information will ordinarily be included in response to a subpoena.

RESPONSIBILITY FOR GENERATING
THE MEDICAL RECORD

The individuals who provide care to the patient are responsible for documenting that care. This responsibility may be specified in state or other requirements. However, in the absence of outside requirements, and usually in addition to them, institutional policies and procedures should specifically address the responsibilities for documentation. Individuals who provide hands-on care are, of course, included. Those who interpret tests and the results of treatment should also be included. Support individuals, such as those providing social services and pastoral care, and those generating patient identification and sociological data should have their documentation responsibilities specified.

Individuals granted the privilege of documentation should be appropriately trained so that non-essential information is excluded. This is important not only for legal purposes but for cost containment as well.

Only those specified in the policies should be allowed to enter data. In teaching institutions the policies should specify whether students can record in the official record, and if so, the requirements for verification of the accuracy of their entries. If information entered by house staff or by nonphysicians requires countersignature, the medical staff rules and regulations should identify which entries are involved.

Entries made by individuals granted documentation privileges should be identifiable by name and title. Signature should be, at a minimum, first initial and full last name. Computer keys are acceptable, if institutional policy allows this type of verification. Authentication of entries by initials should be avoided because of the difficulty in positively identifying the author of an entry based on initials alone and distinguishing that individual from others having the same initials.

AMENDING OR CORRECTING THE MEDICAL RECORD

It is not unusual for mistakes in documentation to occur in the course of entering data in the medical record. Sometimes it happens that information is accidentally written in the wrong record. When information is recorded which is later discovered to be in error, the proper method for correcting it is for the author of the original entry to draw a single line through the incorrect information without obliterating it, and to record the correct information above, below, or beside it. The date of the correction should always be recorded, as well as the name of the person making the correction. The reason for the incorrect recording should also be included.

In the event the patient wants to correct an entry in the medical record, it should always be done as an amendment to the original entry, without changing the original. The amendment should be clearly identified as an additional document or amendment to the original which has been done at the direction of the patient. Once amended, the patient's change is then regarded as a part of the record and released along with other information when a proper release is authorized.

CONFIDENTIALITY OF MEDICAL RECORDS

One of the most important responsibilities of the health information practitioner is to safeguard the confidentiality of medical records. Confidentiality is the underpinning of the legal aspects of medical records. It is the reference point for security measures which affect medical data and is the underlying reason for most of the state and federal legislation regarding medical records.

In its 1993 position paper on disclosure, the American Health Information Management Association makes the following distinctions between confidential and nonconfidential information:

- Nonconfidential information is that which is generally common knowledge, and there is no specific request by the patient to restrict disclosure. Nonconfidential information includes: name of the patient; verification of hospitalization or outpatient services; and dates of service.
- Confidential information is any information that derives from a clinical relationship between patients and healthcare professionals. Confidential information includes, but is not limited to, all clinical data and the patient's address on discharge.

Confidentiality and privacy are terms often used interchangeably in reference to medical data. Although not precisely synonymous, they are quite similar when applied to medical information. Reduced to a simple definition, privacy is the right to be left alone. In the words of the famous turn-of-the-century Supreme Court Justice, Louis Brandeis, the right to privacy is the "right most valued by civilized men." Despite the eloquent simplicity of Justice Brandeis' statement, the right to privacy is a complex social concept with significant ramifications. The right to privacy has been the subject of many scholarly writings.

Medical confidentiality can be viewed as a special case of the right to privacy. Simply defined, confidentiality means keeping a secret. This implies that two people are involved and precludes sharing with a third. Confidentiality becomes an issue, however, only when the third person is involved, that is, only when there is a need to share the secret. Medical confidentiality, then, is concerned with the restrictive use of information obtained from and about a patient.

There is no such thing as absolute medical confidentiality, nor should there be. Information must be shared between health care providers so that quality patient care can be provided. However, ethical if not legal requirements control re-disclosure of information and forbid the unauthorized use of medical information for purposes unrelated to patient care. In some states violations result in civil penalties, such as fine or imprisonment.

The medical record is growing daily in importance as the source of information to meet a wide variety of needs. The health information practitioner has the responsibility of responding to legitimate demands for information while protecting the confidentiality interests of the patient.

Carrying out this dual responsibility requires a knowledge of the laws and regulations affecting disclosure of information, including the conditions under which it can be disclosed without the patient's consent and the circumstances in which patient consent is required. The health information practitioner makes decisions based on this knowledge and in so doing serves as a patient advocate. Because the patient is usually not present when demands for information are made, the health information practitioner stands in place of the absent patient, assuring that confidential information is secure and released only in accordance with legal and institutional requirements.

Safeguarding the confidentiality of medical records has long been the health information practitioner's responsibility. In today's environment, however, it is not as simple to accomplish as in the past. The number and types of demands for information have dramatically increased in recent years. Major reasons include the method of payment for care, increased computerization, and the mobility of the population.

Disclosure of minimal information was sufficient in the past for the provider to receive reimbursement. However, those who pay the bills now want additional data to evaluate the necessity for care, the level of that care, and its quality, before reimbursing the provider.

The increase in computerization of health care presents another potential complication to the preservation of confidentiality. The user-friendly nature of computers and the proliferation of input/output devices result in easy retrieval of information at many sites throughout the facility and the production of copious printouts containing clinical data. Attempts to control dissemination of this information and to assure it is not inappropriately disclosed are challenges for the health information practitioner.

Another fact which affects confidentiality is the need to provide medical services to a highly mobile population. The methods of transmitting data must keep pace with the ability of patients to change location, whether that is a move across the country, a vacation, or the seeking of medical care in a different facility. Technology allows data to be transmitted over telephone and fax lines and other means. Technology makes it possible for patients to carry a credit card-sized, machine-readable, version of their medical record in a wallet or purse. As technological advances occur, consideration must be given to an increased risk of inappropriate disclosure.

In this information-driven society some would say that confidentiality is a thing of the past. A typical teaching hospital has as many as 100 health professionals and administrative personnel with a legitimate need to consult a patient's record during hospitalization. This does not include those who require access following the patient's discharge. Such proliferation of information makes it difficult to claim that confidentiality can be preserved; however, the implications of one disease, AIDS, has taught us not only that confidentiality can and should exist, but that we must redouble our efforts to control unwanted and unauthorized intrusions.

All health care facilities should have policies which address confidentiality and the consequences of improper disclosure of patient information. The policies should apply to all individuals who come in contact with patient information, regardless of whether or not they are paid staff members or members of the

medical staff. The health information practitioner should assure that the health information department staff, volunteers, and others, are properly oriented to the institutional and departmental policies. Statements signed by these individuals will verify their understanding of the policies and the consequences for violation. Periodic in-service programs will reinforce this orientation.

LAWS AND REGULATIONS REGARDING MEDICAL RECORDS

There is no federal law which protects the confidentiality of medical information in all settings or addresses the general subject of information release from medical records. Widely publicized events detailing the invasion of privacy regarding medical information have caused consumers to become concerned about the erosion of their right to privacy. This concern has, in the past, spurred legislatures to introduce legislation at the federal level which specifies constraints on handling confidential health information. However, federal legislation which protects medical information in the private sector has yet to be passed.

There are, however, federal laws and regulations which address medical records in specific circumstances or specific facilities.

PRIVACY ACT OF 1974

This law was enacted to protect the privacy of individuals identified in information systems maintained by federal agencies, and give individuals access to records concerning themselves in these systems. The act includes hospital records of federal government hospitals only. It has no effect on records kept by non-federal government hospitals. The Privacy Act also created the Privacy Protection Study Commission, which undertook a three-year study of privacy provisions needed in other areas of the country. The recommendations of the Commission are contained in their report *Personal Privacy in an Information Society*. The report concludes in part that "the use of medical record data is growing rapidly, with the data being used by more persons and organizations with less control than ever before." Following the passage of the Privacy Act, many states introduced bills on this subject and some were passed.

CONDITIONS OF PARTICIPATION FOR HOSPITALS IN MEDICARE AND MEDICAID PROGRAMS

Conditions of Participation are the requirements that hospitals must meet in order to participate in the Medicare and Medicaid programs. For hospitals wishing to be reimbursed for services provided to Medicare and Medicaid beneficiaries, the *Conditions of Participation* have the effect of law. In determining whether a hospital is in compliance, HCFA may deem a hospital to meet certain conditions by virtue of its accreditation by the Joint Commission or the AOA. The Conditions mandate that a medical record must be maintained for every individual evaluated or treated in the hospital. There are standards for the organization and staffing of the medical record service, for the form and retention of records, and for the content of records. The standard which addresses form and retention has a provision that the hospital must ensure the confidentiality of patient records. "Information from or copies of records may be released only to authorized individuals, and the hospital must ensure that unauthorized individuals cannot gain access to or alter patient records. Original medical records must be released by the hospital only in accordance with federal or state laws, court orders, or subpoenas."

CONDITIONS OF PARTICIPATION FOR LONG TERM CARE FACILITIES

These regulations affect long term care facilities participating in the Medicare and Medicaid program, which includes both skilled nursing facilities (SNFs) and intermediate care facilities (ICFs). They were revised effective August 1, 1989. After October 1, 1990, these facilities are known as nursing facilities (NFs).

The regulations have been extensively revised to focus on facility performance in meeting patients' (referred to as residents) needs in a safe and healthful environment. The sections that affect medical records state that the facility must maintain "clinical records on each resident in accordance with accepted professional standards and practices that are complete, accurately documented, readily accessible, and systematically organized." Generally the faculty must keep confidential all information on a resident's records and must permit each resident to inspect and provide copies of the records on request. The regulations also provide for a transfer agreement with one or more approved hospitals, and for utilization review, and quality assessment.

Health information practitioners should know the general provisions of these regulations, regardless of whether they practice, consult, or oversee transfer of data to a facility of this type. For details, see Chapter 4.

DRUG AND ALCOHOL ABUSE REGULATIONS

The sensitive nature of medical data compiled on drug and alcohol abuse patients was of sufficient federal government concern to result in federal regulations. The regulations implement two laws passed by Congress, one addressing drug abuse treatment and the second addressing alcohol abuse and alcoholism prevention. First promulgated in 1975, the regulations were revised effective August 10, 1987. Many of the provisions which were either unclear or seemingly contradictory, and thus difficult to implement in most hospitals, were clarified or changed in the 1987 regulations. The revised regulations apply to federally-assisted alcohol or drug abuse programs, which are those persons or legal entities which hold themselves out as providing, and which actually provide diagnosis, treatment, or referral for treatment of drug and/or alcohol abuse. Facilities which provide general medical care are bound by the regulations only if they have an identified unit set aside for treatment of drug or alcohol abuse patients or they have personnel whose primary function is providing diagnosis, treatment, or referral. In that case, only records generated on those units or by those personnel are subject to the regulations. General hospitals which do not meet these specifications are not bound by the regulations, even though they may occasionally treat patients who have a diagnosis of drug or alcohol abuse.

Health information practitioners in institutions with covered programs should have a copy of the regulations and assure their institution is in compliance. The penalty for violation is a fine of not more than $500 for the first offense and not more than $5,000 for each subsequent offense. The regulations specify conditions for disclosure with and without the patient's consent. The subpart that provides details for disclosure with the patient's consent includes the form of the written consent and prohibition on re-disclosure. The subpart describing procedures for disclosure without patient consent covers emergencies, research, audit, and evaluation activities. A final subpart addresses the prohibition against responding to a subpoena for records covered by the regulations. An authorizing court order is required, as well as a subpoena, in order to compel disclosure.

Health information practitioners who are not employed in an institution with a covered program should also be familiar with the content of these regulations. It is not unusual to have occasion to provide information on these federal regulations to others, and all health information professionals should be conversant with them.

UNIFORM HEALTH CARE INFORMATION ACT

There is a unique organization that works for the improvement of state laws. Called the National Conference of Commissioners on Uniform State Laws, it is comprised of lawyers, judges, law professors, and government officials who serve as Uniform Law Commissioners. They draft uniform state laws needed where differences in state laws create specific problems, and work for adoption of the proposed laws by all states. Where uniformity in state laws is neither practical nor necessary, they draft and provide states with model acts, which are legislative frameworks adaptable to the state's particular needs and problems.

The uniform state laws drafted by the Commissioners address the private rights of citizens, but only where uniformity between the states is important. Confidentiality of health information meets their criteria. Thus in 1985, the National Conference of Commissioners on Uniform State Laws approved the Uniform Healthcare Information Act (UHIA). Though very few states have passed the legislation as it was written, the UHIA does provide useful information on the legal aspects of medical records.

The UHIA encompasses three principal rules regarding medical information in three contexts. The first prohibits a health care provider from disseminating information to a third party without the patient's consent. The second rule states that medical information is not provided by a health care provider pursuant to compulsory legal process or discovery in any judicial, legislative, or administrative proceeding unless the patient has consented in writing to the release, except in certain defined circumstances. This provision includes a subpoena. The third rule states that patients can have access to their own records and may request that health care providers correct or amend information. The Act specifies the procedure for adding corrections or amendments or statements of disagreement. It also outlines the conditions under which the provider can deny examination and the procedure to be followed when amendment or correction is denied.

PRIVILEGED COMMUNICATIONS' STATUTES

Many states have enacted statutes which recognize a physician/patient privilege with regard to confidential information. They prohibit the physician from testifying in court or other legal proceedings without the consent of the patient. These statutes "seal the physician's lips," under the theory that the privilege belongs to the patient and may be claimed only by the patient, unless specifically waived. A patient can waive the privilege either directly or indirectly by specific actions, such as introducing the subject of the medical condition into evidence.

Although many states have enacted such legislation, the conditions under which the statute is applicable and the exceptions vary widely from state to state.

It is a matter for the court to decide whether the application of a statute which prohibits a physician from testifying in court about information revealed by a patient can be extended to impart a similar status to the patient's entire medical record. In any case, privileged communication statutes apply to testimony in court, and do not address the much broader issue of release of confidential information under other circumstances.

PUBLIC HEALTH LAWS

All states have laws which mandate reporting of certain diseases. In addition, certain occurrences must be reported by state law, such as gunshot wounds as well as births and deaths. Some states have laws requiring the reporting of malignant tumors or other diseases at a central state registry.

Responsibility for reporting usually rests with the health care provider. However, health information practitioners should be familiar with reportable diseases and incidents to assure the responsible individuals in the institution have been designated and are complying with the law. In some instances, this responsibility may be delegated to the health information practitioner.

Although the physician is responsible for providing the medical information for certificates on the births, deaths, and fetal deaths which occur in the health care facility, the health information practitioner can assist in assuring the data is accurate by participating in gathering the required information or reviewing it for accuracy. When possible, a copy of the birth and death certificate should be kept with the medical record and a copy of the fetal death certificate kept with the mother's record.

VOLUNTARY RELEASE OF INFORMATION

CONSENT TO RELEASE INFORMATION

Because the information in the medical record belongs to the patient, the patient may authorize the health care institution to release it to a third party. As in the case of other patient authorizations, consent to release information from the medical record should be in writing, and should be an informed consent. Informed consent means that the patient is aware, in a general way, what information will be released and the use that will be made of the information. The written authorization should contain at least the following data:

- name of institution that is to release the information;
- name of individual or institution that is to receive the information;
- patient's full name, address, and date of birth;
- purpose or need for information;
- extent or nature of information to be released, with inclusive dates of treatment (Note: An authorization specifying "any and all information" should not be honored.);
- specific date, event, or condition upon which the authorization will expire unless revoked earlier;

- statement that authorization can be revoked but not retroactive to the release of information made in good faith;
- date that consent is signed (Note: Date of signature must be later than the date of information to be released.); and
- signature of patient or legal representative (Note: In the case of treatment given a minor without parental knowledge, the institution shall refrain from releasing the portion of the record relevant to this episode of care when responding to a request for information for which the signed authorization is that of the parent or guardian. An authorization by the minor shall be required in this instance.).

The information released should be strictly limited to that which is required to fulfill the purpose of the authorization. Authorizations should be retained as a part of the official medical record. The individual who released the information should make a notation on the authorization following the release showing what information was released, the date released, and sign the entry.

The health information department should have detailed policies regarding the release of information which cover all possible situations which can arise. For example, there should be a policy which covers the situation when a patient is incapable of signing the form, and a policy which requires the individual releasing the information to compare the signature on the authorization with other patient signatures in the record and question gross differences in signatures. Another policy should clearly state the progression of acceptable signatures in lieu of the patient's when the patient is incompetent or deceased.

A patient's written authorization is not required for release of information when release is required by law or when release is to another health care provider currently involved in the care of the patient. Patient authorization is not required when information in the record is used for quality evaluation or for research and education in accordance with the institution's policies for such use.

Health care providers within the institution should satisfy one of the above criteria before being allowed direct access to a patient's record. Routine administrative functions, such as billing or audit, should be permitted only when another means of supplying the required information, other than direct access, is not possible. Employees allowed direct access for such functions should be instructed in policies on confidentiality and be subject to penalties arising from violation.

PROHIBITION ON RE-DISCLOSURE

Re-disclosure of information for purposes which were not authorized in writing by the patient is one of the greatest threats to confidentiality of health data. It is a situation over which the health information practitioner has minimal control. However, all information released should be accompanied by a statement prohibiting re-disclosure, to alert the recipient of the obligation. The re-disclosure statement should state that the recipient is prohibited from using the information for other than the stated purpose, from disclosing it to any other party, and is required to destroy the information after the stated need has been fulfilled.

RELEASE TO GOVERNMENT AGENCIES

Government agencies frequently request information from medical records. Some agencies are empowered by law or regulation to obtain medical information without the patient's authorization. State Workers' Compensation laws are an example. For example, the Iowa Workers' Compensation law states, in part:

Any employee, employer, or insurance carrier making or defending a claim for benefits agrees to the release of all information to which they have access concerning the employee's physical or mental condition relative to the claim and further waives any privilege for the release of such information. Such information shall be made available to any party or their attorney upon request. Any institution or person releasing such information to a party or their attorney shall not be liable criminally or for civil damages by reason of the release of such information. Code of Iowa, chapter 85.27, paragraph 2.

The health information practitioner should receive verification that a claim is pending before the Workers' Compensation board prior to releasing information without the patient's consent.

Law enforcement agencies frequently have need for medical information on patients or former patients. Although prisoners lose some of their rights by virtue of their incarceration, they do not forfeit the right to control their medical information. In the absence of a subpoena, court order, or other legal process, and in the absence of a law or regulation to the contrary, representatives of government agencies, including law enforcement agencies such as the FBI, and state and local police, must have the written authorization of the patient before information from the medical record can be released.

ATTORNEYS

With the exception of the hospital's legal counsel, attorneys must have the patient's written authorization to obtain medical information. Attorneys may claim that a patient has waived the right to confidentiality because a lawsuit was filed and, under the rules of evidence, the defendant's attorney has a right to review the medical record. However, until a subpoena is served to compel production of the record in court, the attorney must have a written authorization before the health information practitioner can release information. This is true for both the plaintiff's attorney as well as the defendant's.

ACQUIRED IMMUNODEFICIENCY SYNDROME (AIDS)

Much has been written about the adverse effect of breaches of confidentiality on patients with acquired immunodeficiency syndrome (AIDS) or with a positive test for the HIV virus. At least 60% of the states have some type of AIDS-related legislation. Attempts to pass federal legislation which deals with the confidentiality aspects of the disease have yet to be successful, although there is still some promise of success. More and more state legislatures are willing to approve AIDS-related laws, and those that are passed have a comprehensive framework for managing the AIDS epidemic, reflecting a growing sensitivity to the complexity and far-reaching effects of the disease as a public health issue of concern to all.

The major issues that health information practitioners are concerned with relating to the disease are reporting requirements, proper documentation including coding, and disclosure. Most of the states rely on existing public health laws, which require the reporting of sexually-transmitted diseases and require reporting of AIDS under these laws. In many cases the existing public health laws have been amended and updated to cover HIV-infected individuals.

In 1993, the American Health Information Management Association published a position statement on "Maintenance, Disclosure, and Redisclosure of Health Information." In it, the AHIMA encourages health information managers to have a policy that no claim for insurance payment is submitted for AIDS patients without the patients' knowledge of the diagnosis and that the diagnosis must be disclosed to obtain insurance payment. AHIMA recommends that facilities ask for written authorization for releasing this information through billing.

In addition to protecting the confidentiality of the medical record itself, the association says diagnostic codes reflecting AIDS-related diagnoses of HIV-positive test results must also be considered confidential.

PATIENT ACCESS TO THE MEDICAL RECORD

In a 1987 survey of the 50 states and the District of Columbia, 51% of the states had no patient access statutes or regulations governing non-psychiatric hospital medical records. In those states with statutes, the content of the laws varied, but the majority allowed inspection with language such as "upon written request" "upon demand," or "within a reasonable period of time."

Health care institutions in states without a law addressing this issue must determine their own internal policies and procedures. Even institutions in states with statutes may require augmentation of their procedures because the law may not address all contingencies.

The American Health Information Management Association, in its position statement on "Maintenance, Disclosure, and Redisclosure of Health Information," asserts that unless prohibited by state law, the patient or the patient's legal representative should have access to health information. In the case of psychiatric records, the patient's physician should be contacted prior to disclosure.

The AHIMA suggest that facilities not charge patients who wish to review their records, but that those who want copies may be charged a sufficient fee to cover costs of copying the record.

If the patient or the patient's representative disputes any information, the AHIMA recommends first discussing the dispute with the practitioner who made the entry. If the practitioner agrees that the entry contains an error, the practitioner should make the correcting entry in the record by drawing a single line through it, recording the correct data, and the signing and dating the correction. If the error is in a computer-based system, the system should preserve both the original entry and amendment, as well as identify the person making the amendment. AHIMA suggest having persons disputing information in the medical record complete a form similar to the one shown in Figure 1.

METHODS OF RELEASING INFORMATION

There are basically four methods of releasing properly authorized information from medical records: direct access, abstracting information, verbal release, or photocopying all or portions of a record. Health information practitioners should have specific policies governing each type of release.

Direct access may be by the patient, or it may be by a representative of the patient. In both instances, care should be taken that the person directly reviewing the record does not alter the contents nor remove any portion of the record. A department employee should sit with the reviewer to assure neither of these occur and to assist the reviewer with locating desired information. Identification of the individual should be required prior to allowing access.

Abstracting information should be delegated to an employee properly trained, so that only essential information (as stipulated on the authorization) is abstracted and that errors of interpretation do not occur.

Verbal release should be limited to those circumstances when other methods of release cannot be used, such as in an emergency situation. The identity of the caller should be verified by returning the call. Only that information required to satisfy the emergency should be released verbally. When feasible, the response should be given by a trained employee, or an appropriate health care provider should provide the verbal information from the record. A record should be made of the verbal release.

Photocopying all or a portion of the record in response to a legitimate request leaves much to be desired, but is used most often because of the convenience and time saved. Care must be taken not to release more information than is covered by the patient's authorization. The record must be carefully reviewed to assure that highly sensitive data is not inadvertently disclosed.

REQUEST FOR CORRECTION/AMENDMENT TO
HEALTH INFORMATION

Patient Name_____ Date of Birth_____

Patient Number_____ Telephone No._____

Date of Entry to be Amended_____

Type of Entry to be Amended _____

Please explain how the entry is incorrect or incomplete. What should the entry say in order to be more accurate or complete?

Would you like this amendment sent to anyone to whom we may have disclosed information in the past? If so, please specify the name and address of the organization or individual.

_____

Signature of Patient or Legal Representative   Date

COMMENTS OF HEALTH CARE PRACTITIONER:

_____

Signature of Health Care Practitioner   Date

"For discussion purposes only. Not for use without advice of legal counsel."

Source: *"Maintenance, Disclosure, and Redisclosure of Health Information,"* AHIMA, 1993.

FIGURE 1. REQUEST FOR CORRECTION/AMENDMENT
TO HEALTH INFORMATION

Health information practitioners are using commercial photocopy services with increasing frequency. Certain legal issues are raised when such services are utilized. It is advisable to enter into a formal contractual relationship which would include a hold harmless clause to ensure the understanding of obligations of both the facility and the service. Policies and procedures, confidentiality statements, training, and supervision of the contract staff are among issues which should be addressed.

Health information departments are using facsimile (fax) machines for quickly responding to requests for information. Fax machines, however, are not perfectly secure means of transmitting confidential information. It is possible to misdirect information, and information can be mishandled at the receiving end. Therefore, the American Health Information Management Association recommends using fax machines to transmit information only when using the original or mailing photocopies of the original will not meet the immediate needs for patient care.

In its position statement, "Maintenance, Disclosure, and Redisclosure of Health Information," the association suggests health information departments accompany each faxed transmission of medical records with a cover letter which includes the following information:

- date and time of transmission (which may be generated from the fax machine),

- sending facility's name, address, telephone and facsimile number, and sender's name,

- receiving facility's name, address, telephone and facsimile number, and authorized receiver's name.

- number of pages sent, including cover letter,

- statement regarding disclosure,

- statement regarding destruction, and

- instructions for authorized receiver to verify receipt of information.

Figure 2, from AHIMA's position statement, is an example of a detailed cover letter. The original cover letter, with a note of the specific information disclosed, should be filed in the health record.

RECORD OF VERBAL DISCLOSURE OF HEALTH INFORMATION

Patient_____ Date of Birth_____

Patient Number _____

Date of Disclosure _____

Information Disclosed to:_____

Reason for Disclosure:_____

Specific Information Disclosed:

_____
Signature of Individual Making Disclosure   Date

"For discussion purposes only. Not for use without advice of legal counsel."
Source: *Maintenance, Disclosure, and Redisclosure of
Health Information,"* AHIMA,1993.
FIGURE 2. RECORD OF VERBAL DISCLOSURE OF HEALTH INFORMATION

THE MEDICAL RECORD IN COURT

ADMISSIBILITY AS EVIDENCE

The presentation of information from medical records as evidence in a court or other duly constituted tribunal, agency, or commission is quite proper. The record is an unbiased chronological report of the patient's treatment in the hospital, and it is made in the hospital's regular course of business.

As a general proposition, any information from the record can be admitted into evidence; because the record is a business record. If the court can be assured that the record is reliable and trustworthy, it will allow all or part of the information to become evidence subject to rules relating to privilege, relevancy, materiality, and competency. Several state statutes relate specifically to the admissibility of medical records into evidence. The New York statute provides an example:

> (a) Generally any writing or record, whether in the form of an entry in a book or otherwise, made as a memorandum or record of any act, transaction, occurrence or event, shall be admissible in evidence in proof of that act, transaction, occurrence or event, if the judge finds it was made in the regular course of any business and that it was the regular course of such business to make it, at the time of the act, transaction, occurrence or event, or within a reasonable time thereafter. All other circumstances of the making; of the memorandum or record, including lack of personal knowledge by the maker, may be proved to affect its weight, but they shall not affect its admissibility. The term business includes a business, profession, occupation and calling of every kind. (New York Civil Practice Law and Rules, Section 4518).

SUBPOENAS

When one of the parties involved in litigation desires to present medical record information to the court, an order of the court will be sent to the facility as custodian of the records. When the facility or health information director receives such an order, there is no recourse but to obey it. Of course, if the subpoena is unclear, proper inquiry may be made; but the subpoena is a court order designed to cause a witness to appear and give testimony. It commands the witness to come before a specified court or officer at a specified time.

The power to issue subpoenas is defined by statute and varies from state to state. In general, subpoena power is usually vested in attorneys, government boards and commissions, judges, and clerks of court.

Court rules in the federal judicial system and in many state systems provide for the use of notary or deposition subpoenas in order to obtain information before the actual trial of a case. These pretrial discovery procedures and the rules for examinations before trial vary widely from jurisdiction to jurisdiction (territorial range of authority or control). It is necessary to become familiar with local practice, but the subpoena used in pretrial discovery is also generally enforceable and should be obeyed.

A subpoena requires the presence of the witness. A subpoena duces tecum requires the witness to come with certain specified documents. The New York statutes says that any person may comply with a subpoena duces tecum by appearing with the requisite books, documents, or items, identifying them, and testifying respecting their origin, purpose, and custody. (New York Civil Practice Law Article 23, Section 2305(b).) In several states the practice has been to allow the custodian of business records to certify a copy of the records and to send them to the clerk of the court. The requirement to appear personally is thus removed. The person to whom the subpoena is issued may be considered in contempt of court if it is not honored or a satisfactory explanation of the reasons why it was not honored is presented.

The admissibility or exclusion of testimony of the witness or the records of the custodian is governed by the rules of evidence. These rules are complicated, varied, and outside the scope of this chapter. One should note, however, that in any case, none, part, or all of the information in the record may be actually admissible. Admissibility will be governed by the particular rules of the state and the issues and subject matter of the case. The judge and opposing counsel have the responsibility to resolve controversy dealing with the rules of evidence. The responsibility of the health information practitioner is to be an objective witness as a representative of the facility. As noted previously, the New York statute expects the judge to determine whether the record was made in the usual course of business. The health information practitioner will be asked questions regarding position in the facility, whether the record is in the practitioner's possession, and whether it was made in the usual course of business.

While the server of the subpoena is still present, or upon first inspection of a subpoena received in the mail, the subpoena should be checked for the type of subpoena, the name of the person or organization upon whom the subpoena is served, the name and location of the court, the name of the attorney, the docket number of the case, the date and time the witness must appear, signature of the court clerk, and the seal of the court. Subpoenas for civil cases should be accompanied by payment of any fees authorized by court rules. If the subpoena is a copy, it should be checked with the original, which the server should have to ensure they match and that the original bears the seal of the court. If the subpoena lacks any of the above information, the attorney who caused the subpoena to be issued should be notified that the subpoena was improperly served. The attorney's name may be obtained from the clerk of the court if not listed on the subpoena.

It is not possible to predict which records will be subpoenaed. Therefore, each medical record must be regarded as potentially subject to courtroom scrutiny. Consequently, a careful quantitative analysis by the health information practitioner of the medical record of every discharged patient is of utmost importance. For example, entries that have been erased or not corrected according to the rules of the facility should be rejected and sent back for proper correction.

PREPARING SUBPOENAED RECORDS FOR COURT

After a subpoena duces tecum is accepted, the requested records must be found and prepared for use as follows:

1. Log in subpoena according to hospital policy.
2. Determine whether the patient has a record at the facility and where it is located; e.g., inpatient, ambulatory care, emergency service, etc.
3. Check the record to make sure it is complete, that signatures and initials are identifiable, and that each sheet contains the patient's name and number.
   a. If the record is incomplete, take steps to expedite its completion.
   b. If the record is on microfilm, notify the attorney who caused the subpoena to be issued so arrangements can be made for either a microfilm reader to be in

court or to pay for having the record reproduced in hard copy. Microfilm records are admissible as primary evidence in place of the original record under the provisions of Public Law 129.

4. Become familiar with the contents of the record, in case called upon to read from the record on the witness stand.

5. Read the record to be sure it is not a potential malpractice suit against the facility or physician. If it is, or might be, notify the administrator and the attending physician.

6. Obtain additional records specified in the subpoena; e.g., x-ray films, bills, etc.

7. Remove all correspondence, duplicate copies of reports, copies of medical records from other facilities, and insurance reports, unless the subpoena specifically calls for such documents.

8. Number the front and back of each page of the record in ink, and record the total on the record folder.

9. Photocopy the record (or make a paper copy of microfilm) and complete a statement certifying that the copy is an exact duplicate of the original. If only portions of the record were subpoenaed, prepare a copy of the whole record as it may be required by the court to admit the subpoenaed portion into evidence.

10. Prepare an itemized listing in duplicate of the record contents which can be used as a receipt if the record is left in court. The copy of the listing should be retained at the facility.

11. Record the type and number of the medical record and the number of pages in the log. If no medical records exist on the patient specified in the subpoena, submit a "no record" statement to the issuer of the subpoena. You may be required to testify in court as to this fact.

CONDUCT AS A WITNESS

Before going to court, it would be well for the health information practitioner to become familiar with the following counsel given in *Legal Aspects of Health Care Administration* by George D. Pozgar:

1. Dress conservatively.

2. Do not be antagonistic towards either counsel. The jury may already be somewhat sympathetic toward the injured party; your antagonism may only serve to reinforce such an impression.

3. Be polite, sincere, and courteous at all times.

4. Be organized in your thinking and recollection of the facts.

5. Do not use the witness box to show how knowledgeable you are. What you think is harmless may be the downfall of the case.

6. Explain your testimony in simple, succinct terminology.

7. Do not overdramatize the facts you are relating.

8. Do not allow yourself to become overpowered by the cross-examiner.

9. Pay close attention to objections either attorney may have as to the line of questioning being conducted by the other counsel.

10. Never deny discussing the case with the institution's attorney when questioned about such practice.

11. Be sure to review any oral deposition you may have participated in during examination before trial.

12. Do not show any visible signs of displeasure regarding any testimony with which you are in disagreement.

14. Be sure to have questions that you did not hear repeated and questions which you did not understand rephrased.

15. When asked questions which you are not qualified to answer about medical facts, state this immediately.

The presiding judge at the trial rules whether all or portions of the hospital record should be received in evidence. If so ruled, the record, according to the general practice of the courts, must be identified by the person representing the hospital. The health information practitioner is qualified to testify that the record was kept in the hospital's regular order of business, to the component parts of the record, and to identify who was responsible for the compilation of each part of the record. For this reason the health information practitioner should be the person to answer a subpoena duces tecum. Testimony on such facts, however, is the extent of responsibility as a witness.

The record is usually marked for identification and then offered in evidence. It may be later used by the physician or other health care practitioner in testimony.

When the health information practitioner is called to the stand, a swearing in takes place. This serves to identify the bearer of the record and answer certain questions to lay the foundation for the introduction of the record in evidence. Subject to objection from opposing counsel, health information practitioners may be asked to read portions of the record. On the other hand, the attorney may merely ask for the medical record, and the health information practitioner may be excused from the stand. The health information department director should obtain a receipt for the record if the original must remain with the court. The judge may permit photocopies to be substituted for the original record.

To avoid leaving the original record, many health information directors photocopy the record and take the photocopy together with the original medical record when answering a subpoena. Many trial judges will accept the photocopy in lieu of the medical record after the latter has been properly identified.

While a receipt may be accepted from the court in case the medical record is retained, there is the possibility that the court may keep the record for an indefinite period; therefore, it is advisable to have the photocopy of the medical record substituted, or to remain during the entire court procedure and recover the medical record whenever possible. For obvious reasons, the original record should be returned to the hospital. If it becomes necessary for the court to retain the record for a long period during court procedure, permission will generally be granted to have a photocopy substituted after comparison with the original. The court or the lawyers for the litigants will usually permit the records to be received promptly in evidence if the health information director requests it. Then it will not be necessary for the health information practitioner to remain in the courtroom for any great length of time.

Occasionally a health information practitioner will receive a warrant, which differs from a subpoena in that it is issued by a judge after hearing testimony that the warrant is proper. Warrants are issued to conduct a search of a person or place or to authorize the arrest of a person. Since it rarely occurs that a health information practitioner is faced with the execution of a warrant, it is sufficient to state that full cooperation when presented with a warrant by a law enforcement officer is recommended. Hospital personnel should not physically impede the officer's activity, even though they may indicate to the officer that they believe the action is beyond the authority under the warrant. Hospital personnel may also advise the officer when in their judgment, the patient's physical condition precludes removal if a patient is arrested and is to be removed from the premises.

SECURITY OF MEDICAL RECORDS

The subject of medical record security has always been an important one. However, due to the ease of data transmittal in computerized systems, the ability to produce multiple printouts of confidential data, and the ever-increasing number of requests for medical data to be used for non-patient care purposes, the subject of security deserves renewed attention.

Medical records, whether in paper form or computerized form, should be subject to the rules of confidentiality. Institutional policy should specifically address the inclusion of computerized records in the confidentiality policies. Additions to the policies and procedures may be necessary to assure computer files are secure and not accessible to unauthorized users.

Medical records must be stored in secure areas accessible only to authorized personnel. Records must be secure at all times, including the time they are circulating for patient care purposes out of the department. The health information practitioner should be aware of the usual storage areas for records on nursing units and the areas where other departments keep records when out of the health information department. These areas should be secure and not accessible to unauthorized individuals. It is not unusual for directors of health information management to maintain a locked file for records the facility considers particularly sensitive, such as records of patients whose health status could be newsworthy or patients involved in legal proceedings, to protect them from unauthorized disclosure as well as tampering.

When the record is required for internal use, the original record should be circulated. When photocopies or printouts are necessary, they should be subject to the same controls as the original record and should be returned to the health information department for destruction.

Virtually all regulatory bodies which address the subject of medical records include a provision for assuring the security of the records.

This is an important responsibility of the health information practitioner; however, it is often thought of as a responsibility relating to the paper medical record. Health information practitioners must be involved in the design of every computerized system in the institution that stores patient or provider identifiable confidential medical data. In addition, the health information practitioner should be knowledgeable about the various types of computer security measures, so the security of the data can be reasonably evaluated. These measures are continuously enhanced by advancing technology, requiring the practitioner to remain current on this subject. In general, security should address who is allowed access to the system, what functions each individual is allowed to execute in the system, and how each person who has gained access is identified. The most common access method is via a password or combination of passwords and security codes. Care must be exercised when passwords are the method of authorizing entry. They should be changed frequently, at least biannually. The system should be programmed to stop responding to repeatedly erroneous passwords, or to continue to ask petty, persistent questions to allow time for tracking. The most effective passwords are those that combine numbers and letters with the letters in a combination of upper and lower case. This type of password is difficult for an unauthorized person to discover accidentally.

Other means of identifying authorized users are cards or badges inserted in the terminal. More sophisticated means of identifying authorized users include identification by fingerprint or by the individual's voiceprint or retinal image. As these methods are more widely used, their cost will be reduced and may become common methods of identification in the near future.

The method of entering the system can also identify the level of function the individual is authorized to perform. For example, certain passwords are reserved for those who can inquire only. A second level of authorization is granted to those who add information to the system. Other passwords or data entry methods may authorize individuals to change data or delete it. Certain passwords may be assigned to identify trainees or supervisors.

The system may allow access to certain parts of the system, but not to specified data in that part of the system. For example, a clerk may have access to all information except the diagnosis on a specified screen.

To assure that security measures are operating correctly, there should be a system to audit activities showing who had access to what data. The audit trail may reveal all activities of a given user, group of users, specific terminal or a physical grouping of terminals. Auditing should be done to determine activity for different time periods. For example it could detect activity on a specific terminal in a department when the department is normally closed. A good audit trail can reveal not only unauthorized use, but can assist in evaluating whether the security systems are adequate or, in some cases, whether they are unnecessary and thus contributing to the cost of the system unnecessarily.

Key factors in determining security needs are the system function, the equipment configuration, the degree of sensitivity of the data involved, and the cost of the security measures.

People, not the system itself, are the greatest threats to computer security. Considerations should include the degree of employee loyalty and judgment, their degree of experience, particularly in handling confidential data and properly using the system, and the degree of involvement of non-employees, such as consultants, auditors, and vendors.

ETHICAL ISSUES

In keeping with increased use of technology in the health care field is an increase in the ethical issues raised by utilizing technology. For example, health care providers are faced with the ethical and medical dilemma of whether given patients should be resuscitated. Before the landmark Supreme Court decision of Roe V. Wade, 410 U.S. 113, (1973), abortion was illegal in virtually every state in the nation. Although now legally sanctioned under certain conditions, it remains a hotly debated ethical issue.

The health information practitioner becomes involved in these ethical dilemmas to the extent that adequate documentation of events in the medical record is required. Institutional policies and procedures should detail documentation requirements when ethical situations are an issue, and health information practitioners should be alert to evolving situations which may require additions to these policies.

SECONDARY RECORDS

The information in this chapter focuses on the primary medical record as a legal document. However, health information practitioners should be cognizant that secondary records also have legal implications. Secondary records are defined as those maintained by the health care institution containing information transferred from the primary record, or duplicate copies of the primary record, which are identifiable by individual patient or provider. Examples are indexes or logs containing medical information, carbon or facsimile copies of the primary record, quality assurance reports, and merged clinical and financial reports.

In its 1994 report on Health Data in the Informational Age: Use, Disclosure, and Privacy, the Institute of Medicine (IOM) predicts that "new uses for and users of data will emerge," raising many privacy issues. The institute, which examines health policy matters in depth, provided numerous recommendations about the proper disclosure, protection, and use of secondary health information.

The American Health Information Management Association also addresses secondary information in its position statement on "Maintenance, Disclosure, and Redisclosure of Health Information." AHIMA says that the facility is responsible for protecting all the data it possesses against loss, defacement, tampering, and unauthorized use of disclosure and gives guidance on how to ensure such protection.

The increased use of computers in health care facilities has resulted in a proliferation of reports containing patient and provider identifiable information. Reports are often produced because it is possible to do so without regard for the utility of the report and its final disposition. This introduces the possibility of breaching the confidentiality of sensitive health care data and presents problems with control of this data. Institutions establish procedures defining who is authorized to request printouts of computerized information. A log or listing should be maintained which specifies individuals by title authorized to receive such documents, and for what periods.

Some secondary records, such as patient or provider identifiable quality management reports, are protected by state law from discovery as legal documents. The extent of protection varies widely. Some states offer no protection to the records while others grant an absolute statutory exemption protecting the records. Health information practitioners should be familiar with the state laws, and assure the institution is in compliance with all requirements and criteria for protection.

In addition to state laws protecting records of quality management activities, the Health Care Quality Improvement Act of 1986 offers some immunity to peer reviewers. This is a federal act which was passed to strengthen the peer review process by protecting participants when they act in good faith to assure the quality of care. The Act provides immunity from damages in legal actions, except in civil rights litigation and litigation filed by the attorney general of a state or the United States. It provides this immunity when legal action is brought as a result of a credentialing decision affecting a physician as long as the process meets certain standards and the health care entity reports decisions adverse to the physician to the appropriate Board of Medical Examiners.

As part of the Health Care Quality Improvement Act, hospitals have a duty not only to report but also to request information. They must request information from the National Practitioner Data Bank concerning a physician, dentist or health care practitioner at the time the individual applies for a position on its medical staff (courtesy or otherwise) or for clinical privileges at the hospital, and every two years thereafter.

SUMMARY

The medical record is a legal document and as such is affected by laws, rules and regulations, and institutional policy.

The medical record is the property of the health care facility while the personal data contained in the record are considered a confidential communication in which the patient has a protectable interest. The record is compiled, preserved, and protected from unauthorized inspection for the benefit of the patient, facility, and physician as required by law in some states and by administrative practice in others.

Since the medical record frequently is used as legal evidence of the patient's care, it can serve as a protection to the facility, physician, and patient only when it clearly shows the treatment given the patient, by whom given, and when given. It must show that the care and service given by the hospital and by the physician were consistent with good medical practice. By the same token, the record may prove to be a potent weapon against the facility or physician in an action by the patient when these standards are not met.

The medical record must be maintained to serve the patient, the health care providers, and the institution in accordance with legal, accrediting, and regulatory agency requirements. The health facility should have a provision for making its procedures regarding disclosure, access, and amendment of health record information known to patients upon request; and the release of information should be closely controlled. A properly completed and signed authorization is required for release of all health information except

     a) as required by law
     b) for release to another health care provider currently involved in the care of the patient
     c) for medical care evaluation
     d) for research and education in certain situations

The health information practitioner must be familiar with the statutes, regulations, and cases governing medical records in general, and those which apply to the state in which employed, and community in particular. In addition, the health information practitioner must take an active role in the development and enforcement of the policies of the facility regarding the proper release of information, whether it be in answer to a subpoena, in response to requests from governmental agencies, from the individual patient, from relatives of patients, or others.

STUDY QUESTIONS

1.   Identify the sources of legal requirements and explain how to obtain information on federal and state law.

2. Define confidentiality and privacy.

3. Describe the circumstances in which the patient may intentionally or unintentionally waive the privilege of consenting to release the medical record.

4. Specify the recommended items to be included in a form for authorization of release of patient information.

5. List the steps to be taken in preparing a patient's medical record for entry into court proceedings in response to a subpoena duces tecum.

6. Discuss redisclosure of medical records.

7. Differentiate between primary records and secondary records of medical care.

REFERENCES

American Health Information Management Association, "Code of Ethics," (1994).

American Health Information Management Association, "Maintenance, Disclosure, and Redisclosure of Health Information," (Chicago 1993).

American Health Information Management Association, *Position Statement on Managing Health Information Relating to Infection with the Human Immunodeficiency Virus,* (Chicago, 1994).

"American Journal of Law and Medicine," Vol. XIII, Nos. 2 and 3, (Boston: American Society of Law & Medicine and the Boston University School of Law, 1987).

American Medical Record Association, "Code of Ethics," (1985).

Banach, Joan, "Legislative Currents: The Uniform Health-Care Information Act: Current Status," Part I, II, *Journal of the American Medical Record Association,* Vol. 59, No. 9/10, (September/October 1988).

Bruce, JoAnne Czecowski, *Privacy and Confidentiality of Health Care Information,* (Chicago: American Hospital Publishing, Inc., 1989).

Buchanan, Robert J. and James D. Minor, *Legal Aspects of Health Care Reimbursement,* (Rockville, MD: Aspen Systems Corporation, 1985).

Buckland, Ann E. and Joelaine Wasson, "Behind the Headlines: Significance for Medical Record Practitioners," *Journal of the American Medical Record Association,* Vol. 59, No. 8, (Chicago: AMRA, August 1988).

Christoffel, Tom, *Health and The Law,* (New York: The Free Press, 1982).

Clark, Laura A., "A State By State Evaluation of Patient Access to Hospital Medical Records," *Journal of the American Medical Record Association,* Vol. 58, No. 6, (Chicago: AMRA, June 1987).

"Comprehensive Alcohol Abuse and Alcoholism Prevention, Treatment and Rehabilitation Act Amendments of 1974," *Public Law,* (May 14, 1974): 93-282 (42 U.S.C. 290dd3), (42 U.S.C. 290ee-3).

Conditions of Participation for Hospitals, U.S. Dept. of Health and Human Services, (Washington, DC: Social Security Administration, June 17, 1986).

"Confidentiality of Alcohol and Drug Abuse Patient Records," *Federal Register,* Vol. 42, No. 110, (June 9, 1987).

Hayt, Emmanuel, Lillian Hayt and August Groeschel, *Law of Hospital, Physician and Patient,* (Berwyn, IL: Physicians' Record Company, 1972).

Health Data in the Information Age: Use, Disclosure, and Privacy, (Washington, D.C.: National Academy Press, 1994).

Hellebust, Lynn, *State Legislative Sourcebook 1986,* (Topeka, KS: Government Research Service, 1985).

Hogue, L. Lynn, *Public Health and The Law,* (Rockville, MD: Aspen Publishers, Inc., 1980).

Hoyt, Eugene M., "Privacy, Confidentiality, Privilege, and the Medical Record, Parts I and II," *Journal of the American Medical Record Association,* Vol. 57, No. 8/9, (Chicago: AMRA, August/September 1986).

Joint Commission on Accreditation of Healthcare Organizations, *Accreditation Manual for Hospitals,* (Chicago: Joint Commission, 1994).

Morgan, Charles, "Patient Access to Medical Records - From Issue to Law, Part I: An Historical Perspective," *Journal of the American Medical Record Association,* Vol. 55, No. 5, (Chicago: AMRA, May 1984).

Morgan, Charles, "Patient Access to Medical Records - From Issue to Law, Part II: A Case Study," *Journal of the American Medical Record Association,* Vol. 55, No. 6, (Chicago: AMRA, June 1984).

O'Gara, Sarah, "Does Patient Access to Health Records Cause Harm?" *Journal of the American Medical Record Association,* Vol. 55, No. 3, (Chicago: AMRA, March 1984).

Pozgar, George D., *Legal Aspects of Health Care Administration,* (Rockville, MD: Aspen Systems, 1987).

"Requirements for federal subpoenas are streamline," *Medical Records Briefing,* (Marblehead, MA, March 1993).

Rowland, Howard S. and Beatrice L. Rowland, *Hospital Legal Forms, Checklists, and Guidelines,* Vol. 1, (Rockville, MD: Aspen Publishers, Inc., 1986).

Smith, Robert Ellis, "Privacy, An Endangered Species in a Computer Age?" *District Lawyer.*

Southwick, Arthur F., *The Law of Hospital and Health Care Administration,* (Health Administration Press, 1978).

"Topics in Health Record Management, Legal Issues, Part I and II," (Rockville, MD: Aspen Systems, June/September, 1981).

U.S. Government Printing Office, Washington, D.C., "The Report of the Privacy Protection Study Commission," *Personal Privacy in an Information Society,* (July 1977).

Willett, Edward, F., *How Our Laws Are Made,* (Washington, DC: U.S. Government Printing Office, 1986).

chapter **16**

THE MANAGEMENT OF QUALITY

The evaluation of the quality and cost of medical care is as old as medicine itself. The Code of Hammurabi spelled out a number of conditions which controlled medical practice and specified the fees that could be charged. In the 1600s, the legal code of the colony of Virginia stated that a physician could be compelled to swear to the "true value and worth of the drugs and medicines prescribed." And in the 1860s, studies were performed which compared hospital size with the probability of survival.

In early hospitals, assurance that the medical care provided was of high quality was indirectly controlled through licensure of health care practitioners, granting of medical staff privileges, and some peer review mechanisms. The American College of Surgeons realized that a system of standardization of hospital equipment and work should be established. Thus in 1918, the American College of Surgeons developed a voluntary accreditation program. This program evolved into what is now known as the Joint Commission on Accreditation of Healthcare Organizations.

Today's health care facilities use a variety of activities to monitor and evaluate quality, including quality assurance, quality improvement, utilization management, recredentialing, and risk management. Each of these activities is discussed separately in this chapter, and each began as a separate activity. Yet the activities are closely related and should be conducted through integrated facility-wide programs.

EXTERNAL AND INTERNAL PRESSURES FOR QUALITY

JOINT COMMISSION ON ACCREDITATION OF HEALTHCARE FACILITIES (JCAHO)

A number of external and internal pressures have changed the way health care facilities monitor and improve care. The Joint Commission on Accreditation of Healthcare Organizations was a forerunner in evaluating medical care strictly from a quality standpoint. There have been several milestones in the development and refinement of standards relating to quality improvement.

- In 1952, the Joint Commission was formed as an outgrowth of the American College of Surgeons. It encouraged voluntary attainment of uniform high standards of care and established a structured set of standards.

- In 1972, the Joint Commission established a requirement for medical audits, and in 1975, it required hospitals to "demonstrate that the quality of patient care was consistently optimal by continually evaluating care through reliable and valid measures." In 1979, the JCAHO began to require hospitals to coordinate and integrate all quality of care activities into a hospital-wide program and committee rather than allowing segmented review activities without central coordination.

- In 1985, JCAHO added a specific chapter on quality assurance to its hospital and other facility standards. In addition standards describing monitoring and evaluation were included throughout the standards. To help facilities, JCAHO introduced what it called the 10-step process for quality evaluation (see Figure 1). At the same time, JCAHO expected hospitals to monitor five activities: blood usage, drug usage, medical records, pharmacy and therapeutics, and surgical cases.

- In 1986, the Joint Commission launched a major new project called the "Agenda for Change." The project's intent was to shift the emphasis of accreditation from review of structures to review of outcomes. Simply put, JCAHO's intent was to replace the question "Can this organization provide high quality health care?" with the question "Does this organization provide high quality health care?"

JCAHO'S 10 - STEP - PROCESS

1. Assign responsibility.

2. Delineate scope of care.

3. Identify important aspects of care or service

4. Identify indicators and criteria.

5. Establish thresholds for evaluation.

6. Collect and organize data.

7. Analyze and evaluate data.

8. Take action to solve identified problems.

9. Assess the actions and document improvement.

10. Communicate relevant information to the organization-wide quality program.

FIGURE 1. JCAHO'S 10 - STEP PROCESS

- In 1994, the *Accreditation Manual for Hospitals* began the first phase of a transition from standards organized around hospital departments to standards organized by functions critical to patient care. For example, standards for the health information department were moved into a chapter on information management that addressed all types of information in the hospital, including information from the pharmacy, library resources, and medical records as well as aggregate clinical information.

- In 1994, the Joint Commission implemented the Indicator Monitoring System. Hospitals that voluntarily participate gather data on their care, send the data to JCAHO, which in turn gives participating hospitals comparison data on the quality of their care. By 1996, JCAHO is likely to require hospitals to participate in the Indicator Monitoring System as part of accreditation.

LANDMARK COURT DECISIONS ON QUALITY

Several landmark decisions have had an effect on establishing a quality improvement and performance program in health care institutions. In each case, the court ruled that the hospital and their medical staff have the right and obligation to oversee quality of professional services rendered by the medical staff.

- In 1965, the Darling vs. Charleston Community Hospital case found that a hospital must assume certain responsibilities for care of the patient.

- In 1973, the Gonzales vs. Nork and Mercy Hospital case found the hospital negligent if it knew or had reason to know or should have known of the surgeon's incompetence. The peer review system at Mercy Hospital was infrequently performed, random, and not critical.

- In 1981, the John vs. Misericordia Hospital case found that the hospital had written requirements for checking the credentials of medical staff members but they did not verify information on the applicants. The court found that the hospital owes a duty to its patients in selecting medical staff members and granting privileges.

GOVERNMENT INFLUENCES ON QUALITY

The federal government has also influenced quality management in health care facilities through the laws, regulations, and required review processes.

- In 1965, the Social Security Amendment Title XVIII (Medicare) and Title IXI (Medicaid) programs were developed. Within two years, in 1976, the government issued a Medicare *Conditions of Participation*.

- In 1986, the government expanded the *Conditions of Participation* to include a quality assurance requirement that the governing body must ensure that there is an effective hospital-wide quality assurance program to evaluate the provision of patient care. The *Conditions* also required a clinical plan that includes evaluation of all organized services related to patient care, nosocomial infections, medication therapy, and all medical and surgical services. The hospital must take and document appropriate remedial action to address deficiencies found through the quality assurance program.

- In 1983, with the establishment of Peer Review Organizations (PROs) came new quality assessment requirements for hospitals. PROs are independent organizations that contract with the federal government to review health care services given to Medicare patients. (See the Utilization Management section for more detail on these organizations.)

- In 1986, the federal Health Care Quality Improvement Act was passed. It provides peer review protection and limited immunity for peer review activities. The law provides immunity from damage suites for persons who give information to professional review bodies, if the activities are being conducted fairly and in good faith.

- The National Practitioner Data Bank was established as a central data bank to provide information on physicians. The data bank contains information on malpractice payments, revocations, suspensions, and voluntary surrendering of licenses, and professional review actions that limit physicians' activities. Information in the database is used by hospitals as part of their medical staff credentialing processes.

INTERNAL PRESSURES FOR QUALITY

Although some quality assurance activities have been performed to fulfill accreditation and Medicare requirements, hospitals and other health care providers also have internal incentives for quality improvement.

Economic constraints, such as decreased Medicare reimbursement or competition from other institutions, force facilities to emphasize productivity and cost-efficiency. In connection with productivity monitoring, facilities develop quality monitors by which to measure the success of their productivity programs. Quality monitoring and evaluation systems can identify areas where poor quality translates into unnecessary expenditures.

Moreover, in today's climate of managed care and competition among facilities, institutions must be able to show that they offer good care at reasonable rates. More and more managed care groups and third party payers expect hospitals to be able to prove that their care is of high quality.

But the most important internal pressure to manage quality comes from the institutions themselves. By their very mission, hospitals and other facilities, physicians and other providers, want to make sure their services and care are appropriate and of high quality.

QUALITY ASSESSMENT AND QUALITY IMPROVEMENT

The Joint Commission gives facilities flexibility in determining the structure and mechanisms they will use to monitor and improve quality. However, two general methods are used most often, and they care described in this section. It is important to note that the descriptions given are general; facilities should and do adapt quality philosophies to their own unique situations and needs.

QUALITY ASSESSMENT

For years, most health care facilities monitored quality through a formal program of quality assurance. In quality assurance activities, the facility develops criteria by which to measure quality of specific diagnoses, procedures, or problems. Data is gathered, generally from medical records, to determine how well the actual care followed the predetermined criteria. If there are problems, whether they are documentation problems, education gaps, or practitioner competency questions, the facility determines how to correct them and monitor the improvement.

Quality assurance is a generic term covering a large number of activities. Regardless of the names given to the efforts the basic components of these programs involve developing criteria (sometimes called indicators), gathering information on whether the care met the criteria, and taking action in areas where the care did not measure up.

The term and the method for this type of quality monitoring have changed over the years. In the 1970s, the Joint Commission, the PSRO program, and hospitals used the term patient care audits of medical care evaluation studies. In its 1979 standards, the Joint Commission said that an acceptable audit must use valid criteria, must measure actual practice against the criteria, use peers to analyze the results, include corrective action and monitoring, and must be documented. At that same time, the JCAHO as well as the PSRO required hospitals to

PSROs also performed multi-hospital audits in hospitals used the same criteria to review care, pooled their results, and obtained comparative quality information.

In the 1980s, the term used was quality assurance (QA), and in 1981 the Joint Commission dedicated an entire chapter of its standards manual to QA. The Joint Commission made its requirement more flexible and stopped requiring a certain number of audits. Instead, it required a written plan for QA, a well-defined and organized program, and evidence of effectiveness.

In the 1990s, quality assurance came to be referred to as the "10-step process" being encouraged by the Joint Commission at that time. The Joint Commission also began to use the term "performance improvement" to describe a wide range of activities hospitals should use to measure and improve care. In addition, hospitals are required to monitor blood and blood components, medication usage, medical records, surgical and other invasive procedures, and utilization.

Facilities may use medical staff departments or individual committees for conducting the various reviews or may assign the quality assurance committee responsibility for many activities. Quality assurance support functions may be organized as a separate department or as a division within the health information department.

QUALITY IMPROVEMENT

Quality improvement (QI), also known as total quality management (TQM) and continuous quality improvement (CQI), is another way facilities monitor and improve care and services. Quality improvement programs often enhance quality assurance and other existing quality efforts.

Quality improvement programs focus on clinical excellence, customer service, and leadership. Instead of fixing problems as they occur, QI is aimed at looking at the ways problems develop and seeking ways to prevent the problems from happening again.

Facilities usually take an institution-wide team approach by involving representatives of all departments or services involved in each aspect of service or in each problem. Incomplete records, for example, are not simply the dilemma of the health

records, for example, are not simply the dilemma of the health information management department. Records completion also involves the medical staff, other providers who document in the records, as well as users of medical record information, such as billing and quality assurance. Thus, a team concerned with records completion would involve persons from a variety of departments and disciplines.

Quality improvement techniques work within a health information department too. Health information managers have, for example, used quality improvement techniques and teams to select new transcription equipment, to implement concurrent coding, and to smooth out the flow of ambulatory records.

Quality improvement involves employees, as the examples above illustrate. Therefore, it is as much a management philosophy as it is a quality strategy. A facility with a QI program in place will likely have the following characteristics:

- The organization makes its mission clear and ensures its policies, plans, and attitude follows its mission.

- Employees are involved. Teams of employees do ongoing problem solving and determine changes that need to occur. The facility rewards and recognizes employees' achievements.

- The facility focuses on its customers. Facilities use surveys of customers as well as bench marking (comparing oneself to others with excellent processes) to determine customer needs and wants.

- Teams make decisions based on data, rather than based on complaints or suspicions. Many common data and statistical tools have been incorporated into quality improvement programs Figure 2 lists 11 common tools, and Figures 3-5 illustrate several of those tools.

QUALITY IMPROVEMENT PIONEERS

Though the developers of today's quality improvement concepts have slightly different theories on their application, the basic techniques remain the same: train and educate employees so they can analyze processes in order to improve services and products. The following summarizes the unique theories of several pioneers in QI.

QUALITY IMPROVEMENT TOOLS

1. **Brainstorming** - used for generating ideas on a specific subject or problem. It can be done in a group or individually.

2. **Customer Satisfaction Survey** - used to collect feedback on a system, process, or activity. Helps to identify what needs to be improved.

3. **Flow Chart** - used to identify all the steps in a process, including activities performed, decisions made, waiting periods, and documentation needed. Helps to identify bottlenecks or track the improvement made.

4. **Cause and Effect Diagram** - used to identify the problems in a process. Helps to see a problem and the causes. It is often referred to as a fishbone diagram because of its shape. Helps to evaluate relationships between a problem and its causes.

5. **Check Sheet** - used to determine how often an event occurs and to identify patterns. Sometimes used as a preliminary tool for a Pareto Chart, Histogram, or Run Chart. Helps to identify key causes and ways to improve problems.

6. **Decision Matrix** - a grid chart used to evaluate, compare, and seek out alternative solutions or problems. Helps to determine the most important alternative by rating it.

7. **Pareto Chart** - is a bar graph used to determine priorities in problem solving. Helps to narrow down the causes of a problem and illustrate how things may affect one another. It plots the causes of a problem and its frequency.

8. **Histogram** - a bar graph used to display data over time. Used to search for problems or changes in a system or process.

9. **Run Chart** - is a simple, plotted chart of data that shows the progress of a process over time. Trends, shifts, or changes in the process can be identified.

10. **Scatter Diagram** - used to show possible relationship between two variables and how they interact with one another. Used when you have two similar variables that are possibly related.

11. **Nominal Group Technique (NGT)** - used when there is a need to identify the most pressing problems or find the function that needs the most improvement. All participants generate ideas and then rate them to determine the item that is most important.

FIGURE 2. QUALITY IMPROVEMENT TOOLS

WALTER SHEWHART

Walter Shewhart was an original pioneer of QI and statistical quality control. In the 1920s, he developed a tool called PDCA or Plan, Do, Check, Act that illustrates the complete QI process. (See figure 6.) PDCA is based on planning, putting solutions into action, checking on progress, and acting on the results. W.

Edwards Deming made this methodology popular when he introduced it to Japanese manufacturers.

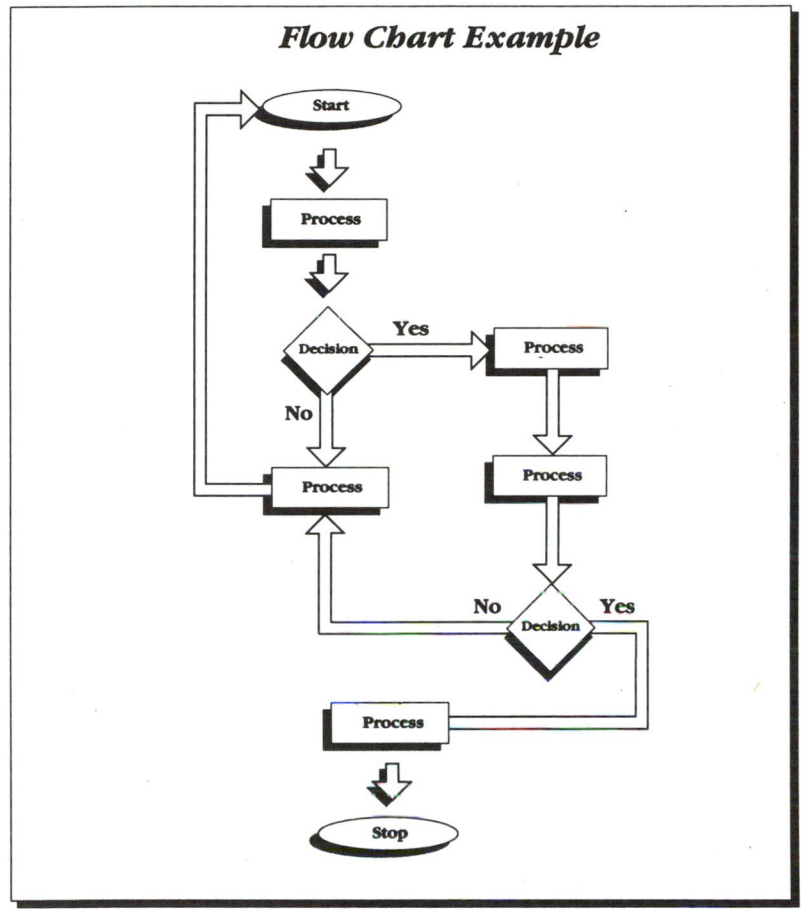

Reprinted with permission from *Quality Improvement Techniques for Medical Records*, Opus Communications, P.O. Box 1168, Marblehead, MA.

FIGURE 3. FLOW CHART EXAMPLE

W. EDWARDS DEMING

Perhaps the most notable and well-known of the quality pioneers is W. Edwards Deming. His concepts were first implemented in Japan during the 1950s. Deming's philosophies, illustrated in what he terms "14 Points," revolve around changing the current style of management to incorporate quality methods, techniques, and tools into everyday work life.

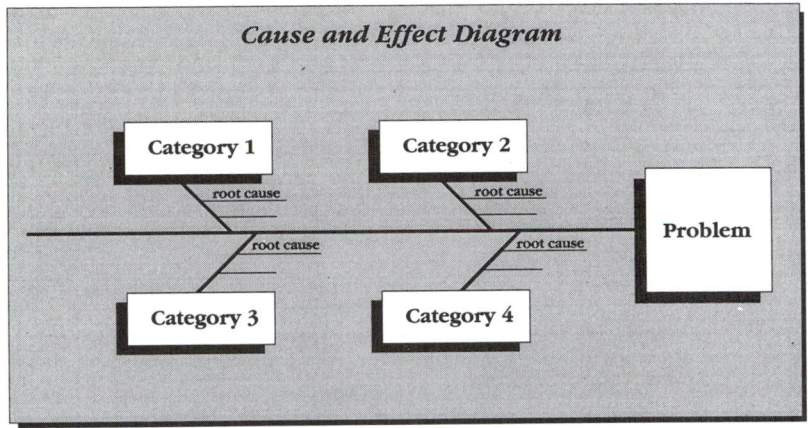

Reprinted with permission from *Quality Improvement Techniques for Medical Records*, Opus Communications, P.O. Box 1168, Marblehead, MA.

FIGURE 4. CAUSE AND EFFECT DIAGRAM

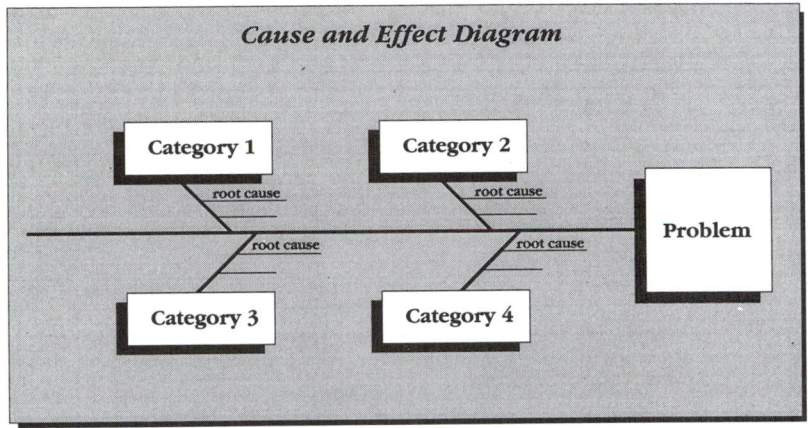

Reprinted with permission from *Quality Improvement Techniques for Medical Records*, Opus Communications, P.O. Box 1168, Marblehead, MA.

FIGURE 5. RUN CHART EXAMPLE

JOSEPH M. JURAN

Joseph M. Juran also helped Japan implement quality concepts to produce better products. Juran cites three main goals that a quality program should encompass: Goal setting based on customers or competition Revising the infrastructure to facilitate change Focusing resources on training and measuring quality

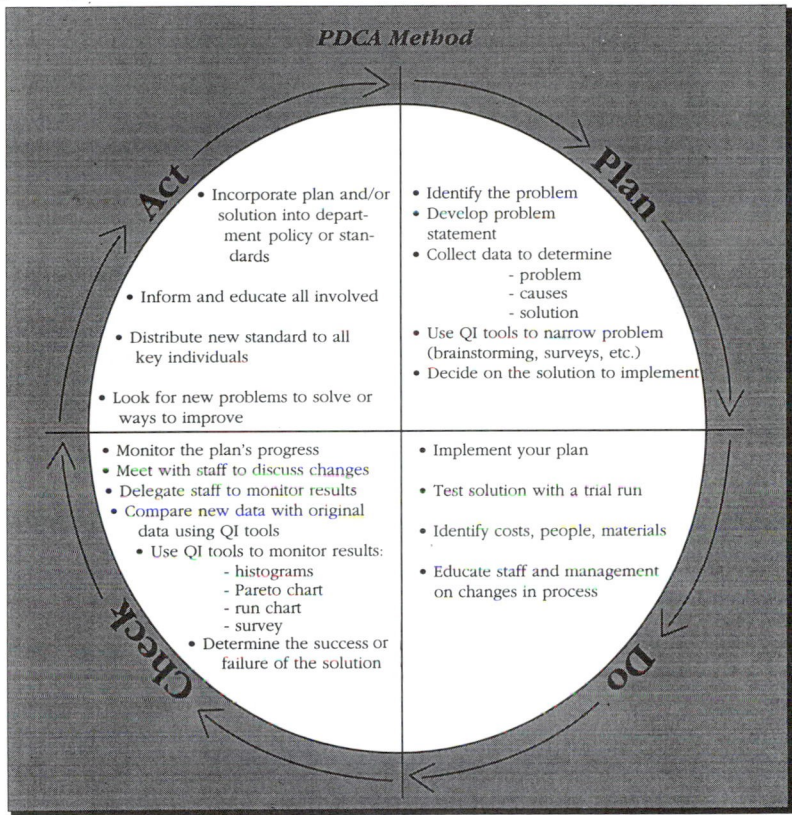

Reprinted with permission from *Quality Improvement Techniques for Medical Records*, Opus Communications, P.O. Box 1168, Marblehead, MA.

FIGURE 6. PDCA METHOD

PHILIP CROSBY

Philip Crosby, a quality consultant, created "four quality absolutes" to improve quality in an organization. He believes that quality should be defined as conforming to requirements, and that organizations should expect "zero defects." His philosophy is based on educating an entire organization, not just management.

BRIAN JOINER

Brian Joiner is a proponent of Deming's philosophies and a quality consultant. He developed the Joiner triangle with these basic elements:

- Quality - Quality ensures customer loyalty and satisfaction.
- Scientific Approach - A scientific approach uses data to identify causes of problems and develop solutions.
- All-one-team - The team approach emphasizes employee involvement in solving problems, thus creating an environment in which employees and management work side by side to develop new ideas, improve the company, and keep morale and enthusiasm high.

UTILIZATION MANAGEMENT

Utilization management, sometimes called utilization review, looks at the facility's efficiency in providing necessary services in the most cost-effective manner possible. It evaluates the level of care required and assesses options, with the goal of eliminating over-and underutilization of services and inefficient scheduling.

The earliest utilization review efforts in hospitals can be traced to the 1950s when guidelines were developed by the Allegheny County Medical Society. This was the first review plan focusing on both the quality and cost of medical care. From these efforts, the Hospital Utilization Project (HUP) was formed to provide data and consulting services for utilization review activities in western Pennsylvania.

Originally, utilization review was conducted by hospital admissions committees. These committees were assigned the task of allocating scarce hospital beds to patients who could demonstrate the greatest need for hospitalization. Before it was mandated by the federal government, only hospitals with frequent bed shortages conducted utilization review.

MEDICARE REQUIREMENTS

Utilization review first became mandatory in 1965 with the passage of Medicare. The Medicare law required that hospitals and extended care facilities establish a plan for utilization review, and that a committee for utilization review be maintained. Even though the law encouraged physician utilization review, it in fact gave fiscal intermediaries the power to deny payment where medical care was determined to be unnecessary.

In 1972, Public Law 92-603 required concurrent review for Medicare and Medicaid patients and set up the Professional Standards Review Organization (PSRO) program. PSROs performed professional review and evaluated patient care services for necessity, quality, and cost-effectiveness. Utilization review committees were required to review all admissions reimbursed by Medicare, Medicaid, and Maternal and Child Health Programs. The law also required extended stay review for covered hospitals and long-term care patients. Physician review committees were required to establish standards and criteria for use in evaluating the necessity of admissions and hospital stays.

In 1977, the UR Act was established for Medicare and Medicaid and included regulations for fraud and abuse. Continued stay review was the act's main emphasis.

In 1982, the Peer Review Improvement Act redesigned the PSRO program, renaming the agencies Peer Review Organizations (PROs). Hospitals began to review the medical necessity and appropriateness of certain admissions even before the admissions occurred. The next year, 1983, the government implemented the prospective payment system for Medicare patients, basing reimbursement on diagnosis related groups.

In 1993, the fourth scope of work was implemented for PROs as part of the government's Health Care Quality Improvement Initiative (HCQII) described later in this chapter.

Professional Standards Review Organizations (PSRO)

In 1972 Public Law 92-603 provided for the establishment of Professional Standards Review Organizations (PSROs), non-profit professional organizations composed of licensed physicians, organized to determine if services provided were medically necessary, and to assure that care was provided in the most economical setting consistent with the health needs of the patient. The PSROs also had quality objectives.

All hospitals were required to have a written utilization review plan which outlined their involvement in utilization review and the norms and standards by which utilization review was to be performed by the physician utilization review committee. The PSROs monitored hospital utilization review activities to assure compliance with the requirements.

During the 1970s, the scope of utilization review activities changed. Review of all admissions was found to be costly and without significant benefit. Some hospitals were allowed to discontinue 100 percent Medicare review and encouraged to focus on known utilization problems only. Other hospitals discontinued concurrent review altogether and participated only in long stay and retrospective reviews. Serious questions were raised about the cost-effectiveness of PSROs as experience with the program accumulated. While isolated instances of cost-savings could be documented, the expenditure of dollars for inpatient health care was dramatically increasing, threatening to bankrupt the medical trust fund. The incentive for stringent utilization control did not exist. Hospitals were paid for the services they provided and the incentive for reducing these services was nonexistent. Many hospitals participated in "paper exercise" utilization review programs which did little to reduce Medicare outlays.

In the early 1980s, the Health Care Financing Administration began to phase out the PSRO program and to increase reliance on fiscal intermediaries to perform utilization review functions. In response to the growing concern about the adequacy of utilization review under the Medicare program, a redesigned program was passed as the Peer Review Improvement Act of 1982. This legislation coincided with the Prospective Payment System, which changed the Medicare payment system from a cost-based system to a diagnosis-related group system.

Peer Review Organization (PRO)

Peer Review Organizations (PROs) perform many utilization-oriented activities including review of the appropriateness of admissions, discharges, and transfers; the completeness and quality of care provided; and the appropriateness of care for which additional payments are sought (outliers). Health Care Financing Administration (HCFA) contracts with PROs to carry out the above work. These contracts delineate the scope of work the PRO will perform during the year and hospitals must comply with the PRO review.

The PRO program was enacted to ensure that services provided to Medicare beneficiaries and reimbursed through Title XVII are:

- Reasonable and medically necessary
- Of a quality which meets professionally recognized standards of health care
- Provided in the most effective and economic setting

Skilled nursing facilities have also been subject to Medicare utilization review since 1972. These requirements include admission review to determine the appropriateness of admission; and continued stay review to determine the need for continued stay. The PROs are involved in monitoring compliance with these requirements but have not assumed the responsibility for review, as they have in hospitals. The same is true for other nonhospital participants in the Medicare program (hospice, psychiatric facilities, alcohol and drug rehabilitation, etc.).

Each PRO has conducted medical peer review in different ways under flexible Medicare contracts. The lack of consistent practices has led to variation in review decisions between PROs and within PROs. In the next PRO contract, reliability and consistency in review decisions will be a primary goal.

Under the new contracts, known as the Fourth Scope of Work, PROs will be participating in the Health Care Quality Improvement Initiative (HCQII). This represents a major effort to increase the impact of PROs on the quality and cost of care. PROs will use medical peer review and other tools to identify patterns of care and outcomes that need improvement. They will then work cooperatively with facilities and individual physicians to improve care.

The goal of the HCQII is to change the focus of review from dealing with individual clinical errors to helping providers improve the mainstream of care for Medicare beneficiaries. HCFA established a comprehensive program in which PROs will use a data-driven approach to monitoring care and outcomes and a cooperative approach for working with the health-care community to improve care.

A set of clear, complete, and mutually exclusive categories for classifying quality concerns have been developed. The categories correspond to the components of quality care provided to a patient. (See Figure 7).

In conducting peer review, the PRO physician reviewer will review for three different issues: utilization concerns, quality concerns, and DRG concerns.

For utilization concerns, the physicians reviewer assesses the appropriateness of the level of care provided the patient. These categories define medically unnecessary admissions, length of stay, and services. The special categories of inappropriate read-missions and transfers called prohibited actions are included. For quality concerns, the physician reviewer assesses the quality of care provided the patient. For DRG concerns, the physician reviewer assesses the medical issues related to the DRG assignment: was the principal diagnosis selected correctly? Are diagnoses and procedures substantiated by the medical record?

If the physician feels that there is potential concern, the PRO will issue an inquiry letter to both the physician and the facility asking for information. They encourage the physician and facility to prepare a joint response. A PRO physician reviewer will then determine whether or not a concern exists. If there is an adverse determination, both parties are offered an opportunity to request reconsideration of a medical necessity denial or to request rereview of a quality concern or DRG change. The beneficiary is also notified of a medical necessity denial and may request reconsideration.

The PRO will analyze data to discover patterns and trends in care and outcomes. PRO pattern analysis is to be the foundation for peer education and guidance and will be used to examine how average care or average outcomes in one place or at one time differ from average care of outcomes in other places or other times. This pattern analysis will include:

The Medicare Hospital Information Project - this includes evaluation of the HCFA Mortality data to target opportunities for significant improvement of medical care.

The Cooperative Cardiovascular Project - this will be the first of a series of projects on special medical conditions used to

FOURTH SCOPE OF WORK CATEGORIES FOR CLASSIFYING CONCERNS

RESOLVED CONCERNS

0   Concern is resolved

UTILIZATION CATEGORIES

A.1.   Medical condition appears not to require inpatient hospital level of care

A.2.   Services rendered appear not to require hospital level of care

A.3.   Admission solely for a procedure that appears unnecessary (also consider C.7.)

A.4.   Apparent unnecessary days of stay in a non-PPS admission or PPS day-outlier case

A.5.   Patient whose admission was initially noncovered subsequently developed a condition requiring covered inpatient care (assign a deemed date of admission)

A.6.   Apparent medically unnecessary days/items/services in a PPS cost-outlier case

A.7.   Hospital-issued notice of noncoverage level of care determination appears to be inappropriate

A.99. Other utilization concern not elsewhere classified (i.e., procedure denied - admission approved)

PROHIBITED ACTION

B.1.   Readmission apparently resulted from a previous premature discharge (also report the inappropriate/premature discharge as quality concern for first admission)

B.2.   Readmission for services that should have been rendered during previous admission

B.3.   Apparent inappropriate transfer from PPS unit to non-PPS unit or vice-versa in same hospital

QUALITY CATEGORIES (PHYSICIAN, NURSING, OR OTHER)

C.1.   Apparently did not obtain pertinent history and/or findings from examination

C.2.   Apparently did not make appropriate diagnoses and/or assessments

C.3.   Apparently did not establish and/or develop an appropriate treatment plan for a defined problem or diagnosis which prompted this episode of care [(excludes laboratory and/or imaging (see C.6. or C.9) and procedures (see C.7 or C.8) and consultations (see c.13 and c.14.)]

C.4.   Apparently did not carry out an established plan in a competent and/or timely fashion (e.g., omissions, errors of technique, unsafe environment)

C.5.   Apparently did not appropriately assess and/or act on changes in clinical/other status

C.6.   Apparently did not appropriately assess and/or act on laboratory tests or imaging study results

C.7.   Apparently did not establish adequate clinical justification for a procedure which carries patient risk and was performed

C.8.   Apparently did not perform a procedure that was indicated (other than lab and imaging, C.9)

C.10. Apparently did not develop and initiate appropriate discharge, follow-up, and/or rehabilitation plans

C.11. Apparently did not demonstrate that patient was ready for discharge

C.12. Apparently did not provide appropriate personnel and/or resources

C.13. Apparently did not order appropriate specialty consultation

C.14. Apparently specialty consultation process was not completed in a timely manner

C.40. Apparently did not follow-up on patient non-compliance (HMOs only)

C.99. Other quality concern not elsewhere classified

DRG CATEGORIES (Requires referral to a physician review only if medical decision is needed)

D.1.   Principal diagnosis not present at admission

D.2.   Principal diagnosis not treated/evaluated during stay

D.3.   Principal diagnosis not principal reason for hospitalization

D.4.   Principal diagnosis not billed as attested

D.5.   Complication/comorbidity/secondary diagnosis attested but omitted from claim

D.6.   Complication/comorbidity/secondary diagnosis billed but not attested

D.7.   Complication/comorbidity/secondary diagnosis billed as attested but not substantiated by record

D.8.   Complication/comorbidity/secondary diagnosis is substantiated in record but not attested or billed and changes the DRG

* D.9.   Procedure attested but omitted from claim

* D.10. Procedure billed as attested but not substantiated by record

D.11. Procedure is substantiated in record but not attested or billed and it changes DRG

* D.12. Procedure determined medically unnecessary is billed and must be removed from DRG

D.13. Disposition statute code is incorrect and changes the DRG

D.14. Patient's age is incorrect and changes the DRG

* D.15. Correct diagnosis or procedure is incorrectly coded

D.16. Deemed date of admission established which changes the DRG

D.99. Other DRG concern not elsewhere classified

*These categories also apply to ambulatory review and HCPCS coding, even though the category may mention an attestation or DRG assignment

FIGURE 7. FOURTH SCOPE OF WORK CATEGORIES FOR CLASSIFYING CONCERNS

analyze clinical data on Medicare patients hospitalized for heart attacks, bypass surgery, and angioplasty.

Trend Analysis - this includes analysis of distributions of significant events (e.g. admissions, readmissions, transfers) by provider for each diagnosis related group (DRG).

Special Local Analysis and Feedback Projects - this includes development of projects to target variations in care in their areas.

The feedback and/or cooperative project process will be used when a pattern of concerns or interest is identified and there is a potential for improvement in the pattern of practice and outcomes of care provided to Medicare beneficiaries and/or efficiency of operation to the Medicare program.

The Uniform Clinical Data Set (UCDS) will be used for case screening on a national basis. Clinical Data Abstraction Centers (CDACs) will abstract data from the hospital medical records using the UCDS direct data entry software.

The PRO will look to a health care organization for cooperation in successful implementation of the Health Care Quality Improvement Initiative. A collaborative effort of national organizations has made an integrated medical peer review system possible.

This new approach should improve reliability and help reviews to record their decisions clearly and easily.

JCAHO Utilization Review Requirements

The Joint Commission has required utilization review since the early 1970s. Physicians were required to periodically review bed utilization and the diagnostic, nursing, and therapeutic resources of the hospital with respect to both the availability of these resources to all patients in accordance with their medical needs. In 1980, the Joint Commission separated the utilization review requirements from the overall Quality of Professional Services standard by developing a Utilization Review standard which required the hospital to demonstrate appropriate allocation of its resources through an effective utilization review program. This new emphasis on utilization review by the Joint Commission paralleled Medicare and other third-party payer interests in decreasing inappropriate hospital utilization. The medical utilization review requirements focused only on Medicare beneficiaries. The Joint Commission requirements expanded the utilization review concept to all hospital patients, regardless of payment source.

Hospitals were required to implement a utilization review program. The program must be delineated in a written plan that describes the methods for conducting review of the appropriateness and medical necessity of admission, continued stays, and supportive services, and for providing discharge planning. The standard specified that retrospective monitoring of the hospital's utilization of resources would be ongoing, and concurrent review would be focused on those diagnoses, problems, procedures, and/or practitioners with identified or suspected utilization related problems. The Joint Commission emphasized discharge planning as a method of ensuring timely discharge at that point in time when an acute level of care is no longer required. The Joint Commission required that the hospital's utilization review program include the written plan, criteria, and length of stay norms be reviewed and evaluated annually and revised as appropriate to reflect the findings of the hospital's utilization review activities.

Organization Of A Hospital Utilization Management Program

A hospital's utilization management program is based on its utilization management plan which outlines the purpose; lines of authority; committee organization, responsibilities, and functions; reporting mechanisms; administrative support; relationship to other quality improvement activities; and the procedure for updating the plan.

The utilization management program's administrative support may be a utilization management department, a quality improvement department, or the function may be assigned to the health information management department. Regardless of the organizational pattern utilized at a particular hospital, the health information management practitioner's expertise in data collection and data analysis is needed to develop an efficient utilization management program. The data requirements of the utilization management program must be integrated with other data requirements to ensure that quality data are maintained and that each data element is collected only once.

Utilization Review Process

The utilization review process consists of certain basic procedures in all hospitals. Preestablished objective screening criteria are used for all reviews. The time frames for completing reviews are specified in the utilization management plan. The types of review most commonly performed are:

Preadmission review - Review prior to admission to determine if the procedure and reason for potential admission is appropriate and necessary in an acute setting. It is designed to identify patients who do not qualify for inpatient benefits prior to admission and refer them to the appropriate health care setting.

Admission review - Review at time of admission to determine if the admission is medically necessary and appropriate.

Continued stay review - Review for continued medical necessity and appropriateness and utilization of beds and facilities. Review is done at specified intervals throughout the inpatient stay.

Discharge review - Review done at discharge to determine if the patient meets discharge screens. Timely discharge planning is also required.

Retrospective review - Review done by the PRO on a retrospective basis for evaluation of quality issues, cost and day outliers, as well as utilization and appropriateness of admissions and resources. Designed to identify trends or utilization related problems such as overutilization, underutilization, inefficient scheduling, and patterns of nonacute days.

At any time during the review if there is not enough documentation to support the admission or continued stay, a physician advisor is contacted for review of the case. If it is determined that there is not enough supporting documentation, a notification of the denial is provided in writing to the business office, patient, attending physicians, and PRO. The patient and attending physician are informed of their right to reconsideration of the decision.

Screening Criteria

Screening criteria are used by most utilization management programs and the PRO for review of appropriateness of admission and continued stay. There are two types of criteria sets available. 1) diagnostic/procedure-specific and 2) severity of illness/intensity of service. Most facilities and PROs utilize the latter category because it measures the level of intensity of resources used. (Figures 8 and 9 illustrate such criteria).

---

1. GENERIC

SEVERITY OF ILLNESS

VITAL SIGNS
Temperature above 102° F (38.9° C) with WBC above 15,000/
cu. mm or bacteria by smear
Pulse below 40/minute
Pulse above 140/minute

BLOOD PRESSURE
Systolic below 80 mm Hg
Systolic above 250 mm Hg
Diastolic above 120 mm Hg

LABORATORY – BLOOD
Serum Sodium below 123 mEq/L
Serum Sodium above 156 mEq/L
Serum Potassium below 2.5 mEq/L
Serum Potassium above 6.0 mEq/L
Blood pH below 7.30
Blood pH above 7.45 (newly discovered)
Presence of toxic level of drugs or other chemical substance

FUNCTIONAL IMPAIRMENT (sudden onset)
Sight loss
Hearing loss
Speech loss
Loss of sensation or movement any body part
Extreme weakness without paralysis
Impaired breathing
Unconsciousness
Disorientation

PHYSICAL FINDING
Gross, continuous hemorrhage from any site
Wound disruption (requiring reclosure)
Vomiting/diarrhea with any one of the following:
• Serum Sodium above 150 mEq/L
• Hematocrit above 55%
• Hemoglobin above 16 grams
• Urine specific gravity above 1.026
• BUN above 35
• Creatinine above 2 mg%
• Ileus

OTHER
Incapacitating pain

Reprinted with permission of InterQual from "ISD-A Review System"

FIGURE 8. SCREENING CRITERIA - SEVERITY OF ILLNESS

Outcomes of Utilization Management

In order to survive and grow, a hospital must render quality care while increasing its efficiency, decreasing its costs, and responding effectively to marketplace pressures. Hospitals have had to establish alternative utilization services to meet

---

1. GENERIC

INTENSITY OF SERVICE

MONITORING (at least every two hours)
Special care unit (refer to CCU/ICU/PCU criteria, pp. 4-6 to 4-11)
Vital signs (T,P,R)
Blood pressure
Orientation to time and place
Urine output
Pupil reaction to light
Central venous pressure
Electrolytes
Blood gases

MEDICATIONS
Intravenous therapy if n.p.o.
Intravenous medications
Continuous intravenous chemotherapy or chemotherapy requiring parenteral medications for control of nausea and vomiting
Initial Insulin therapy/Insulin pump regulation
Parenteral analgesics three or more times daily

TREATMENTS
Respiratory assistance (e.g., ventilator, Bird, MAI)
Implantation of radioactive materials in doses greater than 30 millicuries*
Plasma phoresis requiring hospitalization

PROCEDURE (scheduled within 24 hours)
Surgery or procedure not on ambulatory surgery list and requiring general or regional anesthesia (refer to Ambulatory Surgery Guidelines, pp. 3-6 to 3-9)

PROCEDURE (NOT scheduled within 24 hours)
Surgery or procedure requiring preoperative preparation in the hospital (2 days only):
- Bowel preparation (except colonoscopies and sigmoidoscopies)
- Nutritional supplementation (refer to TPN criteria, p. 5-12)
- Medication adjustment (potassium, glucose, etc.)
- Obtain blood products (cardiac and thoracic admissions)
- Dialysis for living related renal transplant admissions

*See Nuclear Regulatory Commission Requirements.

DISCHARGE SCREENS

Temperature below 99° F/37.2° C for last 24 hours without antipyretic such as aspirin, Tylenol, Bufferin
Prescribed diet tolerated for 24 hours without nausea or vomiting
Passing flatus/fecal material
Voiding or draining urine (at least 800 cc) for last 24 hours
Type/dosage of major drug unchanged for last two days
No parenteral analgesics/narcotics for last 24 hours
Wound(s) healing
Able to clean and care for drainage tubes

Reprinted with permission of InterQual from "ISD-A Review System"

FIGURE 9. SCREENING CRITERIA - INTENSITY OF SERVICE

the demands of the government and managed care. Some of these include preadmission review, 23 hour observation beds, hotel accommodations, same day surgery, furlough days, discharge planning, outpatient day surgery (free standing), skilled nursing facilities, swing beds, and home care services.

To remain competitive, hospitals must determine the most efficient way to provide care in the most cost effective manner while providing the highest quality of care. Constantly evaluating and monitoring services and outcomes will help hospitals to survive the 1990s.

CREDENTIALING

Credentialing has become very important to hospitals to ensure quality care is being provided to patients.

Credentialing involves the review, verification, and evaluation of the key factors that determine an individual's ability to carry out certain patient care activities.

Credentialing is designed for licensed independent practitioners who provide patient care without supervision or direction. Credentialing is the granting of permission to provide medical or other patient care services in the institution, within well-defined limits, based on the individual's professional license and experience, competence, ability, and judgment.

The importance of effective credentialing includes delineation of clinical privileges. Clinical privileges are defined by JCAHO as "authorization granted by the governing body to a practitioner to provide specific patient care services in the hospital within defined limits, based on an individual practitioner's license, education, training, experience, competence, health status, and judgment." Clinical privileging is a specific component of the credentialing process.

The medical staff members are subject to medical staff bylaws, rules and regulations and the hospital's quality improvement program. Therefore the medical staff monitoring activities must be coordinated with the medical staff credentialing function.

The key processes of credentialing are:

– Initial appointment to the medical staff
– Initial delineation and granting of clinical privileges

- Periodic reappointment to the medical staff

- Periodic renewal or revision of clinical privileges

In granting medical staff membership, information regarding the applicant's licensure, specific training, experience, and current competence must be verified by the facility from the primary source(s) whenever feasible. Based on the requirements of the Health Care Quality Improvement Act, facilities must query the National Practitioner Data Bank. Facilities are also encouraged to consider additional information concerning the applicant from other sources, including the American Medical Association's Physician Masterfile and the Federation of State Medical Boards Physician Disciplinary Data Bank. These databases and other sources may provide the facility with information that is new or inconsistent when compared with the individual's application.

In addition, the granting of medical staff membership is based on information regarding previously successful or currently pending challenges to any licensure or registration (state or district, Drug Enforcement Administration) or the voluntary relinquishment of such licensure or registration. Voluntary or involuntary termination of medical staff membership or voluntary or involuntary limitation, reduction, or loss of clinical privileges at another facility should also be investigated.

Clinical privileges are often delineated along specialty board certification lines. Privileges, as related to an individual's clinical privileges, include the limitations, if any, on an individual's privileges to admit and treat patients or direct the course of treatment for the conditions for which the patients were admitted.

When appropriate, temporary clinical privileges may be granted for a limited period of time by the chief executive officer on the recommendation of the chairman of the applicable clinical department/service or the president of the medical staff. A process for reappointment to the medical staff and reappraisal of clinical privileges must also be described in the medical staff bylaws and rules and regulations. The mechanism for reappointment to the medical staff and/or reappraisal and renewal of clinical privileges is hospital specific; approved by the governing body; and described to each applicant seeking reappointment or the renewal of clinical privileges.

Reappointment and/or the renewal or revision of clinical privileges is based on a reappraisal of the individual at the time of reappointment and/or the renewal or revision of clinical privileges. The reappraisal includes information concerning the individual's current licensure; health status; professional performance; judgment; clinical and/or technical skills, as indicated in part by the results of quality improvement activities; previously successful or currently pending challenges to any licensure or registration (state or district, Drug Enforcement Administration) or the voluntary relinquishment of such licensure or registration; voluntary or involuntary termination of medical staff membership or voluntary or involuntary limitation, reduction, or loss of clinical privileges at another hospital; and other reasonable indicators of continuing qualifications. At a minimum, final judgments or settlements of professional liability actions involving the individual are reported.

All individuals with delineated clinical privileges must participate in continuing education activities that relate, in part, to the privileges granted. Each individual's participation in continuing education must be documented; and considered at the time of reappointment to the medical staff and/or renewal or revision of individual clinical privileges.

Departmental and peer recommendations are also a part of the basis for the development of recommendations for continued membership on the medical staff and/or for the delineation of individual clinical privileges.

The governing body is responsible for the final decision, based on medical staff recommendations, regarding an individual's reappointment and/or renewal or revision of individual clinical privileges.

Figure 10 is an example of how quality improvement may be incorporated in a Physician's Credentialing Profile.

Medical Staff Office

In some hospitals, a health information management staff member serves as the individual responsible for maintaining a credentials file for each staff member. This is a very appropriate responsibility for the health information management department, since the results of staff monitoring and evaluation activities are readily available.

PHYSICIAN'S PERFORMANCE PROFILE			
Physician ID: 1234		Department Code:	99
<u>Indicators Not Met</u>			
		YEARS	
	1992	1993	1994
Complications of Outpatient Management	2	1	1
Readmission Within 30 Days	0	1	1
Transfer to Care Unit	2	5	4
Unplanned Return to OR	2	1	0
Neurological Deficit at Discharge	1	0	0
Unplanned Injury to Organ	0	0	0
Nosocomial Infection	2	3	1
Drug Utilization	0	1	1
Normal Tissue Review	0	0	1
Death	1	1	2
Complications	3	5	4
TOTAL	**13**	**18**	**15**

FIGURE 10. PHYSICIAN'S PERFORMANCE PROFILE

Basic information which should be included in the credentials file of each practitioner includes: education, state licensure expiration date, previous practice, prior malpractice claim history, denial of medical staff privileges at other institutions, suspension or revocation of licensure, narcotics number, third-party payment program participation, reference letters, acknowledgment of Medicare fraud notice, and privileges granted with renewal dates. A separate file with quality improvement data should be kept for each physician. This will protect the quality improvement information from discoverability.

Computer support is very helpful in maintaining credentials files for a large staff because many items must be updated regularly, such as licensure expiration dates and privilege delineations. Continuing education attendance records for each practitioner may also be maintained via computer.

Controls are necessary, however, to maintain such a system. Only authorized personnel should enter data; all input data should have supporting documentation in the credentials file, and no documentation should be put into the file until it has Been entered in the computer. In addition, access to credentials files must be strictly limited to authorized individuals. For this reason, the medical staff often prefer a stand-alone microcomputer to be used for credentialing files.

Credentialing is a key mechanism in maintaining high quality professional services provided to patients. The hospital has the obligation to select its medical staff carefully and grant appropriate privileges in order to ensure quality services are rendered by the medical staff.

RISK MANAGEMENT

More than 1,600 years before the development of the Oath of Hippocrates (circa 400 B.C.), the Code of Hammurabi made provisions for defining physicians' liability in the case of certain injuries they might inflict upon their patients. This code stated: *"If a surgeon has made a deep incision in the body of a free man and has caused the man's death or has opened the caruncle in the eye and so destroys the man's eye, they shall cut off his forehand."*

From this beginning, the fundamental principle of physician liability and accountability for iatrogenic patient injury became an integral part of each subsequent society's medical practices. As civilization and the practice of medicine evolved, physician liability and accountability expanded to include nonphysicians who provide medical care to patient and later to include health-care institutions that deliver patient care. Today, if a patient experiences, or is believed to have experienced, an adverse medical occurrence in a hospital, the patient may attempt to hold both the private physician and the hospital liable. The extension of liability to hospitals occurred in 1965, with the court case of Darling vs. Charleston Community Memorial Hospital. In this instance, the court upheld the patient's right to recover damages for malpractice from both the physician and the hospital. This ended the long-standing philosophy that hospitals were exempt from liability because of charitable immunity and established the hospital's duty to supervise the action of independent staff physicians and established the theory that hospitals "know or should have known" about care that was of unacceptable quality.

Hospital Liability

From the malpractice crisis of the 1970s came the development of hospital-based risk management programs, which included risk financing as well as loss prevention and control. Health care organizations designed risk management programs to combat high premium costs and attempted to reduce the frequency and severity of losses.

In the fall of 1986 the American Society for Hospital Risk Management (ASHRM) described risk management in a publication *Perspective in Hospital Risk Management*. Their definition states "Health care risk management is an insurance and quality control-related discipline comprising activities designed to minimize adverse effects of loss upon a health care organization's human, physical, and financial assets through identification and assessment of loss potential, loss prevention and reduction, loss funding and risk financing, and claim control (including professional/general liability and workers' compensation."

Health care facilities must develop strategies to minimize adverse effects of loss resulting from medical professional liability claims.

Today, hospitals are corporately liable for:

– Exercising reasonable care in providing proper medical equipment, supplies, medication, and food for their patients.

– Exercising reasonable care in providing safe physical premises for their patients.

– Adopting internal policies and procedures reasonably estimated to protect the safety and interest of their patient.

– Exercise reasonable care in the selection and retention of hospital employees and in the granting of medical staff privileges.

– Exercising reasonable care to guarantee that adequate patient care is being administered.

Risk Management Program

There are three basic objectives that a health care organization risk management program must have: 1) To create and maintain a safe, healthy environment and enhance the quality of care, 2) To minimize risk of medical or accidental injuries and losses, 3) To provide cost-effective techniques to insure against financial loss.

An effective risk management program incorporates the identification, analysis, evaluation, and elimination or reduction of possible risks to patients, visitors, and employees.

Components of a Risk Management Program

A comprehensive program contains three components:

1. **Risk Identification** - areas of potential or existing loss must be identified. Risk management has the responsibility of determining the potential extent of liability and the financial impact of an incident on the facility. The primary tool used in the identification of risk is the incident report (Figure 11). Mechanisms through which incidents can be identified are:

   a. Incident reporting - provides for early detection of problems or potential compensable events (PCE) and provides a mechanism for an early investigation of serious incidents.

   b. Occurrence screening - allows for concurrent or retrospective identification of physician and hospital-related adverse patient occurrences. They are used to identify specific events that occur during a patient's hospitalization. Examples of occurrence screens are:
      - Return to Operating Room
      - Unplanned Injury
      - Neurological Deficit at Discharge
      - Hospital Incident (Failure of Equipment, Falls, Medication Errors)

   c. Reports of patient dissatisfaction

   d. Results of QI activities

   e. Medical staff minutes

   f. Infection control reports

2. **Risk Control** - The loss prevention and control aspects of risk management were designed to control preventable risks and keep to a minimum the incidents for which the institution might be held liable. Loss prevention focuses on the individual case and the potential for a claim to arise from it. Some of the risk control programs include:

   a. Preventive maintenance and equipment control

Incident Report

An incident is any occurrence which is not consistent with the routine operation of the institution or the routine care of a particular patient. It may involve an injury or damage to property. It may involve visitors, in-house staff, or patient.

—USE ADDRESSOGRAPH IF PATIENT—

CONFIDENTIAL REPORT OF INCIDENT
(Not a part of Medical Record)

Hospital   LARS Loc. Code

PERSON INVOLVED:

(Last Name)	(First Name)	(Middle Initial)
☐ Child ☐ Male	☐ Female Age:	

Exact Location of Incident   Date of Incident   Time of Incident   ☐ A.M. ☐ P.M.

EMPLOYEE: Department   Job Title

VISITOR: Home Address   Home Telephone

OTHER: Home Address   Home Telephone

PATIENT: Room Number   State Cause of Hospitalization

Patient's condition before incident
☐ Normal   ☐ Senile   ☐ Disoriented   ☐ Sedated   ☐ Other

Were Bed Rails present   Other Restraints
☐ Yes   ☐ No   ☐ Up   ☐ Down   ☐ Ordered

Name, Address and Telephone Number of Witness(es)

Describe exactly what happened. (Facts, no opinions):

Date of Report   Person Preparing Report

FIGURE 11. INCIDENT REPORT

b. Hazard surveillance

c. Claims management

d. Development of appropriate policies and procedures, and rules and regulations

e. Staff training and education

f. Good patient assessment techniques

3. **Risk Financing** - A health care facility must plan for the following types of funds to cover losses:

    a. Self-insurance

    b. Insurance pools

    c. Commercial insurance

Elimination or Reduction of Possible Risks

The incident report is also used as a tool to eliminate or reduce future adverse occurrences. In many instances, the event is discussed with those involved and serves as an educational device to prevent future problems. The data from incident reports are also collated and analyzed to identify high risk areas which may require more intensive education and/or restructuring to eliminate future risks. By constant surveillance of the most frequent areas of injury or risk, risk control programs can be targeted to the problem area.

The hazard surveillance function is used to identify areas of potential environmental risk prior to an adverse occurrence. In this way, liabilities may be prevented entirely.

They physician-related adverse patient occurrences identified through an occurrence screening procedure are usually coordinated with the medical staff peer review and credentialing function. Disciplinary action, including loss of staff privileges, may occur if data indicates a pattern or trend of unacceptable physician practices.

Organization and Operation of a Risk Management Program

The organizational structure of an institutional risk management program varies. Larger facilities may employ a risk manager with a staff of specialists to maintain an effective program. In other facilities the health information manager may be responsible for the risk management program through a committee. In either structure, the health information management department may perform occurrence screening, analyze and display incident reports and occurrence screening data, and assist the risk management or quality improvement committee with follow-up activities.

To be effective, the risk management program should be integrated with the facility's quality improvement program. The Joint Commission requires medical staff, governing body, and management participation in risk management activities. The medical staff must identify general areas of potential risk and evaluate the cases, correct problems in the clinical aspects of patient care, and design programs to reduce risk in the clinical aspects of patient care.

The governing body and the administration must support appropriate medical staff involvement in clinical aspects of risk management, operational linkages between quality improvement and clinical aspects of risk management. Without such integration, inadequate communication, duplication of effort, excess costs, and questionable impact on the quality of care can occur. With the quality improvement program having moved away from periodic audits of patient care and into quality monitoring and evaluation, the functions of risk identification and analysis are being easily integrated with those of quality improvement.

SUMMARY

The health information management professional with a knowledge of health care information systems and data systems can provide invaluable leadership in quality management functions. This leadership may be manifested by accepting responsibility for directing the hospital-wide quality improvement program or coordinating any or all aspects of the program (i.e. quality improvement, utilization management, credentialing, or risk management).

The primary data source for the quality improvement activities is the medical record. Health information management personnel routinely analyze each patient record. No other department is so closely involved with the documentation in the record. While others may write patient care notes in the medical record, only the health information management professional evaluates the record in total. By evaluating the documentation in the record, health information management professionals can identify unrecorded diagnoses, over- or underutilization of services or resources, complications or other inappropriate patient care, inadequate documentation, medical errors, or other procedural problems. For risk management, the health information management professional may identify patient complaints, patient incidents, equipment failures, deficiencies in informed consents, inappropriate record alterations, or other documentation problems which may increase liability.

Many health information management departments are actively involved in identifying patient care problems through the use of generic screening mechanisms or other systematic record monitoring. Through the efficient use of health information management professionals in the problem identification phase of quality improvement, duplicative record review by others is eliminated.

The records management expertise of the health information management professional is invaluable in the problem resolution phase of quality improvement. If documentation is a problem, the health information management professional can suggest methods for improvement. In-service programs on the legalities of record documentation may be prepared by the health information management professional. If new forms are proposed, the health information management professional should be involved in the format design.

Health information management professionals also play an important role in the follow-up phase of problem resolution. Once a problem in patient care has been identified and steps taken to resolve the problem, the health information management professional can assist in monitoring to assure satisfactory problem resolution. This assistance may take the form of ongoing record review or a one-time collection of patient care information. The data obtained by the health information management department are then shared with the medical staff committees or departments interested in resolving the problem.

Health information management professionals play a key role in all aspects of a facility-wide quality improvement program. Intra-departmentally they monitor to insure efficiency and effectiveness of their procedures. More importantly, they assist all other components of the program in the problem identification and problem resolution phases. By virtue of their expertise in data collection, record documentation, and forms design, health information management professionals may enhance the overall effectiveness of the health care quality improvement.

Figure 12 is the Position Statement of the Quality Assurance Section of the American Medical Record Association (American

---

POSITION STATEMENT OF THE QUALITY ASSURANCE SECTION AMRA ON CONTINUOUS QUALITY IMPROVEMENT IN HEALTHCARE

PURPOSE

This statement has been prepared to assert the position of the American Medical Record Association's Quality Assurance Section[1] on the use of continuous quality improvement[2] (QI) philosophies and methods in healthcare institutions, and on the integration of QI methods and philosophies with existing quality management (QM)[3] systems and programs. Healthcare providers and leaders are not faced with an either/or decision relative to quality improvement and quality management. Rather, the industry is presented with an opportunity to build upon the best of these approaches to reach the goal of continual improvement of healthcare quality.

STATEMENT

The Quality Assurance Section of AMRA recognizes that the multiple dimensions of quality in healthcare dictate the need for integrated quality management systems which consolidate the components of clinical quality; patient and customer service; appropriateness, cost-effectiveness and efficiency; the reduction of clinical risk; and patient and employee safety. The Section further recognizes that adoption of QI philosophies and successful implementation of QI methods offer resolution of many current barriers to effective quality management for the healthcare institution. The Section therefore endorses and supports the application of continuous quality improvement philosophies and methods in healthcare institutions. The decision to adopt QI philosophies and implement QI methods should be based upon recognition and acceptance of all of the following premises by the institution's leadership.

The effective long-term process of quality improvement must be preceded by commitment of the leadership to continuous quality improvement.

Each endeavor of quality improvement must be continually driven by:

- leadership commitment,
- customer expectations and
- process variation reduction.

QI and healthcare quality management approaches are not synonymous and are not mutually exclusive. Adoption of QI philosophies and methods does not preclude the use of or eliminate the need for existing quality management systems and programs.

Strengths of the institution's current quality management systems should be employed as the foundation for developing totally integrated quality management and improvement programs.

---

1.   The Quality Assurance Section of the American Medical Record Association is a national organization of healthcare professionals employed directly or indirectly in healthcare quality management roles, and individuals interested in healthcare quality management issues and developments.

2.   The term quality improvement is used to identify philosophies adopted and processes undertaken by an organization to achieve continual improvement in product and service quality, continual improvement in the quality of operations and elimination of waste in all functions of the organization. Quality improvement is not a program, a system, or a set of activities. Quality improvement is a set of philosophies and methods which may be used to guide the organization in continual improvement in all aspects of its business. Philosophies and processes are also frequently referred to as: Total Quality Control (TQC), Total Quality Management (TQM), and Total Quality Improvement (TQI).

3.   The term quality management (also commonly referred to in Healthcare as Quality Assurance) refers to the collective components and functions enacted by the healthcare institution to assist in achieving the goals of delivering high quality, cost-effective healthcare services.

Courtesy of The American Medical Record Association

FIGURE 12. POSITION STATEMENT

Health Information Management Association) on Continuous Quality Improvement in Healthcare that was written in 1990. All health information management professionals must ensure that they are the type of leader that is needed in today's

---

Position Statement
AMRA Quality Assurance Section
Page 2

Implementation of QI should not occur separate from, but in coordination with the institution's quality management program.

The institution's medical staff must be supported in developing leadership and member motivation to enable effective participation in institution quality improvement processes.

Operationalizing QI is a long-term endeavor that will over time result in sustained quality improvement.

The institution implementing QI will be an institution undergoing long-term, significant organizational and behavioral change.

Adoption of QI is adoption of a new management style.

Leadership's commitment to quality must be constantly demonstrated through decisions made and actions taken, not solely through the provision of training.

Leadership must not be insulated from quality problems, issues and quality improvement processes.

Employees must be empowered through training, support and delegation of appropriate authority to take actions to improve quality.

QI requires appropriate structural organization and support.

The Section further encourages use of the term "quality management" over "quality assurance" to describe the collective components and functions enacted by the healthcare institution to assist it in continually improving clinical quality, appropriateness, cost-effectiveness, patient and customer satisfaction, patient and employee safety, and clinical risk reduction.

DISCUSSION

Both quality management and quality improvement offer strengths, techniques, assumptions and philosophies which, if properly merged and adapted can forge the optimal quality system for healthcare. Strengths of current quality management provide a foundation to bolster the success of quality improvement efforts. These strengths include the following:

- acknowledgment that optimal results will be realized through a focus toward clinical process,

- experience in the development of indicators to evaluate healthcare structure, process and outcome,

- identification of high priority areas for improvement,

- analysis of appropriateness, effectiveness and efficiency of clinical care,

- identification of educational needs,

- identification of specific approaches needed for improvement of care/services,

---

Courtesy of The American Medical Record Association

FIGURE 12. POSITION STATEMENT (continued)

healthcare environment to assist with all phases of Quality Improvement. Quality Improvement is a key to ensuring the high quality care can be provided to patients in the most efficient and cost effective manner. All phases of the QI Pro-

---

Position Statement
AMRA Quality Assurance Section
Page 3

- expansion of the ranks of professionals knowledgeable about the theory and methods of quality assessment and improvement,

- development of quality information systems, and

- identification of professionals knowledgeable about information systems and data management.

QI brings strengths in its philosophies and techniques which offer resolution of long-standing and current obstacles to effective healthcare quality management. These strengths include the following:

- unquestioned and constantly demonstrated commitment to quality by the institution's leadership,

- stronger reliance on the institution's organizational structure for improvement of processes,

- elevation of the support function for managing quality, with appointment of a senior officer for quality, reporting directly to the institution's Chief Executive Officer,

- integration of quality into total management of the institution, such that quality management is not viewed as being separable from the management of operations, clinical care processes, finance, and business planning for the institution,

- reliance on scientific management techniques and tools for evaluating and improving quality of services,

- employee ownership of quality, with delegation of authority to evaluate, plan improvements, and take corrective measures within the scope of the individual's identified responsibilities, and

- focus on systems for service delivery and on performance of the average provider, versus focus on identification and correction of outlier performance.

CONCLUSION

Quality improvement and quality management are complementary endeavors for attaining continual improvement in healthcare quality. Improvement of the quality of care provided, is and has always been the fundamental goal of healthcare quality management. Attainment of that goal can be advanced through building on the strengths of traditional quality management efforts and adopting philosophies and methods of quality improvement. The Quality Assurance Section of AMRA supports and encourages the adoption of QI philosophies, tools and techniques as core forces of the healthcare providers' quality management programs.

September, 1990
Board of Directors
Quality Assurance Section
American Medical Record Association

Courtesy of The American Medical Record Association

FIGURE 12. POSITION STATEMENT (continued)

gram play an important role in monitoring and evaluating the quality of patient care and assuring the patients and the public that high quality care is the primary concern for health care facilities and providers.

STUDY QUESTIONS

1. Describe four different ways hospitals can monitor quality.

2. What external influences have caused hospitals to monitor quality?

3. Name the quality improvement pioneers.

4. What is the purpose of Peer Review Organizations?

5. What are the five different types of review performed in a utilization management program?

6. Identify the purpose of credentialing and explain how it is tied to other quality management activities.

7. Describe the use of an incident report.

8. What are the factors involved in an effective risk management program?

9. What is the role of the health information department in quality management?

REFERENCES

American Medical Record Association: Quality Assurance Section, "Continuous Quality Improvement in Health Care" *Position Statement*, (Illinois: American Medical Record Association, 1990).

Andrews, Susan L., "QA vs. QI: Then Changing Role of Quality in Health Care", *Journal of Quality Assurance,* (January/February 1991): 14-15, 38.

Berwick, Donald M., A. B. Godfrey, and J. Roessner, *Curing Health care: New Strategies for Quality Improvement,* (California: Jossey-Bass Publishers, 1990).

Cofer, Jennifer I. and Hugh P. Greeley, *Quality Improvement Techniques for Medical Records*, (Massachusetts: Opus IV Communications, 1993).

Conner, Melody, Gloria Mach and Eugene Handelman, *Dynamics of Utilization Management*, (Chicago: American Hospital Association, 1983).

Crosby, Philip B., *Quality is Free*, (New York: McGraw-Hill, Inc., 1979).

DeMuth, William E., "Health Care Coss: One Surgeon's Perspective", *Colloquim*, Vol., No. 1, (Greenwich, CT: CPC Communications, February 1982).

Donabedian, Avedis, "Criteria and Standards for Quality Assessment and Monitoring," *Quality Review Bulletin 12*, (March, 1986): 99-108.

Feature of the Month, "Total Quality Management", *Commitment Plus*, Vol. 5, No. 4, (March, 1991): 1-4.

Feature of the Month, "TQM: What the Leaders Are Doing", *Commitment Plus*, Vol. 5, No. 6, (April 1990): 1-4.

Gagne, James, "America's Quality Coaches", *Advertisement*: 1-4.

Glazier, Don C., "How to Deal with the Impact of Alternate Providers," *Hospital Forum,* (September/October 1984): 57-59.

Greenspan, Jack, *Accountability and Quality Assurance in Health Care*, (The Charles Press Publishers, 1980).

Health care Financing Administration, "Medicare Program; Peer Review Organizations: New PRO Contracts for All States and Territories and the District of Columbia", *Federal Register*, Vol. 58, No. 39, (March 2, 1993): 12042-12047.

Health Care Financing Administration's Quality Review Task Force, "The Integrated Peer Review Process: Medicare's Foundation for Improving Quality of Care", *Health Care Quality Improvement Initiative,* (Washington D. C.: Health Care Financing Administration, 1993).

Imai, Masaaki, *Kaizen - The Key to Japan's Competitive Success*, (New York: McGraw-Hill, Inc., 1986).

Ishikawa, Kaoru, *What is Total Quality Control? - The Japanese Way*, (New York: McGraw-Hill, Inc., 1985).

Joint Commission on Accreditation of Healthcare Organizations, *1994 Accreditation Manual for Hospitals*, (Illinois: Joint Commission on Accreditation of Healthcare Organizations, 1993).

Joint Commission on Accreditation of Healthcare Organizations, *Medical Staff Credentialing: Questions and Answers About the Joint Commission's Standards*, (Illinois: Joint Commission on Accreditation of Healthcare Organizations, 1993).

Joint Commission on Accreditation of Healthcare Organizations, "The Joint Commission Newsletter - Special Issue on the 1994 Accreditation Manual for Hospitals", *Perspectives*, (1993): 1-15.

Joint Commission on Accreditation of Healthcare Organizations, *The Joint Commission Guide to Quality Assurance*, (Illinois: Joint Commission on Accreditation of Healthcare Organizations, 1988).

Joint Commission on Accreditation of Healthcare Organizations, *The Measurement Mandate*, (Illinois: Joint Commission on Accreditation of Healthcare Organizations, 1993).

Joint Commission on Accreditation of Healthcare Organizations, *Transitions: From QA to CQI - Using CQI Approaches to Monitor, Evaluate, and Improve Quality*, (Illinois: Joint Commission on Accreditation of Healthcare Organizations, 1991).

Joiner, Brian L. and Marie A. Gaudard, "Variation, Management, and W. Edwards Deming", *Quality Progress*, (December 1990): 29-37.

Juran, J. M., "The Quality Trilogy: A Universal Approach to Managing for Quality", *Quality Progress*, (August 1986): 19-24.

King, Bob, "Healthcare as Quality Trendsetter", *Healthcare Forum Journal*, (July/August, 1990): 17-18.

Kraus, Gary P., *Health Care Risk Management: Organization and Claims Administration*, (Owings Mills, MD: Rynd Communications, 1986).

Lamprey, Joanne and Charles Jacobs, *ISD - A Review System of Adult Criteria,* (North Hampton, NH: InterQual, Inc., 1987).

Spath, Patrice L., "Critical Paths: A Tool for Clinical Process Management", *Journal of American Health Information Management Association*, (March 1993): 48-58.

Walton, Mary, *The Deming Management Method*, (New York: Dodd, Mead, & Company, Inc., 1986).

chapter 17

HEALTH INFORMATION DEPARTMENT MANAGEMENT

OVERVIEW OF MANAGEMENT

Management has been defined as the process of getting things done through and with people. It is the effective utilization of resources toward the accomplishment of specific objectives. Four basic components emerge from any definition of management: effectiveness, functions, resources, and objectives (see Figure 1).

First, the term "management" should be synonymous with effectiveness. Effectiveness ensures that the utilization of resources accomplishes the objectives. In general, an organization will define its objectives in terms of producing a certain number of products or services at a specified level of quality with a specified amount of resources. Effectiveness embodies productivity, performance, and efficiency. Productivity is the measure of the number of items created or the number of services accomplished per staff hour that meet established levels of quality. Performance is the execution of work. Performance results in a level of productivity. Efficiency is the utilization of appropriate resources to achieve performance that is productive at the desired level.

The process of utilizing resources to accomplish objectives is defined as specific managerial functions. These functions are planning, organizing, directing, and controlling. Planning is the definition of objectives and the devising of a course of action to accomplish the objectives. Organizing brings together resources in an orderly manner and arranges people in an acceptable pattern so they can perform activities to accomplish the

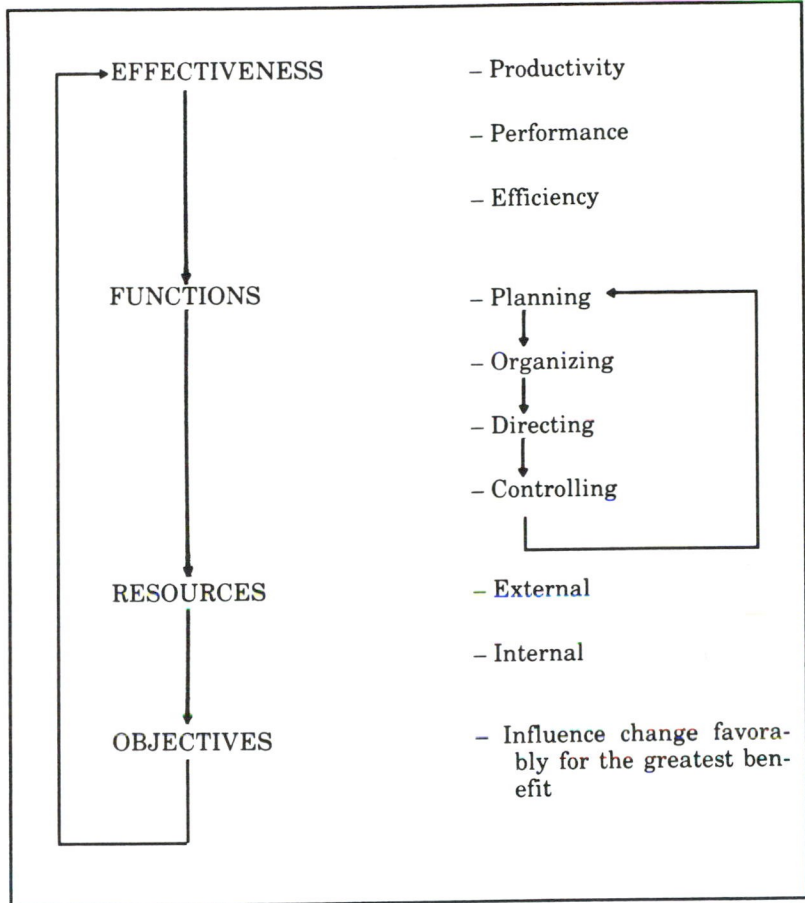

FIGURE 1. MANAGEMENT DEFINED

objectives. Directing deals with stimulating members of a work group to perform work in such a manner that the objectives are met. Controlling is the feedback mechanism to the planning function. It is guiding operations in accordance with plans and ensuring that desired results (objectives) are achieved.

The third component of management is resources, which are both external and internal to a manager. External resources include manpower, money, materials, methods, and machinery. Internal resources include the managerial traits of creativity, coordination, cooperation, communication, common sense, and many other behavioral characteristics.

Finally, objectives exist because underlying all of management is the existence of change. Objectives direct an organization in the face of change - in human attitudes, technology, legislation, and all aspects of the environment. A manager is one who monitors an organizational environment to anticipate change and to bring about the necessary adaptive responses to ensure that the organization's objectives are met.

As can be seen by its definition, management is a complex of interrelated conceptual, human, and technical components. The management challenge is a demanding one. The abilities needed to become a manager must be developed not only through study but through experience and the cultivation of one's own innate talents. A chapter in a text designed to define the roles and functions specific to health information practice cannot fully cover every aspect of management. Thus, this chapter identifies pertinent aspects of management for achieving a department's objectives. The next chapter covers the specific managerial task of personnel supervision. To gain full knowledge and understanding of the concepts and techniques presented, the reader is expected to study additional references, such as those provided at the end of the chapter and others.

THE PLANNING FUNCTION

It has been suggested that planning is "something you do before you do something, so that when you do it, it's not all mixed up" (A. A. Milne, Winnie the Pooh). Planning is the process of determining a desired outcome and defining a course of action to achieve the outcome.

Planning is the most important management function, yet often the most neglected. Managers may not allow enough time for planning or may procrastinate over its decision-making component with the result being "crisis" management. The "crisis" manager takes action on problems only when the efficient operation of the department is hampered. By this time, problems have to be solved rapidly; there is no time for investigation of their causes or careful consideration of alternative solutions. While planning cannot foresee or prepare for all problems which may arise, it can certainly reduce the number of crises a manager faces.

PLANNING HIERARCHY

Planning is performed at many levels. In an organization the mission is the driving force behind all planning. From the mission a strategic plan is developed by the organization as a whole. Then specific objectives and goals are set at the overall organization level and the individual department level. Finally, these objectives and goals are used to develop daily, weekly, and monthly tactical plans and schedules.

Mission

The mission of an organization is a statement of its overall purpose and philosophy. For example, one hospital's mission may be to serve all health care needs of the community in which it exists. Another's may be to excel in medical research, or specialize in treating children or cancer patients.

Mission embodies environment, resources, values, and responsibilities. Environment refers to demographic, economic, natural, technological, political, and cultural factors. The aging population, changing family structure, and quality of education are some demographic factors that define a health care facility's resources and responsibilities. On a broad scale, economic factors such as the national debt influence the availability of resources for a facility. The accelerating pace of technology has dramatically influenced the health care delivery system. Legislation, regulation, enforcement, and public-interest and consumer groups are a major influence in reassessing a health care facility's mission. Finally, "culture" refers to an organization's relationship to itself, others, and society as a whole. The culture of managers individually and as a group influences the values set forth in a facility's mission.

Although a health care facility's mission is defined with these changing influences in mind, a mission is not changed frequently. While reassessed periodically, the mission is reaffirmed more often than changed. It should be the stable force in the changing environment. Only a major change in governing philosophy, often due to significant changes in the environment, should cause an organization to modify its mission.

Strategic Plan

A strategic plan is one developed by top management for a period of three to five years, and is directed at accomplishing the organization's mission in the face of change. A strategic plan should address the following deceptively simple questions: 1) Where is the organization now? 2) Where does it want to go? 3) How does it get there?

Response to these questions does not guarantee the development of the "right" plan, for executives may disagree in difficult strategic situations. The result of a systematic approach to strategic planning, however, provides the logic and assumptions underlying the plan, making it more explicit and clear to all.

Tactical Plans

Tactical plans are short term (usually annual) descriptions of operations, programs, and finances. Individual managers develop these plans, which are then brought together as a whole for the organization. They are reviewed in light of the mission and strategic plan and approved by top management.

Operational Plans

Operational planning addresses objectives relating to the ongoing activities of a department. Objectives are specific, reality-oriented, verifiable, and time-oriented. In the health information department, objectives identify specific categories of services to be performed, such as "provide medical record retrieval service daily" or "transcribe reports for inclusion in the medical record within two days of their dictation."

Operational planning through objective setting is very important and much research has gone into developing techniques to assist the process. Two of the most commonly used techniques and their advantages and disadvantages are management-by-objectives (MBO) and goal-setting. These may be used to develop both the operational plan for the department and for the individual employee.

MBO, originally designed in the mid-50s as a participative management tool, is a technique in which the flow of planning moves from the bottom of the organizational hierarchy up. In MBO managers first provide subordinates with a framework reflecting their own purposes and objectives. Then subordinates propose objectives for themselves, which are discussed with managers, modified, and agreed upon. Finally, subordinates review their own progress and describe it periodically to their managers.

The benefits of MBO have been cited as directing work activities toward organizational goals, aiding planning, providing clear standards for controlling, improving motivation among managers, improving use of human resources, reducing role conflict and ambiguity, providing more objective appraisal criteria, identifying problems better, and improving personnel development.

In practice, the benefits of MBO are not always realized. MBO often becomes a paperwork ritual that reflects no serious commitment on the part of management. A frequent complaint is the considerable time that can be spent in individual objective-setting sessions. Another difficulty relates to quantification. Not all valuable results and performances lend themselves to being quantified. Overemphasis on results as being too short-term is another flaw. MBO has also been criticized for being a technique used within an authoritarian philosophy to provide the appearance of being participative. Finally, it has been observed that MBO can lead to excessive emphasis on the individual rather than on team building.

Goal setting is a technique for operational planning that many research studies have shown is probably the most effective. The idea of assigning employees a specific amount of work to be accomplished - specific task, quota, performance standard, objective, deadline - is not new. It has been found to work more successfully, however, than any other technique developed to modify it. There are three primary steps in goal-setting:

1. Setting the goals - Goals should reflect the same characteristics as those described for objectives. They should be challenging yet reachable. In general, difficult goals have been found to lead to better performance than easy goals. Further information on development of goals is included in the section on controlling in this chapter.

2. Obtaining goal commitment - for goal setting to work, subordinates must accept and remain committed to goals. Simple instruction backed by positive support and an absence of threats have been found to ensure goal acceptance in most cases. Subordinates must perceive goals as being fair and reasonable, and they must trust management. Supportive rather than punitive management is more linked to goal acceptance than participation in goal-setting. A subordinate gets a feeling of pride and satisfaction from reaching a challenging but fair goal and the recognition that provides, not only from the manager but from peers as well. Although setting up formal competition is not recommended because it can lead to employees placing individual goals ahead of organizational goals, informal competition can reinforce commitment and may lead employees to raise goals spontaneously. Success in reaching a goal tends to reinforce acceptance of future goals. A significant aspect of goal-setting is to raise goals as original ones are achieved. Starting out with slightly easier goals known to be attainable may be necessary for subordinates with low self confidence or ability, or those who appear to reject goal setting.

3. Providing support elements. Effective goal-setting must begin with capable employees, who must be given adequate resources - equipment, time, help, budget - as well as the knowledge and freedom to utilize them in attaining goals. Regular and honest feedback is also a necessary support element.

Programmatic Plans

The second major type of tactical plan is the programmatic plan. It addresses objectives relating to special projects or programs, such as "install a medical record tracking system on a personal computer." The organization may contract with an independent consultant to design and implement a project or program. The consultant draws up a programmatic plan which the organization accepts or rejects. When programs or projects are to be accomplished internally the organization draws up the programmatic plan. A programmatic plan is highly formalized, explicitly documenting each step of the planning process. Depending on the scope and nature of the program, any number of planning techniques may be utilized, such as interviews, forecasts, flowcharts and so forth. Programmatic planning may frequently take the form of systems analysis (described in Chapter 13).

Financial Plans

Financial plans are the third major type of plan. Financial plans are those expressed in monetary terms. The most common financial plan is the budget. It outlines the objectives for a specific period of time and the resources required to achieve those objectives.

BUDGET

The budget describes in monetary terms the activities that should occur in a future period in order to meet specified objectives. As a plan, the budget is also a tool for controlling - setting limits on spending and evaluating the results of activities and the financial condition of the organization.

There are two types of budgets that managers of health information departments may develop. These are the capital budget and the revenue and expense budget.

Capital Budget

The capital budget is a plan that shows the major expenditures and sources of funds for plant and equipment. Because purchase (or sale) of land, buildings, and equipment impacts the type and number of services rendered by the facility, the capital budget drives the forecasts upon which all other budgets are developed. For example, the plan to purchase a new piece of medical equipment may mean a change in the volume of patients, a shift from inpatients to outpatients, or the addition of patients to a particular medical staff service. The purchase of equipment in the health information department may reduce staff or allow for provision of additional services to other departments thus generating revenue for the health information department.

A capital expenditure is defined as one that will have an impact on services performed by the department for a period exceeding a year and whose total investment exceeds a financial limit established by the governing board. The justification for a capital budget may include the following:

1. Statement of purpose - This identifies the reason for the capital expenditure request, such as replacement of old equipment, improvement in productivity and/or quality of service; meeting accreditation, licensure, or certification requirements; offering new or expended services; or reducing costs.

2. Identification of alternatives - Different means of accomplishing the same objectives should be analyzed. The analysis generally includes the identification of strengths and weaknesses of the present means as well as alternative means. For example, improving productivity in medical transcription may be accomplished by using an outside service, obtaining new equipment, or instituting an alternative compensation system. If new equipment is an alternative, lease versus purchase should be evaluated.

3. Request for proposal - (RFP) This obtains detailed information on costs and benefits of alternatives from vendors. The RFP includes a statement of purpose and authorization for requesting the proposal, a brief description of the facility, a detailed explanation of the project the proposal is to address, a description of the proposal's expected contents, a timetable, and the criteria upon which proposals will be evaluated.

4. Benefit analysis - Benefits to the various project alternatives are analyzed to ensure that each alternative considered meets the minimum expectations. A weighted benefit analysis, such as in Figure 2 is helpful. Each benefit element is ranked in importance. Then each alternative is rated in its ability to meet the element. The ratings are

ELEMENT	RANK	ALTERNATIVE 1		ALTERNATIVE 2		ALTERNATIVE 3	
		RATE	VALUE	RATE	VALUE	RATE	VALUE
1. XXXXXX	5	3	9	4	20	4	20
2. XXXX	2	3	6	1	2	2	4
3. XXXXX	2	2	4	2	4	3	6
4. XX	4	3	12	4	16	5	20
TOTAL			37		42		50

FIGURE 2. WEIGHTED BENEFIT ANALYSIS

multiplied by the rankings for a total score for each alternative.

5. Cost analysis - Cost analysis is the determination of the net financial results of the capital expenditure. The total cost of project including purchase price, installation charges, and so forth are identified. Revenues or cash savings that result from the project are determined. Specific financial calculations involving the time value of money may be performed.

6. Recommendation - Upon completion of the cost and benefit analyses, one alternative is recommended.

7 Priority ranking - because all capital expenditures may not be feasible for a facility, each department submitting a capital budget should prioritize each expenditure.

8. Time phasing - because the health care facility may not have the resources to make all budgeted capital expenditures at once at the start of the budget year, departments are asked to identify the time period in which the capital expenditure is planned.

Capital budgets are approved by the governing board. Approval of the budget, however, does not constitute approval for expenditure. Each expenditure must be reviewed by administration at the time it is to be made and approval granted if the planned resources are actually available.

Revenue and Expense Budget

In a health care facility, the revenue and expense budget includes estimates of gross patient revenue; allowances for cost-based and contractual payers and uncollectable accounts; expenses for personnel, supplies, depreciation, interest, and insurance; and other nonpatient care operating and non-operating revenue and expenses. This budget is based on statistical estimates for occupancy, patient or case mix, ancillary services, and other level-of-activity projections.

The revenue and expense budget may be developed in a number of ways. For health care facilities, the two most common are the standard budget (by responsibility or function), and zero-based budget. A standard responsibility budget is one that is organized by cost center or group of cost centers over which a single manager is responsible. A standard functional budget is organized along functions, services, or departments in order to identify such functional costs as nursing, housekeeping, and medical records.

A zero-based budget is one which is created as if all activities were entirely new. Each activity is evaluated for funding or elimination. Appropriate funding levels are determined by priorities established by top management according to the overall availability of funds. This type of budget instills accountability into the manager, because all activities must be completely justified, not just increases over the previous year's appropriation as in the standard type of budget. A zero-based budget may be based on either responsibilities or functions.

In a health information department, the revenue and expense budget generally is prepared in three parts: revenues, personnel, and expenses.

A revenue budget may be prepared if the department generates revenues. For example, a health information department may perform transcription, photocopy, or other services for other departments. A health information department may obtain fees from the release of information function or special studies in which it participates. It may conduct training seminars or continuing education workshops. Because the revenues generated by a health information department are generally very small - less than 1 percent of overall facility revenues - administration may consider them immaterial and not require the department to prepare a revenue budget.

The personnel, or wage and salary, budget is the most important expense budget. This budget should be based on staffing projections for the forecasted service activity levels (see information on work distribution in the section on directing in this chapter) and administrative guidelines.

General projections for service activity levels are obtained from administration at the start of the budget process. This includes information such as anticipated changes in numbers of patients, changes in case mix, new programs requiring medical record services, and so forth. The health information department director utilizes these data to project services that will be performed in the department. For example, an increase in Emergency Department visits may mean a proportional increase in procedure coding and filing functions. The department director must also observe trends in departmental functions that cannot be predicted from overall facility projections but can be projected using statistics regularly kept in the department. For example, changes in release of information volume may not be related specifically to numbers of discharges or visits. External events should also be monitored. Changes in the PRO's scope of work or new accreditation requirements, can significantly impact the work of the health information depart-

PERSONNEL BUDGET WORKSHEET

SERVICE	Current Data				Forecast			
	UNITS OF SERVICE ACTIVITY	FTES	PERFORMANCE STANDARD	ACTUAL PRODUCTIVITY RATE	UNITS OF SERVICE ACTIVITY	PERFORMANCE STANDARD	PRODUCTIVITY RATE	FTES
ASSEMBLY ANALYSIS								
ABSTRACTING	20,500 records	2.0	10 min. per record	91%	21730 records	10 min. per record	100%	1.9
INPATIENT CODING								
OUTPATIENT CODING								
INCOMPLETE RECORDS								
FILING RETRIEVAL								
CORRESPONDENCE								
STATISTICS								
TOTAL FTES								

Calculations:

$$\text{Productivity} = \frac{\text{Service Units} \times \text{Time Standard} \div 60 \text{ min./hr.}}{\text{Actual Hours}} = \frac{\text{Earned Hours}}{\text{Actual Hours}}$$

$$= \frac{20,500 \text{ Records} \times 10 \text{ min./record} \div 60 \text{ min./hr.}}{40 \text{ Hrs./wk.} \times 47 \text{ wks./yr.*} \times 2 \text{ FTEs}} = \frac{3,417 \text{ Hours}}{3,760 \text{ Hours}}$$

$$= 91\%$$

*52 weeks per year less 2 weeks vacation, 1 week sick leave, and 10 holidays is 47 weeks per year, or 1,880 hours.

A 6% increase in volume (21,730 records) should not increase the required number of FTEs if the employees improve their productivity.

FIGURE 3. PERSONNEL BUDGET WORKSHEET

ment. Productivity must be measured on a regular basis and steps taken to ensure that standards are met and progress is made toward constant improvement. The department that can demonstrate trends in service activities and regular productivity improvement stands a much better chance of obtaining needed staffing than one that does not. Figures 3 and 4 display worksheets and sample calculations which may be of assistance in developing the personnel budget.

PRODUCTIVE TIME CALCULATION WORKSHEET

Employee	Wage/ Salary	Exempt/ Non-Exempt	Regular Hours	Overtime Hours	Anniversary Date	% COLA	% Merit	19YY Budget
12345	$6.70	N-E	1,880	0	April 1	2%	4%	$13,160
Total								

Calculations:

Jan. - Mar. = 25% time at 19XX rate:	.25(1,880 hrs.) = 470 hrs. X $6.70 =	$ 3,149
Apr. - Dec. = 75% time at 19YY rate:	.75(1,880 hrs.) = 1,410 hrs. X [$6.70 X 1.06*] =	$10,011
		$13,160

Non-Productive time including paid vacation, sick leave, and holidays is calculated separately from productive time

* 2% COLA and 4% merit increases equal total of 6% increase

FIGURE 4. PRODUCTIVE TIME CALCULATION WORKSHEET

Administrative guidelines must be used in developing the personnel budget. These guidelines delineate any cost-of-living adjustments, merit increases, and requirements about staffing. The personnel/human resource department regularly conducts or receives information on salary surveys to use in setting salary ranges for each classification or grade of personnel. Where ranges change, cost-of-living adjustments may be made to ensure equitable pay. Merit increase guidelines usually specify the types of merit increases that can be given. For example, an overall maximum may be set, as well as maximums for employees with specified numbers of sick days used, productivity levels, and so forth. Unless otherwise specified, the overall maximum should be used across the board in the budget plan, because the actual amount each employee will earn cannot be anticipated in advance. Because merit increases may be given on anniversary dates instead of one standard time per year, this factor may be included in the budget. Staffing level guidelines may address a variety of factors including replacement of personnel lost through attrition, use of overtime and/or temporary services, policies on part-time employees, shift differentials, layoffs, and so forth. Hospitals with unions must also observe union guidelines in preparing personnel budgets.

The format of the final personnel budget differs from one facility to another. Figure 5 is an example.

	19XX Budget	19XX Year End Projection	19XX Variance(%)	19YY Hours	19YY F.T.E	19YY Budget	19YY Change(%)
Productive time: non-shift							
Productive time: shift							
Non-productive: sick							
Non-productive: vacation							
Non-productive: holiday							
Non-productive: other							
Total regular time							
Overtime							
Total wages & salaries							
Social Security taxes							
Other benefits							
Total Personnel Expenses							

FIGURE 5. PERSONNEL BUDGET

Because budgets are prepared as much as six to nine months in advance of their implementation, facilities usually require a year-end projection and estimate of variance from budget for the current year's budget, as well as the information for the next year. Comparisons between last year's budget and the proposed budget may also be required as part of the budget submission. Social security taxes and benefits are often added by the personnel/human resources department later.

Administrative guidelines also specify the types of justifications which must accompany the budget. Certainly all new positions must have a separate justification. Other changes, such as going to an incentive pay plan, may also require separate justification and approval. These are often done before the final personnel budget is submitted.

The operating, or non-wage and salary, expense budget is the third part of the revenue and expense budget. This delineates all other expenses. Labor expense for other than the facility's own employees should be categorized in the operating expense budget as "purchased services" or "contracted services."

Every facility may have a slightly different categorization of expenses. Figure 6 shows an operating expense budget with typical categories.

In order to plan an operating expense budget, the unit of service activity, the expense type, the unit cost, and the projected service activity level must be known.

Books	Units of Service Activity/s	Expense Type (F/V)	19XX					19YY			
			Unit Cost	Projected Serv. Act. Level	Budget	Projected Actual	Vari-ance %	Projected Serv. Act. Level	Unit Cost	Budget	Change %
Contractual services											
Data processing											
Forms - purchased											
Meeting and travel											
Membership dues											
Minor equipment											
Office supplies											
Printing - in house											
Professional fees											
Postage — Corre-spondence		V	$.40	10,000	$4,000	$4,200	5%	11,000	$.40	$4,400	10%
Rental											
Repair service											
Storage and microfilming											
Total Operating Expenses											

FIGURE 6. EXPENSE BUDGET

The unit of service activity for each budget category is the function for which the expense is incurred. For example, the

COST	BEHAVIOR	
	IN TOTAL	PER UNIT
VARIABLE	Increases and decreases in proportion to changes in activity level.	Remains constant per unit.
FIXED	Not affected by changes in activity level.	Decreases per unit as activity level rises and increases per unit as activity level falls.

FIGURE 7. BEHAVIOR OF EXPENSES

postage budget category may include expenditures primarily for the release of information function.

Each expense is categorized as either fixed or variable. Figure 7 defines these terms and shows how they act when they are viewed in aggregate or as a unit cost. The postage expense is a variable cost because the expense for one unit (of the same weight) is the same whether one piece of mail is sent or hundreds of pieces are sent.

A unit cost is the expense associated with performing one service unit or purchasing one item. Thus, in this context, the unit cost for the release of information function is the cost to mail one item. The unit cost multiplied by the projected service activity level (which is the total number of units of service to be performed for the function) is the budget amount. So, if the health information department determined that, on average, each piece of correspondence mailed cost 40 cents (unit cost equals 40 cents), and there were estimated to be 10,000 requests for release of information (service activity level equals 10,000 units), the amount to budget would be $4,000.

Often a facility will want to have the present year's service activity level, unit cost, budget, year-end projection of actual expenses, and variance between budget and actual reported on the next year's proposed budget, as well as the forecasted unit cost, service activity level, and budget. The facility can then determine the percent change between the present year's budget and the proposed budget.

To accurately compile an operating budget, a health information department manager must keep good records of work performed. Some budget categories may comprise several items each with their own unit cost. For instance, the postage expense may actually be broken down for several areas of the department: correspondence/release of information, incomplete control, tumor registry, general office, and so forth.

The manager must also obtain accurate estimates of unit cost. For example, the projected unit cost for medical record covers - a variable expense - can be obtained from the vendor, or the current unit cost can be adjusted for the anticipated rate of inflation provided in administrative guidelines to the budget.

Although a variable expense, office supplies is a category for which it is more difficult to develop unit costs and volumes. In this case, the previous year's budget, actual expenses to date, and projections may be used instead of a unit cost. For example:

	Budget	Actual to Date (9.mos.)	Year End Projection	Variance to Date
Supplies	$7,000	$5,400	$7,200	$150

Variance calculation:

$$\frac{\$7,000}{12 \text{ mos.}} \text{ annual budget} = \$583.33 \text{ budget/mo.}$$

$$\frac{\times 9 \text{ mos.}}{\$5,250 \text{ budget to date}}$$

$5,400 - $5,250 = $150 variance (over budget to date)

Projection calculation:

$$\frac{\$5,400}{9 \text{ mos.}} \text{ actual to date} = \$600 \text{ actual/mo.}$$

$$\frac{\times 12 \text{ mos.}}{\$7,200} \quad (\$200 \text{ over budget})$$

The manager must determine if variances from budget will continue across the year or not. For example, a larger volume of supplies may have been purchased mid-year, so that purchases at the end of the year may be less. Alternatively, volumes may have increased in other areas so supplies increased as well, suggesting a trend.

Minor equipment may be an example of a fixed cost. One piece of equipment purchased may be used for any amount of service units. To budget for fixed cost categories, estimates of next year's prices must be obtained from vendors, or in some instances from the facility's accountants.

Some expenses may be fixed or variable depending on how the facility treats them. For example, data processing may be variable if charges are applied for processing time. Some facilities may simply charge a flat fee irrespective of usage.

PLANNING TOOLS

In addition to formal planning, tools must also be in place to allow for ad hoc planning. These tools include policies, rules, procedures, standards, and time and project management schedules. Techniques of problem analysis and decision making are also important.

Policies

Policies are plans within which objectives may be set and decisions made. An effective policy requires judgment but not complex interpretation. Policies translate overall objectives into comprehensible and practical terms. An example of a policy is "promote from within whenever possible." The phrase "whenever possible" allows the manager to look outside the organization for a qualified candidate if, in the manager's judgment, none exists within.

Policies within an organization should be consistent. Policy making is thus generally limited to upper management and approved by the chief executive officer. Department managers may develop policies specific to their department, but must be limited to the activities of the department and not conflict with any organizational policies.

A health care facility should have a policy manual. Policies pertaining to personnel issues should be included in an employee handbook. Policies are sometimes implied. For example, it may be generally allowed that employees may leave their work area for a few minutes at any time, not just during formal breaks. The danger with implied policies is that they are not officially approved, are difficult to enforce, and may be applied inconsistently. Exceptions to rules (see below) are often the impetus for creating policies.

Rules

Rules are plans that delineate a required or prohibited course of action. Rules allow for no decision making or interpretation but, rather, require or limit specific action authoritatively and officially. Examples of rules include "sign in when work is begun" and "no smoking except in designated areas." Within an organization, rules should be reasonable, known to all, and applied equally to all.

When rules are appealed, the consequences of exception should be evaluated carefully. "Rules are made to be broken" is not a rule; yet rigid adherence to rules which circumstances may have negated is also wrong. When an exception is made to a rule, a specific delineation of the exception should be made. This exception should then be used as a policy for carrying out the rule in the future, or for taking formal action to change the rule.

Procedures

Procedures are plans for action. They are a series of related steps designed to accomplish a specific task. Procedures are developed for repetitive work in order to specifically define the task, to achieve uniformity of practice, and to facilitate training. An example of a procedure is displayed in Figure 8.

PROCEDURE: *Assembly of Medical Records*	PAGE: *1* OF: *1*
PREPARED BY: *Mary Martin, RRA*	REVISION: *7-7-89*
PURPOSE:	*Arrange the contents of the medical records of discharged patients to facilitate later review and permanent filing.*
RESOURCES:	*Medical records from Discharge Area* *Hole punch, black pen*
DETAILS:	*1. At 9:00 am and 1:00 pm visit the Discharge Area to obtain medical records of discharged patients to assemble.*
	2. Assemble all sheets pertaining to the hospitalization period in accordance with the Filing Arrangement of Medical Records (see Appendix A).
	3. Each group of like forms (e.g., all progress notes) should be filed in date order, from admission date to discharge date.
	9. Attach all sheets in the correct order to the top set of prongs in the medical record. Punch holes if necessary.
	10. Deliver assembled records to Analysis Work Station immediately.

FIGURE 8. SAMPLE PROCEDURE

The health information department manager is responsible for developing the department's procedures and keeping them up-to-date.

The following steps are included in writing procedures:

1. Determine all of the steps required. Use only the minimum number needed for carrying out the procedure.

2. Determine the best sequence for the performance of these steps. Those which are similar or closely related to each other should be grouped together.

3. Review procedures which might be affected by changes in other procedures.

4. Test a procedure before putting it into everyday use; try to discover its flaws.

5. Evaluate the procedure after it has been used for several weeks. Employees who work with the procedure are good sources for identifying its possible problems and offering suggestions for its improvement.

It is important to record procedures in writing, describing each of their phases in step-by-step detail and including correctly completed samples where appropriate.

Once procedures in the department have been planned and tested, any employee should be able to follow the procedure with a minimum of questions after initial on-the-job training is completed.

In addition to giving the employees a copy of the procedures they perform, all procedures should be filed in a procedure manual for easy reference at any time. Using word processing to type procedures is helpful for updating them. Any change in a procedure should be incorporated into the formal document as soon as finalized. It is also necessary to review procedures against actual performance regularly, as changes can creep into procedures easily. These changes may or may not be appropriate. Steps must be taken to ensure that procedures are as simple and straightforward as possible. Regular review is one way to ensure work is performed correctly and completely and in the most efficient manner.

Standards

Standards are measures established to serve as criteria or levels of reference for determining the accomplishment of objectives. Because standards are so closely tied to the controlling function, they are fully described under the topic of controlling later in this chapter.

Time and Project Management Schedules

Time management is one of the major problems facing a manager. This is often because the manager must perform a wide variety of functions. Every manager needs a calendar, or daily schedule. Managing time, however, means more than scheduling - it means using time effectively and efficiently. It is often necessary to formally plan and control time.

Planning time requires prioritizing activities. It is helpful to make a "to do" list and assign priorities: top/urgent, important-non-delegatable, important-delegatable, and not important. When there is uncertainty about a priority, the manager should request clarification from administration. The important element in planning time is following the established priorities. Top priority/urgent work must be performed first. Delegation is described in the section on directing in this chapter. The manager must accept the fact that unimportant activities must be foregone. (Managers must learn how to say "no.")

Understanding personal peak times and work habits is also important. It may be necessary to schedule a "meeting" with yourself in order to gain the quiet time needed to accomplish a difficult task. Managers need to evaluate the "open door" policy,

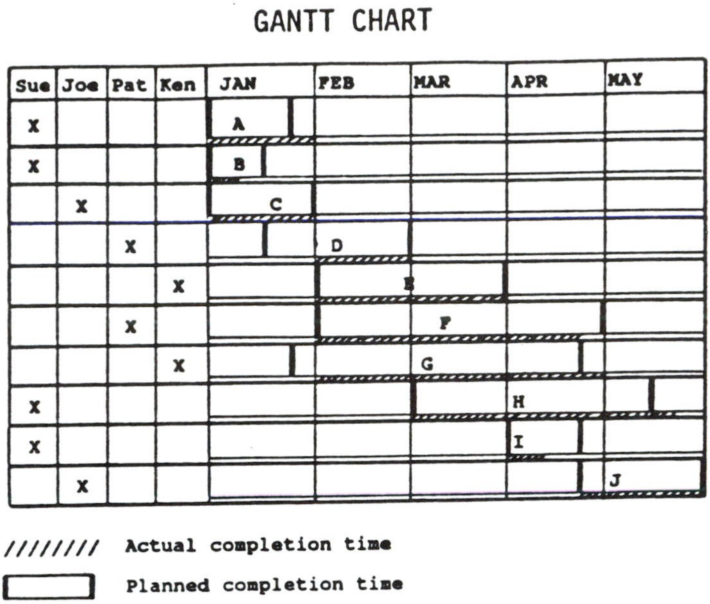

GANTT CHART

Sue	Joe	Pat	Ken	JAN	FEB	MAR	APR	MAY
X				A				
X				B				
		X		C				
			X		D			
			X			E		
			X			F		
			X			G		
X							H	
X							I	
		X						J

////////   Actual completion time

[ ]   Planned completion time

FIGURE 9. GANTT CHART FOR PROJECT MANAGEMENT

and may have to designate a period of time each day for ad hoc consultation. Effective time managers often schedule "telephone" time when they will return all telephone messages. The needs of the department must be evaluated in light of not only accessibility to the manager, but ability of the manager to complete both routine and project work.

Project management schedules are formal tools used to delineate steps in major projects, such as implementing a new computer system, moving an office, and so forth. The Gantt chart is a simple tool which displays both a project's time line and progress. Figure 9 displays an example of a project, such as installing a new dictation system, with 10 components or steps. The project extends over a period of five months. Four employees are involved in the project. Thus Sue is responsible for component A which is planned to be completed by the third week of January. The hash marks below show the actual length of time it took to complete this component (a full month). By evaluating planned and actual timelines during the project, adjustments can be made to better control the project's completion.

Problem Analysis and Decision Making

Problem analysis and decision making are the steps taken to carry out plans in the face of change. These plans may be formal project steps or daily operations. Unanticipated events occur all the time. In any department employees get sick, service activity levels change, errors are made, and so forth. As a result, steps must be taken to understand the problem and to make decisions that resolve the problem. Decision-making is the choice that precedes action in the face of change that does not allow plans to be carried out precisely as defined. Ensuring the right/best choice - that is, making the right/best decision - depends first on problem analysis and second on issues of confidence, creativity, authority, and conviction.

Problem analysis is the identification and understanding of deviations from defined objectives. The steps in problem analysis are:

1 Identify objectives in which change is causing a deviation.

2. Collect complete data about all factors surrounding the problem.

3. Analyze data fully to understand the problem and how it occurred.

Decision-making then, is the selection of the best course of action given various alternatives. The steps in decision-making include:

1. Identify the requirements and constraints surrounding the objective.

2. Develop alternative solutions to the problem to meet the objective.

3. Select the alternative which meets as many requirements and constraints as possible in accomplishing the objective.

4. Define how and when the alternative will be accomplished.

5. Develop a system for follow-up to evaluate the progress of the objective's accomplishment.

Some decision-making situations require less formal attention than others. Making decisions about minor changes may appear to be made without thought. These are situations where the manager has had similar changes take place in the past and experience and intuition guides a prompt decision.

Many decisions require the manager to formalize problem analysis and decision-making - the extent of formality depending on the importance of the problem.

A manager may perform problem analysis and decision-making without the aid of others. Using a group to help make some decisions, however, has advantages. A group may generate more ideas, and, if the group will be involved in implementing the decision, may be more supportive of it. Several group process techniques are available:

Consensus - A group gets together, discusses the issues, looks for areas of agreement, and resolves areas of disagreement, ultimately reaching the one best solution. Hasty agreement or bargaining is avoided, and only when all attempts to reach a consensus have failed does voting take place.

Brainstorming - This technique elicits creative suggestions without inhibition. In the Delphi approach to brainstorming, group members are asked to write their position with respect to the information presented to them. The written positions are collected and tallied. If a consensus does not result, the reasons for each position are made known to all, often in writing, and another round of written position-taking takes place until consensus is reached or a vote must be taken. In the Nominal Group Technique participants meet face-to-face to talk, but in a carefully controlled situation. Once initial ideas are generated on paper, all ideas are listed on a flip chart. Each idea is discussed. Then each participant records a rank-ordering of the ideas. The decision is the idea that emerges in first place.

Considered opinion and devil's advocate are similar techniques. In the first, a panel of experts assesses alternatives and develops arguments for and against each. The resulting comparison helps the decision-maker clarify all courses of action. In devil's advocate the decision-maker requests an individual or group to delineate all negative aspects of each alternative. The decision-maker has the advantage that every alternative is frankly assessed.

Specific tools also exist which aid decisions-making. In a factor analysis matrix all elements concerning the problem are ranked in importance and each alternative's ability to satisfy each element is rated. The result is a weighting of the alternatives. (This is very much like the benefit analysis in Figure 2.) A decision tree is a tool used to depict the possible directions actions may take from various decision points. Forecasting techniques, simulation, model building, and other operations research techniques employ sophisticated mathematics and probability theory to aid in decision-making.

Decision-making also involves some social/psychological factors that influence a manager's ability to make decisions and the quality of those decisions. Some of these factors include creativity in generating ideas, confidence in one's knowledge of the issues that form the basis for the decision, risk-taking in reaching a decision quickly or easily, and conviction that one is certain of the chosen path. The health information department manager must also have the ability to overcome personal prejudice or bias, fear of failure, and resistance to change. Organizational factors of authority and responsibility (discussed in the next section) also influence decision-making ability.

THE ORGANIZING FUNCTION

Organizing is the management function of distributing or allocating resources toward the accomplishment of the objectives defined in the plans. Organizing requires an understanding of the concepts of staffing and work distribution. Organizing, however, also includes the allocation of material, machine, and space resources.

STAFFING AND WORK-DISTRIBUTION CONCEPTS

The allocation of work among staff has both horizontal and vertical components. The horizontal components of organization include the concepts of departmentalization, line-staff responsibility, and coordination, since they involve dividing work into departments, assigning tasks to departments, and coordinating these departments. Levels and span of control, authority, and delegation make up the vertical components.

Departmentalization and Coordination

Departmentalization is the efficient and effective grouping of jobs into meaningful work units to coordinate efforts. The major means of departmentalization are by purpose or process. Purpose departmentalization is most common in the industrial/product sector, where work is divided by specific products, customers, or geographic locations. This type of departmentalization emphasizes an external, "market" orientation. Traditionally, health care facilities have not been market-oriented.

The prospective payment system, however, has encouraged health care facilities to use marketing techniques such as product lines (e.g., cases, DRGs, etc.), differentiating specific customer groups (i.e., acute care, long term care, ambulatory care, intensive care, etc.), and providing services in alternate locations (e.g., mobile units, ambulatory care centers).

This philosophy has filtered down to the department level. Some health information departments may adopt a concept of "department without walls," and focus service activities along "product lines." For example, management of medical record content is enhanced through concurrent review of medical records on the nursing station. Medical information now flows throughout the entire organization via computerization so central archiving may take new forms. As with other facility functions certain health information services may be contracted out of the facility (e.g., transcription, microfilming, correspondence, photocopying). Services may be performed in remote locations and communicated via modem. Many health information departments treat medical records of Medicare patients differently than other inpatient records. Health information "outreach" departments may provide services for outpatient care or other areas. Thus, departmentalization is taking new forms.

The more traditional means of departmentalization for health care organizations has been by process. Process departmentalization focuses on building departments around functions. Thus a hospital has one medical record or health information department, dietary department, finance department, etc. Traditional departmentalization also occurred within a department, where subdepartments or subunits were formed by purpose or process. Within the health information department, process subdepartmentalization might result in a transcription area, filing area, discharge processing area, etc.

Departmentalization in either form results in units that are highly differentiated, in that they develop different goals, points of view, and organizational structures within themselves. Yet no organization can meet its overall objectives unless all departments work together. Coordination is the process that integrates the differentiated, yet interdependent, departments. Organizations use rules, plans, and the authority hierarchy to coordinate work units; but as problems facing the organization become more numerous and complex, rules, plans, and referral up the organizational hierarchy become insufficient. The manager then must create lateral relationships to reduce and solve problems.

Formal coordinating mechanisms include committees, liaison roles, and independent integrators. Committees, task forces, or teams are the most common means of trying to achieve coordination, where members meet to discuss and resolve problems common to several departments. Less commonly, a liaison (a person from one department, such as medical records, who works with or in another department, such as billing) handles communication between two departments where problems are frequent but can be resolved quickly with the liaison's expertise. An independent integrator is another means of coordination in which an individual or department coordinates activities which cross several departmental lines. An example is the patient representative in a large hospital who works with several departments, as well as the patient, to see that the patient's needs are met. Formal means of coordination have limited effectiveness without a cooperative spirit on the part of the respective departments. Developing informal coordination is difficult and dependent on the personalities involved.

Responsibility and Authority

Dividing work into departments and then coordinating the departments is only one aspect of organizing. Each department must also be assigned responsibility for certain tasks and the authority to see these tasks to their completion. Responsibility is the obligation of an individual to carry out assigned activities to the best of the individual's ability. Within an organization, responsibility is usually defined by the relationship of the position to the accomplishment of the organization's objectives. In an organization there are two major types of relationships - line and staff. Line positions have direct responsibility for accomplishing the objectives of the organization. They form a hierarchy within an organization with each position reporting to the level above. There are generally four main levels: top management, middle management, supervisors, and line workers.

The term "manager" is used in both a generic and title sense. In a generic sense it refers to any member of the management team from supervisor to chief executive officer. In the title sense it refers to the person who is at an organization level below an executive (title for top management persons) and above a supervisor (person who has front-line responsibility for workers). (This distinction has been used to divide the topics of management and personnel supervision in this book.) Thus the distinguishing characteristic of a manager is responsibility for a division or department. Managers spend more of their time in planning and organizing and less time in directing and controlling.

At any level of management the concept of span of control exists. Span of control refers to the number of immediate subordinates who report to a manager. Proper span of control is determined by a number of factors. The type of work is the most important factor. In situations where the work is essentially simple and repetitive, the manager may have a wide span of control (as many as eight to fifteen subordinates); whereas in highly dynamic and complex activities a more narrow span of control (four to eight subordinates) is customary. Thus, at lower levels of the organization where day-to-day operations occur, managers generally have wider spans of control than at higher levels where they must deal with more strategic issues. Other factors which can influence the span of control are the necessity for frequent and involved communication, the amount of subordinate training, and the level of planning which can anticipate and propose solutions for subordinate problem solving.

The principle of unity of command is also operative in the organizational hierarchy. The principle essentially states that the more complete an individual's reporting relationship to a single superior, the less the problem of conflicting instructions and the greater the feeling of personal responsibility for results. Although it is possible for a subordinate to report to two people, there are often problems of conflicting priorities, imbalance of loyalty, and so forth.

Staff positions within the organizational hierarchy are those positions which assist and advise the line manager in accomplishing the objectives. Staff positions are sometimes considered "less important;" however, these positions usually are ones with a high degree of specialization and are afforded esteem for their level of expertise.

In addition to the relationship between a position and its responsibility for accomplishment of the organization's objectives, each position must have a degree of authority commensurate with its responsibility. Authority is the right given to each position holder to command the behavior for which the position is responsible. It gives managers the right to carry out their tasks by giving orders to their subordinates and to expect compliance. Equally important, but sometimes overlooked, authority also gives subordinates the right to carry out their duties as assigned and to expect support from their superiors when those activities are carried out within their scope of authority.

Delegation

The conveyance of responsibility and authority from superior to subordinate is delegation. Delegation involves determining the results expected, assigning the tasks, granting the authority for accomplishment of the tasks, and holding the subordinate responsible for their accomplishment. Delegation is critical to an organization, for one individual cannot accomplish an organization's objectives single-handedly. In addition, delegation allows a manager to better utilize time, increases promotional opportunities for both management and subordinate because the subordinate is prepared to take over, provides the manager with satisfaction in developing people, and provides the subordinate with self-esteem, motivation, and increased confidence.

Most managerial failures result from poor delegation, and much of the reason for poor delegation lies in personal attitudes toward delegation. There are many reasons why managers do not delegate, among them a desire to dominate, a sense of indispensability, an unwillingness to accept risks, and an insecurity in their own positions. There are some things which cannot be delegated - accountability, powers other than authority, responsibilities regulated by law, and certain activities which have representational or long-lasting effects (e.g., formulating policy, approving budget, representing top management at a meeting). But a manager who is receptive to a subordinate's ideas, willing to let go of the right to make decisions within the scope of delegated authority, able to let others make mistakes, trusting of subordinates, and establishes broad controls as a means of feedback, will find enhanced success in accomplishing the organization's objectives through delegation.

Informal Organization

In staffing and distributing work the manager must also be aware of the informal organization. Whenever people work together, informal groups form. These have both advantages and disadvantages. The informal organization affords its members status which may provide a sense of belonging that contributes to personal satisfaction, resulting in a happier, more productive employee. Social values of the informal group, however, may work against the objectives of the formal organization when restrictive membership makes individuals feel outcast or when perpetuation of social values creates resistance to change. The informal organization also promotes communication, with members helping one another. This may lighten management's workload and act as a safety valve for members to relieve their frustrations. When such communication includes unfounded rumors or frustrations become self-fulfilling, the informal organization can undermine morale. The informal organization also provides social control by influencing and regulating members' behavior. Such conformity may keep members in line with formal organizational goals or may stifle initiative and creativity.

STAFFING AND WORK DISTRIBUTION TECHNIQUES

A department manager has overall responsibility for staffing and work distribution. Staffing refers to the identification of the number and types of employees needed to carry out the work of the department.

Organization Chart

The kinds of employees are depicted in an organization chart (see Figure 10). Each position is shown, typically, from the top

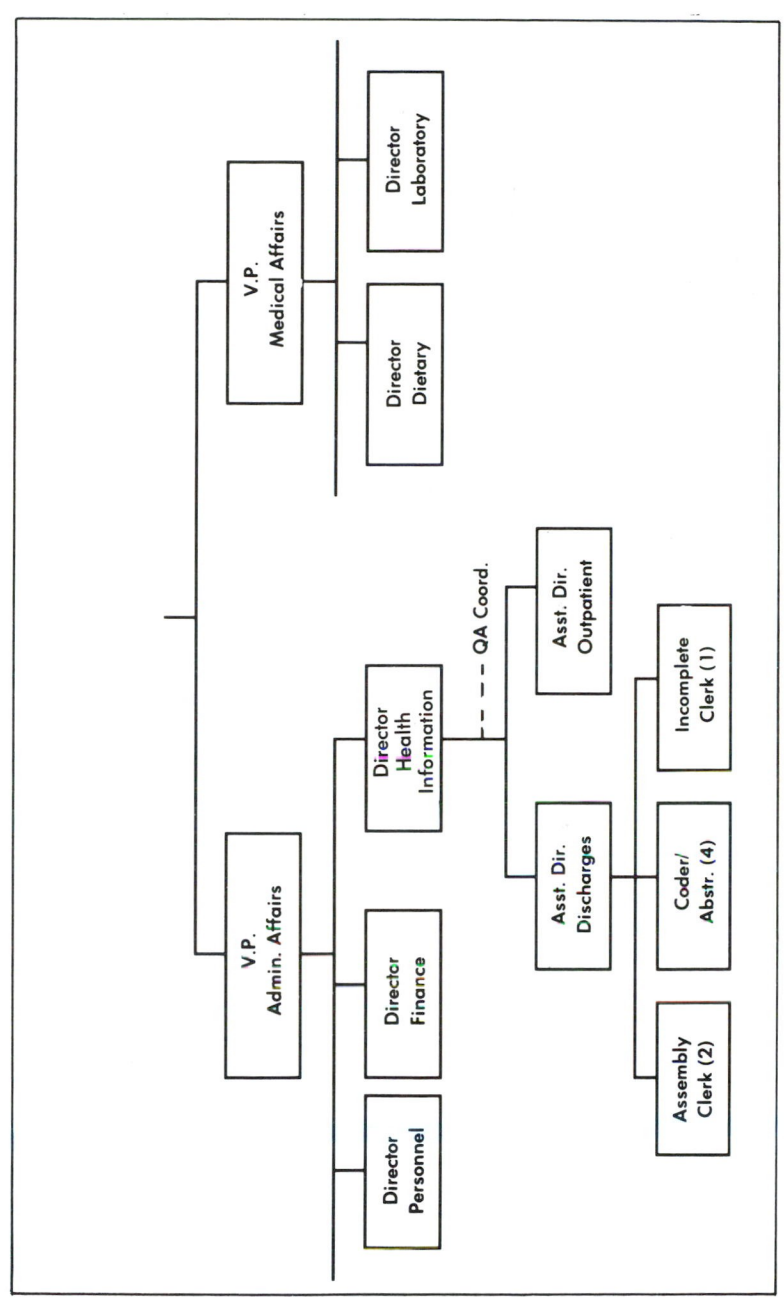

FIGURE 10. PORTION OF HOSPITAL ORGANIZATION CHART

of the authority hierarchy down. Line relationships are shown as solid lines and staff as dotted lines. An organization chart shows the limits of each position's authority and responsibility. It aids the manager in discovering confused lines of authority, duplication of functions, inefficient allocation of personnel, too large a span of control, and lack of intermediate supervisory levels. Separate charts may be drawn in an attempt to depict informal relationships, although they become out of date quickly. Organization charts should be drawn carefully so authority relationships are not confused with status. For instance, if a manager's secretary is shown closer to the manager than the assistant manager, there can be confusion over who has more authority.

The organizational chart contains job titles or functions. A job is made up of tasks and responsibilities which, when considered together, are regarded as the regular assignment of an individual.

Service Activity Level

The number of individuals, or full time equivalents (FTE), needed to perform each task is determined overall by service activity levels. Service activity levels relate to the volume of services and the productivity level that can be achieved in performing those services. (See also previous section on budgets.) Productivity is the number of service units performed per staff hour that meet established levels of quality. Thus to determine, for instance, the number of FTEs required to code medical records of discharged patients for a given period, the manager must know how many discharges are expected for the period and the performance standard. If an employee can be expected to accurately code 7 records in an hour, and 20,500 discharges are expected in a year, 1.56 FTEs are required. The calculation is shown below. The standard of 6 records accurately coded in an hour has been adjusted for personal time, fatigue, and delay (PF&D - a factor which accounts for breaks, inservices, and other time during which the employee is legitimately not performing the task). It is also assumed that the employee's regular productive time is 1,880 hours per year (after deducting for non-productive time for vacation, sick leave, and holidays).

$$\frac{20,500 \text{ medical records of discharged patients to be coded/year}}{7 \text{ records/hour (adjusted for PF\&D) X 1880 hours paid per year}} = 1.56 \text{ FTEs}$$

Work Distribution

Frequently the number of FTEs required to perform any one task is not a whole number. Once staffing levels are determined for all tasks in a department, overall staffing must be established. This is work distribution and can be aided by a work distribution chart. A typical work distribution chart is shown in Figure 11. It records, generally for a period of a week, the activities performed, the time it takes to perform them, the individuals who are working on the activities, and the amount of time spent by each person on each activity.

Activity	Total Hours	MARY SMITH	Hours	SUSAN JONES	Hours	
Chart Assembly	10	Assembly	9	Assembly	1	
Chart Analysis	50	Analysis	20	Analysis	20	
Chart Controls	5	Secure All Charts	2			
Maintenance and Filing Activities on Recent Discharges	8	Chart Repair Filing Loose Reports Chart Location	1 4 1	Chart Repair Chart Location	1 1	
Phone	1	Answer	1			
Statistics	12	Fill Out Work Sheets	2	Fill Out Work Sheets Daily Re-Sort	3 4	Fill Out Daily
Coding	12			Coding	3	Cod
Indexing	23			Indexing	6	
Total	121		40		39	

FIGURE 11. WORK DISTRIBUTION CHART

A work distribution chart is prepared by having each employee keep daily task lists of the major activities performed. (The number of days recorded will depend on the cyclical nature of the work, but usually a week is adequate). At the end of the data collection period, the manager summarizes the time spent on all activities by each employee. Each employee's time may not add to the total number of hours in the work day because of interruptions for minor tasks, and other PF&D types of activities. A 10 to 15 percent margin of discrepancy is often found.

The work distribution chart lays out work assignments in a form that facilitates critical questioning of the existing situation. It does not provide solutions, but makes finding them easier. Analysis of the work distribution chart answers questions such as what activities take the most time? Are unnecessary activities being performed? Are employee skills being properly utilized? Are employees doing too many unrelated tasks? Are tasks being spread too thinly throughout the department or unit? Is work in the unit being distributed evenly?

The traditional work distribution chart can also be modified to show needed staffing levels and skill requirements (Figure 12). Using this modification fractional FTEs can be smoothed out so the total number of employees required can be found. For instance, the analysis function and incomplete control func-

Task	Skill Requirements						Staff Requirements	
	Coding	Medical Term.	Typing	Inter-personal	Filing	General Clerical	FTEs	Persons
Assembly					x		0.73	1½
Analysis		x		x			1.20	
Coding	x	x					1.56	2
Abstracting			35 wpm		x	x	0.82	
Inc Chart Cont		x		x			0.84	4
Correspondence			35 wpm		x	x	0.68	
Transcription		x	70 wpm				2.45	
. . .								etc.
Total							8.28	

FIGURE 12. DETERMINING STAFFING LEVELS

tions may have similar skill requirements. Thus the employee designated "incomplete control clerk" could take on the extra workload of the "analyst."

Layout

Organizing the physical environment of the department is also the responsibility of management. The physical environment must be laid out so the work flows smoothly through the department.

The most common means to physically arrange the work environment is to use a layout. This is an architectural chart, drawn to scale, which depicts the location of furniture and equipment within available space. Constraints in designing a layout include permanent physical structures such as walls, posts, and windows, and the location of electrical outlets, water, and drains. Environmental factors such as lighting, color, air conditioning, heat, and sound must be considered when designing a layout. The nature of the furniture and equipment itself puts constraints on their placement. Finally, the policies of the department or organization with regard to private offices, space commensurate with position or tenure, and other elements play a part in the layout. The ideal layout provides for an effective work flow, safety, space that is ample and well utilized, employee comfort and satisfaction, ease of supervision, favorable impression on visitors (if applicable), ample flexibility for varying needs, and balanced capacity of equipment and personnel at each stage in work flow.

One of the greatest problems in designing a layout where work is performed in a sequence of steps passing from one employee to another, or where one employee must move to different work stations, is planning an efficient work flow. Much time can be wasted in backtracking and crisscrossing throughout the work area. A movement diagram (Figure 13) is a simple tool which can check that furniture and equipment are placed effectively by superimposing the flow of work on the layout.

Important points in layout include:

1. Equipment should be near the user.

2. Employees' desks should face in the same direction with two and one-half to three feet between desks.

3. As a general guideline, each clerical employee should be allowed 60 square feet, including space for filing cabinets, additional work area, and aisles for each employee.

4. It is best not to place the file room near the main office entrance, in order to reduce the accessibility of medical records to unauthorized personnel.

5. Since medical transcription is one of the noisier activities, it should be confined to one area. Soundproof booths or partitions help to reduce the noise from transcription equipment.

6. Coders generally require a quiet work area conducive to their focused tasks.

7. Employees who most often deal with patients or other hospital personnel should be placed near the entrance of the department.

8. Main aisles should be at least 5 feet wide; secondary aisles should be at least 3 feet wide.

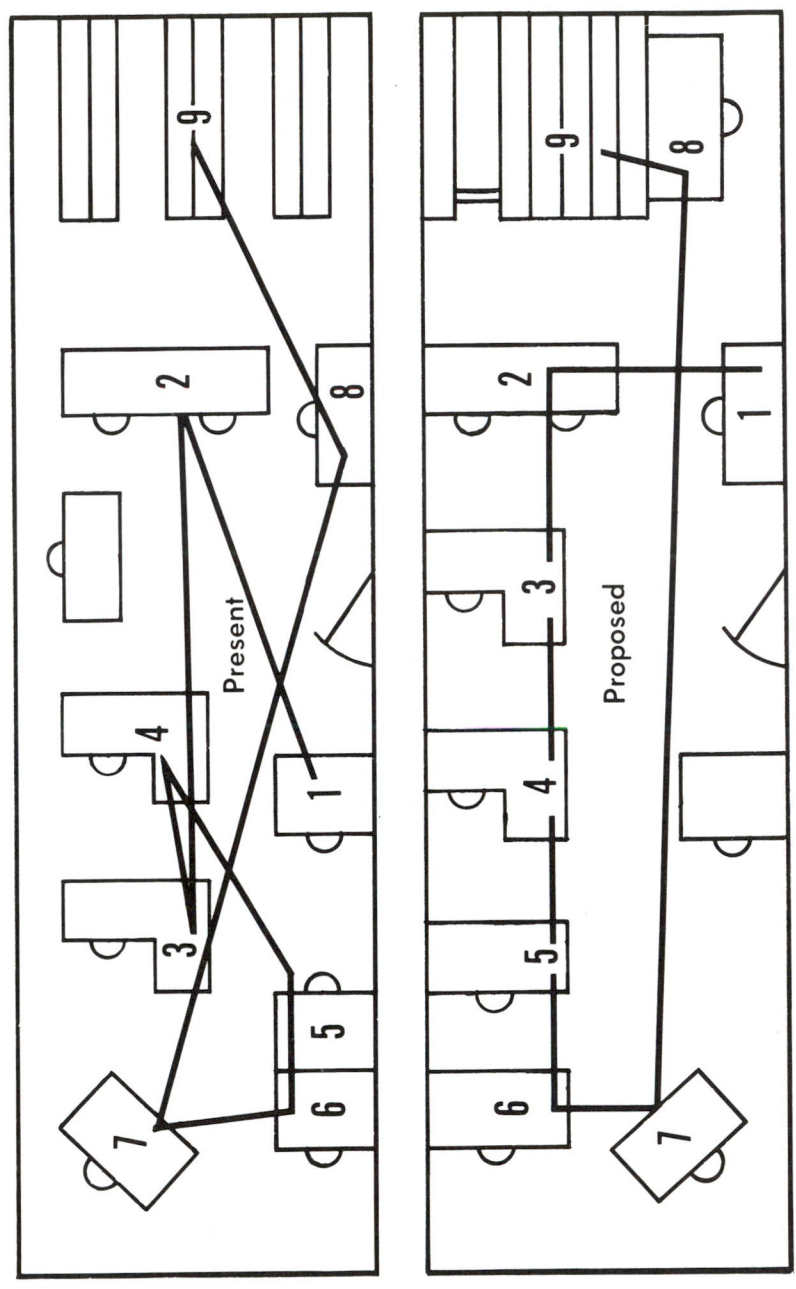

FIGURE 13. MOVEMENT DIAGRAMS SUPERIMPOSED OVER LAYOUT

9. Private offices have both advantages and disadvantages. The disadvantages include the loss of some esprit de corps and a lessening of supervisory control. Private offices offer a quiet place in which to ponder complex problems, complete projects, and to confer with staff, physicians, and employees.

A configuration chart may aid in organizing equipment such as computers and dictation systems. The need for a configuration chart arises when there are many pieces of interrelated equipment, located in several physically separate areas. The configuration chart helps to keep track of the location and type of equipment and how each is connected. Standard symbols or pictures are used to depict the equipment. Lines connecting the symbols or pictures delineate the flow of data, materials, or work through the equipment.

Finally environmental factors such as temperature, humidity, and ventilation must also be considered in office layout. This is especially true as employers become more concerned about employee health and departments acquire more computerized equipment.

Temperature and humidity control and adequate ventilation have been proven to have a direct effect on employee productivity and effective operation of computer equipment. The ideal office temperature is about 70 degrees Fahrenheit with a relative humidity of 40% to 60%. Air circulation via central air conditioning, window fans, and ventilators is important.

The proper use of color is an important consideration. Color not only spruces up an office but improves working conditions. Psychologically color can affect human emotions, senses and thought processes, and an individual's ability to relax. Some colors have a favorable psychological effect, others a negative effect. Some colors give a lift; others can depress mental action.

Lighting is important especially in health information departments where considerable reading is done. Light sources on the ceiling can usually provide enough light for the entire office area at a prescribed level of illumination. However, task or ambient light, maybe more energy efficient. Task lighting is that provided directly over a work surface. Light shining on a surface can produce glare, and should be avoided, especially with respect to computer display screens.

THE DIRECTING FUNCTION

The directing function of management involves getting all members of a work group to contribute effectively and efficiently to the achievement of the organization's objectives. The terms "directing" and "actuating" are sometimes used synonymously. The dictionary definition of direct is "to set straight, to show or point out, to regulate the activities or course of." The definition of actuate is "to move to action." The slight but distinct difference in these two terms relates to two, often-competing aspects of management - the scientific approach of directing, using tools of work simplification or methods engineering, and the humanistic aspects of actuating, including leadership, motivation, and communication.

However, the quality improvement programs currently being implemented by many healthcare organizations emphasize the critical importance of synchronizing measurement processes and human factors to achieve desired results from any group of people within an organization or from the organization as a whole.

WORK SIMPLIFICATION

Work simplification is commonly referred to as the organized use of common sense to find easier and better ways of doing work. Work simplification, however, is not a speed-up system, or a new way of working harder or faster. It means doing a better job with less effort, in less time, without hurrying, with greater safety, and with lower costs. This is accomplished by eliminating unnecessary parts of the work, combining and rearranging other parts of the work, and simplifying the necessary parts of the work. Work simplification does not change the basic tenets of a procedure, but changes the methods employed to accomplish it. This may involve new supplies, equipment, a new arrangement of materials, or new operations.

Several tools are available to gather facts, question these facts, and consider alternative ways to perform the work. A flow process chart is the most common tool (Figure 14). While it is possible to simplify without a formal chart, a chart ensures that as much data as possible about the work have been recorded. It permits the analyst to see the whole task at one time and compare alternatives. It provides documentation to implement the task. The flow process chart is prepared by listing every

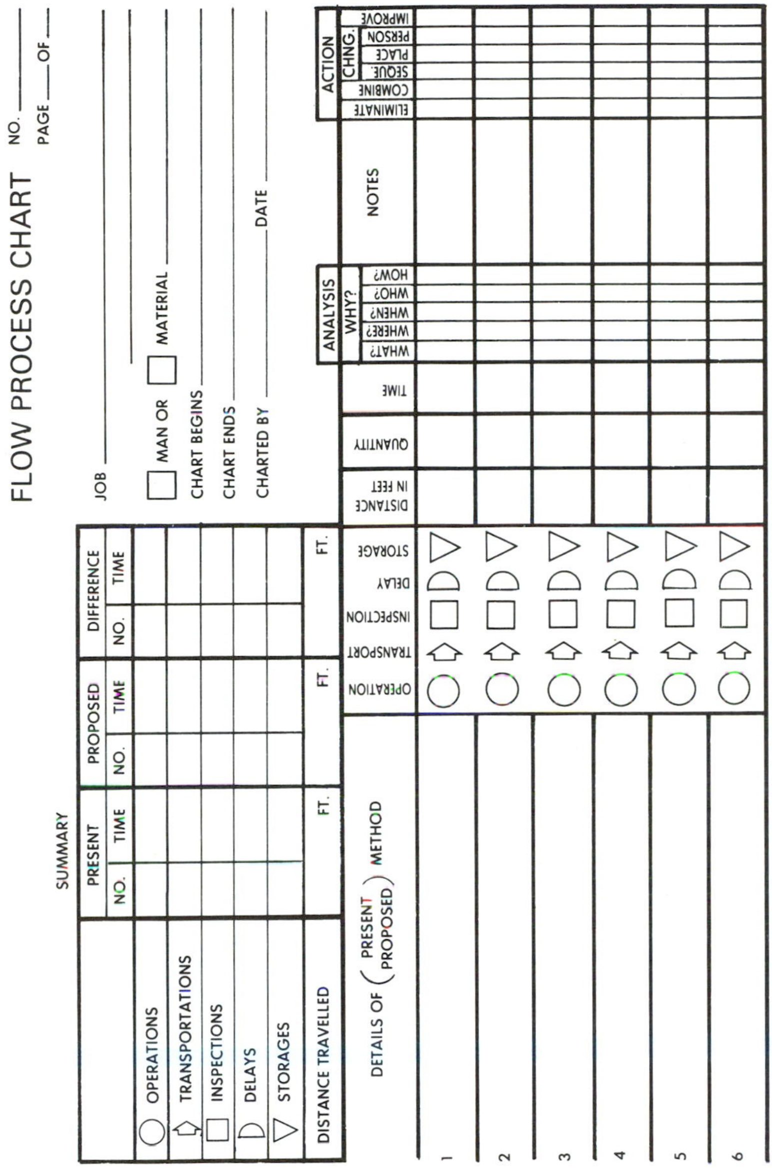

FLOW PROCESS CHART

NO. _____
PAGE _____ OF _____

JOB _____

☐ MAN OR ☐ MATERIAL _____

CHART BEGINS _____

CHART ENDS _____

CHARTED BY _____ DATE _____

SUMMARY

	PRESENT		PROPOSED		DIFFERENCE	
	NO.	TIME	NO.	TIME	NO.	TIME
◯ OPERATIONS						
⇧ TRANSPORTATIONS						
☐ INSPECTIONS						
◗ DELAYS						
▽ STORAGES						
DISTANCE TRAVELLED	FT.		FT.		FT.	

DETAILS OF (PRESENT / PROPOSED) METHOD

	DISTANCE IN FEET	QUANTITY	TIME	OPERATION	TRANSPORT	INSPECTION	DELAY	STORAGE	ANALYSIS						NOTES	ACTION					
									WHAT?	WHERE?	WHEN?	WHO?	HOW?	WHY?		ELIMINATE	COMBINE	SEQUE.	PLACE	PERSON	IMPROVE
																				CHNG.	
1				◯	⇧	☐	◗	▽													
2				◯	⇧	☐	◗	▽													
3				◯	⇧	☐	◗	▽													
4				◯	⇧	☐	◗	▽													
5				◯	⇧	☐	◗	▽													
6				◯	⇧	☐	◗	▽													

FIGURE 14. FLOW PROCESS CHART

step in the work in the sequence performed; classifying each step according to type; and recording distance, time, and/or quantity related to each step. Then, every step is challenged - asking why the step is done, why at that location, at that time, by that person, and in that manner. Finally, an improved method that eliminates or combines; changes places, sequences, or persons; and simplifies should result.

The result of work simplification is change. Yet most people tend to resist change. Change disturbs complacency and disrupts habits. One of the most critical reasons for resistance to change is that change implies criticism. Every way of doing something was devised by somebody; so when someone else tries to recommend a change, persons related to the previous method often feel their ideas and efforts are being criticized. Another factor related to change is the feeling of insecurity which often results. People may feel they will be unable to perform as well with the new method or machine or may not be able to learn the new method. A major goal of work simplification is to develop open-mindedness toward work methods in everyone - managers and employees alike. The manager's role in work simplification is one of guidance and assistance, while it is the employee's role to initiate the improvements. An atmosphere in which work simplification is a team effort requires a manager who is an effective leader, who understands factors which motivate people, and who can develop a climate conducive to action.

LEADERSHIP

Leadership is an important managerial trait. Leadership is the interpersonal influence directed toward attainment of a specific goal or goals. Influence infers power; but power comes in several forms, some of which are more desirable in managerial leadership than others. French and Raven, in a classic work on power, suggest six sources of power:

1. Coercive Power - Based on a follower's perception that an influencer has the ability to inflict punishment.

2. Reward Power - Based on a follower's perception that an influencer has the capacity to administer some reward.

3. Legitimate Power - Based on a follower's internalized values which convince the follower that an influencer has the right to influence and the follower is bound to accept.

This base of power endows leadership positions with formal authority.

4. Referent Power - based on a follower's desire to identify with a charismatic leader, who is followed out of blind faith. This is maintained only so long as the follower behaves as the leader directs.

5. Expert Power - Based on a follower's perception that the leader has special knowledge or expertise which can be useful in satisfying the follower's needs.

6. Representative Power - Based on followers democratically delegating power to the leader for the purpose of representing their interests and making decisions on their behalf.

A manager's source of power often determines the type of effectiveness of leadership. Rensis Likert, one of many researchers in leadership theory, is a proponent of participative management. He believes an effective manager is one who is strongly oriented to subordinates and relies on communication to keep the organization running. Likert defined four systems of management (see Figure 15). These form a hierarchy, with the fourth system the one which Likert believes describes the manager who can most successfully direct the work of others. A manager might perform self-appraisal to determine the need to move to a higher system.

Another approach to understand one's leadership style and thus one's ability to direct work has been proposed by Robert Blake and Jane Mouton, whose primary concern was that interest in people must be coupled with interest in production. They displayed this concept on a managerial grid (Figure 16). The grid is a useful tool for classifying managerial styles, although the underlying cause of a classification is not directly evident. Personality, training, environment, and other situational factors influence the manager's position on the grid, and must be considered before a manager attempts to alter personal style.

THE CONTROLLING FUNCTION

While all of the four functions of management are interrelated, the functions of controlling and planning are more di-

TITLE	CHARACTERISTICS				
	LEADER'S POWER BASE	LEVEL OF CONFIDENCE IN EMPLOYEES	MOTIVATION TECHNIQUE	DIRECTION OF COMMUNICATION	LEVEL OF PARTICIPATION
SYSTEM 1 Exploitive – Authoritative	Coercive	Little	Fear and Punishment	Downward	Decision Making at Managerial Level
SYSTEM 2 Benevolent – Authoritative	Reward Legitimate	Patronizing	Some Fear and Punishment, Some Reward	Permit Upward	Some Delegation with Close Control
SYSTEM 3 Consultative	Referent Expert	Substantial	Reward with Occasional Punishment	Up and Down	General Decisions at Top–Specific at Bottom
SYSTEM 4 Participative – Group	Representative	Complete	Reward and Involvement	Up, Down and with Peers	Encourage Decision Making

FIGURE 15. LIKERT'S SYSTEM OF MANAGEMENT

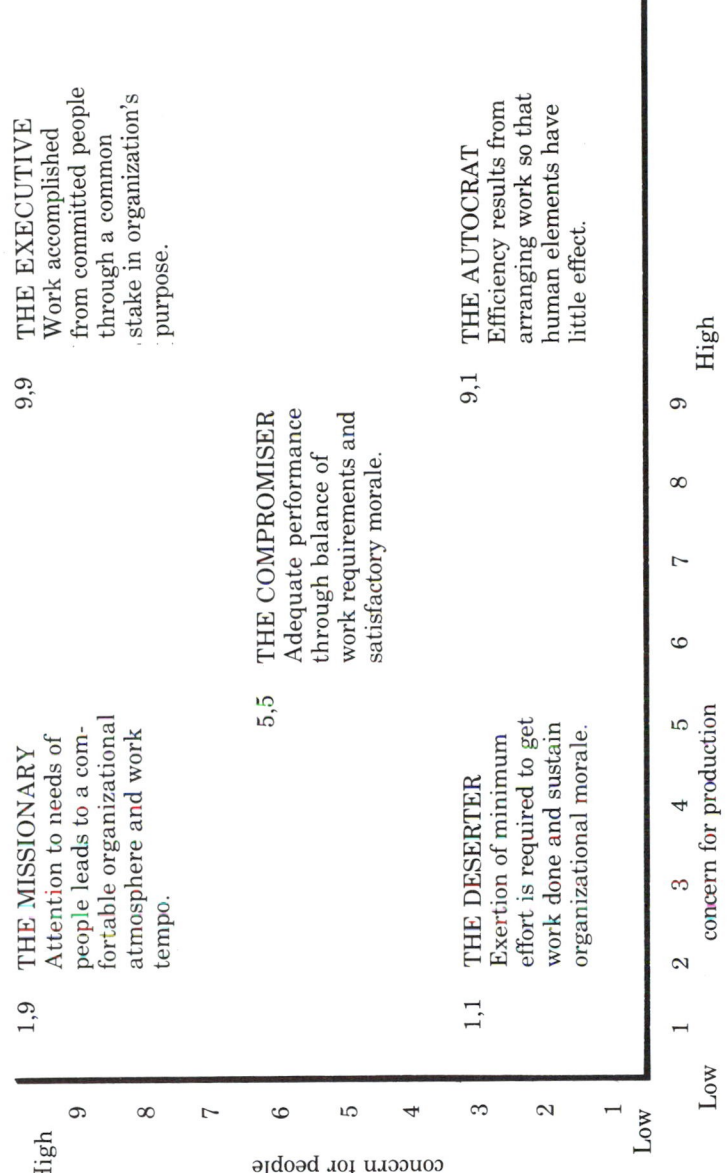

FIGURE 16. MANAGERIAL GRID

rectly related to one another than any other functions. Controlling is the feedback mechanism for planning. Controlling is determining whether planning has been effective and taking steps to ensure that objectives and goals are met. Controlling can be viewed as detecting and correcting significant variations in the results obtained from planned activities.

Controlling requires an understanding of what is necessary to meet the standards defined in objectives and goals. It requires monitors to determine and compare actual performance with the expected. It also requires mechanisms to ensure that adequate resources exist to meet standards (staffing and budgeting) and that corrective action is taken so performance will meet standards.

STANDARDS

Standards are embodied in the objectives and goals set in the planning function of management. Frequently, however, standards are not so explicitly defined that they are easily usable as controls. For instance, the objective "transcribe basic reports for inclusion into the medical record within two days of their dictation" does not define how many lines of transcription are expected to type, the number of FTEs required for the volume of dictation, or the level of transcription quality expected.

Standards are developed for a particular task by measuring all aspects of the work, and evaluating the results for their reliability and validity for use as a standard. Once the most reliable and valid measure is found, it becomes the official criterion or reference point for staffing, budgeting, and ensuring that performance meets the standards. As previously discussed under goal-setting, standards should be challenging yet reachable. Although participation of employees in setting goals or standards has not been found to be the most critical element in the success of goal setting, working with employees to set standards contributes to their reliability and validity and ensures that they are realistic. Employees may also feel they are controlling their own destiny, which will improve their compliance with the standards.

Measuring work in order to define a standard first requires the definition of a unit of measurement. For example, "basic hospital reports" is quite vague when discharge summaries, operative reports, and history and physical examination reports differ greatly in their length and complexity. A measurement unit for quantity must define the precise item which will be counted - number of reports by type, number of lines, or number of lines by type of report. A measurement unit for quality must also be defined - number of errors or number of omissions. In defining the quality component the consequences of errors on patient care and financial status of the facility can serve as guidelines. A unit of measurement is important not only for consistency but for ease in subsequent use of the standard. The unit of measurement, however, should not be too cumbersome to use continually (for example, hand counting keystrokes transcribed may be very precise but not practical over time).

Once the unit of measurement is defined, there are several ways to accomplish the measurement. These include primarily the use of scientific method, simulation, past performance records, and benchmarking.

Scientific Method

Applying scientific method in measuring work results in the highest degree of accuracy. Scientific method refers to the use of stopwatch time studies and work sampling to study different workers in different organizations performing essentially the same task to arrive at "standard time data" for each element in a task. Managers then compile the standard time data for each element, comprising the task performed in a given situation to arrive at an overall task standard.

Unfortunately, most of the work in this area has been done for setting time standards for workers in departments other than health information, such as those in laboratories.

Simulation

Another method for measuring work to define a standard is simulation. This method is used when defining a standard for new work. In simulation, one person performs the task several times as if it were actual work and (the same person or preferably another person) records the time it takes to complete the task and the number and types of errors made. The "someone" to perform the task for the simulation is difficult to choose. Persons generally available for this are the manager, an "average" employee, the "best" employee, or an outsider. With each person there are problems which may influence the reliability of the standard, including how well the person knows the task, how comfortable they are in performing the task, and their attitude about what they are doing. In addition to these problems, until the standard is instituted, there is no means to verify it against actual practice.

Past Performance Records

Using past performance records is the third, and most common method of work measurement. These refer to data collected, by a variety of means, on actual work performed previously. Several problems with this method exist. Standards set on past performance will not be valid if a change in procedure, methods, or qualifications of personnel takes place. If such change does not take place, and the intent is to institute standards where none previously existed, or where only the volume and frequency of work are expected to change, then the only caution about using past performance records is their appropriateness. One would not want to base future standards on poor performance.

Benchmarking

Benchmarking is the fourth method of measuring the performance of a health information department. Benchmarking involves comparing one's department to other departments or organizations known to be excellent in one or more areas. It is more than merely comparing one's department to another, however. The success of benchmarking involves finding out how the other department functions and then incorporating their ideas into the health information department.

Benchmarking may be internal or external. If internal, the health information department compares itself to its own averages from the past, similar to past performance records described above. The purpose of internal benchmarking is to find out what the department was doing right when productivity or quality was especially high. Or a health information department might use internal benchmarking to look at similar activities in different departments of the hospital, for example, reviewing the processes used in the radiology department to find out how their staff achieve a fast turnaround time for transcription.

External benchmarking involves comparing the department to state-of-the-art departments or organizations. A health information manager might investigate how an outstanding medical center handles the flow of medical records, for example. Or a health information department might go so far as to benchmark with a hotel, bank, or other business to find out how their staff handle large volumes of phone calls or files.

The key to benchmarking, however, is not to compare one department with another, but rather to use that comparison to improve the department's processes.

MONITORS

Past performance records are used not only to define standards but also to monitor productivity. Monitoring the quantity component of productivity is generally easier than monitoring quality. Because productivity is the number of items produced per staff hour that meet established levels of quality, monitoring both quantity and quality, if only on a sampling basis, is critical. There are several different types of monitors.

Quantity Monitors

One of the most widely used quantity monitors is the employee-reported volume log, which collects data on how much work comes in and how much work is produced. To collect data on "input," each unit of work entering the work area is represented by a hash mark on a log. This may be combined with an "output" log to demonstrate backlogs (see Figure 17). Such logs are quite reliable because their data can usually be verified against other records. However, these logs are only useful for identifying trends in workload.

An employee-reported time log is a past performance record in which the employee notes on a time sheet the time spent on each activity (see Figure 18). A time log is used with other pertinent data such as the daily census or volume logs to produce information on how much time is spent on each function. This is not the most accurate means of determining productivity, since the time log can be disruptive to work. Employee cooperation in reporting all work as well as personal time must be obtained in order for this type of record to be reliable. However, time logs serve a useful purpose in pointing out such things as constant interruptions or where adjustments could be made in work duties or procedures so the employee can accomplish the work expected.

Stopwatch time study is a more accurate method of studying productivity. This involves observing work and timing each

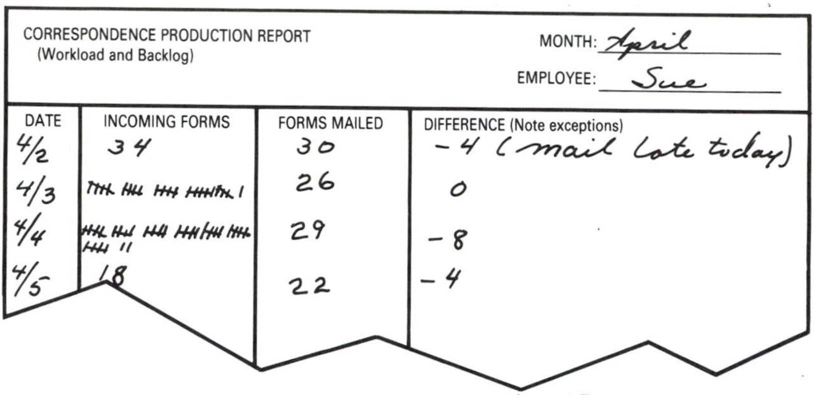

CORRESPONDENCE PRODUCTION REPORT
(Workload and Backlog)

MONTH: April
EMPLOYEE: Sue

DATE	INCOMING FORMS	FORMS MAILED	DIFFERENCE (Note exceptions)
4/2	34	30	−4 (mail late today)
4/3	~~||||~~ ~~||||~~ ~~||||~~ ~~||||~~ ~~||||~~ I	26	0
4/4	~~||||~~ ~~||||~~ ~~||||~~ ~~||||~~ ~~||||~~ ~~||||~~ ~~||||~~ II	29	−8
4/5	18	22	−4

FIGURE 17. EMPLOYEE-REPORTED VOLUME LOG

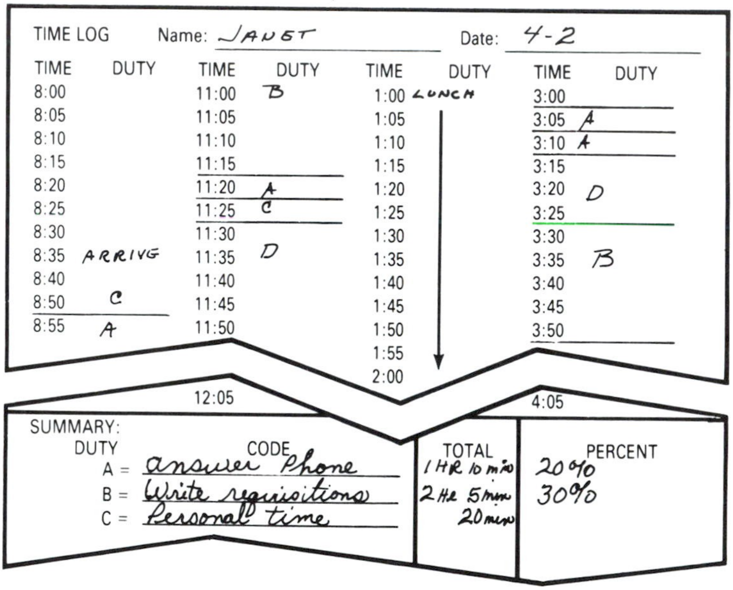

TIME LOG Name: JANET Date: 4-2

TIME	DUTY	TIME	DUTY	TIME	DUTY	TIME	DUTY
8:00		11:00	B	1:00	LUNCH	3:00	
8:05		11:05		1:05		3:05	A
8:10		11:10		1:10		3:10	A
8:15		11:15		1:15		3:15	
8:20		11:20	A	1:20		3:20	D
8:25		11:25	C	1:25		3:25	
8:30		11:30		1:30		3:30	
8:35	ARRIVG	11:35	D	1:35		3:35	B
8:40		11:40		1:40		3:40	
8:50	C	11:45		1:45		3:45	
8:55	A	11:50		1:50		3:50	
				1:55			
				2:00			
		12:05				4:05	

SUMMARY:

DUTY CODE	TOTAL	PERCENT
A = answer Phone	1 HR 10 min	20%
B = Write requisitions	2 Hr 5 min	30%
C = Personal time	20 min	

FIGURE 18. EMPLOYEE-REPORTED TIME LOG

element with a stopwatch (see Figure 19). Such a study may be performed where one wants to determine if the employee is performing a given task at an acceptable speed, or it can replace the time log to determine time spent on all activities. As a quantity control device the stopwatch time study can pinpoint problems, such as too much time spent on one component of the task, wasted time in not performing components uniformly, proving to an employee that a task can be performed in the established time, or finding that a task cannot be done as originally expected.

Stopwatch time study, while being very precise, is the weakest technique psychologically. Having someone watch your every move is quite unsettling to most people. While it may seem more likely with the time log, both techniques allow for the same amount of employee manipulation. In the time log the employees are on their own to record whatever they feel is

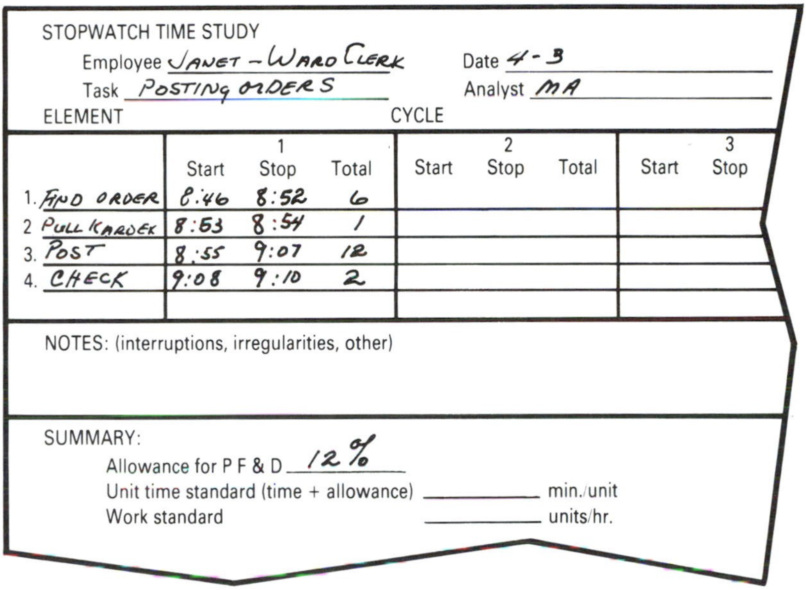

STOPWATCH TIME STUDY

Employee _JANET – WARD CLERK_   Date _4 - 3_

Task _POSTING ORDERS_   Analyst _MA_

ELEMENT   CYCLE

ELEMENT	1			2			3	
	Start	Stop	Total	Start	Stop	Total	Start	Stop
1. FIND ORDER	8:46	8:52	6					
2. PULL KARDEX	8:53	8:54	1					
3. POST	8:55	9:07	12					
4. CHECK	9:08	9:10	2					

NOTES: (interruptions, irregularities, other)

SUMMARY:

Allowance for P F & D _12 %_

Unit time standard (time + allowance) _____ min./unit

Work standard _____ units/hr.

FIGURE 19. STOPWATCH TIME STUDY

"right," but employees can also pace themselves in front of a stopwatch analyst. Other problems with the stopwatch time study relate to the analyst. The supervisor performing this function can instill feelings of insecurity or defensiveness. An outsider will need explanation as to what is being done, thus automatically slowing the employee. To be effective as well as precise, this tool must be used with a great deal of employee cooperation and, perhaps, is only reliable in its use as a technique for establishing standard time data where employees understand that their results will be pooled with others' results.

Work Sampling

Work sampling is spot checking work and drawing conclusions from it. Although work sampling is generally used to monitor quantity, the principle may also be used in monitoring quality. Work sampling is based on probability - that a sample taken at random will tend to resemble the actual work. The key to accuracy in work sampling is in the number of observations made and how they are made. Elements in determining the number of observations required to make the sample statistically significant are:

Population - The full range of activities from which a sample will be drawn should be defined. For instance, if sampling the file area functions, the population may include filing medical records, pulling medical records, answering the phone, filing loose sheets, and miscellaneous activities performed on the day shift.

Sample - The part of the population to be studied. The sample must contain a large enough number of observations to be valid and small enough to be cost effective. Statistical formulas are available to calculate sample size for a desired degree of accuracy. An alignment chart may also be used. In using an alignment chart, the percent of activity constituting the work and the desired degree of precision are decided upon; then the result of alignment through these points on the chart is the number of observations. In Figure 20, the element of work being sampled constitutes 80% of a job and the degree of precision is 4% (i.e. the probability that the sample will not represent the population is + 4% from 80%). Thus, 400 observations must be made. Note that if it were desired to be twice as precise, (+ 2% from 80%) 1,500 observations would have to be made.

Random - The condition that every activity has an equal chance of being observed. In order to ensure randomness, a random number table found in most statistics textbooks can be used. Tables of random observations, such as displayed in Figure 21, can either be designed from a random number table or found in some management textbooks. Such a table identifies times for making observations.

Once all observations are made, the percentage of each type of observation out of the total number of observations is applied to the volume of work and hours in a workday to

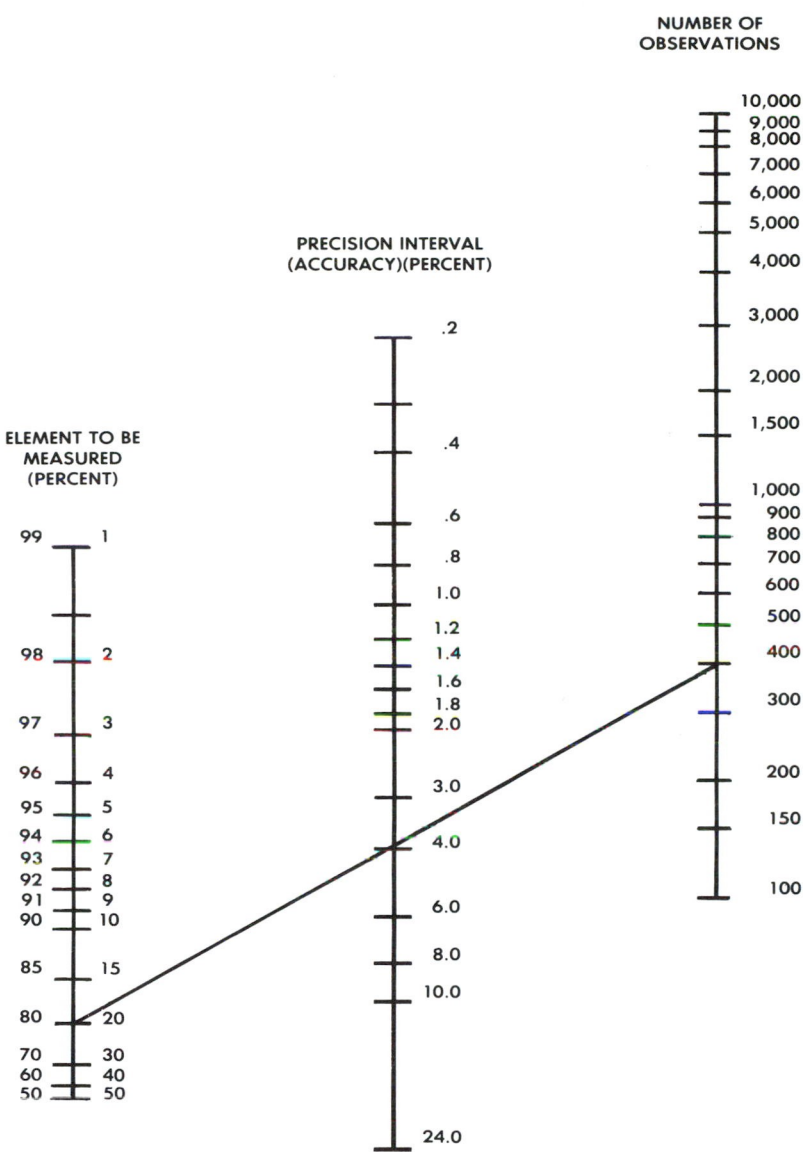

NUMBER OF
OBSERVATIONS

PRECISION INTERVAL
(ACCURACY)(PERCENT)

ELEMENT TO BE
MEASURED
(PERCENT)

Figure 20. Alignment Chart

determine the standard time. For instance, if in the total 400 observations, 140 observations were made of one employee filing records, this would represent 35% of the employee's time. If the employee works 7 hours a day (420 minutes), then the employee spends 147 minutes filing per day. If during the day the employee averages filing 100 records, then it took 1.47 minutes per record to file.

While observations may yield the best data if they are unannounced, this is not suggested because most employees discover the observation and are rightfully upset. Employees do not need

---

TABLE OF RANDOM OBSERVATIONS

Employee _MARY_   Job _CLERK_   Time Period _APRIL_

	Week 1			Week 2		Week 3
Monday	8:20 A	1:00 B	8:05	1:20	8:40	1:23
	8:25 B	2:45 A	8:40	1:30	9:20	1:40
	9:15 B	2:47 D	8:43	3:50	11:15	2:12
	11:07 B	3:06 D	9:20	3:55	11:16	3:56
	12:13 C	4:08 D	10:50	5:00	12:19	4:20
Tuesday	8:30 D	1:20 A	8:15	1:01	8:12	1:05
	8:35 D	1:30 B	9:00	2:15	9:12	2:20
	9:35 A	3:19 D	10:00	4:49	10:02	3:46
	10:15 A	4:40 D	11:43	4:50	10:30	4:08
	12:09 A	5:00 D	11:50	5:17	12:00	5:10

SUMMARY: TASK   CODE   PERCENT OF TOTAL OBSERVATIONS

A = Filing   MR
B = Pulling MR
C = Answering Phone
D = Filing   Loose sheets

FIGURE 21. WORK SAMPLING

---

to be notified every time an observation is made, but must be told they will be observed and the purpose of the observation. An effective manager should be able to put employees at relative ease with work sampling. All work measurement depends on the rapport between the manager and employees, but work sampling can become the most deceptive and disliked.

Quality Monitors

Direct inspection is the technique of actual verification of all or selected work performed by an employee to determine its accuracy. In inspection, the manager, or another employee, either retrospectively performs or concurrently observes the work in its entirety. If the work cannot be repeated, inspection must be done concurrently with the work, making this monitor very similar to the stopwatch study for recording production. Direct inspection is most useful when quality can be quantified, either as a single generally accepted practice, or as a range of normal values. For instance, this monitor would be used to count the number of typographical errors in transcription, the number of diagnoses coded incorrectly, etc.

The checklist is a monitor for direct observation of the quality of work performed when the quality is less easy to quantify. The checklist provides a specific listing of factors to be observed. The factors may be evaluated as simply "yes" or "no," or on a rating scale. An example of an application for the checklist monitor is in defining standards and evaluating the work of the insurance clerk - observing factors such as "did the clerk greet the patient respectfully?"

Audit is a formal quality monitoring technique patterned from the production industry. Generally, the audit is tailored to fit the area being studied and involves a comparison of the present operations against the intended. The primary objective of an audit is to reveal variations in any of the elements examined and to identify areas for corrective action.

Questionnaires are an indirect method of evaluating quality of work performed. A questionnaire is completed by the persons who receive the service, rather than by those who manage it (for example, physicians may be asked questions about health information department personnel). Questionnaires should not be used as the only quality assurance monitor, but they can provide information about performance which is not observed by the manager or cannot be evaluated directly in an audit.

Reports are records of work or work characteristics made by persons other than the manager (but not the consumer of the service as in the questionnaire type of monitor). Reports may be anecdotal, describing an incident, in the form of letters of commendation, complaints, or requests that reflect on the work of the department or employees. Reports may also be regular records that demonstrate level of work and variations from planned activities. Such reports include department budget variance reports, personnel statistics (such as sick time, vacation, and overtime usage, etc.), results of the Medicare Peer Review Organization's DRG validation, feedback on abstracting errors from the abstracting computer service, and many others.

In selecting the monitor or monitors to use for evaluating productivity in the health information department, several points should be kept in mind. First, monitors should measure significant tasks. It may not be appropriate or necessary to establish standards and evaluate certain types of tasks, for instance, those performed infrequently. Monitors should not only aid in setting standards and comparing actual work but should also aid in analyzing the cause of deviations from the standards so preventive as well as corrective action can be taken. Monitors should be objective - this is especially true of those which attempt to measure less quantifiable aspects of performance. Monitors should be flexible in the face of changed plans - there should be room to identify and explain variations when this is the case. Monitors should be cost effective. They should be evaluated to ensure that the cost of their implementation does not exceed the benefit of their implementation.

PRODUCTIVITY

As a result of standard setting and monitoring performance, productivity levels can be determined. It is important to distinguish between activity and productivity. Activity is purely quantitative and refers to the number of units of work completed. This is the number of units reported on employee-reported volume logs, time logs, and so forth. Activity does not address whether the work has been performed satisfactorily. In order to make a statement about the number of units of work that meet established levels of quality it is necessary to assess the quality of a sample of work performed to determine an overall productivity level. For example:

Standard: 20 units/hour with no more than 2 errors per unit.	
Work received	160 units
Work completed	144 units
Activity level (144/160 units)	90%
Backlog	16 units
Work sampled for quality (amount completed in 1 hr)	18 units
Work meeting quality standard	16 units
Productivity level (16 units/20 units standard)	80%

Both the quantity and quality of work are accounted for when a productivity level is calculated.

VARIANCE ANALYSIS

Determining productivity levels for individual employees, work units, and the department overall is one aspect of variance analysis. Variance analysis is the critical review of deviations from standards found via the monitoring activity. Variances from standards should be regularly analyzed for their rate of occurrence, severity, and cause.

A minor variance that happens infrequently probably can be ignored. Alternatively, a major variance should be investigated immediately, and corrective steps taken so it will not be repeated. Minor variances that are frequent, or that follow a pattern of occurrence, should also be investigated so their

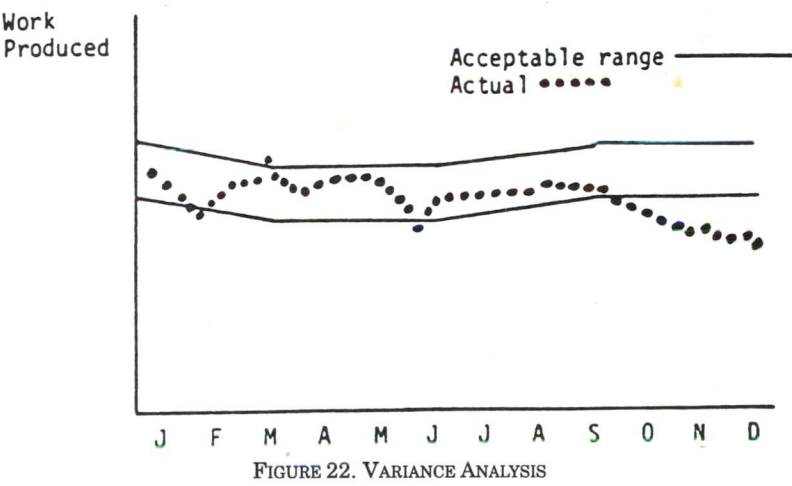

FIGURE 22. VARIANCE ANALYSIS

cumulative effect is minimized. In order to analyze the rate of occurrence of variances, data collected from productivity records should be plotted on a table or graph. For instance, in the graph displayed in Figure 22 variance from the range of acceptable productivity occurs three times in the first three quarters: twice slightly below range and once slightly above. These are probably not significant. However, during the fourth quarter, all productivity is below range and there is a downward trend which should be investigated. The rate of occurrence of variances can also be evaluated by comparing quantity and quality. If quality deteriorates when quantity increases, it may be that workload has increased and work simplification or additional staffing may be necessary. Yet if quality remains the same as quantity increases, the standard may be too low, or the employee may be demonstrating improved productivity.

The severity of the variance depends on the nature of the task for which the standard is set and the degree of deviation from the standard. A small deviation in a very critical task may be very important, whereas a moderate deviation in a less critical task may not be as important. Defining standards within an acceptable range is useful in evaluating the severity of deviations.

Analysis of variance also includes the determination of the cause of the deviation. It is necessary to evaluate the data from monitors with respect to the procedure, job description, or work method in order to determine the cause of a variance. For instance, the procedure may be out of date, the employee now performing the task may not be qualified, or the employee may have changed the work method. Aggregate production and performance records may also have to be separated by employee, or by smaller units of time to determine the specific attributes of the problem.

Variance analysis is also applied to financial plans. As shown earlier, a variance amount or percent difference between actual expenditures and budget is generally calculated. This is not only used in preparing a budget, but in monitoring budgetary performance. In budgetary variance analysis, a range of acceptable variance may be used, or other considerations may apply. For instance, a manager may be expected to meet the budget's "bottom line" - the overall total expenses while variance within categories is allowed. Alternatively, managers may vary in certain categories and not others. A flexible budget is one that is prepared with a range of activity levels so adjustments can be made throughout the year if changes in activity levels occur. Thus, variances truly reflect poor managerial control rather than changes outside of a manager's control.

CORRECTIVE ACTION AND FOLLOW-UP

Viable solutions to the problems that are identified in variance analysis should be developed and implemented. Solutions are many and varied, depending on the problem. In finding solutions, however, increases in staffing or additions to the budget should be a last resort. Too often, more staff and more money have been used to attempt to solve problems, yet the problems remain because their real cause has not been determined. Instead of more staff and money, procedures may need to be revised or updated, methods may need to be improved, work may need to be redistributed, employees may need additional training or counseling, and, of course, management is never exempt from the need to improve.

Controlling does not end with corrective action taken on a problem or set of problems. Corrective action must be followed up to ensure that it was appropriate and effective. A new set of monitors must also be implemented for ongoing productivity evaluation. As with all the functions of management, controlling is a continual, integrated process.

SUMMARY

Efficient management of the health information department is an important factor in the effective functioning of health care facilities. The health facility exists for the benefit of the patient; and the health information department is responsible for the completeness, accuracy, safekeeping, and availability of the medical record at all times. The department can discharge these responsibilities only when it is well managed.

Management is the effective utilization of resources toward the accomplishment of specific objectives. Good management is facilitated by carefully made plans, a chart of organization, proper analysis of each job, a study of the work flow with simplification when necessary, adoption of necessary internal controls, and adequate written procedures for each individual job and for the health information department as a whole.

The health information department director must not only create and manage the organization but must also provide the leadership to ensure that all functions are properly executed.

Because of higher educational and professional standards during the past few years, health information practitioners have earned recognition as trusted and responsible partners in the successful administration of health care facilities. As department managers they are responsible for certain functions which support the proper care of the sick and injured. To be successful in one's position, the health information practitioner must unceasingly analyze the procedures, delegate duties, supervise personnel, and display enthusiasm for work while keeping the department in step with the ever-changing health care environment.

STUDY QUESTIONS

1. What are the four components of management, and the four functions?
2. Explain the hierarchy of planning and the processes of management by objectives and goal-setting.
3. Describe budgetary planning.
4. List the steps in problem-solving and decision-making.
5. Distinguish between policies, procedures, standards, and rules.
6. Describe the importance of time management.
7. Define the components of organization.
8. Why is it important for the manager to delegate authority?
9. Define service activity level, and describe tools used in analyzing and developing staffing patterns, work distribution, and work environment.
10. Describe work simplification.
11. How does a manager acquire leadership skills?
12. List the major requirements of the controlling function.
13. Define productivity and describe the various types of quantity and quality monitors.
14. Describe the importance of variance analysis.

REFERENCES

Amatayakul, Margret K., *Finance Concepts for the Health Care Manager,* (Chicago: American Medical Record Association, 1985).

Amatayakul, Margret K. and Lou Ann Schraffenberger, *Productivity - A Handbook for Health Record Departments,* (Chicago: American Medical Record Association, 1988).

"Benchmarking gives managers a chance to learn from the best," *Medical Records Briefing,* March 1993, pp. 4-5.

Christensen, C. Roland, Norman A. Berg, Malcolm S. Salter, Howard H. Stevenson, *Policy Formulation and Administration,* (Homewood: Richard D. Irwin, Inc., 1985).

Dessler, Gary, Organization Theory - *Integrating Structure and Behavior,* (Englewood Cliffs: Prentice-Hall, Inc., 1980).

Herkimer, Allen G., *Understanding Health Care Budgeting,* (Rockville: Aspen Systems Corporation, 1988).

Liebler, Joan Gratto, *Managing Health Records - Administrative Principles,* (Germantown: Aspen Systems Corporation, 1980).

McConnell, Charles R., *The Health Care Supervisor's Casebook,* (Rockville: Aspen Systems Corporation, 1982).

Metzger, Norman, *The Health Care Supervisor's Handbook,* (Rockville: Aspen Publishers, Inc., 1988).

Spendolini, Michael J., *The Benchmarking Book,* American Management Association, New York, 1992.

Umiker, William, *Management Skills for the New Health Care Supervisor,* (Rockville: Aspen Publishers, Inc., 1988).

chapter 18

MANAGEMENT OF HEALTH INFORMATION
DEPARTMENT PERSONNEL

Getting things done through people is an important and challenging aspect of health information management. This chapter focuses on two of the most important traits required for effective management of medical record and health information personnel — motivation and communication. It also describes the job analysis, coaching and counseling employees, and several laws that affect managers in all settings.

MOTIVATION

Motivating employees is a critical concern of the health information professional. Because the health information department employs workers to perform routine tasks as well as workers for technical functions, the manager must adopt different motivational techniques for each situation.

Motivation Theories

Need satisfaction and motivation are highly complex and have been researched extensively. One of the most well-known psychologists in the area of motivation, Abraham Maslow, defines a needs hierarchy. This hierarchy begins at the lowest level with basic physiologic needs, such as hunger, and moves through security, acceptance, esteem, and self-actualization. The last four depend on the environment, and thus they may be useful motivators. Maslow's hierarchical theory has been the subject of much research without very much support; but the needs themselves are widely accepted, and the suggestion that there are two groups of needs seems to have been borne out by other research.

The concepts behind self-actualization were perhaps best expressed by Douglas McGregor, who presented two opposite sets of assumptions he believed basic to most managers. Summarized in Figure 1, one set was labeled Theory X and the other

THEORY X	THEORY Y
• People dislike work and will try to avoid it.	• People do not inherently disklike work
• People have to be coerced and threatened with punishment if goals are to be met	• People do not like rigid control and threats
• Most workers like direction and will avoid responsibility	• Under proper conditions, people do not avoid responsibility
• People want security above all in their work	• People want security but also have other needs such as self-actualization and esteem

FIGURE 1. MC GREGOR'S THEORY X AND THEORY Y

Theory Y. McGregor felt that managers typically held one of these sets of assumptions about human nature and acted in keeping with those assumptions. It is important for a health information manager to recognize that people in general are more like Theory Y than Theory X. A key point in McGregor's Theory Y is that work is itself a motivator of most people.

Frederick Herzberg and associates also defined two categories which they called maintenance factors and motivators, and proposed within each category those things which might satisfy needs, i.e., serve as motivators or maintenance factors. These, and Maslow's hierarchy, are shown in Figure 2.

In health information departments where advancement often depends on additional (formal) education, and where there are limited resources for educational assistance, the manager must ensure appropriate recognition and status for subordinates who may be unable to obtain further education. Employee training programs and in-service education help provide growth opportunities. Identifying the importance of their jobs can also help employees assume responsibility for and find challenge in their work. For instance, the importance of the medical record being available for patient care may help motivate file clerks.

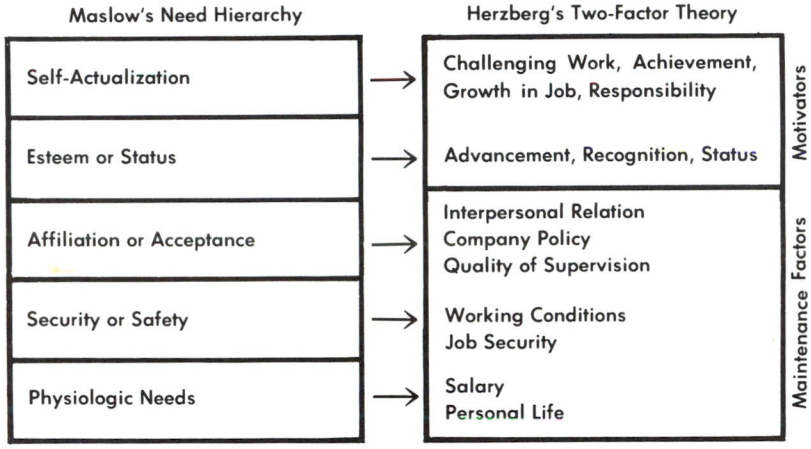

FIGURE 2. MASLOW'S AND HERZBERG'S MOTIVATION THEORIES

Finally, a fourth approach to motivation and human behavior recognizes that people are "complex." The complex view suggests that, because each person is different, a variety of items may prove to be motivating, depending upon the needs of the individual, the situation the individual is in, and the rewards the individual expects for the work done. Theorists who hold to this view do not attempt to fit people into a single category, but instead accept human differences. In health information departments there are frequently several types of people employed. A transcriptionist, for instance, is often one who prefers to work independently, while a physician's incomplete record clerk may depend on human interaction as a motivator. Even within groups, each individual is unique.

Victor Vroom noted that individuals act to obtain goals. But whether they will act at all depends on whether they believe their behavior will help them achieve their goal. In charting a path to a goal, people choose among various actions based upon their prediction of the outcome of each action. For example, some people think that hard work leads to more money and others think it does not, depending upon past experiences. Another critical element is how much the person wants the expected outcome. To put it another way, a person's motivation depends on the expectation that a particular behavior will result in a desired outcome or goal, and the value the person assigns to that outcome.

Lyman Porter and E.E. Lawler proposed that the value a person places on a desired goal includes a perception of fairness, or equity as fairness is called in management, and that this perception influences job behavior. Perception is the way an individual views the job. This view is further affected by what

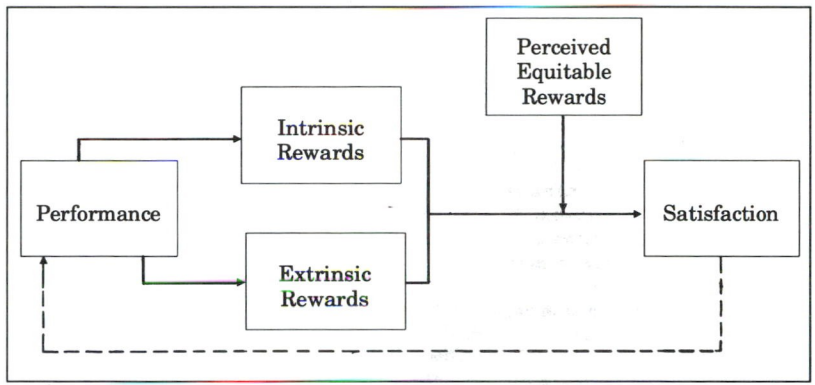

FIGURE 3. THE PORTER AND LAWLER MODEL OF THE COMPLEX VIEW OF MOTIVATION

people expect to receive from their jobs. If their expectations are not met, they may feel that they have been unfairly treated, and they may become dissatisfied. In addition, if a feedback loop is present, performance leads to satisfaction rather than satisfaction leading to performance. Figure 3 contains a simplified Porter and Lawler model.

A part of the complex view of motivation is that equity is a motivator. People want to be treated fairly; not just in the rewards they receive, but also in such areas as vacations, work assignments, and penalties assessed. Equity relates to what a person brings to the organization (education, age, experience, productivity, and other skills or efforts) with the rewards obtained in exchange. These include pay, benefits, recognition, achievement, prestige, and others.

The individual's view of fair value is critical. Perception - correct or incorrect - significantly affects the valuation. Thus the health information manager cannot rely solely on the belief that all treatment is equal, but must check perceptions as well.

One view of equity theory research suggests that if a worker is under-rewarded, the worker will tend to reduce the inequity. Reactions include some or all of the following: increasing dissatisfaction, attempting to get compensation raised, quitting the job for a more equitable one, reducing productivity, or changing the perceptual comparison.

Alternatively, if the worker is over-rewarded the inequity must also be resolved so the worker will either put forth more effort or recompare, in which the worker decides that efforts were evaluated inaccurately and that overpayment really is not true. Research evidence on the type of action most likely to be taken in either situation is mixed. Because they may affect motivation, feelings of inequity have important implications for the design and administration of compensation programs, staffing, training, and performance appraisal in health information departments.

Diagnostic Signs of Motivational Problems

Some diagnostic signs of deteriorating morale or motivation that may be observed in health information department employees are:

1. signs of boredom
   - idle conversation, excessive socializing, (e.g. comparing family pictures)
   - frequent absences from work area (e.g., long breaks or lunch hours)
   - wandering around work area, horseplay
   - daydreaming, yawning, stretching
   - personal non-work related activities (e.g., checkbook balancing)
2. excessive turnover
3. decreased productivity or work quality
4. increased gossip
5. an increase in complaints, grievances, or sabotage
6. an increase in disciplinary problems (e.g., absenteeism, tardiness, insubordination)

An effective manager must recognize the signs of motivational problems and determine what aspects of motivation are missing and try to replace them. Studies have shown that managers and subordinates do not see eye-to-eye on what workers want most. Employees who start a new job bring with them a caring attitude and a high level of motivation. The subsequent lack of productivity and efficiency is usually caused by the organization, which by its inherent noncaring style destroys an employee's natural desire to care about work and to do it well. A manager cannot get so caught up in the day-to-day activities or other management functions that employee concerns are overlooked or not addressed.

Motivational Techniques

Many techniques have been developed to solve motivational problems, or limit motivational problems from occurring in the first place. Some popular motivational techniques are described here.

Positive reinforcement, also known as behavior modification, is a technique made famous by B.F. Skinner. In this technique, specific goals are set with employees, regular feedback is provided, and other recognition and praise is awarded. Even where performance does not meet the goal, the action on the part of management is a positive one - coaching and finding something about the employee to praise. While it has doubters who suggest it is too simple or morally wrong, research conducted in several organizations has found the approach beneficial. Plotting a graph to show the department's advancement in completing records for billing, for instance, can easily provide feedback. Something as simple as bringing pizza when an intermediary goal is reached can provide praise. Individual performance can be recognized with a few complimentary words, a note of commendation placed in the person's personnel file, and so forth.

Job enrichment is a technique which is believed to make work challenging and meaningful, and thereby satisfy some of the higher level needs. Job enrichment must be distinguished from job enlargement, which adds jobs to make an employee's work more varied and less dull and routine. Job enrichment gives the employee more opportunities for decision making, participation, responsibility, and involvement without more work. Job enrichment may be accomplished by encouraging interaction between workers; giving workers a sense of personal responsibility for their tasks; taking steps to see that workers know how their tasks contribute to a finished product and the welfare of the organization; giving people feedback on their job performance; and involving workers in analysis of the work environment. In health information departments there are always new medical terms, new coding problems, new release of information situations, etc. A simple example of job enrichment is the sharing of the new information among employees which adds to everyone's knowledge and improves the quality of work.

There are limitations, however, in job enrichment. One of these is technology which may make it impossible to enrich some jobs. There is also some question as to whether workers really want job enrichment. Various surveys of worker attitudes have shown that a high percentage of workers are not dissatisfied with their jobs and that few want "more interesting" jobs. There is a tendency for managers to apply their own scale of values of challenge and accomplishment to other people's personalities. Some people are challenged by jobs that would appear dull to many managers. Another difficulty is that job enrichment is usually imposed on people; they are told about it, rather than asked whether they would like it and how their jobs could be made more interesting. Also, there has been little or no support of job enrichment by union leaders. If job enrichment were so important to workers, one would expect it to be translated into union demands.

The limitations of job enrichment apply primarily to jobs requiring low skill levels. The jobs of highly skilled workers, professionals, and managers already contain varying degrees of challenge and accomplishment. Such jobs can be enriched by modern management techniques such as management by objectives, goal setting, utilizing more policy guidance and delegation of authority, introducing more status symbols in the form of titles and office facilities, and tying bonus and other rewards more closely to performance.

A broader vehicle for participation is a quality of working life (QWL) program. This is a systems approach to job design and job enrichment. In developing a QWL program, a labor-management steering committee is set up, ordinarily with a QWL specialist, with the charge of finding ways of enhancing the dignity, attractiveness, and productivity of jobs through job enrichment and redesign. The participation of workers in the effort is thought to be very important, not only because of the exercise of democracy but also the practical advantage that people on a job are best able to identify what would enrich the job for them and make it possible for them to be more productive. This typical QWL technique tends to solve the problem encountered in many job enrichment cases where workers have mistakenly not been asked what would make the job more interesting for them.

Out of the deliberations of the QWL committee, a number of changes may be suggested in the design of jobs and in the entire working environment. The recommendations of the committees may extend to such matters as the organizational structure, communication mechanisms, technical modifications, quality control, and other things that might improve organization health and productivity.

Teamwork or participation is another technique that enjoys strong support. Quality improvement programs, as described in Chapter 16, are motivating because they involve employees in making decisions about their jobs and the way they do them. Some hospitals have used teams, including health information staff as well as others in the facility, to improve records completion or to decide on new equipment. Within the health information department, teams are useful for addressing specific problems, such as backlogs or work flow.

The quality improvement literature reveals many different names for quality improvement teams. Whatever these employee-based teams are called, their objectives are generally to analyze and solve problems or to investigate, in detail, a specific work activity in order to redesign it more efficiently.

While most quality improvement teams have a life-cycle limited to a specific project or task, some healthcare organizations are carrying the philosophy even further by implementing functional long-term teams which manage themselves. Generally, such self-directed teams:

- manage and coordinate work schedules, productivity, purchasing, and performance appraisals among the team members themselves.
- make decisions through consensus building within the team; resolve conflicts internally; use peer pressure as a

strong motivational force for change in individual team member behavior.

- are empowered as a work group to continuously improve day-to-day operations.
- participate on an ongoing basis in both formal and informal educational processes.

In the context of self-directed teams, the traditional management role changes from a directive approach to one which primarily utilizes facilitation and coaching techniques.

COMMUNICATION

Communication Model

Creating a climate in which motivational techniques will be successful, and thus reducing resistance to change depends on effective communication. The Hay's communication model in Figure 4 is commonly used to depict the communication process. The significance of this model is that it displays communication

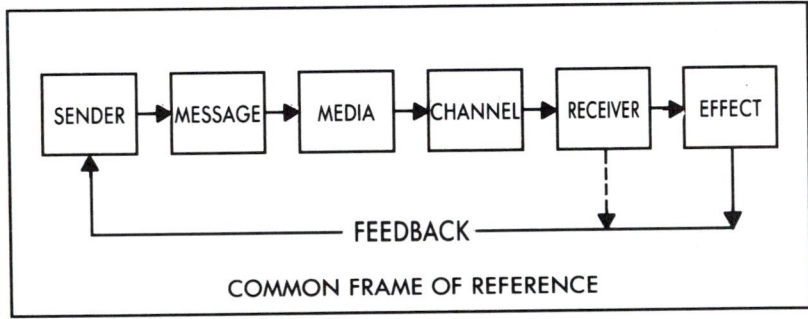

FIGURE 4. HAY'S COMMUNICATION MODEL

as an interaction between two parties which takes place by means of several factors and within a common frame of reference. In addition to the manager simply speaking or writing words, the manager must be aware that there are factors which can alter the intent of a message or even block a message totally. For instance, a reprimand given to a file clerk orally in front of all other file clerks has a different effect than if it is given in private and face-to-face, and still different than if it is given in writing. Effective communication is that which comes closest to conveying the intended message and no other.

The first factor that may alter or block the intended message is the way in which the message is conveyed. Communication media are spoken words, written words, pictures, and graphics. A second factor in conveying a message is the channel through which it is conveyed. Spoken words may be conveyed face-to-face; in person in front of a group; or over telephone, television, or radio.

Channels vary for written messages as well, from letters, memos, and computer screens, to bulletin board announcements and billboards. The message sender selects the medium and the channel and in so doing has some control over the ability to convey the intended message. Other factors over which the message sender has varying degrees of control include the frequency, accuracy, completeness, and timeliness of the message.

For there to be effective communication, the sender and receiver must also have a common frame of reference. It is not enough to speak the same language; the background, education, emotional state, and other aspects of both the message sender and receiver make a difference in how effective communication will be. For instance, one person who is embraced by the manager may feel very uncomfortable, while another of a different culture may feel satisfied or consoled by the same gesture. The message sender has little or no control over the frame of reference of the receiver; so instead must attempt to understand the receiver's frame of reference and adjust the communication in view of it.

Because communication is an interaction between sender and receiver, it is possible to obtain feedback on the message by observing the effect of, or reaction to it. It should be understood, however, that the nature of the feedback frequently depends on the communication medium and channel used by the sender, with less immediate feedback from some. Also, feedback is essentially another communication; so it also goes through a medium and channel and depends on the frame of reference. For instance, the effect of a message of good news may be happiness for two different people, but one may be very open about the happiness and another more quiet and reserved.

Steps for Improved Communication

The health information manager should constantly monitor the effectiveness of communication in order to take steps to improve it. Some symptoms of communication problems in the work environment include increased rumors, unaccountable increases in mistakes, confusion in the implementation of decisions, increased demands of subordinates for personal contact, and the need to repeat communications frequently. Some steps the message sender may use to improve communication include:

1. Gain a positive self-concept. If the sender is insecure, timid, or is convinced that no one wants to hear the message, these factors will be manifest. Monitor feedback for ways to improve.

2. Form a clear idea of what, where, when, and how you want to communicate. Communicate not only the content of the message but its context - explain as concisely as possible why it is being delivered, where it fits in, and what its implications are likely to be.

3. Invest some of yourself in the message. Effective communication requires courage to reveal one's honest thoughts and feelings. Hold the receiver's attention through the character of the message. This also means communicating in an appropriate atmosphere free of distractions.

4. Balance self-disclosure with a sense of propriety and courtesy that maintain a positive image. Maintain control over the communication - check that the message has been received, understand its effect, and make adjustments for different frames of reference.

Listening

Listening (or concentrating on the written communication) is as important in communication as is the conveyance of the message. Every message sender is ultimately a receiver. Steps which improve listening (or reading) improve the effectiveness of the overall communication. The receiver should avoid distractions; hear or read the full message before making judgments about it; evaluate the sender and make adjustments for a different frame of reference; seek to sort out the major theme and key points of the message to cut down the amount of information that must be remembered and thus aid memory;

consider the factors surrounding the message to learn its full meaning; reflect on what is being heard or read; seek further clarification if necessary; and then respond to the message thoughtfully.

Written Communication

As more and more communication becomes verbal, effective writing may be the exception rather than the rule. Education and intelligence do not guarantee good writing. In health care, many people fall into the habit of using technical jargon that can be understood only by health care experts. Common problems in written communication are that writers omit the conclusion or bury it in the report, are too wordy, and use poor grammar, ineffective sentence structure, and incorrect spelling. A few guidelines may do much to improve written communication:

- Use simple words and phrases.
- Use short and familiar words.
- Use personal pronouns (such as "you") whenever appropriate.
- Give illustrations and examples; use charts.
- Use short sentences and paragraphs.
- Use active verbs such as "The manager plans . . ."
- Avoid unnecessary words.

Writing style should fit the situation and the effect to be achieved. Specifically, a forceful style may be used when the writer has power or wants to convey power; the tone should be polite, but firm. This style may be appropriate for notices to physicians about incomplete records. The personal style is recommended for communicating good news and making persuasive requests for action. A memo sent to employees asking them to identify vacation requests may be written in the personal style. The impersonal style is generally right for conveying negative information, such as a letter explaining why medical record information cannot be provided without patient authorization. The lively or colorful style is also suitable for good news items and persuasive letters. On the other hand, a less colorful style, combining the impersonal with the passive, may be appropriate for common business writing.

Communication in Meetings

Health information managers spend a great deal of time in meetings. There are interdepartmental or section meetings. Health information professionals may also serve on various medical staff and hospital-wide committees. Although frequently a member of a group, health information professionals may also chair committees - to design a computerized health information system module, plan community service activities for the health care facility, and so forth. The use of the meeting is not only due to the democratic tradition in American social life, but also to a growing emphasis on group management and participation in organizations and the team approach in health care delivery. In attempting to overcome some of the disadvantages of meetings, managers may find the following guidelines to more effective communication useful.

Authority - The group's authority should be spelled out so members know whether their responsibility is to make a decision, make a recommendation, or merely to deliberate and to give the chairperson some insights into the problem under discussion.

Size - The size of the group is very important. As a general rule, a group should be large enough to promote deliberation and include the breadth of expertise required for the job but not so large as to waste time or foster indecision. An analysis of small-group research indicates that the ideal group size may be five when the five members possess adequate skills and knowledge to deal with problems facing the group.

Membership - The members of the group must be selected carefully. If a meeting is to be successful, the members must be representative of the interests they are intended to serve. They must also possess the required authority, and be able to perform well in a group. Finally, the members should have the capacity for communicating well and reaching group decisions by integrating group thinking rather than by inappropriate compromise.

Subject matter - The subject matter must be carefully selected. Certain kinds of subjects lend themselves to group action, while others do not. Jurisdictional disputes - perhaps over which section of the health information department is responsible for a specific function - and strategy formulation - possibly brainstorming about ways to ensure prompt return of medical records - are examples of subjects suitable for group deliberation. Certain isolated, technical problems such as a medical record coding question may be better solved by an expert in the specialized field. To make meetings effective, an agenda and relevant information should be circulated well in advance so the members can study the subject matter before the meeting.

Chairperson - The selection of the chairperson is crucial for an effective meeting. Such a person can avoid the drawbacks of meetings by planning the meeting, preparing the agenda, seeing that the results of research are available to the members ahead of time, formulating definite proposals for discussion or action, and conducting the meeting efficiently. The chairperson sets the tone of the meeting, integrates the ideas, and keeps the discussion from wandering.

Minutes - Effective communication in meetings usually requires circulating minutes and checking conclusions. At times, individuals leave the meeting with varying interpretations as to what was agreed. To avoid this, it is good to take careful minutes of the meeting and circulate them in draft form for correction or modification before the final copy is approved by the committee.

Cost effectiveness - The meeting must be worth its cost (consider the hourly salaries of the attendees for the duration of the meeting). It may be difficult to count the benefits, especially such intangible factors as morale, enhanced status of committee members, and the committee's value as a training device to enhance teamwork. But the committee can be justified only if the costs are offset by tangible and intangible benefits.

PERSONNEL SUPERVISION

Managers motivate and communicate in every aspect of their jobs, from analyzing and staffing jobs to performance appraisal. Personnel supervision must be understood from many perspectives - including organizational, legal, and social.

EQUAL EMPLOYMENT OPPORTUNITY

Before any action is taken to organize work; recruit, select, and develop staff; and appraise and compensate employees, equal employment opportunity (EEO) laws must be understood by every manager.

Over the past several decades, various laws have been passed that require employers to provide equal opportunity for people to be employed and to progress in their employment.

Laws have been passed prohibiting discrimination against individuals on the following bases:

Race/ethnic, origin/color (Black, Hispanic, Oriental, Pacific Islanders, American Indians, Eskimos)

- Gender (women, including those who are pregnant)
- Age (individuals over 40)
- Disability (physically and mentally disabled and limited)
- Military experience (Vietnam veterans)
- Religion (special beliefs and practices)

The term *discrimination* has been used in many ways. The dictionary definition is neutral and identifies discrimination as the ability to recognize the difference between, or the ability to differentiate between, items or people. Thus, discrimination involves choosing among alternatives. For example, employers must discriminate (choose) among applications for a job on the basis of job requirements and each candidate's qualifications. However, discrimination also is used to mean preferential treatment being given to members of a particular group. Individuals who are covered under equal employment laws are referred to as "members of a protected class" or protected group members.

Figure 5 contains a listing of the major EEO laws and regulations affecting employers.

To implement laws barring discrimination, several regulatory agencies have developed guidelines and regulations. The two most prominent agencies which have the power to investigate illegal and discriminatory practices are the Equal Employment Opportunity Commission (EEOC) and the Office of Federal Contract Compliance Programs (OFCCP).

The EEOC, created by the Civil Rights Act of 1964 (Title VII), is responsible for enforcing the employment-related provisions of the act. The agency initiates investigations, responds to complaints, and develops guidelines to enforce Title VII regulations.

Whereas the EEOC is an independent agency, the OFCCP is part of the U.S. Department of Labor. The OFCCP was established by executive order to ensure that federal contractors and subcontractors have nondiscriminatory practices. A major

ACT	YEAR	PROVISION
Wagner Act	1935	Prohibits firing because of union membership
Equal Pay Act	1963	As a part of amendments to the Fair Labor Standards Act in 1963, 1968, and 1972, this Act requires equal pay for men and women performing substantially the same work.
Title VII, Civil Rights Act	1964	Section 703A prohibits discrimination in employment on basis of race, religion, color, sex, or national origin. Title III, as amended by the Equal Employment Opportunity Act of 1972, the Civil Rights Act covers employers of 15 or more persons who are employed 20 or more weeks per year.
Executive Orders 112446 and 11375	1965	Requires federal contractors and subcontractors to eliminate employment discrimination and prior discrimination through affirmative actions.
Age discrimination in Employment Act (as amended in 1978 and 1986)	1967	Prohibits discrimination against persons over age 40 and restricts mandatory retirement requirements.
Executive Order 11478	1969	Prohibits discrimination in various government agencies on the basis of race, color, religion, sex, national origin, handicap, or age.
Vocational Rehabilitation Act, Rehabilitation Act of 1974	1973 1974	Prohibits employers with federal contracts over $2,500 from discriminating against handicapped individuals.
Vietnam-Era Veterans Readjustment Act		Prohibits discrimination against Vietnam-era veterans by federal contractors and the U.S. government and requires affirmative action.
Pregnancy Discrimination Act	1978	Prohibits discrimination against women affected by pregnancy, childbirth, or related medical conditions; requires they must be treated as all other employees for employment related purposes, including benefits.
Immigration Reform & Control Act	1966	Establishes penalties for employers who knowingly hire illegal aliens; prohibits employment on basis of national origin or citizenship.
State and Local Employment Laws		Many states and municipalities have passed their own laws prohibiting discrimination on a variety of bases.
		"Public Policy" and "Implied Contract" cases prevent or reverse firings on certain situations.
Americans with Disabilities	1990	Prohibits discrimination against disabled persons in employment, public accommodations, transportation, and communication.
Family Medical Leave Act	1993	Provides certain workers with the prerogative to take up to 12 weeks of unpaid leave per year for (1) the birth of or adoption of a child; (2) the care of a seriously ill spouse, child, or parent; or (3) the employee's serious health condition.

FIGURE 5. EEO LAWS

thrust of OFCCP efforts focuses on requirements that federal contractors and subcontractors take affirmative action to overcome the effects of prior discriminatory practices.

Affirmative action means that an employer sets goals and takes positive steps to guarantee equal employment opportunities for protected group members. Affirmative action focuses on the hiring, training, and promoting of protected groups where there are deficiencies. An affirmative action plan (AAP) is a formal document available for review by employees and enforcement officers. It contains utilization analysis, which identifies the number of protected group members employed and the types of jobs they hold, and availability analysis, which identifies the number of protected group members available to work in the appropriate labor market. From these analyses it can be determined whether underutilization exists within an organization.

In addition to the AAP, employers must maintain EEO records. An Annual Reporting Form must be filed with EEOC by all employers with 100 or more employees, federal contractors who have at least 50 employees and contracts of $50,000, and other specified employers.

Under various laws, employers also are required to post an "officially approved notice" in a prominent place where employees can see it. This notice states that the employer is an equal opportunity employer and does not discriminate. Usually this notice is posted on a bulletin board next to a time clock or in another prominent place.

Although the personnel/human resource department of the health care facility is generally responsible for maintaining EEO records, all managers must comply with the regulations and guidelines as they deal with employees.

AMERICANS WITH DISABILITIES ACT (ADA)

The Americans with Disabilities Act also affects employers' hiring and management practices. The ADA was passed in 1990 and went into effect in July 1992. It gives basic legal rights to individuals with impairments that limit a major life activity. Its purpose is to prevent discrimination against disabled persons in employment, public accommodations, transportation, and communication.

The law says that employers must not discriminate against a "qualified individual" because of a disability. The law defines a "qualified individual" as one who is able to accomplish the essential functions of the position with or without reasonable accommodations, and without causing undue hardship to the employer.

It is important to spell out the essential functions of each position in a job description and to judge each employee's ability to perform those tasks. Employers are also prohibited from requiring applicants to have a physical examination before the job offer is made. Other preemployment tests are legal under the ADA, as long as the function being tested is clearly essential to the job.

THE FAMILY AND MEDICAL LEAVE ACT (FMLA)

The Family and Medical Leave Act provides certain workers with the prerogative to take up to 12 weeks of unpaid leave per year for (1) the birth or adoption of a child; (2) the care of a seriously ill spouse, child, or parent; or (3) the employee's serious health condition. The FMLA, which applies to for-profit and not-for-profit organizations with 50 or more employees was effective in August 1993.

To be eligible for a leave, an employee must have worked at least 12 months for the employer (not necessarily consecutively) and 1,250 hours in the 12 months immediately preceding the leave. If possible, employees must provide at least 30 days notice in advance of the leave and arrange for a schedule that minimizes disruptions to the employer's operations. Employers may require certification of a serious health condition.

On returning to the job, the employee must be reinstated to the same job or a job with equivalent status and pay. Although leaves under the FMLA are unpaid, the employee may choose or the employer may require the employee to use up all paid vacation and personal or sick leave time before using unpaid leave.

JOB ANALYSIS AND JOB DESCRIPTION

Although personnel supervision is ongoing, the process may be thought to begin with job analysis and job description.

To ensure that tasks and responsibilities are organized properly, a job analysis is performed. Jobs are analyzed to determine their content, including the skills, knowledge, abilities, and responsibilities required of the worker. Job analysis provides the manager the opportunity to clarify lines of responsibility and authority. Job analysis can ensure that tasks are grouped and responsibilities are assigned appropriately, resulting in efficiency and quantifiable standards of performance. Wage and salary administration is also facilitated by job analysis. Comparing tasks within jobs across organizations can provide a basis for establishing or realigning a salary structure. A job description is the written result of job analysis and is a listing

---

DEPARTMENT: *Health Information*

POSITION: *File Clerk*   GRADE: *I*

HOURS: *8:00 am – 4:30 pm*   DAYS: *M–F*

JOB SUMMARY: *Files and retrieves medical records; receives, sorts, and files clinic appointment slips, sends and receives medical records to and from Outpatient Department and Admitting Office.*

JOB DUTIES:

    1. Retrieves, as requested, from straight numerical file, medical records for OPD and Admitting Office.

    2. Retrieves and sorts medical records for OPD by appointment slips.

    8. Performs other duties as assigned.

EXPERIENCE: *No experience required, will train on job. High school diploma preferred, but not essential. Must be able to arrange numbers in numerical sequence.*

PHYSICAL: *Standing, stooping, walking 90%; sitting 10% of time. Must be of physical build to permit travel through closely aligned files.*

ENVIRONMENT: *Works in clean, moderately lighted, well-ventilated room.*

REPORTS TO: *File Area Supervisor.*

FIGURE 6. SAMPLE JOB DESCRIPTION

---

of duties and responsibilities of a particular job as an average incumbent might fulfill it (see Figure 6).

Job descriptions facilitate personnel selection and placement. The personnel department uses them in recruiting job applicants. On the job, descriptions can enable the manager to prepare job orientation plans and training manuals. Job descriptions are necessary for an effective performance-evaluation system for they provide formal documentation of the standards against which an employee will be rated. The list of duties can also be used in investigating grievances regarding the nature of the employee's responsibilities.

RECRUITMENT AND SELECTION

The objective of the recruitment process is to provide a sufficient group of candidates with qualifications as described in the job description so satisfactory employees can be selected. General recruitment is performed by the personnel/human resource department. A variety of internal and external means are used. Internal means include job posting and bidding, recruiting through current employees, promotions, and transfers; and recruiting former employees and applicants. External sources of candidates include schools and colleges, labor unions, professional and trade associations, temporary help agencies, employment agencies, search firms, and media (newspapers, magazines, TV, radio, billboards).

If an adequate candidate pool is not generated by general recruitment, special techniques may have to be used. The manager may find that personal contacts with colleagues, or networking may be necessary. The manager may also have to make decisions about changing the job to a different shift, allowing flexible working hours or working at home, and using part-timers, students, and senior citizens.

Whatever source is used for recruitment, the most critical factor is realistic portrayal of the job. Some managers oversell jobs and choose to make them appear better in recruitment literature than they are in actual practice. Realistic job previews however, help reduce motivational problems once on the job and ultimately turnover. From an ethical standpoint, realistic presentation of the job is preferable to misrepresentation, even if fewer candidates are the result.

Selection is the process of picking the individual who has the relevant qualifications to fill the job. The selection process begins in the personnel/human resources department. This department receives applicants, interviews them, administers tests, conducts background investigations, arranges for physical examinations, places and assigns new employees, coordinates follow-up of these employees, performs termination interviewing, and maintains adequate records and reports.

The final selection decision, however, rests with the manager, and usually entails a selection interview. There are seven key steps in the selection interviewing:

1. Preparation - the manager must review the job description, read the applicant's resume and/or application form, prepare a list of questions, and prepare the environment (block out time, arrange for a conference room if necessary, hold telephone calls, etc.)

2. Welcome/warm-up - the manager should establish rapport with the applicant. This not only puts the applicant at ease for more effective communication, but also portrays a desirable image of the organization.

3. Applicant-talking - many managers begin the main part of the selection interview by asking a general question requiring the applicant to provide information about previous positions, interest in the position, or other open-ended questions. This provides insight into an applicant's character and experience, as well as communication experience.

4. Questioning - using the plan devised in the preparation step, the manager should seek answers to questions that pertain to how well the candidate matches the qualifications of the job. There are several forms of questions which may be used.

   - *"Who?" "what?" "when?" "where?" "why?" and "how?"* questions are useful in most interviewing situations.

   - *Probing questions:* These are incisive and specific questions used to obtain more detail about a specific activity or area.

   - *Situational questions:* With these, the manager poses hypothetical problems and encourages the applicant to answer, so that knowledge and understanding of a subject are revealed.

   - *Clarification and reflection questions:* This type of questioning essentially "mirrors" the applicant's answers. It is used to get a fuller understanding of a question previously answered.

   - *"Yes" - "No" questions:* This type of question should be used sparingly. A yes-no question cannot stand alone, since the form of the question does not give the applicant the opportunity to expand the answer.

- *Leading questions:* Too often these questions move the applicant to give an answer the manager wants. Leading questions are discouraged, but they may be used to control the interview or to stop digressions.

In any part of the interview it is important to remember that asking questions on the following subjects violates the rules of the Equal Employment Opportunity Commission (EEOC).

- age, nationality, and marital status
- Spouse's occupation or place of employment
- pregnancy or plans for pregnancy
- children or babysitting arrangements (it is acceptable to ask if there are potential problems with getting to work)
- military record, except as related to the job being filled
- arrest record (it is acceptable to ask if the person has ever been convicted of a crime, but not about arrests)
- membership in organizations other than work-related ones
- religious affiliation
- personal finances
- handicaps unrelated to the demands of the job
- history of mental illness
- Issues that affect only men, women, certain age groups, or nationalities

To comply with the Americans with Disabilities Act, employers should not question applicants about disabilities. If the applicant is disabled, the manager should focus on the applicant's ability to do the essential functions of the job and not, for example, on how the employee might get to work or how the employee might cope with nonessential tasks.

The successful interviewer speaks far less than the applicant, even when giving information about the job. This often gives the applicant an opportunity to ask questions and make comments that can be evaluated.

In the questioning stage, the manager should give the applicant the impression of genuine interest in the applicant. If the applicant appears to be holding back information or not telling the complete truth, it may be best to avoid a confrontation and to assume a sympathetic posture.

5. Employer information - managers often forget that there are two decisions to be made in an interview. Not only is the manager determining if the applicant fits the job, but the applicant must determine if the job is right.

The manager provides the applicant with all pertinent information concerning the job itself and the institution in general. Too many times newly hired employees find that the job to which they are assigned is quite different from the job explained to them in the interview. Answering questions about the job can be a most revealing part of the interview since the applicant's questions often are indicative of the applicant's value system.

6. Close - knowing when and how to conclude an interview is important. Sometimes an applicant takes a long time to warm up, and initial negative perceptions change later in the interview. The manager should give the candidate a fair chance to reveal a complete picture of qualifications, motivation, and aspirations. It is also important that the interview not drag on. It should be closed at the right time, end on a positive note, and leave the applicant with a positive impression of the institution.

7. Documentation/Report - as soon as possible, certainly before an interview with another applicant, a report on the interview should be prepared. Any additional information that must be obtained such as references or credentials should be noted. The candidate's apparent assets and liabilities should be listed and the applicant rated overall. A summary statement that presents major points for and against hiring this particular person is helpful.

The final decision to hire or not hire a particular applicant should be based on established criteria including previous experience, education and training, manner and appearance, and emotional stability and maturity.

In addition to the application, resume, and interview, results of tests may be evaluated, and references may be checked.

Although tests can be beneficial, employers must be sure that the tests are essential and reliable. There must be a significant relationship between skills tested and performance required on the job, and the test must measure the performance trait consistently.

REFERENCES

Reference checking is another area which has undergone scrutiny by the EEOC. Background references can be obtained from academic sources, prior employers, financial institutions, and personal friends of the candidate.

Personal references often are of little value. No applicant will ask somebody to write a recommendation who is going to give a negative response.

Several federal and state laws have been passed to protect the privacy of personal information. The most important is the Federal Privacy Act of 1974, which applies to federal agencies and organizations supplying services to the federal government. This Act addresses issues with respect to employees' right to:

- access personnel information
- respond to unfavorable information
- correct erroneous information
- be notified when information is given to a third party
- know how the information is being used internally
- reasonable precautions, assuring the individual that the information will not be misused

Similar state laws somewhat broader in scope have also been passed regulating private employers. Some laws define the contents of the "personnel file," such as Pennsylvania; which states it includes:

> applications for employment; wage or salary information; notices of commendations, warning, or discipline; authorizations for a deduction or withholding of pay; fringe benefit information; leave records; and employment history with the employer; including salary information, job title, retirement record, attendance records, and performance evaluations.

Most lawyers recommend that only basic employment history such as job title, dates of employment, and ending salary data be released to third parties from personnel files. Many employers will not let reference checkers talk to current employees. There have been cases where an employer who gave information that could not be documented and which prevented an applicant from obtaining a job has been successfully sued.

In spite of the potential privacy problems, organizations increasingly are finding candidates who falsify their credentials. Organizations are also finding themselves targets of lawsuits that charge negligence in hiring workers who commit violent acts on the job. Lawyers say that an employer's liability hinges on how well it investigates an applicant's fitness. Prior convictions and frequent moves or gaps in employment should be a cue for further inquiry.

Several methods of obtaining reference information are available to a potential employer. Telephoning a reference is the most widely used and preferred method. Some organizations

---

1. Before responding, telephone the inquirer to check on the validity of the request.
2. Do not volunteer any information. Respond only to specific questions.
3. State that the information being provided is confidential. Use qualifying statements such as "information is provided upon request" to imply that it is not presented to damage a person's reputation.
4. Provide only reference data that pertain to the job in question.
5. Avoid vague statements such as "John was careless at times."
6. Document all released information.
7. Identify all subjective statements as being personal opinion.
8. When providing a potentially negative statement, add the reason or explain the incidents that led to the event.
9. Do not answer questions such as "Would you rehire this person?"
10. Avoid answering questions "off the record."

FIGURE 7. GUIDELINES FOR REFERENCE-GIVING

---

have pre-printed reference forms that they send to individuals who are giving references for applicants. Specific or general letters of reference are requested by some employers and/or provided by applicants.

Figure 7 provides some guidelines for defensible reference-giving. These guidelines emphasize that dealing with references requires reliance on factual and verifiable information.

ORIENTATION AND TRAINING

Once hired, employees need to learn organizational policies and procedures and how to perform their jobs. Orientation is the process of acquainting new employees with the organization and their jobs. The orientation process should create an initial favorable impression, enhance interpersonal acceptance, and aid adjustment. During orientation, the personnel/human resources department has the employee complete all necessary forms. For health information department employees these should include a confidentiality statement. The work area should also be prepared with adequate supplies, an employee handbook if not distributed by the personnel/human resources department, and copies of relevant procedures. Next, essential information about the normal workday, and policies, rules, and benefits should be provided. One common problem in orientation is information overload, so it may be necessary to spread out the orientation over time. Providing written material helps. Because we are a visually oriented society, a videotape is very effective for describing the organization. An orientation checklist can be used to ensure that eventually all necessary information has been provided.

Follow-up is an essential element to orientation. This may entail a visit with a personnel/human resources representative, the manager of the health information department, and/or the manager. Some organizations use a questionnaire especially for evaluating the socialization process. A test on content of the employee's handbook may help ensure understanding and identify areas for clarification.

Training provides the employee with specific knowledge and skills to perform a job. Training should be an ongoing process as changes in the job take place or as cross-training is performed. Although training can be time-consuming and costly, it is an investment in the human resources of the organization. A good training program with a positive environment ensures productivity, stronger loyalty, lower turnover, and higher job satisfaction. Some employers are reluctant to provide advanced training for fear the employee will leave for a better job. The organization risks losing employees through advanced training only when positive motivation and communication are lacking.

Effective training considers the psychology of the learning process including the learning curve (rate at which people can learn a particular skill or mental task), needs assessment (appraisals of job performance, analyzing organizational factors, identifying employee needs, prioritizing training programs, and setting objectives), and teaching strategies (training methods, media, and evaluation systems).

Human resource development is often used to describe a specific type of training that enhances an employee's capacity to handle greater responsibilities. This can also include career path development. Human resource development is often a combination of formal education (conceptual learning) and training (task and skill learning). Current trends in human resource development include shared responsibility between employee and organization, more emphasis on horizontal movement to provide breadth as organizations trim the depth of their organizational structures, increased use of mentors, and the concept of continuous improvement (postulated by Americans, W. Edwards Deming and M. Juran, and popularized by Japanese management systems in the form of kaizen - meaning gradual, unending improvement, doing "little things" better, and setting and achieving ever higher standards). (For more information, see Chapter 16.)

COACHING AND COUNSELING

Coaching involves many processes including: training, delegating, facilitating, disciplining, counseling, evaluating, and mentoring. Use of praise and criticism are the dichotomous components of coaching.

Positive feedback helps people feel like winners and causes them to act like winners. A manager should be on the alert for things about which praise can be offered, such as when employees work beyond the call of duty, produce work that is right on target or that exceeds previous performance even if not yet up to par, and when they offer good suggestions. Although praise should be given liberally, praise must be honest, not on a set schedule, and only when truly deserving. An expression of gratitude may substitute for praise sometimes. For example, if an employee gets behind but stays late to make up the work, the manager may thank the employee while not necessarily offering praise for performing at the level expected. When an employee deserves special praise, a thank you note from the manager, a word of praise from an upper level manager, and even a token such as a flower in a vase, or a few hours time off is appropriate.

Criticism is also a component of coaching and must be offered at times. Recipients seldom regard criticism as "constructive." Instead, they are likely to: regard it as demeaning, react defensively, try to shift blame, feel that their initiative is stifled, or look to informal leaders for support.

In order to minimize the negative aspect of criticism, a manager should:

1. avoid global criticism (i.e., criticizing general behavior or characteristics such as work habits or attitudes, or criticizing a group when only certain individuals are deserving).

2. depersonalize criticism by directing it at behavior, not at personality, character, or attitude.

3. substitute "enhancing value" instead of criticism. The manager should start by commenting on what is right about the subordinate's performance and then make specific suggestions on ways to improve it. The secret is to make the subordinate feel that the manager wants to help, not to judge.

4. avoid being judgmental; use expressions as "What concerns me ...," "I am worried about ...," and "Let us see if we can overcome the problem of ...."

Coaching requires a fine balance of praise and criticism. Whereas coaching tends to identify and encourage positive behavior, counseling deals with employee behavior that has deviated from the expected. This may be a violation of policies, rules, or procedures; or it may be unsatisfactory productivity. The goal of counseling is to correct the deviant behavior while preserving the self-esteem of the person. When unsuccessful, counseling progresses to disciplinary measures.

The role of the manager is to recognize performance problems, to take prompt action, and to assist employees in solving their problems.

Counseling should be conducted privately in a formal interview process. If possible, it is best to counsel early in the day and at the beginning of the week so that the employee has time to observe that the manager is concerned about behavior and not with individual personality.

In the counseling interview, the manager should greet the employee in a business-like manner and immediately state the problem, using the guidelines as previously suggested for offering criticism. Organizational psychologists recommend stating, in a business-like manner, personal feelings the manager may have about the situation. For example, "I am concerned that your excessive use of the telephone is against hospital policy, keeps you from meeting your performance standards, and ties up communication lines to the department. This makes me angry and puts me in the embarrassing position of having to explain excessive telephone costs to administration."

After statement of the problem, the manager should obtain the employee's explanation, agreement that there is a problem, and acceptance of a solution. These may not be easy to elicit. It is important for the manager to anticipate ways the employee may respond and prepare to deal with them. For example, anger or tears can be therapeutic and should be allowed until the employee calms down, or the manager may have to reschedule the interview. Refusal to talk requires further probing questions, or also rescheduling the interview. Minimizing the problem, suggesting that other employees are also guilty, or becoming defensive requires the manager to restate facts and redirect attention to the employee and the behavioral problem. Some employees blame personal problems which can be legitimate or simply an excuse. The manager must stand firm on the problem, but offer referral to expert counseling if needed. Finally, some employees act as though they are in agreement but in reality are not. This situation may be the most difficult to identify and solve, but the manager should pursue counseling if there is any question of the validity of the employee's statement or actions.

During the interview the manager may offer to help, but it should be made clear that the employee must assume responsibility for corrective action. Once resolution takes place, the interview should be closed on a positive note in which the manager expresses appreciation for cooperation.

Counseling interviews should be documented. This is necessary to further identify problems and to provide grounds for disciplinary action if necessary. Initial documentation should not be made in the employee's personnel file. A simple note in the manager's file should suffice. If repeated problems necessitate more formal action, documentation to be placed in the employee's personnel file then must be shown to the employee and attempts made to obtain signature verifying the discussion. The employee must be allowed to write a rebuttal and must be told how the report can be deleted from the file.

Finally, counseling requires feedback to the employee, hopefully by expression of appreciation for improvement, but obviously further counseling if expected results are not achieved.

TERMINATION OF EMPLOYEES

Terminating employees for poor performance (and occasionally for budget constraints) is a necessary, although sometimes difficult management chore.

To make termination less onerous, the manager should set a goal of not arguing with the employee being terminated. A termination is not a negotiation session, so the manager must communicate clearly that the termination is final. It is also useful to make a list of what is to be covered in the termination discussion to ensure all relevant points are explained thoroughly. Also, make sure the employee's personnel file contains complete documentation of all counseling sessions and all incidents that led to the termination.

During the termination discussion, the manager should briefly describe the reasons for the termination and tell the employee the decision is final. The session should be brief, because a long session allows the employee to argue and gives the impression that the termination decision is not final.

When the termination is due to downsizing and not due to poor performance, it may be helpful to express regrets about the situation and explain in general terms how the downsizing decisions were made. As with other terminations, the manager should cover the specifics of leaving the facility, for example, what to do about keys, personal belongings, computer passwords, and salary checks.

HEALTH AND SAFETY

Employers are obligated to provide employees with a safe and healthy environment. Being on the alert for potential hazards and cautioning employees may be considered a special form of coaching and counseling.

The Occupational Safety and Health Act was passed in 1971 and requires that an employer must provide safe and healthy working conditions using national standards where available or general practice standards of a trade association. Safety refers to protection of the physical health of people. Health is a more subjective concept, referring to a general state of physical, mental, and emotional well-being.

While most health information departments do not maintain obviously unsafe conditions or substances hazardous to one's health, hospitals, in general, do have areas where specific cautions are necessary and do handle hazardous substances such as radiation, laboratory reagents, and so forth. It is often the unsuspecting, however, that can result in accidents or health problems. In the health information department, for example, an employee can trip over a step stool in the file area, bump into an open file drawer in the physicians' incomplete area, and so forth.

While accidents resulting in injuries or "occupational illnesses" have been the focus in the past, employers are becoming much more concerned with general health issues as well. Employers recognize the cost of health problems (and injuries) both directly in workers' compensation and indirectly in lost work time. Many employers are instituting programs that address four major health problems: physical illness, emotional illness, alcoholism, and drug abuse. Employers may sponsor physical exams, wellness programs, smoking cessation seminars, and so forth. As stress may be related to many physical illnesses, emotional health concerns are being added to employers' agendas for health programs. Alcoholism and drug abuse are important problems that require special guidelines and supervisory training, both in counseling and discipline.

The Occupational Safety and Health Act, which established the Occupational Safety and Health Administration (OSHA), requires standard reporting of injuries and illnesses resulting from a work accident or exposure in the work environment. It is, thus, important for every manager to monitor operations, routinely coach employees about safety and health precautions, and appropriately report work-related injuries and illnesses.

DISCIPLINING AND COMPLAINTS

When expected results are not achieved, disciplinary action is necessary. As unpleasant and as detail-oriented as it may be, employers have the responsibility to discipline. Unproductive or disruptive behavior is costly to the organization and unfair to other employees. EEO laws and employee rights greatly influence the disciplinary process. It is important for the manager to understand their provisions and obtain assistance from the personnel/human resources department if there are any questions. Employee rights defined in various state laws are

---

Minor Problems:

Discipline:

First offense	Oral warning
Second offense	Written warning
Third offense	One-day suspension
Fourth offense	Three-day suspension

Examples:
Unsatisfactory performance
Discourtesy
Attendance problems

More Serious Problems:

Discipline:

First offense	Written warning
Second offense	Three-day suspension
Third offense	Discharge

Examples:
Conducting of personal affairs during working hours
Violation of smoking, safety, fire, or emergency regulations
Unauthorized absence

Serious Problems:

Discipline:

First offense	Written warning
Second offense	Discharge

Example:
Insubordination
Fighting on the job
Negligence
Improper release of confidential or privileged information

Major Problems:

Discipline:

First offense	Discharge

Example:
Absence without notice for three consecutive days
Falsification of employment application
Theft
Intoxication or use of alcohol or drugs on premises
Willful damage to organizational property
Outside criminal activities
Possession of weapons

FIGURE 8. GUIDELINES FOR DISCIPLINARY ACTIONS

---

divided into three major categories:

1. Rights affecting the employment agreement
   - Employment at will
   - Implied employment contracts

- Due process
- Dismissal for just cause

2. Employee privacy rights
   - Employee rights to records
   - Substance abuse and drug testing
   - Polygraph and honesty testing

3. Other employee rights
   - Rights in workplace investigation
   - Rights to know of potential hazards and unsafe working conditions
   - Employee free speech and whistle-blowing

Discipline is actually a form of training that enforces organizational rules. Although discipline should not be negative and should lead to self-discipline, there are circumstances when punishment is corrective. The key to discipline is to have documented duties, performance standards, policies, rules, and procedures and explicit actions to be taken when variances occur.

A formal system of progressive disciplinary actions must also be in place. These actions include verbal warnings, written warnings, suspension and discharge. Figure 8 provides some guidelines for disciplinary actions.

Complaints and grievances are the "other" side of discipline. A complaint is an expression by an employee of dissatisfaction. When a complaint becomes a formal dispute between an employee and management over conditions of employment, it is a grievance.

When appropriate motivators are in place, complaints should be minimized and there should be evidence that employees feel free to air their complaints to their managers. While the environment should be conducive to handling complaints in an informal manner, it is essential to have a formal system. Employees and managers should know the steps for bringing a complaint first to the manager; then a human relations department counselor, arbitrator, or review committee; and then full-scale grievance procedure. Every complaint should be heard, documented, investigated, and the decision regarding the complaint should be made known, implemented, and feedback obtained. Handling grievances in a union situation requires application of special procedures which managers must be familiar with for their own situation.

Approaching complaints and grievances from the standpoint of resolving underlying problems is the best overall solution.

PERFORMANCE APPRAISAL AND COMPENSATION

Performance appraisal is the evaluation of work performed by an employee. It may be done at the completion of a probationary period for a new employee, at the end of a training program, in an ad hoc manner as needed, in counseling sessions, and in periodic formal reviews.

Whenever performance appraisal is performed, EEO regulations must be observed so the appraisal is job-related and valid, based on a thorough job analysis, standardized for all employees, objective, not biased, and performed by managers who have adequate knowledge of the person and the job.

Performance standards are the key element in performance appraisal. How performance standards are set and how they are monitored are explained in Chapter 17.

For the formal appraisal review, information from the performance standards monitoring system is gathered and used in an overall performance appraisal.

Formal appraisal review is often done on the anniversary of the employee's hiring, though it may be done at any time; and it may be done more often than once a year. Because this is a formal evaluation of work, however, it should not be done so frequently as to lose its impact. The completion of a performance appraisal form usually initiates the evaluation. This may be done by the manager or by both the manager and the employee. When both participate in the form's initial completion, the nature of the form and the process of its final completion should be made clear to all concerned prior to the start of the performance appraisal.

The performance appraisal form reflects the aggregate results of performance standards monitoring. It may also describe various attributes such as attitude and behavior (as measured by attendance, interpersonal relations, etc.), knowledge and skills (demonstration of technical competence in meeting performance standards, ability to learn new tasks, etc.), personal impression (such as appearance, poise, etc.), and, if for a supervisory employee, supervisory traits (including communication skills, motivational ability, etc.). Performance appraisal sometimes is conducted without the use of a form. However, forms identify for employees the factors to be evaluated. They are also used to document the appraisal function and serve as a reference for comparison over time.

Discussion of the performance appraisal form with the employee is the second step in the process. This should be done in a private interview. As with other personnel interviews, careful planning ensures a successful appraisal interview. The interview should begin with a summary of past performance. If all other aspects of personnel supervision have been in place, the past performance information gathered for the review should be no surprise. In fact, review of this information should be able to be dispensed with rather quickly. The major part of the interview should be spent discussing the future and needed improvements. Specific goals should be mutually set. The final completion of the form involves the employee commenting on the appraisal and acknowledging, in writing, that it has been discussed with the employee.

Performance appraisal is an art as well as a tool. Many managers and employees alike are uneasy about performance appraisal. For the manager, it requires a strong understanding of human relations, complete information about the employee's performance, and, above all, objectivity. The manager must avoid some of the common errors in performance appraisal. These include using different standards for employees performing similar jobs; giving greater weight to recent occurrences; introducing bias; rating all employees too leniently or all in a narrow band in the middle (central tendency error); rating a person high or low on all items because of one characteristic (halo effect); or rating an employee in contrast to all others rather than on the basis of standards (contrast error).

For the employee, performance appraisal requires maturity, an honest appraisal of one's self, and the conviction to state one's own viewpoint. If appraisal is done regularly and in good faith, it can be an effective human relations tool.

At the conclusion of the appraisal interview the major points should be reviewed. Reassurance may be offered. Even if performance does not meet expectations, the employee can be thanked for cooperation in the appraisal process. Follow-up should also be scheduled. Follow up matters may include salary discussion, in-depth counseling, training appointments, and feedback on progress. The appraisal form also needs to be completed.

Many organizations prefer that salary not be discussed during the performance appraisal, believing that such discussion is contradictory to the purpose of the appraisal - especially if it has any negative components. There are many factors that go into compensation, including the employee's new objectives, availability of persons with certain qualifications, pay schedules of competitors, and budgetary constraints.

While the performance appraisal does not depend on adjustments to compensation, compensation does depend on performance in addition to the factors mentioned above. Health care facilities usually have a compensation scale which sets compensation guidelines in accordance with performance and other factors. In addition, there are legal considerations on compensation systems.

The major law affecting compensation within most government and private employers is the Fair Labor Standards Act of 1938 (FLSA) which has two objectives relevant to health care facilities: to establish a minimum-wage floor and to encourage limits on the number of weekly hours employees work through overtime provisions.

The FLSA sets a minimum wage to be paid to the broad spectrum of covered employees. The actual minimum wage must be changed by Congressional action.

The FLSA also sets overtime pay at one and a half times the regular pay rate for all hours in excess of 40 per week, except for employees who are not covered by the law. The workweek is defined as a consecutive period of 168 hours (24 hours X 7 days) and does not have to be a calendar week. Hospitals are allowed to use a 14-day period instead of a 7-day week as long as overtime is paid for hours worked beyond 80 in a 14-day period.

Under the FLSA, employees are classified as exempt or nonexempt. Exempt employees are those who hold positions identified as executive, administrative, professional, or outside sales. Employers are not required to pay overtime to these employees. Three major factors are considered in determining whether or not an individual holds an exempt position. They are:

- Discretionary authority for independent action

- Percentage of time spent performing routine, manual, or clerical work
- Earnings level

Under provisions of the FLSA, compensation for jobs can be categorized in three groupings:

- Hourly
- Salaried nonexempt
- Salaried exempt

Hourly jobs are those that require employers to pay wages directly calculated on the number of hours worked, including overtime. Each salaried position must be identified as salaried exempt or salaried nonexempt. Employees in positions classified as salaried nonexempt are covered by the overtime provisions of the FLSA, and therefore must be paid overtime. Salaried nonexempt positions may include secretarial, clerical, or salaried blue-collar positions.

In addition to pay, compensation may take two other forms: incentives are rewards designed to encourage and reimburse employees for efforts beyond normal performance expectations, and benefits are rewards available to an employee as a part of organizational membership. Incentive pay plans are being investigated by many health care facilities as a way to improve productivity. Incentive pay systems are more fully described in Chapter 17 under budgeting.

Benefits are an increasingly important form of compensation. Employees are demanding more benefits and employer costs for them are rising. In health care facilities benefits to represent an average of 24 percent of organizational total payroll with health insurance benefits representing the greatest proportion. Other benefits include pension plans, vacation time, sick leave, profit-sharing, service awards, bonuses, and tuition expenditures.

In addition, there are three types of benefits which employers are required by law to provide. State and federal workers' compensation laws require employers to provide cash benefits, medical care, and rehabilitation services to employees for injuries or illnesses occurring within the scope of employment.

Another benefit required by law is unemployment compensation, which was established as part of the Social Security Act of 1935. Each state operates its own unemployment compensation system, and provisions differ significantly from state to state.

Employers finance this benefit by paying a tax on a portion of annual earnings of each employee to state and federal unemployment compensation funds. The payment percentages for employers are based upon "experience rates," which reflect the number of claims filed by workers who leave. If an employee is out of work and is actively looking for employment, the employee normally receives up to 26 weeks of pay, at the rate of 50 to 80 percent of normal pay. Most employees are eligible. However, workers fired for misconduct or those who are not actively seeking employment are generally ineligible.

Another part of the Social Security Act established a system providing old age, survivor's, disability, and retirement benefits i.e., Social Security. Administered by the federal government through the Social Security Administration, this program provides benefits to previously employed individuals. Both employees and employers share in the cost of Social Security by paying a tax on the employees' wages or salaries.

While compensation may not be a "motivator" it is still very important to employees. Because comparison is such a critical part of how employees view compensation, some advocate the need to "open up" pay systems by providing more pay information to employees. Pay information kept secret in "closed" systems includes how much others make, what raises others have received, and pay grades and ranges in the organization. One reason for closed pay systems is the fear that open pay systems will create discontent, petty complaining, and tension. Also, a closed pay system does not force managers to explain and justify pay differences.

A growing number of organizations are opening up their pay systems to some degree. Information that some organizations supply to employees includes compensation policies, a general description of the basis for the compensation system, and where an individual's pay is within a salary grade. By being given pay information, employees have the necessary information to make more accurate equity comparisons. Many believe that policies that prohibit discussion of individual pay are likely to be violated anyway. Co-workers share pay information and may feel that an open pay system recognizes this fact. By having the pay system explained in the open, employers can avoid distortions and other misinformation carried by the "grapevine."

SUMMARY

Personnel supervision is an important, yet difficult task for the health information professional. As a part of the management team, health information managers must manage effectively. To accomplish this they must understand what motivates employees and know how to communicate with all levels in the organization. Managers are responsible for analyzing and describing the jobs to be performed; recruiting and selecting appropriate people to fill the jobs; orienting and training employees so they have the knowledge and skills necessary to perform the jobs; coaching and counseling employees to enhance job performance ensuring a safe and healthy workplace; disciplining and reserving complaints or grievances where necessary; and administering effective performance appraisals and compensation programs. All aspects of personnel supervision must be conducted within applicable legal requirements.

STUDY QUESTIONS

1. Define motivation, and describe four major theories of motivation.

2. Describe popular motivational techniques.

3. Discuss the importance of effective communication and steps which may be taken to improve it.

4. What are the special factors that make communications in meetings effective.

5. List and define the major laws applicable to supervision.

6. Define discrimination and affirmative action.

7. State the components of a job description.

8. List the steps to take for conducting a successful interview.

9. Describe the importance of recruitment, selection, orientation, and training.

10. Identify the key element in performance appraisal.

11. Distinguish between: exempt and nonexempt, hourly and salary incentives and benefits.

REFERENCES

Berwick, Donald M., "Sounding Board-Continuous Improvement as an Ideal in Health Care," *New England Journal of Medicine*, (January 5, 1988): p. 53-56.

Drucker, Peter F., *The Effective Executive,* (New York: Harper Colophon Books, 1967).

"Follow these points to make termination less difficult," *Medical Records Briefing*, November 1991.

"Get ready for yet another new law — the Americans with Disabilities Act," *Medical Records Briefing*, July 1992.

Hampton, David R., Charles E. Summer, and Ross A. Webber, *Organizational Behavior and the Practice of Management*, Fourth Edition, (Glenview, IL: Scott, Foresman and Company, 1982).

Karpel, Jane, et al., "Record Ring: Moving Toward Solutions - A Quality Control Circle in A Medical Record Department," *Journal of the American Medical Record Association*, (January 1983): 15-20.

Liebler, Joan Gratto, *Managing Health Records - Administrative Principles*, (Germantown: Aspen Systems Corporation, 1980).

"Manager's notebook: ADA requires shift in personnel policies," Briefings on Practice Management, March 1994.

McConnell, Charles R., *The Health Care Supervisor's Casebook,* (Rockville, MD: Aspen Systems Corporation, 1982).

Mathis, Robert L. and John H. Jackson, *Personnel / Human Resource Management,* Fifth Edition (St. Paul, MN: West Publishing Company, 1988).

Metzer, Norman, *Personnel Supervision in the Health Services Industry,* 2nd Edition, (New York: SP Medical and Scientific Books, 1979).

Metzer, Norman, *The Health Care Supervisor's Handbook,* 3rd Edition, (Rockville, MD: Aspen Systems Corporation, 1988).

Quality Improvement Techniques for Medical Records, Opus Communications, Marblehead, MA, 1992.

Smith, Len Young, et al., *Smith and Roberson's Business Law,* 5th Edition, (St. Paul, MN: West Publishing Company, 1982).

Terry, George R. and Stephen G. Franklin, *Principles of Management*, 8th Edition, (Homewood, IL: Richard D. Irvin, Inc., 1982).

"The Family and Medical Leave Act," *Respiratory Care Manager*, July 1993.

Towers, Mark, *The ABC's of Empowered Teams: Building Blocks for Success,* MTVT Publications, 1993.

LIST OF ILLUSTRATIONS

INDEX